Current Topics in Microbiology and Immunology

246

Editors

Springer
Berlin
Heidelberg
New York
Barcelona
Hong Kong
London
Milan
Paris
Singapore
Tokyo

Mechanisms of B Cell Neoplasia 1998

Proceedings of the Workshop held
at the Basel Institute for Immunology
4th-6th October 1998

Edited by F. Melchers and M. Potter

With 111 Figures and 28 Tables

Springer

Fritz Melchers, Ph.D.
Basel Institute for Immunology
Postfach
Grenzacherstr. 487
CH-4005 Basel
Switzerland

Michael Potter, M.D.
Laboratory of Genetics
Building 37, Room 2B04
National Cancer Institute
National Institutes of Health
37 Convent Drive MSC4255
Bethesda, MD 20892-4255
USA

Cover Illustration:
SKY image prepared by E. Schröck and T. Ried (for further details see T. Ried, this volume) of a human myeloma cell provided by M. Kuehl. Superimposed are some display illustrations used in the workshop discussions to describe various properties of the products of a hypothetical gene with three domain-separated binding sites. Possible real examples are on the left.

Cover photograph:
Bea Pfeiffer, Basel Institute for Immunology, Basel, Switzerland

Cover design:
Hanspeter Stahlberger, Basel Institute for Immunology, Switzerland, and Design & Production GmbH, Heidelberg, Germany

Editorial assistance:
Leslie Nicklin, Basel Institute for Immunology, Basel, Switzerland

Cover:
Design & Production, GmbH, Heidelberg, Germany

ISSN 0070-217X
ISBN-13: 978-3-642-64283-8 e-ISBN-13: 978-3-642-60162-0
DOI: 10.1007/978-3-642-60162-0

Softcover reprint of the hardcover 1st edition 1999

Library of Congress Catalog Card Number 15-12910

Typesetting: Camera-ready by authors
SPIN: 10723919 27/3020 - 5 4 3 2 1 0 - Printed on acid-free paper

Preface

Workshops on the mechanisms of B cell neoplasia have been organized alternatively in Bethesda and Basel since 1983. Progress in our understanding of the development and responses of B lymphocytes is presented and discussed with the aim and hope to understand what might go wrong when B lymphocytes are transformed into malignant cells. Such knowledge might lead to better diagnosis, prevention and even cure of these terrible diseases. The presentations at the Bethesda workshops are published as papers in volumes of *Current Topics in Microbiology and Immunology*, while the presentations and discussions in Basel were transcribed and published in *Editions Roche*. For the first time, a Basel workshop (held 4th-6th October 1998) that has been recorded and, in part, transcribed is being published as papers and discussions within *Current Topics*. This volume is the latest of a long series which documents the excitements of ground-breaking discoveries as well as the frustrations of our inability to fully understand the mechanisms leading to B cell neoplasia.

The papers at the workshop are presented when possible in the sequence in which they were given. However, to facilitate the organization and reading of the book and to highlight general topics and themes, the papers are organized into five sections:

I B Cell and Plasma Cell Development
II Chemokines and Chemokine Receptors
III Chromosomal Translocations, DNA Rearrangements and Somatic Hypermutations
IV Biology of Lymphomagenesis, B-CLL, Autoimmunity
V Myeloma, Plasmacytomas and Related Subjects.

We thank the long list of investigators who have continued to participate, present and discuss at our workshops, making them the successes for which they are known in the world. We thank Peter Hannel for the video recordings; the students of the Basel Institute – Christoph Schaniel, Marijke Barner, Tilman Borgreffe, Maurus Curti, John Gatfield, Jan Kisielow, Hinchi Kong, Anna Krotkova, Erika Meier, Thomas Seidl, Sabine Stotz, Greg Terszowsli, Claudia Waskow and Dheepika Weerasinghe – for projecting the slides; Michel Delétraz, Michel Dekany, Jean-Paul Rudloff and Peter Menini for the catering; Bea Pfeiffer for the photography, and, last but not least, and again, Leslie Nicklin, for organizing the meeting in Basel, transcribing some of the papers and all of the discussions, and for the tremendous help in editing the papers and discussions. Finally we thank F. Hoffmann-La Roche, the company which fully supports the Basel Institute for Immunology, and thus fully supported this workshop.

Fritz Melchers,
Michael Potter

Table of Contents

II Chemokines and Chemokine Receptors

III Chromosomal Translocations, DNA Rearrangements and Somatic Hypermutations

IV Biology of Lymphomagenesis, B-CLL, Autoimmunity

V Myeloma, Plasmacytomas and Related Subjects

List of Contributors

(Their addresses can be found at the beginning of their respective chapters.)

Speakers at the B Cell Neoplasia Workshop 1998

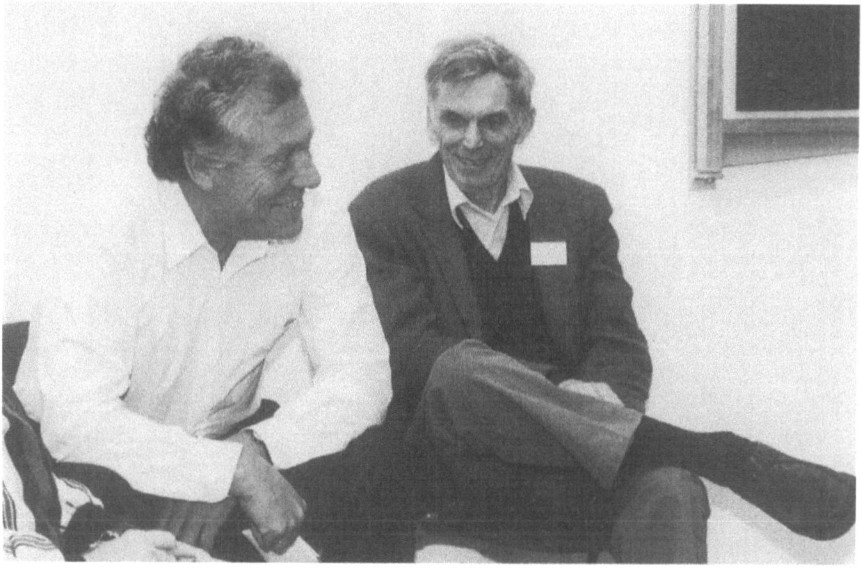

Fritz Melchers and Michael Potter

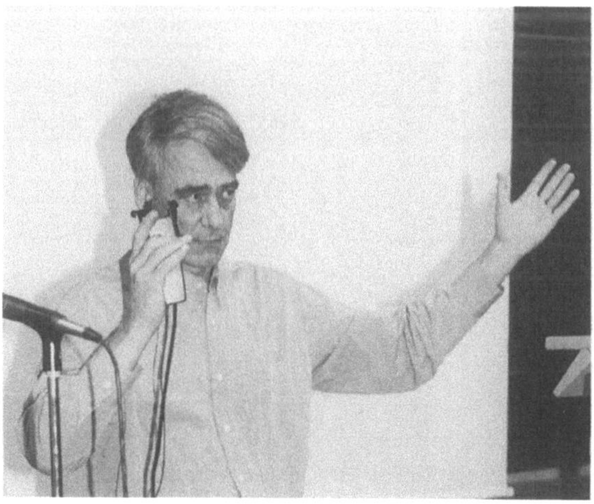

Jan Andersson

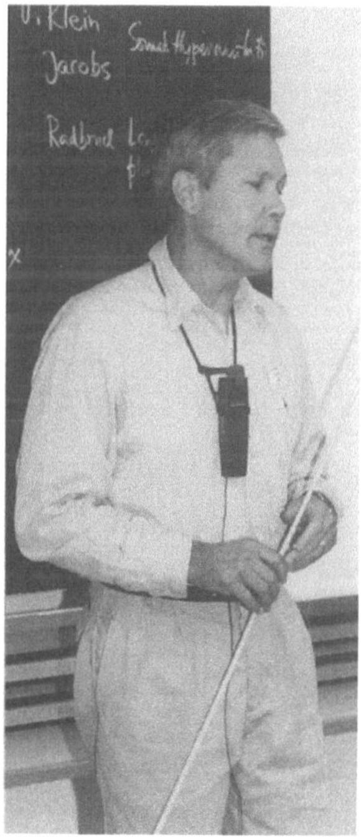

Michael Carroll

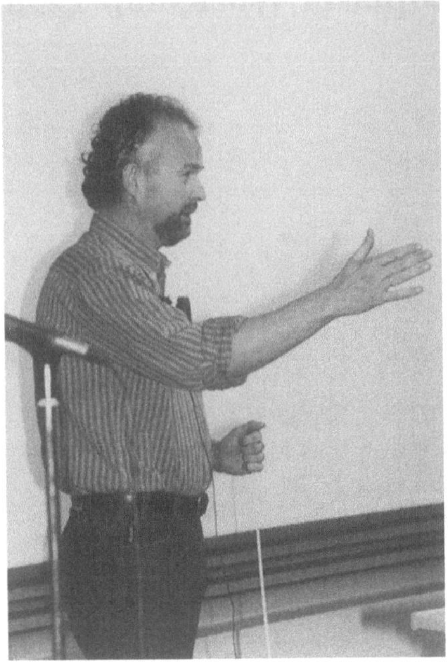

Steven Pals

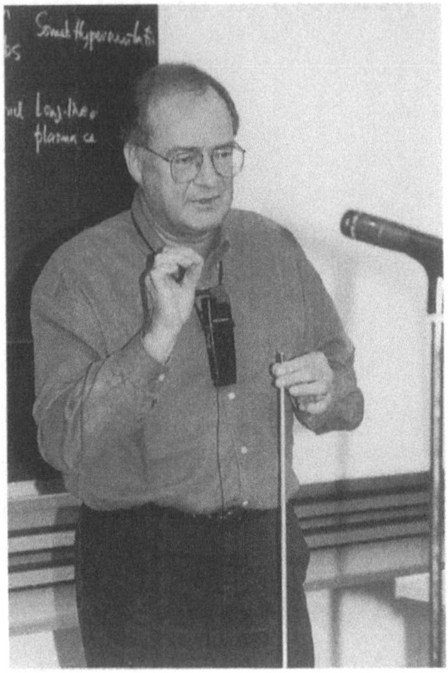

John Kearney

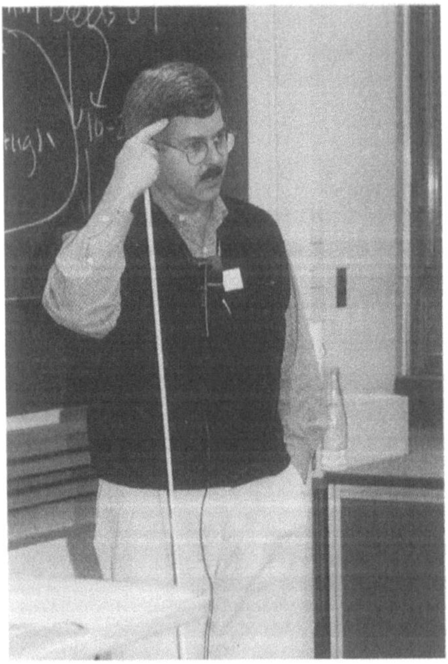

Garnett Kelsoe

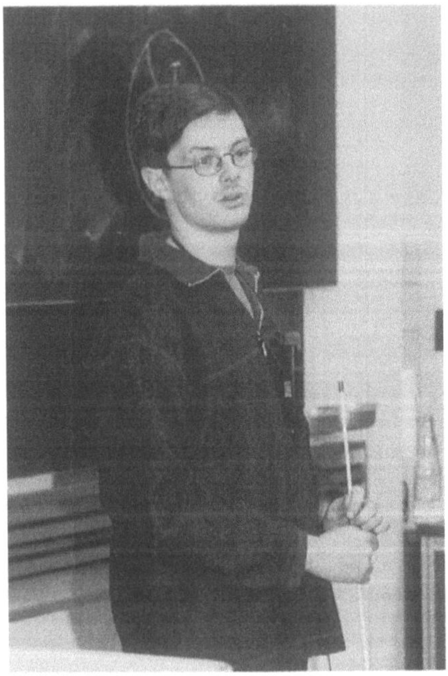

Christoph Schaniel

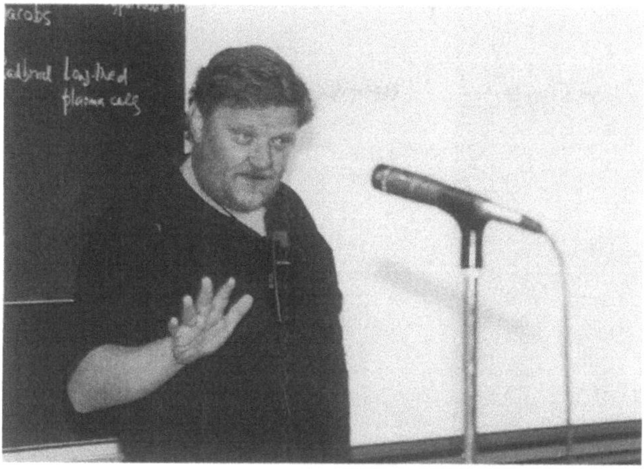

Ton Rolink

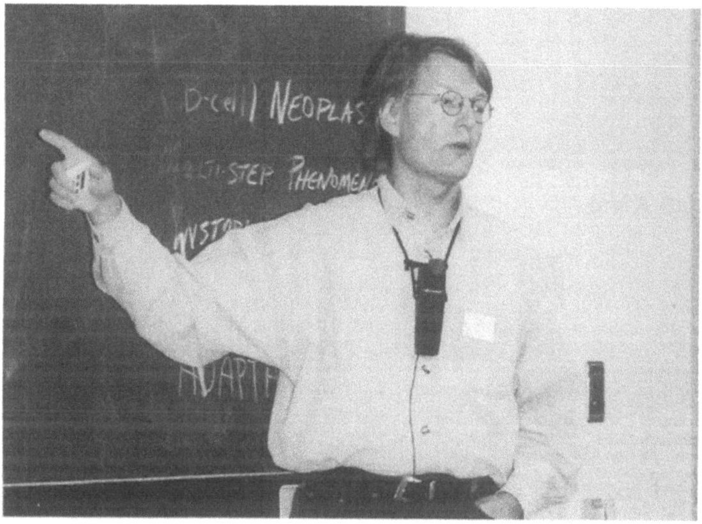

Martin Lipp

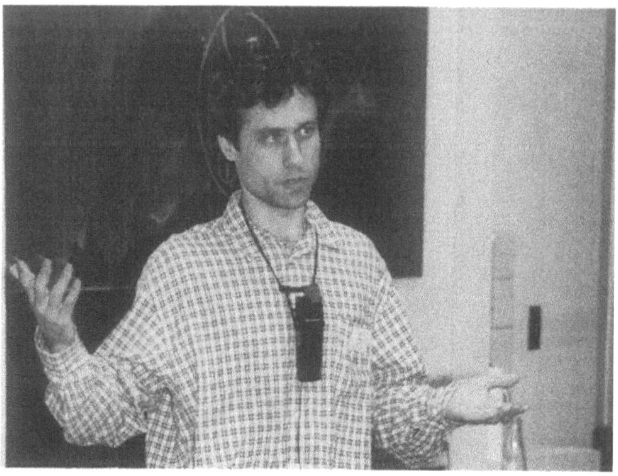

Jason Cyster

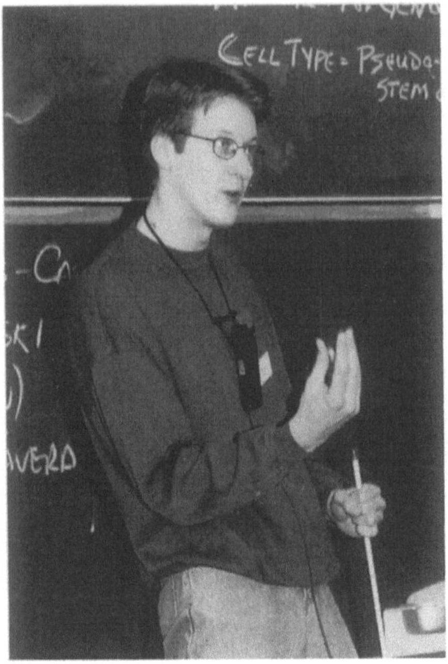

Ulf Klein

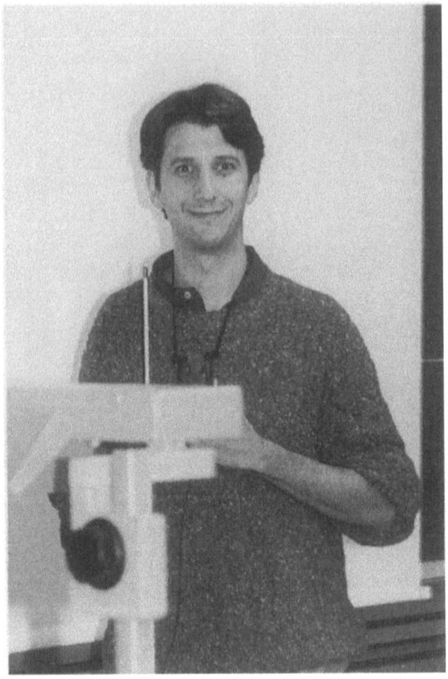

Paolo Ghia

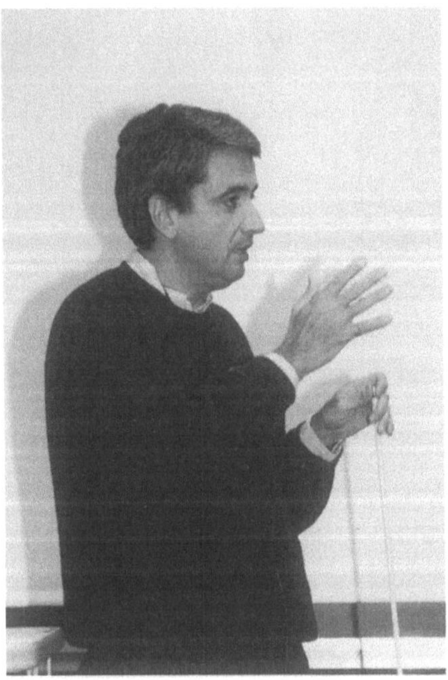

Riccardo Dalla-Favera

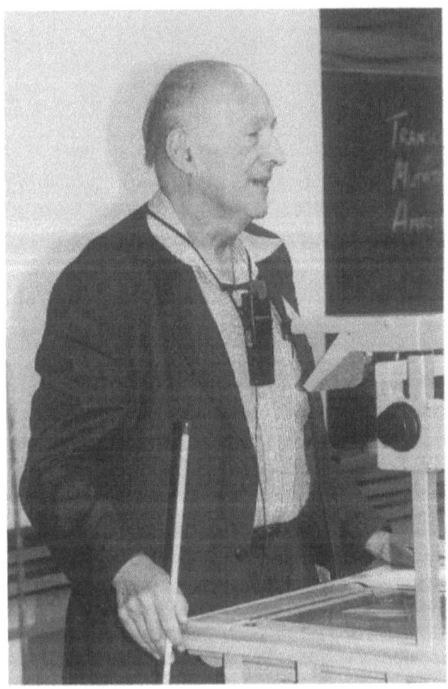

George Klein

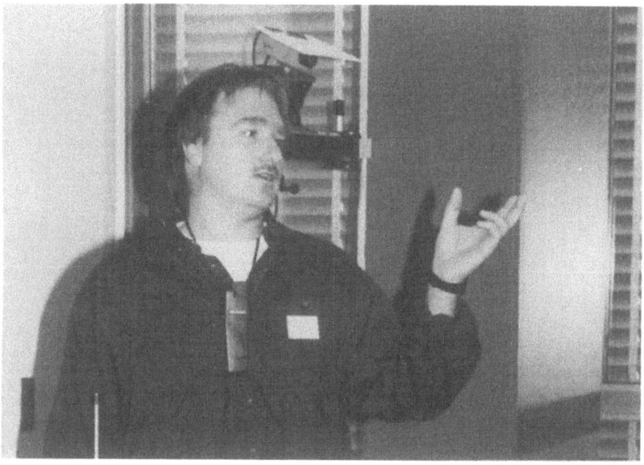

Heinz Jacobs

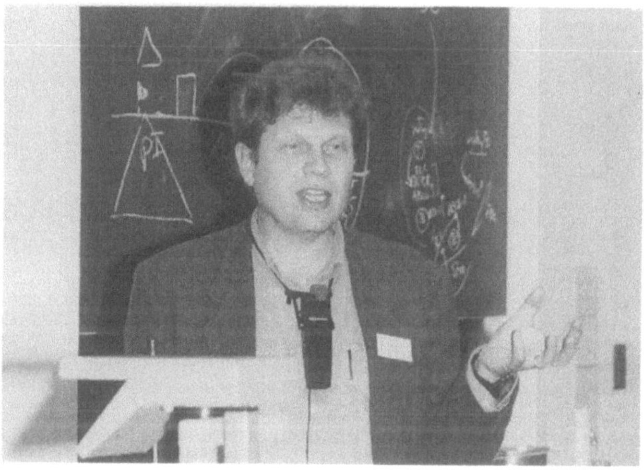

Andreas Radbruch

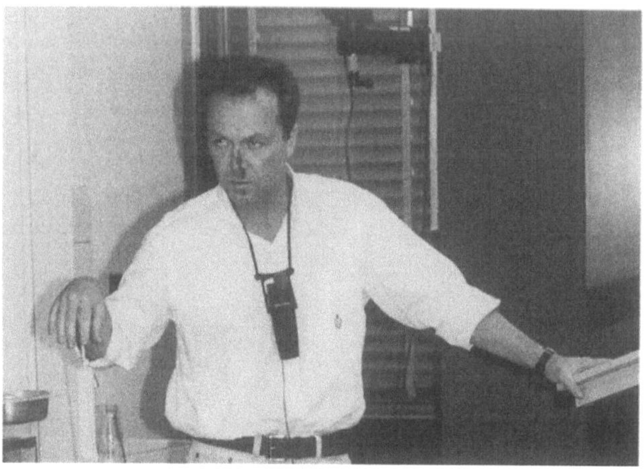

Thomas Ried

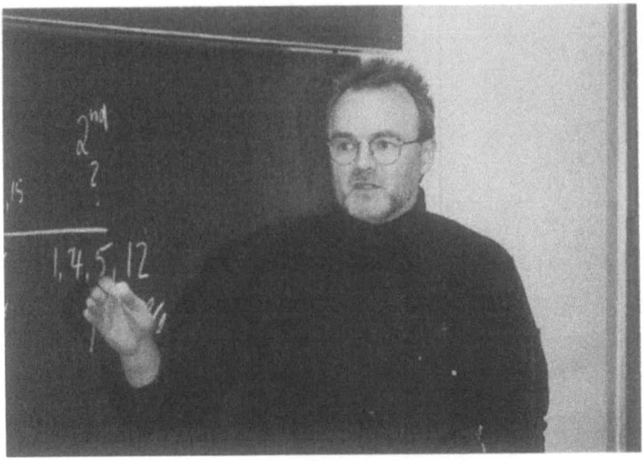

Siegfried Janz

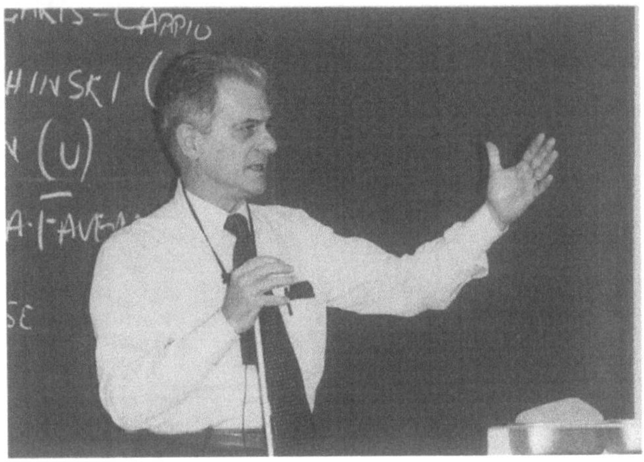

Federico
Caligaris-Cappio

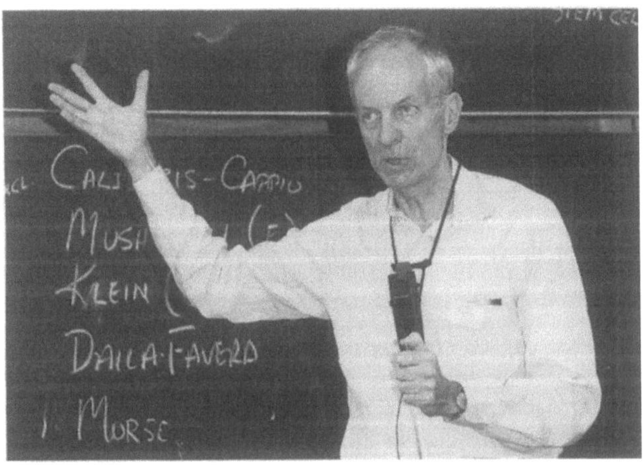

Fred Mushinski

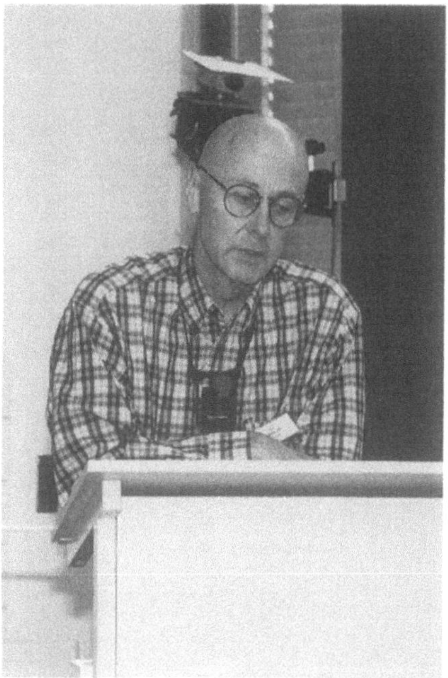

Bart Barlogie

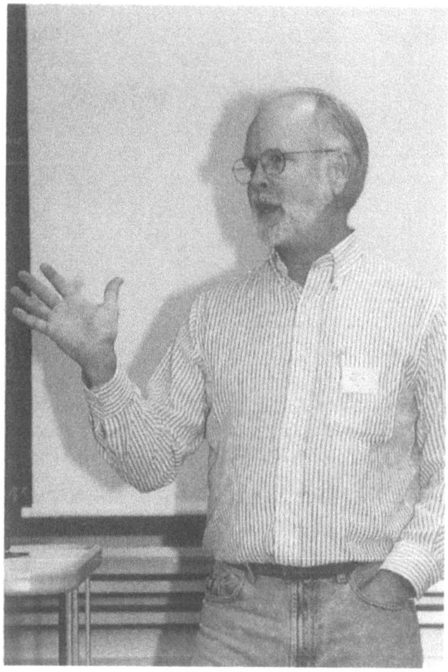

Sandy Morse

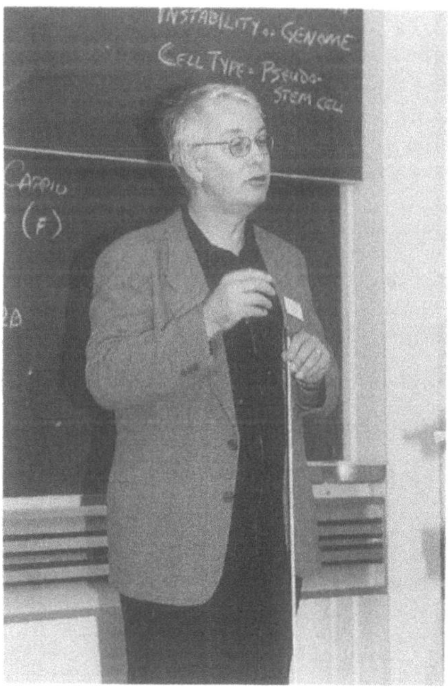

Kenneth Nilsson

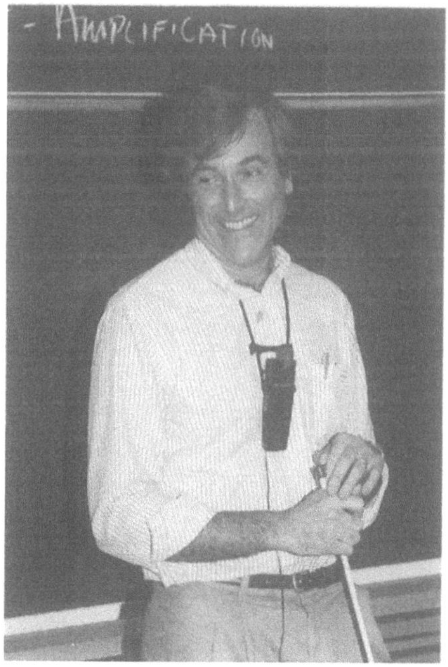

Charles Rabkin

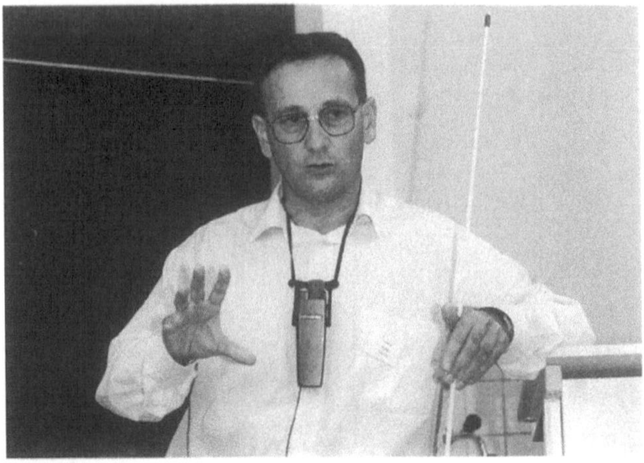

Bernard Klein

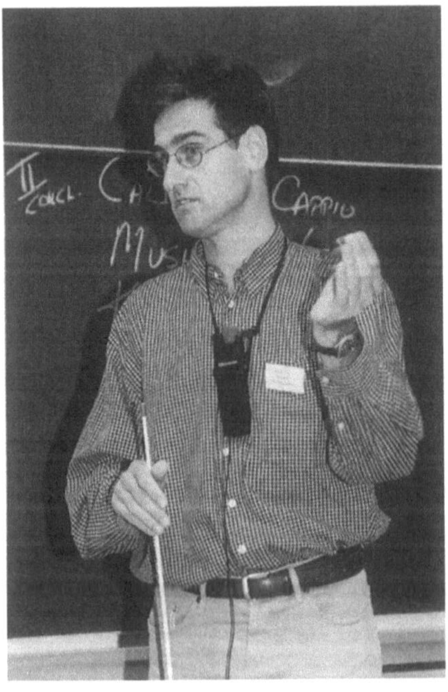

Frans Kroese

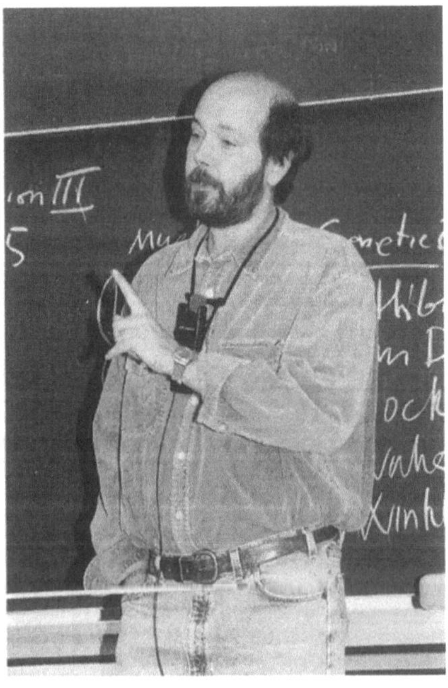

Gary Rathbun

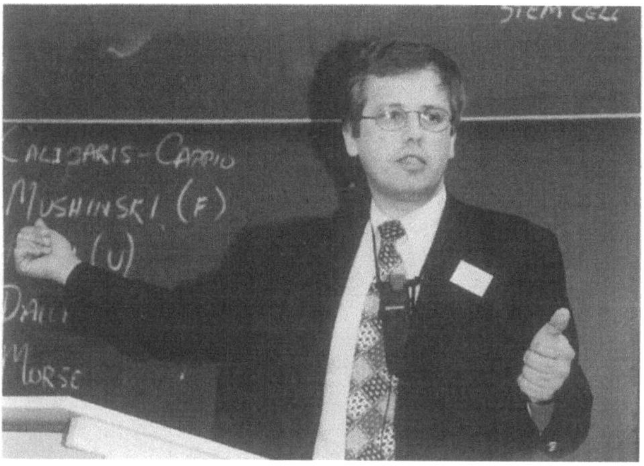

Jacques van Dongen

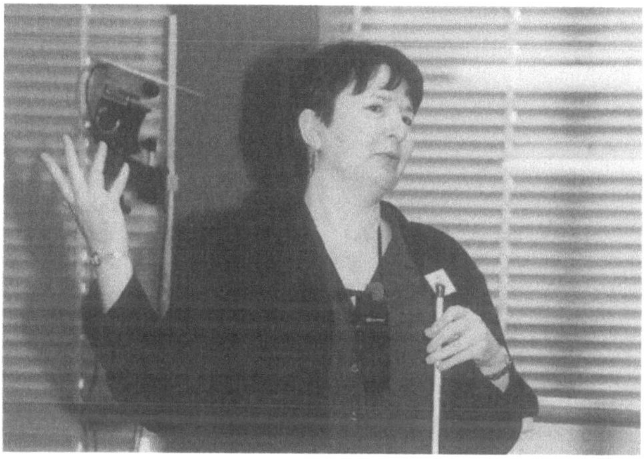

Cathy Siminovitch

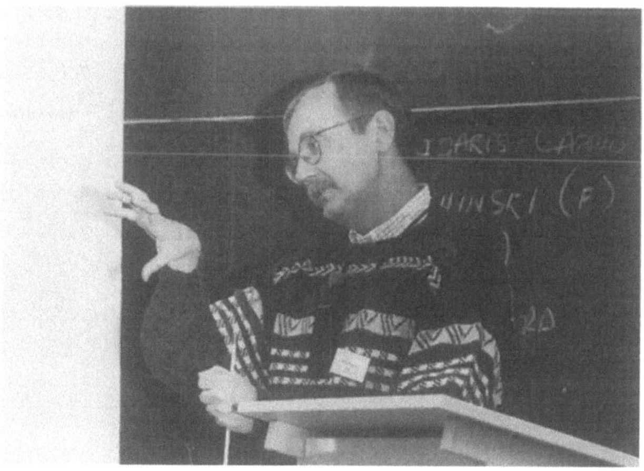

Edward Wakeland

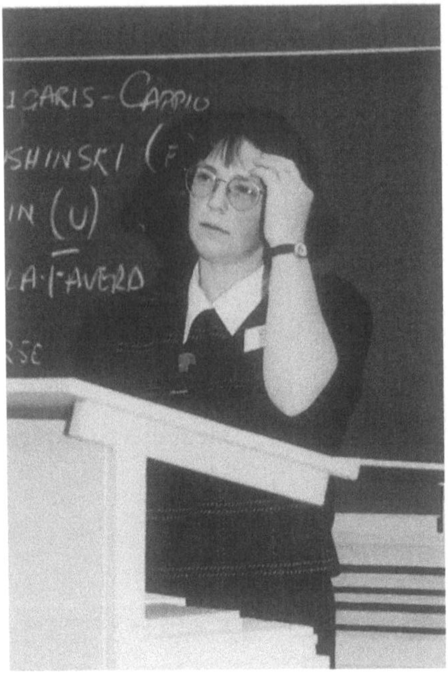

Beverly Mock

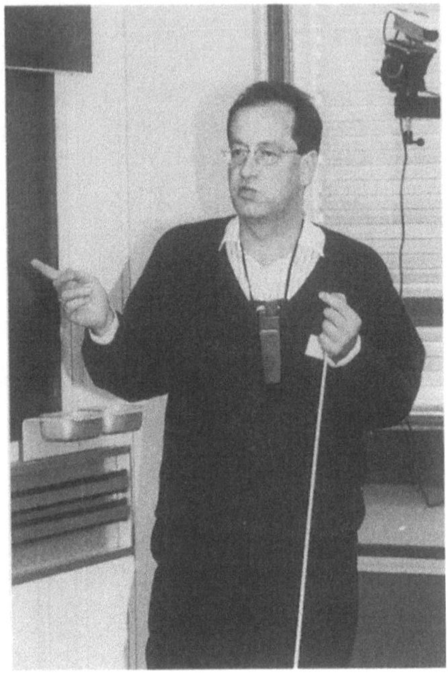

Thomas Winkler

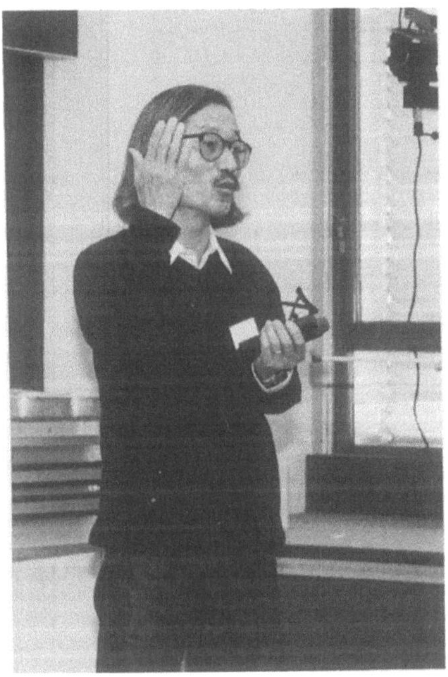

Shozo Izui

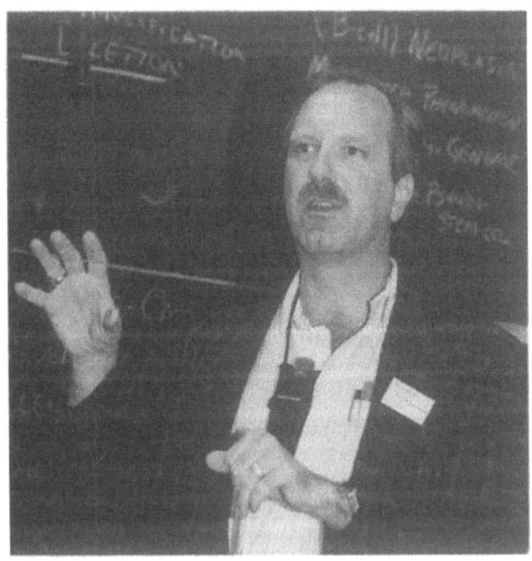

Richard Scheuermann

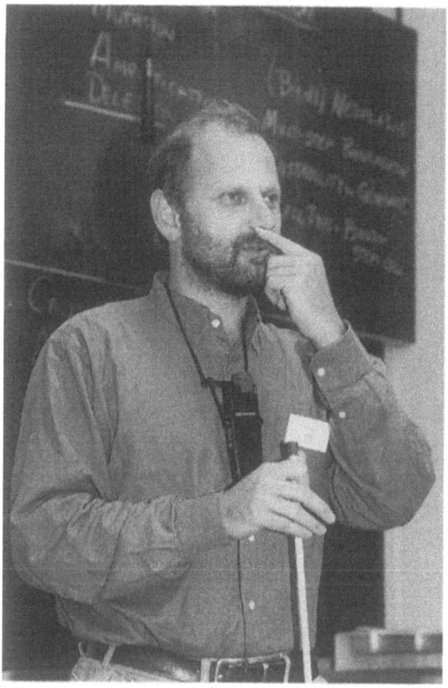

Michael Reth

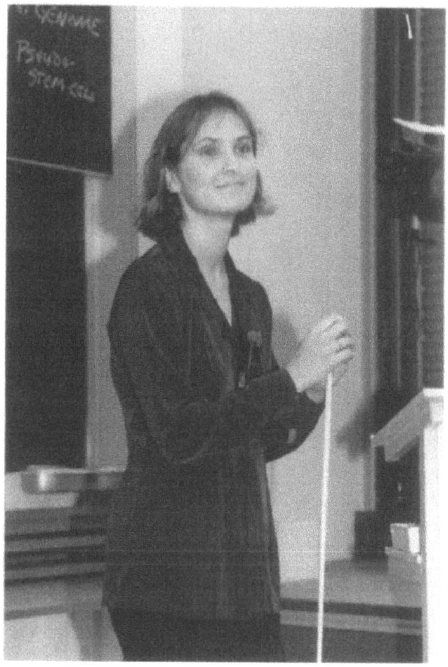

Mijntje Aarts

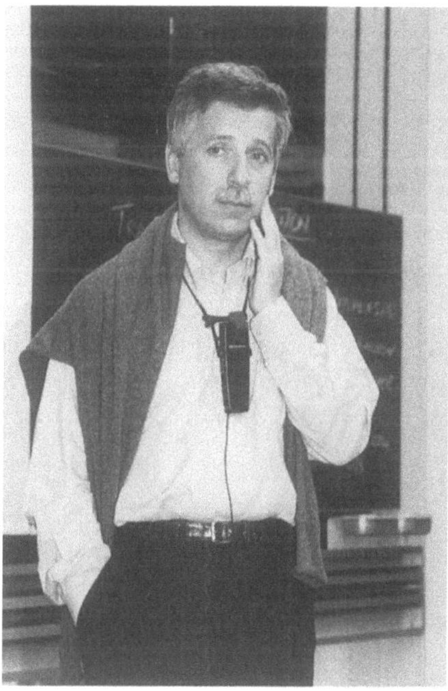

Antonio Lanzavecchia

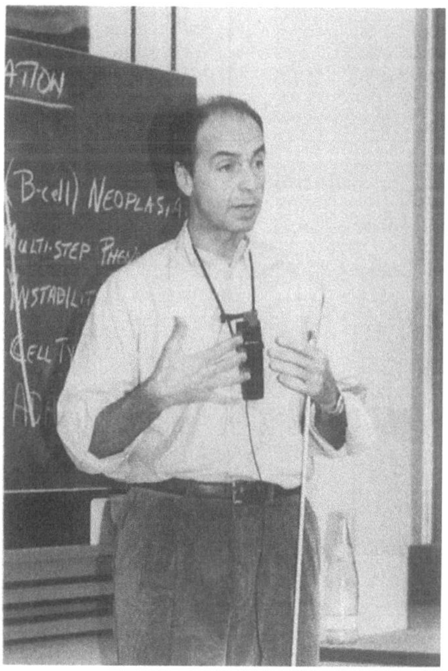

Francesco Sinigaglia

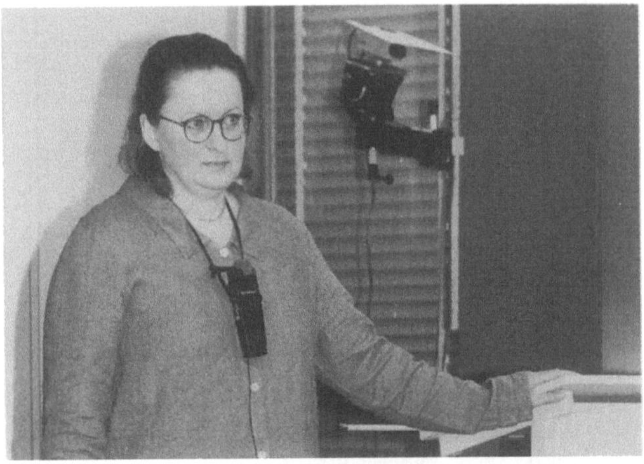

Ursula Günthert

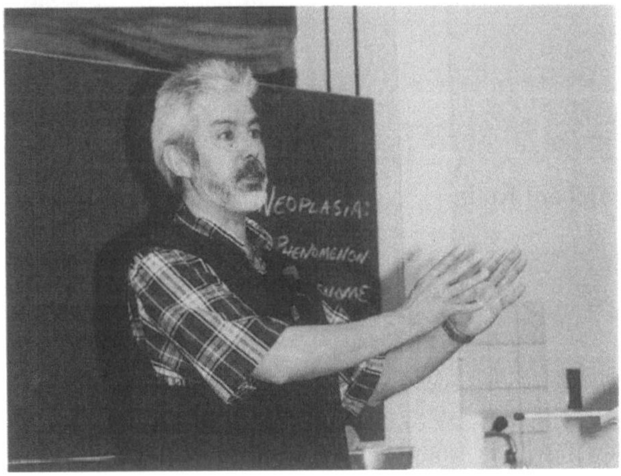

Santiago Silva

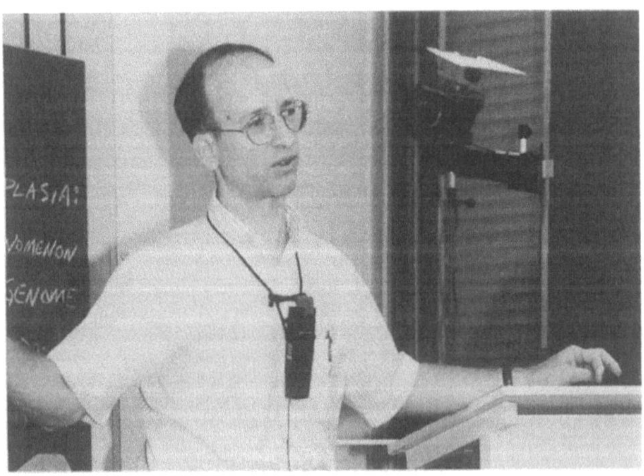

Westley Reeves

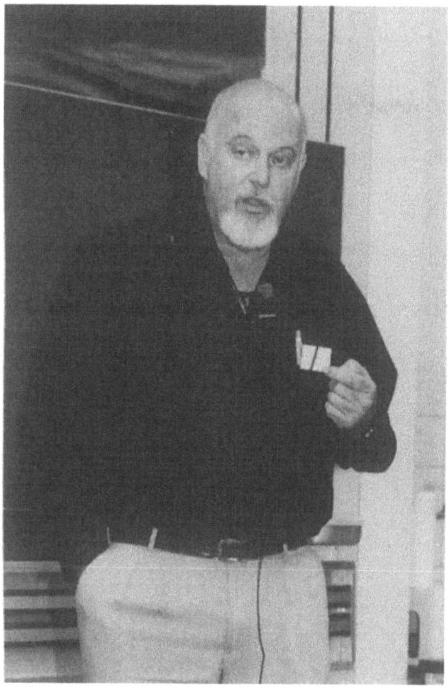

Isaac Witz

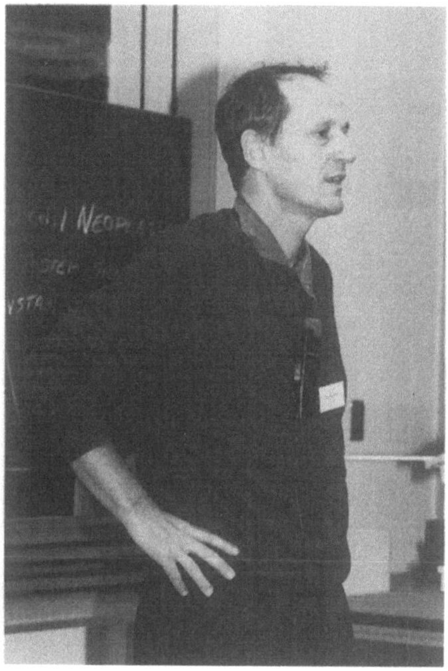

Georg Bornkamm

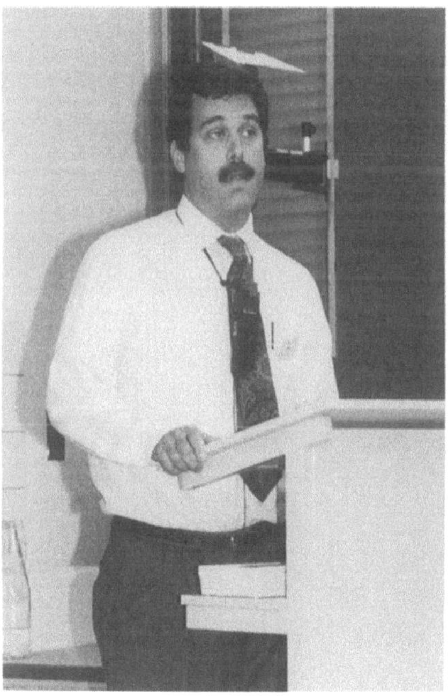

Robert Vescio

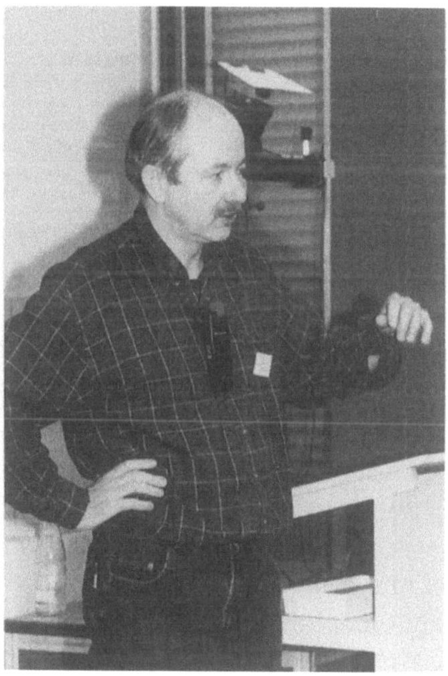

Dirk Eick

I

B Cell and Plasma Cell Development

The Formation and Selection of Cells Expressing PreB Cell Receptors and B Cell Receptors

E. ten Boekel, T. Yamagami, J. Andersson, A.G. Rolink and F. Melchers
Basel Institute for Immunology, Postfach, 4005 Basel, Switzerland

Introduction

The repertoires of B cell receptor (Ig)-expressing B cells are generated during B cell development in a stepwise fashion (Tonegawa 1983). First, D_H segments are rearranged to J_H segments on the H chain locus at the transition from $B220^+CD19^-$ proB cells to $B220^+CD19^+ckit^+$ preB-I cells. In most preB-I cells both H chain alleles are D_HJ_H-rearranged (Rolink et al. 1995). PreB-I cells, as proB cells, express the V_{preB} and λ_5 proteins of the surrogate L chain (Melchers et al. 1993) and the preB cell – and B cell – receptor-anchoring proteins Igα and Igβ (Reth 1994). Next, V_H segments are rearranged to D_HJ_H segments (Alt et al. 1984) at the transition from preB-I to preB-II cells (ten Boekel et al. 1995). Whenever this rearrangement occurs in-frame, a μH chain can be expressed. Productive $V_HD_HJ_H$-rearranged H chain alleles are found in large, cycling $ckit^-$ $CD25^+$ preB-II cells which, like all subsequent stages of B cell development, all express an H chain in their cytoplasm (Rolink et al. 1994). One fifth of all large preB-II cells express the μH chains as complexes with surrogate L chains as so-called preB cell receptors on their surface (Winkler et al. 1995). In these cells the L chain loci remain in germline configuration, and are not transcribed. The other portion of the large preB-II cells appears further progressed in development. They no longer express the preB cell receptor, in fact, they have the expression of the surrogate L chain genes downregulated, and begin to transcribe L chain loci (Grawunder et al. 1995). A small fraction of preB-II cells expressing μH chains in their cytoplasm continues to express ckit and surrogate L chain, but fails to express preB cell receptors on their surface. Their properties are described below.

The expression of a preB cell receptor on the surface of preB-II cells allows the cell to enter between 2 and 7 cell cycles and, hence, expand by proliferation. In this way productively H chain gene-rearranged cells are positively selected over those non-productively rearranged preB cell receptor-negative cells. This preB receptor-dependent proliferative expansion is abolished in mice with a defective preB cell receptor, such as the λ_5-deficient ($\lambda_5^{-/-}$), transmembrane μH chain-deficient, or J_H-defective mice (Kitamura et al. 1992; Rolink et al. 1993; Karasuyama et al. 1994; Rolink et al. 1995).

Large preB-II cells which no longer express surrogate L chain eventually fall into a resting state to become small $CD25^+$ preB-II cells. At this cellular transition they begin to rearrange κL and λL chain gene loci, in the mouse at the characteristic ratio of 5:1 (ten Boekel et al. 1995). Again, rearrangements can occur in- and out-of-frame so that only a part of all cells express an L chain protein. If H and L chains can form a B cell receptor (Ig) it is deposited on the surface of an immature B cell. Immature B cells can recognize antigens (in fact autoantigens in the primary lymphoid organs) and respond by being induced to programmed cell death. Consequently the emerging B cell repertoire is purged of autoreactive B cells specific for antigens present in the primary lymphoid organ.

While the rearrangement machinery, i.e. the RAG1 and RAG2 genes, are downregulated as soon as a preB cell receptor is expressed, and the H chain loci are closed for further rearrangements before the L chain loci are opened (Grawunder et al. 1995), the rearrangement machinery remains active in small preB-II and immature B cells (Rolink et al. 1993; Ghia et al. 1995). This allows continued, i.e. secondary, tertiary, and so on, rearrangements at the L chain of the two H chain alleles. Primers were developed which detect three major V_H families, V_H7183 and V_HQ52, at the D_H-proximal, 3' end of the V_H cluster, and V_HJ558 at the D_H distal, 5' end. The two D_H-proximal V_H families have previously been found overrepresented early in B cell development (Yancopoulos et al. 1984; Perlmutter et al. 1985; Wu and Paige 1986; Alt et al. 1987; Malynn et al. 1990). In particular, the V_H81x segment within the V_H7183 family predominates in early repertoires (Marshall et al. 1996). By contrast, the V_H representation in the adult, mature repertoires appeared to represent, in approximation, the representation of the V_H segments in the germline (Dildrop et al. 1986; Schulze and Kelsoe 1987; Jeong and Teale 1988; Yancopoulos et al. 1988; Sheehan and Brodeur 1989). By contrast, V_H81x has been found to decline in frequency during development (Marshall et al. 1996) and to be almost absent in peripheral B cell repertoires (Huetz et al. 1993, Decker et al. 1995). Furthermore, those V_H81x rearrangements found in the peripheral repertoires are mostly on nonproductively rearranged H chain alleles (Decker et al. 1991; Carlsson et al. 1992; Huetz et al. 1993).

The results of the PCR analyses of the H chain alleles of single cells of the ckit$^+$ cytoplasmic μH chain$^+$ preB cells of wildtype and $\lambda 5^{-/-}$ mice, of the large ckit$^-$ CD25$^+$ preB-II cells of wildtype mice, and of the peripheral, mature B cells of wildtype and $\lambda 5^{-/-}$ mice are summarized in Table I. In all compartments of wildtype and $\lambda 5^{-/-}$ mice a ratio of 1:1 between VDJ/DJ and VDJ/VDJ-rearranged cells is established from the beginning and maintained throughout development. We think that the VDJ/VDJ-rearranged cells arise from first a nonproductive, followed by a productive V_H to D_HJ_H-rearrangement, while in the VDJ/DJ-rearranged cells the first rearrangement was productive. Productive rearrangements resulting in preB cell receptor formation and deposition on the surface terminates rearrangements at the second, D_HJ_H-rearranged allele.

Representation of V_H segments of the 7183 and Q52 families, in particular of V_H81x appears normal in the ckit$^+$ cytoplasmic, μH chain$^+$ precursors of wildtype and $\lambda 5^{-/-}$ mice, but becomes suppressed in large preB-II cells (and all subsequent differentiation stages) of wildtype mice loci. A secondary rearrangement may be able to rescue a cell with a previously nonproductively rearranged L chain locus. It also may delete a productive, but autoreactive V_L region, and replace it with a productive but not autoreactive L chain, thus rescuing the immature B cell from apoptosis. The latter process has been termed "receptor editing" (Radic et al. 1993; Tiegs et al. 1993; Hertz and Nemazee 1997).

Finally, the immature sIgM$^+$ B cells are transferred from the primary lymphoid organ (e.g. bone marrow) to a secondary lymphoid organ (e.g. spleen) and are induced to develop to antigen-reactive, mature B cells. Here, we review recent experimental evidence how the H chain and L chain repertoires are formed and selected during B lymphopoiesis in the mouse (ten Boekel et al. 1997, 1998; Yamagami et al. submitted).

Table I Single cell PcR analyses, and tests for pairing or non-pairing with surrogate L (SL) chain of the productively rearranged H chain alleles found in B lineage cells of wildtype and of $\lambda 5^{-/-}$ mice.

Mouse strain	Cells	Number of cells analyzed	Identifiable VDJ/DJ cells	Identifiable VDJ/VDJ cells *	VDJ^+/VDJ^+ cells	V_H usage in productive H chain alleles of VDJ/DJ and VDJ/VDJ cells							
						V_H81x		V_H7183 ***		V_HQ52		V_HJ558	
						p	np	p	np	p	np	p	np
Wildtype	$ckit^+$ cytoplasmic μH^+			33 (33)	0	0	7	5	0	0	3	9	9
	Large preB-II	1020	86	81 (70)	5*	0	0	5	0	1	1	14	0
	Mature B			39	2**								
$\lambda 5^{-/-}$	$ckit^+$ cytoplasmic μH^+	760	67	59 (47)	4**	0	3	3	0	1	2		
	Mature B	576	43	30 (26)	1**	0	0	3	0	1	0	17	0

* cell numbers in brackets are those tested for pairing with SL

** all VDJ^+/VDJ^+ cells were found to produce one SL pairing, and one SL-non-pairing μH chain (ten Boekel et al. 1998)

*** excluding V_H81x

p = pairing/ np = non-pairing

V_H to D_HJ_H rearrangements at the H chain locus generate pairing and nonpairing μH chains

When V_H to D_HJ_H rearrangements occur at the transition from preB-I to preB-II cells two types of precursor B cells become discernible which both express μH chains in the cytoplasm. One is a cell which still expresses ckit and does not yet express CD25, nor does it display preB cell receptor on its surface. Their pool in mouse bone marrow consists of approximately $5x10^5$ cells. In $\lambda 5^{-/-}$ mice they are two to three times as frequent and are, in fact, the only precursor B cell population which can be found in $\lambda 5^{-/-}$ bone marrow after the D_HJ_H-rearranged preB-I cells. The other cell is the large preB-II cell, found in wildtype, but not in $\lambda 5^{-/-}$ mice, forming a pool of $5x10^6$-10^7 cells which is $ckit^-$, $CD25^+$ and initially expresses the preB cell receptor on the surface.

In these precursor populations of wildtype and $\lambda 5^{-/-}$ mice the usage of V_H segments has been determined by single cell PCR analysis and in peripheral, mature B cells of $\lambda 5^{-/-}$ mice. When the μH chains expressed in the different B lineage compartments were tested for their capacity to pair with surrogate L chain and to form a preB cell receptor on the surface membrane, practically all of those found in large preB-II cells of wildtype, and of mature B cells of $\lambda 5^{-/-}$ mice could do so. Surprisingly, however, almost half of all H chains with V_HJ558 segments found in the $ckit^+$ precursors, and in particular almost all those carrying either a V_H81x or a V_HQ52 segment could not pair. In other words, almost half of all H chains originally generated by VDJ-rearrangements do not participate in the build-up of the small preB-II, immature and mature B cell pools, because they do not expand by proliferation as a consequence of their inability to form a preB cell receptor.

More than one structural reason may account for the inability to pair with surrogate L chain. V_H81x and V_HQ52 may contain structural elements encoded in the V_H segments which are incompatible for pairing, while V_HJ558 may often be found together with CDR3 regions which are incompatible for pairing. It remains to be understood why the mouse carries V_H segments in the germline which, most often, it is unable to use in the emerging repertoire of preB cell receptors and, hence, in B cell receptors.

The capacity to pair may not be all-or-none. Especially for the V_HJ558 family, where different CDR3 regions might generate H chains with varying affinities for surrogate L chain, it might be expected that preB cell receptors with difference fitness might be generated. This, in turn, might determine the fitness of the preB-II cell to live and to expand by proliferation. Maybe the preB cell receptor does not recognize a ligand at all, but signals the cell by its mere existence – the better the fit, the stronger the signal.

Precursor B cells showing H chain allelic inclusion display allelic exclusion at the level of preB cell receptor surface expression.

The extensive single cell PCR analyses of the H chain alleles in precursor and mature B cells of wildtype and $\lambda 5^{-/-}$ mice revealed that, in contrast to a previous report by Löffert et al. (1996), between 4% and 8% of all VDJ/VDJ-rearranged cells had both H chain alleles productively rearranged. However, in all these cells only one H chain could pair with surrogate L chain, the other not. Hence allelic exclusion is maintained at the level of surface expression of the preB cell receptor. Surprisingly this is also the case for $\lambda 5^{-/-}$ cells which cannot form a proper preB cell receptor which allows the preB-II cells to enter proliferative expansion. It suggests that V_{preB} and μH chains may form an alternative, incomplete form of a preB cell receptor which may still function to ensure allelic exclusion, or that allelic exclusion operates with a different mechanism.

V_L to J_L rearrangements

Rearrangements at the κL and λL chain loci first occur at the transition from large to small preB-II cells. They continue in the $4x10^7$ small preB-II cells and $2x10^7$ immature B cells in bone marrow since the rearrangement machinery continues to be expressed. Primers have been developed which detect over 85% of all Vκ segments (Schlissel and Baltimore 1989) in rearrangements to either Jκ1, Jκ2, Jκ4, Jκ5 or RS (Yamagami et al., submitted). In addition, Vλ to Jλ-rearrangements at the λ1, λ2 and λ3 ioci can be detected. This has allowed an extensive analysis of L chain gene rearrangements in single, small preB-II cells, immature and mature B cells of mice with either two or one rearrangeable κL chain allele(s), i.e. in wildtype and $c\kappa^{-/-}$, as well as in wildtype/$Jc\kappa^-$ F1 and $c\kappa^-/Jc\kappa^-$ F1 mice (Chen et al. 1993; Zou et al. 1993).

The results of these analyses allow a number of conclusions for the generation and maintenance of L chain gene repertoires expressed in these B lineage cells (Yamagami et al., submitted). Rearrangements at the κL chain locus occur around five times more frequently than at the λL chain loci. Cells with a first productive rearrangement, most often VκJκ1-rearranged on one allele (in wildtype mice with the other κL chain allele in germline configuration) are found to preferentially enter the immature and mature B cell pool, but only when these rearrangements lead to κL chain production (in wildtype cells) and not when these κL chains cannot be made (in $c\kappa^{-/-}$ mice). Multiple κL chain gene rearrangements on single alleles accumulate more frequently in precursor B cells than in immature or mature B cells, and independently of κL chain expression. Small preB-II cells of wildtype and $c\kappa^{-/-}$ mice contain productively and nonproductively rearranged VκJκ segments at a ratio of 1:2, a sign of random generation of multiple rearrangements at one allele. Surprisingly, around a quarter of these sIg^- small preB-II cells expresses an L chain (κ:λ ~ 5:1) in the cytoplasm, together with a μH chain. The lack of surface expression of the L chain/H chain combination as sIg might either be a consequence of downregulation of surface expression after exposure of an immature, sIg^+ B cell to autoantigen. Alternatively some L chains might be incapable of pairing with a given H chain present in a particular preB-II cell. As with the inability of a large portion of all H chains originally generated at the V_H to D_HJ_H rearrangements there might be a large part of all VκJκ (VλJλ) productive rearrangements leading to L chains which are not fit to be included in the repertoires of sIg^+ B cells. At the level of H and L chain pairing fitness may well determine the capacity of a B-lineage cell to turn off the rearrangement machinery and be selected into the mature compartments of the periphery. Again, as with the preB cell receptor, the B cell receptor may provide a signal by its mere fitness and not by a putative ligand which it has to recognize.

Acknowledgements

The Basel Institute for Immunology was founded and is supported by F. Hoffmann-La Roche Ltd., Basel, Switzerland.

References

Alt F, Blackwell K, Yancopoulos G (1987) Development of the primary antibody repertoire. Science 238 1079-1087

Alt F, Yancopoulos G, Blackwell T, Wood C, Thomas E, Boss M, Coffman R, Rosenberg N, Tonegawa S, Baltimore D (1984) Ordered rearrangement of immunoglobulin heavy chain variable region segments. EMBO J 3 1209-1219

Carlsson L, Övermo C, Holmberg D (1992) Developmentally controlled selection of antibody genes: characterization of individual V_H7183 genes and evidence for stage-specific somatic diversification. Eur J Immunol 22 71-78

Chen J, Trounstine M, Kurahara C, Young F, Kuo C-C, Xu Y, Loring JF, Alt FW, Huszar D (1993) B cell development in mice that lack one or both immunoglobulin κ light chain genes. EMBO J 12 821-830

Decker DJ, Boyle NE, Klinman NR (1991) Predominance of nonproductive rearrangements of V_H81X gene segments evidences a dependence of B cell clonal maturation on the structure of nascent H chains. J Immunol 147 1406-1411

Decker DJ, Kline GH, Hayden TA, Zaharevitz SN, Klinman NR (1995) Heavy chain V gene-specific elimination of B cells during the pre-B cell to B cell transition. J Immunol 154 4924-4935

Dildrop R, Krawinkel U, Winter E, Rajewsky K (1985) V_H-gene expression in murine lipopolysaccharide blasts distributes over the nine known V_H-gene groups and may be random. Eur J Immunol 15 1154-1156

Ghia P, Gratwohl A, Signer E, Winkler TH, Melchers F, Rolink AG (1995) Immature B cells from human and mouse bone marrow can change their surface light chain expression. Eur J Immunol 25: 3108-3114

Grawunder U, Leu TMJ, Schatz DG, Werner A, Rolink AG, Melchers F, Winkler TH (1995) Down-regulation of RAG1 and RAG2 gene expression in preB cells after functional immunoglobulin heavy chain rearrangement. Immunity 3: 601-608

Hertz M, Nemazee, D (1997) BCR ligation induces receptor editing in IgM^+IgD^- bone marrow B cells in vitro. Immunity 1997 6 429-436

Huetz F, Carlsson L, Tornberg U-C, Holmberg D (1993) V-region directed selection in differentiating B lymphocytes. EMBO J 12 1819-1826

Jeong HD, Teale JM (1988) Comparison of fetal and adult functional B cell repertoires by analysis of V_H gene family expression. J Exp Med 168 589-603

Karasuyama H, Rolink A, Shinkai Y, Young F, Alt FW, Melchers F (1994) The expression of V_{preB}/λ_5 surrogate light chain in early bone marrow precursor B cells of normal and B-cell deficient mutant mice. Cell 77 133-143

Kitamura D, Kudo A, Schaal S, Müller W, Melchers F, Rajewsky K (1992) A critical role of λ5 in B cell development. Cell 69 823-831

Löffert D, Ehlich A, Müller W, Rajewsky K (1996) Surrogate light chain expression is required to establish immunoglobulin heavy chain allelic exclusion during early B cell development. Immunity 4 133-144

Malynn BA, Yancopoulos GD, Barth JE, Bona CA, Alt FW (1990) Biased expression of J_H-proximal V_H genes occurs in the newly generated repertoire of neonatal and adult mice. J Exp Med 171 843-859

Marshall AJ, Wu GE, Paige CJ (1996) Frequency of V_H81X usage during B cell development. J Immunol 156 2077-2084

Melchers F, Karasuyama H, Haasner D, Bauer S, Kudo A, Sakaguchi N, Jameson B, Rolink A (1993) The surrogate light chain in B-cell development. Immunol Today 14: 60-68

Perlmutter RM, Kearney JF, Chang SP, Hood LE (1985) Developmentally controlled expression of immunoglobulin V_H genes. Science 227 1597-1601

Radic MZ, Erikson J, Kitwin S, Weigert M (1993) B lymphocytes may escape tolerance by revising their antigen receptors. J Exp Med 177 1165-1173

Reth M (1994) B cell antigen receptors. Curr Opinion Immunol 6 3-8

Rolink A, Grawunder U, Haasner D, Strasser A, Melchers F (1993) Immature surface Ig+ B cells can continue to rearrange κ and λ L chain gene loci. J Exp Med 178: 1263-1270

Rolink A, Grawunder U, Winkler TH, Karasuyama H, Melchers F (1994) IL-2 receptor α chain (CD25, TAC) expression defines a crucial stage in preB cell development. Int Immunol 6: 1257-1264

Rolink A, Andersson J, Ghia P, Grawunder U, Haasner D, Karasuyama H, Ten Boekel E, Winkler TH, Melchers F (1995) B-cell development in mouse and man. Immunologist 3 125-151

Rolink A, Karasuyama H, Grawunder U, Haasner D, Kudo A, Melchers F (1993) B cell development in mice with a defective λ5 gene. Eur J Immunol 23 1284-1288

Schlissel MS, Baltimore D (1989) Activation of immunoglobulin kappa gene rearrangement correlates with induction of germline kappa gene transcription. Cell 58 1001-1007

Schulze DH, Kelsoe G (1987) Genotypic analysis of B cell colonies by in situ hybridization. Stoichiometric expression of three V_H families in adult C57BL/6 and BALB/c mice. J Exp Med 166 163-172

Sheehan KM, Brodeur PH (1989) Molecular cloning of the primary IgH repertoire: a quantitative analysis of V_H gene usage in adult mice. EMBO J 8 2313-2320

ten Boekel E, Melchers F, Rolink A (1995) The status of Ig loci rearrangements in single cells from different stages of B cell development. Int Immunol 7: 1013-1019

ten Boekel E, Melchers F, Rolink A (1997) Changes in the V_H gene repertoire of developing precursor B lymphocytes in mouse bone marrow mediated by the pre-B cell receptor. Immunity 7 357-368

ten Boekel E, Melchers F, Rolink A (1998) Precursor B cells showing H chain allelic inclusion display allelic exclusion at the level of pre-B cell receptor surface expression. Immunity 8: 199-207

Tiegs SL, Russell DM, Nemazee D (1993) Receptor editing in self-reactive bone marrow B cells. J Exp Med 177 1009-1020

Tonegawa S (1983) Somatic generation of antibody diversity. Nature 302 575-581

Winkler TH, Rolink A, Melchers F, Karasuyama H (1995) Precursor B cells of mouse bone marrow express two different complexes with surrogate light chain on the surface. Eur J Immunol 25 446-450

Wu G, Paige C (1986) V_H gene family utilization in colonies derived from B and pre-B cells detected by the RNA colony blot assay. EMBO J 5 3475-3481

Yancopoulos GD, Desiderio SV, Paskind M, Kearney JF, Baltimore D, Alt FW (1984) Preferential utilization of the most J_H-proximal V_H gene segments in pre-B cell lines. Nature 311 727-733

Yancopoulos GD, Malynn BA, Alt FW (1988) Developmentally regulated and strain-specific expression of murine V_H gene families. J Exp Med 168 417-435

Zou Y-R, Takeda S, Rajewsky K (1993) Gene targeting in the Igκ locus; efficient generation of λ expressing B cells independent of gene rearrangement in Igκ. EMBO J 12 811-820

Discussion

Michael Carroll: It seems very wasteful that some heavy chains are not pairing with surrogate light chain, as this is such a fundamental event to get the preB receptor on the surface. Does this suggest anything about the evolution of these separate molecules? Perhaps there was a family of V_Hs that were doing something on their own before the light chains.

Fritz Melchers: We distinguish two types of non-pairing chains. One would be the 81X, or maybe also Q52, where no matter what DJ rearrangement with whichever N has been rearranged productively, the resulting H chain seems not to fit. So there you begin to think that it is the variable region itself, the structural properties of V_H 81x or Q52 to be peculiar, that do not allow pairing. If you talk to structural biologists they say that one of the essential elements of V_H-V_L pairing is near the CDR3. Non-fitting CDR3 of H chains may be as many as half of the J558 V_H rearrangements. You may call all of that wasteful but the system goes through a lot of other waste to make a few diverse antibodies. The first case is an interesting one because we really do not have a good explanation as to why the germline would carry variable region segment genes that are unable to pair in most cases. Any suggestions or speculations are welcome. We think that they may be "openers" of the V_H locus.

John Kearney: Is this all studied so far only in adult bone marrow?

Fritz Melchers: This is also in fetal liver, I am sorry to say.

John Kearney: You were saying that in the fetal liver the most proximal V_H genes are rearranged and expressed at a higher frequency. Have you looked at a TdT knockout mouse, because there is a big difference in the rearrangements including the absence of N regions in the fetus and adult?

Fritz Melchers: I do not think we have looked with the same detailed pairing analysis at the H chains from TdT knockouts.

Ton Rolink: There was not a big difference: the V_H81x H chains expressed in the TdT knockout also did not pair.

Fritz Melchers: The numbers are not yet complete, but it seems as if fetal liver looks a lot like bone marrow.

Jim Kenny: There was an experiment that Dan Schulze and I did where we looked at the 81X expression in the adult nude mouse, and found that functional VDJ rearrangements for 81X survived in the nude out to 2 or 3 months. It was only when the nude mice started to become leaky for T cell development that those B cells disappeared. So the 81X and the type of thing that John Kearney is showing in his 81X transgenic suggests that 81X is restricted to a small number of clones. Associations of light chains with the 81X in his system would suggest that there is potentially some type of autoreactive phenomenon selecting on the 81X.

Fritz Melchers: The only thing I can say is that these changes in repertoires are detected at the earliest possible stage of VDJ rearrangements and occur clearly before the light chains are made. We have never been able to see any autoreactivity of a preB cell receptor. We have tried hard to see whether autoantigens would inhibit or stimulate, but we have never seen a positive or negative influence on large preB-II cells, for instance in fetal liver organ cultures.

Garnett Kelsoe: The numbers of L chain gene rearrangements that I deduced from the slide are interesting, but they are also the same numbers that Yamagichi's group and David Nemazee published: a third in-frame. It has always been striking to me that informative models, such as Nemazee's where autoreactivity is the informative principle, the number of in-frame and out-of-frame rearrangements are almost always stochastic. That was certainly true in Yamagichi's data. Is that just coincidence? The alternative is that there is repeated V(D)J rearrangement for good or ill.

Fritz Melchers: That is what it looks like. Since L chain rearrangements per cell are higher in the small preB-II compartment than in the immature and mature compartments, it looks as if the preB-II cells are frustrated by lack of success. This lack of success might be the consequence of out-of-frame rearrangements. On the other hand, if a productive rearrangement was made that cannot pair with H chain, that would be another frustration. Finally, the rearrangement may have been productive and pairing, but autoreactive. That would induce editing.

Thomas Winkler: So how do you explain cells with κ rearrangement on one allele and germline configuration on the other?

Fritz Melchers: Positive selective of cells that have made one productive, pairing rearrangement.

Michael Potter: We will probably discuss later on if one of the cardinal findings in B cell neoplasias is the formation of illegitimate recombinations and those last few slides you showed made it look as if the bone marrow is a battlefield of debris and open-ended DNAs and recombinations. Do you think that is a logical place where the myc/Ig translocations could occur?

Fritz Melchers: For a long time it has been known that a transgenic mouse with an E_μ-myc translocation as a transgene renders the bone marrow very active in the preB-II compartment, so that the number of proliferating preB cells is very much increased. In normal B cell development myc expression goes down as large preB-II cells become small preB-II cells. Hence, if myc expression is kept up by this translocation, the prediction is that it does something functionally either to keep the cells in cycle or not to let them go out of cycle. I agree with your suggestion that the $V_H \rightarrow D_HJ_H$ and $V_L \rightarrow J_L$ rearranging compartments of precursor B cells might be prime sites of B cell development where such illegitimate recombinations might occur.

Fetal Liver Organ Cultures as a Tool to Study Selection Processes During B Cell Development

R. Ceredig[1, 2], A.G. Rolink[1], F. Melchers[1] and J. Andersson[1]
[1] The Basel Institute for Immunology, Basel, Switzerland
[2] Université Louis Pasteur, Strasbourg, France.

Introduction

Recent studies concerning B cell development in the mouse embryo have indicated that the first cells committed to the B cell lineage arise in the para-aortic splanchnopleura at a time prior to the hematopoietic colonisation of the fetal liver [1]. The B lymphoid potential of such cells was revealed by *in vivo* transfer experiments, and has recently been confirmed by analysis *in vitro* [2]. Whether and in what way the mature B cell progeny of such progenitors contribute to the B cell repertoire in the developing embryo is less clear. This also raises the question of the quantitative and qualitative contribution of splanchnopleura and fetal liver-derived cells to the pool of developing B cells.

In 1974 and 1975, Owen and colleagues, using a fetal liver organ culture (FLOC) system, conducted an elegant series of experiments to address the question of the fetal liver's capacity to generate B cells. Several key findings came from these experiments. Firstly, they showed that the fetal liver was a primary lymphoid organ [3]. Secondly, they demonstrated that B cell differentiation could be manipulated *in vitro.* Thus, unlike mature B cells, engaging the BCR on immature cells led to their elimination [4]. Thirdly, they identified cells expressing μH molecules exclusively in their cytoplasm [5].

More recently, analysis of developing B cells using monoclonal antibodies (mAbs.), flow cytometry and single cell PCR has led to a more detailed understanding of B cell development *in vivo* at the cellular and molecular level [6]. Thus, following D_H to J_H rearrangements at the transit from the pro-B cell stage and V_H to DJ_H rearrangements at the transit from the pre-BI cell stage, some IgH molecules are expressed on the cell surface in association with pre-existing surrogate light (SL) chains. The SL chain is a protein complex composed of the V_{pre-B} and lambda-5 (λ_5) proteins which, when expressed on the cell surface together with the IgH molecule, forms the pre-B cell receptor (pre-BCR). The pre-BCR and associated membrane and cytoplasmic proteins are responsible for delivering signals to the B cell which result in their proliferation and continued differentiation. The B cell, which now expresses IgM molecules both at the surface in association with SL and as IgM molecules in the cytoplasm, enters the pre-BII compartment. Initially, pre-BII cells are large cycling cells but after several rounds of division, become small and resting. At this point, IgL chain genes rearrange and the corresponding κ or λ proteins replace the SL chain on the cell surface. The cell is now an immature B cell expressing the conventional BCR composed of IgM and IgL proteins.

Several cell culture systems have been developed in order to try to recapitulate B cell differentiation sequences *in vitro*. Such culture systems, including so-called Whitlock-Witte [7] and stromal cell/IL-7 cultures [8; 9] are essentially single cell in nature. Although all stages of B cell development can be recapitulated in such systems, their efficiency has been relatively modest so far. In addition, it could be argued that the maintenance of a three-dimensional architecture may be important for processes such as BCR repertoire selection, if such exist, in primary lymphoid organs such as the fetal liver. It should be recalled that studies of T cell development have clearly shown that differentiation is more efficient when the three-dimensional architecture of the thymus is preserved, as for example in fetal thymus organ cultures (FTOC) [10; 11]. In addition, FTOC can be used for studying the processes of positive and negative selection of the T cell receptor repertoire [12]. We have, therefore, attempted to explore a three-dimensional B cell developmental system by using pieces of fetal liver as fetal liver organ cultures (FLOC).

Materials and Methods

Fetal Liver Organ Cultures (FLOC)

The method of setting up and analysing fetal liver organ cultures has been previously reported [13] and is basically that described by Owen et al. [3].

Results and Discussion

Preliminary Observations

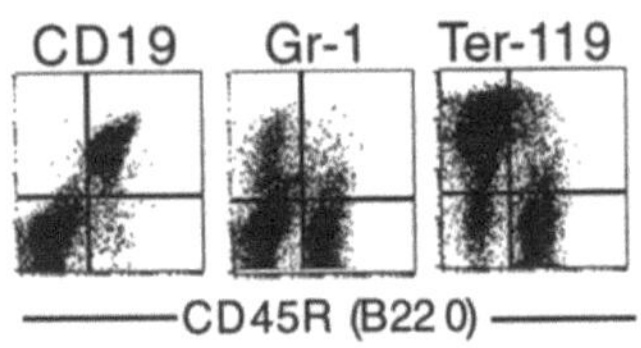

Fig. 1. FACS™ analysis of FLOC. After 6 days of culture, cells were double-stained in two colours for CD45R (B220) and mAbs to CD19, Gr-1 or Ter-119 as described in [16].

Preliminary experiments with mAbs and flow cytometry were carried out in order to see whether mature B cells arose in FLOC initiated with fetal liver fragments from embryos at 14 to 15 days of gestation. Using expression of CD19 as a marker for B cells, Gr-1 as a myeloid marker and Ter-119 as an erythroid marker, it was evident that cells other than B cells developed in FLOC (Fig. 1). FLOC maintained for 6 days *in vitro* contained cells capable of fully reconstituting the hemopoietic system as revealed by injecting $5x10^5$ cells into lethally irradiated RAG-deficient recipients. Six months after reconstitution, the bone marrow B and thymus T-lymphoid lineages were fully reconstituted (data not shown). It should be pointed out that the development of non-B lineage cells in FLOC poses some restrictions on reconstitution experiments. Thus, unlike in FTOC, where residual T lineage cells can be eliminated by the addition of deoxyguanosine (dGua.) to the culture medium [14], B lineage cells in FLOC are resistant to dGua.. Therefore alternative procedures will have to be developed to create "empty fetal" liver fragments for reconstitution experiments.

We carried out a detailed phenotypic analysis of B cells developing in FLOC from endogenous progenitors (Fig. 2). Using expression of *c-kit* for the identification of pro and pre-BI, CD25 for pre-BII cells and surface IgM for immature B cells, it was evident that immature IgM⁺ B cells arose in FLOC from an initial population of pro/pre-BI cells (Fig. 2, left panels). Importantly, for these experiments, care was taken to quantify the number of CD19⁺ cells in FLOC fragments established from one fetal liver and to compare this number to that in cell suspensions of individual livers from age-matched embryos freshly isolated *ex vivo* These preliminary experiments indicated that within a factor of 2-3, the development of B cells in FLOC paralleled that seen *in vivo*. [13]. Thus in FLOC, the development of B cells was accompanied by proliferative expansion of pre-BII cells. In mice in which the λ_5 gene has been inactivated (λ_5T) bone marrow and fetal liver B-lymphopoiesis is characterised by an abscence of pre-BII proliferative expansion. Indeed, FLOC established from λ_5T embryos showed the same defect [13]. Surprisingly, B cells developing in FLOC expressed MHC Class II, CD23 and IgD. However, in FLOC, the number of CD23⁺ cells was consistently less than the number of IgM⁺ cells by a factor of 3-5 [13] implying that many immature B cells were IgM⁺/CD23⁻.

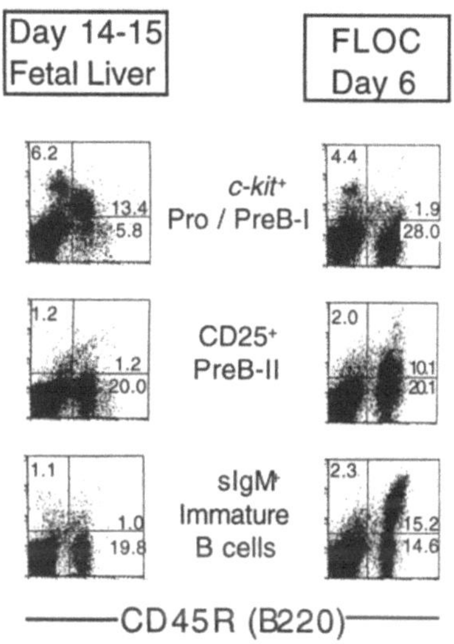

Fig. 2. B cell development in FLOC. Fresh day 14 BDF_1 fetal liver (left) or FLOC cultured for 6 days (right) were stained as described in Fig. 1 legend and analysed by FACS™.

No detailed functional analysis had previously been carried out with FLOC-derived B cells. Therefore, cells positively or negatively selected according to surface expression of the mature B cell marker CD23 were stimulated at limiting dilution with the B cell mitogen LPS and the development of B cell clones secreting IgM molecules detected by ELISA. CD23 was used as a marker for the positive selection of mature B cells in order to avoid BCR engagement with anti-IgM reagents. Such sensitive assays revealed that the frequencies of clonable B cells amongst FLOC-derived CD23⁺ cells was about 1 in 5 [13], similar to that of splenic mature B cells. Generally, such high frequencies of clonable B cells are not seen amongst the few mature B cells developing in single cell suspension cultures [15].

By RT-PCR analysis, no transcripts encoding terminal deoxynucleotidyl transferase (TdT) could be detected in FLOC [13] indicating that the IgH repertoire of FLOC B cells is fetal in type. Taken together, we conclude that a cohort of B cells develop in FLOC and undergo both proliferative expansion and phenotypic as well as functional maturation similar to that of developing B cells *in vivo*. It still remains to be determined whether commitment to the B lymphoid lineage takes place in FLOC. The FLOC system, therefore, allows the study of proliferative expansion of large pre-BII cells which is not seen in single cell IL-7/stroma cell cultures.

Manipulating B Cell Development with mAb

Given that the efficiency of B cell development in FLOC was close to that observed *in vivo,* it was decided to attempt to manipulate their development using mAbs. As a model system, an antibody to the IL-7Rα chain which had already been shown to specifically inhibit IL-7R function *in vivo* and *in vitro* was used [16]. When added at μg/ml concentrations to FLOC, a dose-dependent inhibition of B lymphopoiesis was observed [13]. The specificity of the anti-IL-7R effect was demonstrated by cross titration experiments with the corresponding ligand, IL-7 [13]. It should be stressed that such cross-titration experiments provide a powerful experimental tool for the manipulation of B lymphopoiesis and further demonstrate that molecules ranging in size from IL-7 to antibodies penetrate FLOC, reach their corresponding ligand and mediate their biological effect. In conclusion, such experiments show that the development of a cohort of B cells can be manipulated in FLOC with cytokines and mAbs.

Engaging the BCR complex in FLOC with mAbs

In order to exploit the ability of mAbs to influence B cell development in FLOC, it was decided to carry out a series of experiments using a panel of mAbs to components of the pre-BCR and BCR. Initial antibody titration experiments carried out with three anti-IgM mAbs showed that at μg/ml concentrations, all three had a profound effect on the development of surface IgM$^+$ B cells. Polyclonal anti-IgM antisera had a similar effect, as was previously shown by Raff et al. [5] although at slightly higher concentrations. By using Fab fragments of the rabbit anti-mouse IgM reagent it was demonstrated that these inhibitory effects were not due to binding of antibodies via Fc receptors (data not shown). In these experiments, antibodies used for the detection of surface IgM molecules were specific for independent epitopes from the ones added to FLOC. The phenotype of the remaining B220$^+$, IgM$^-$ cells was that of pre-BII cells as revealed by surface expression of CD19 and CD25 (Fig. 3) as well as by cytoplasmic staining for IgM (data not shown).

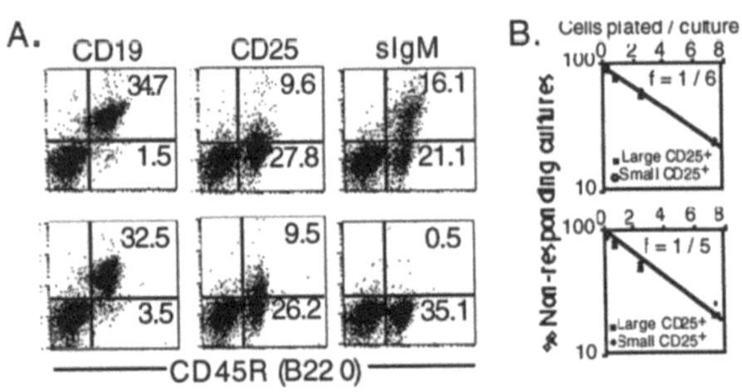

Fig. 3. Phenotypic and functional analysis of FLOC treated with anti-IgM. A. FACS™ analysis of control (upper) and mAb-treated FLOC (lower). B. Frequency analysis of clonable B cells among positively selected large and small CD25$^+$ pre-BII cells.

To demonstrate that treatment with anti-IgM had not irreversibly prevented differentiation beyond the pre-BII stage, CD25$^+$ pre-BII cells were positively selected from anti-IgM-treated FLOC (Fig. 3) and cultured at limiting dilution in the LPS plus irradiated thymus filler cell system. The frequency of clonable B cells capable of maturing to IgM-secreting clones was about 1 in 5-6 cells in both the CD25$^+$ large and small pre-BII compartment. These results also indicate that the arrest of B cell development is relieved once cells are removed from the influence of the anti-IgM reagent.

These experiments also strongly suggest that engagement of the pre-BCR by anti-IgM reagents does not prevent the development of pre-BII cells. In order to confirm this, mAbs to other components of the pre-BCR were added. Using anti-SL, anti-V_{preB} and anti-λ_5 mAbs, development was again normal up to the pre-BII stage. In conclusion, these experiments suggest that in FLOC, engaging developing B cells with mAbs specific for the pre-BCR does not result in inhibition of cellular development to the transitional state between small pre-BII and immature B cells.

Negative selection in FLOC

Two approaches were taken to study negative selection in FLOC. The first used the Sp6 transgenic BCR introduced into RAG-KO (RAG-2T, G2) mice. The Sp6 IgM was initially described to be specific for TNP [17]. However, when transgenes encoding both Sp6 heavy and light chains were introduced onto the RAG-2T background, Sp6G2 B cells were arrested in their differentiation at the transit from small pre-BII to immature B cells in the bone marrow [18]. This might be due to the action of double stranded DNA (dsDNA), since Sp6 IgM could be shown by ELISA to have crossreactivity with dsDNA. In wild-type, RAG-competent, Sp6 Ig transgenic mice, most B cells emerging from the marrow contained endogenous L chains in association with the Sp6 heavy chain. Phenotypically, immature B cells in the bone marrow of Sp6G2 mice showed profound down-modulation of surface IgM, again suggesting that they had been subjected to signals associated with arrested differentiation, apoptosis and, hence negative selection [18].

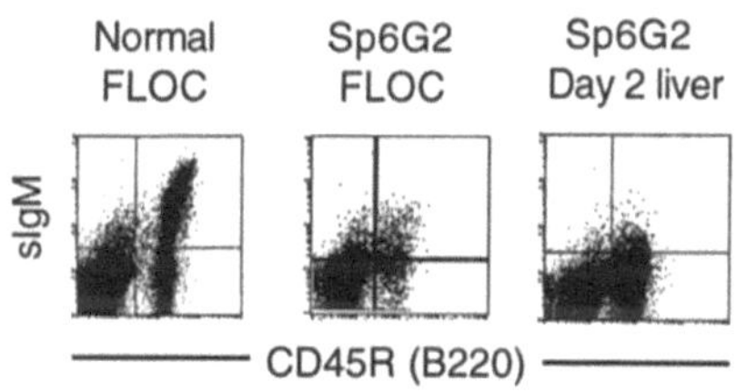

Fig. 4. Negative selection in Sp6G2 newborn liver and FLOC. Shown are FACS™ profiles of cells from the indicated sources. See text for details.

In order to see whether a similar phenomenon associated with negative selection was observed at the fetal liver stage of B-lymphopoiesis, FLOC were established from Sp6G2 embryos. As shown in Fig. 4, IgM expression on Sp6G2 cells either in FLOC (middle panel) or in the newborn liver *ex vivo* (right panel) was down-modulated. The CD19 profiles of normal and Sp6G2 FLOC differed in that the former, but not the latter, contained $CD19^{bright}/B220^{bright}$ immature B cells (data not shown).

Negative selection was also tested in the system of so-called Ig allotype suppression [19]. For these experiments, embryos from IgM allotype heterozygous, (C57Bl/6xDBA/2)F1 ($IgM^b xIgM^a$) mice, were used (Fig. 5). With the availability of a panel of anti-IgM allotype mAbs recognising different epitopes on IgM^a or IgM^b molecules, and IgM allotype-specific ELISA, this system was internally controlled for any non-specific effects of antibody addition. Titration experiments indicated that at 5μg/ml of either anti-IgM^a or anti-IgM^b mAbs phenotypically, >98% of the corresponding IgM allotype-positive cells had disappeared. Importantly, there was no increase in either the percentage or the absolute number of IgM^+ cells expressing the opposite IgM allele (Fig. 5). This result argues against any non-specific effect of antibody addition to FLOC.

In order to verify the efficiency of negative selection and to attempt to define the developmental stage at which negative selection was occurring, $CD23^+$ mature and $CD25^+$ pre-BII cells from treated FLOC were positively selected and subjected to LPS stimulation at limiting dilution. For these experiments, it was again decided not to use surface IgM as a marker for positively selecting cells, in order to avoid any deleterious effect on plating efficiency that this might entail. Supernatants from individual wells, seeded with graded doses of cells, were analysed for total IgM secretion and for IgM allotype. Care was taken so that the sensitivities of all three ELISA's were comparable.

Addition of 5μg/ml anti-IgM allotype mAbs to FLOC resulted in the elimination of >98% of the corresponding allotype-secreting clones from the CD23⁺ mature B cell compartment as measured by LPS responsiveness and IgM secretion (data not shown). Importantly, CD25⁺ pre-BII cells from cultures treated with anti-IgM-allotype mAb were still capable of generating clones secreting the suppressed IgM allotype at frequencies identical to those of the non-suppressed allele. Taken together, these results indicate that the negative selection step mediated by anti-IgM allotype-specific mAb, like the anti-μ-mediated inhibition occurs after the CD25⁺ pre-BII stage and before entry into the IgM⁺/CD23⁺ compartment. It remains to be determined whether deletion occurs in the IgM⁺/CD23⁻ sub-population.

The experiments described above were carried out with anti-IgM mAb as BCR ligands. One technical limitation of such an approach is that mAbs do not diffuse out once they are inside FLOC. Relief from the inhibitory effects is however obtained by disrupting the tissue fragments. In conclusion, our observations suggest that FLOC provide a powerful experimental tool for manipulating the BCR repertoire of normal, as well as Ig transgenic B cells *in vitro*.

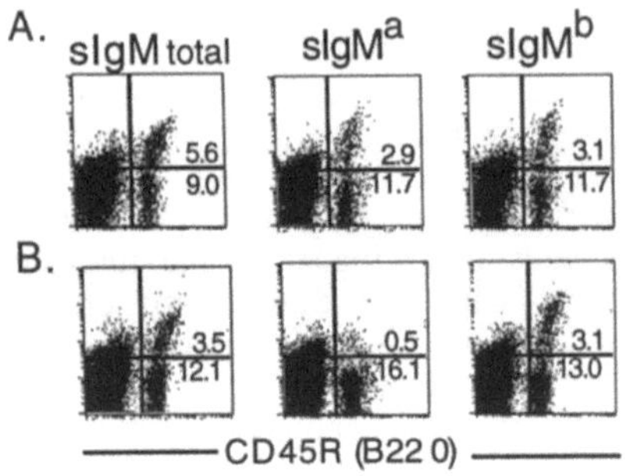

Fig. 5. IgM allotype suppression in FLOC.
Shown are the two colour FACS™ profiles of A. Control or B. Anti-IgMª-treated FLOC stained with CD45R(B220) FITC and PE-labelled mAb to the indicated determinants.

Acknowledgements

The Basel Institute for Immunology was founded and is supported by F. Hoffmann-La Roche Ltd., Basel, Switzerland. This work was carried out whilst Rh. C. was on leave of absence from INSERM Strasbourg.

References

1. Cumano A, Dieterlen-Lievre F, and Godin I. (1996) Lymphoid potential, probed before circulation in mouse, is restricted to caudal intraembryonic splanchnopleura. Cell 86: 907-916
2. Nourrit F, Doyen N, Kourilsky P, Rougeon F, and Cumano A. (1998) Extensive junctional diversity of Ig heavy chain rearrangements generated in the progeny of single fetal multipotent hematopoietic cells in the absence of selection. J Immunol 160: 4254-4261
3. Owen JJT, Cooper MD, and Raff MC. (1974) In vitro generation of B lymphocytes in mouse fetal liver, a mamalian "bursa equivalent". Nature 249: 361-363
4. Raff MC, Owen JJ, Cooper MD, Lawton A, Megson M, and Gathings WE. (1975) Differences in susceptibility of mature and immature mouse B lymphocytes to anti-immunoglobulin-

induced immunoglobulin suppression in vitro. Possible implications for B-cell tolerance to self. J Exp Med 142: 1052-1064
5. Raff MC, Megson M, Owen JJT, and Cooper MD. (1976) Early production of intracellular IgM by B lymphocyte precursors in mouse. Nature 259: 224-226
6. Melchers F, Rolink A, Grawunder U, Winkler TH, Karasuyama H, Ghia P, and Andersson J. (1995) Positive and negative selection events during B lymphopoiesis. Curr Opin Immunol 7: 214-227
7. Whitlock CA, and Witte ON. (1982) Long-term culture of B lymphocytes and their precursors from murine bone marrow. Proc Natl Acad Sci USA 79: 3608-3612
8. Hayashi S, Kunisada T, Ogawa M, Sudo T, Kodama H, Suda T, Nishikawa S, and Nishikawa S. (1990) Stepwise progression of B lineage differentiation supported by interleukin 7 and other stromal cell molecules. J Exp Med 171: 1683-1695
9. Rolink A, Kudo A, Karasuyama H, Kikuchi Y, and Melchers F. (1991) Long-term proliferating early preB cell lines and clones with the potential to develop to surface-Ig positive mitogen-reactive B cells "in vitro" and "in vivo". EMBO J 10: 327-336
10. Ceredig R. (1988) Differentiation potential of 14-day fetal mouse thymocytes in organ culture: Analysis of CD4/CD8-defined single positive and double negative cells. J Immunol 141: 355-362
11. Jenkinson EJ, and Anderson G. (1994) Fetal thymic organ cultures. Curr Opin Immunol 6: 293-297
12. Bevan MJ. (1997) In thymic selection, peptide diversity gives and takes away. Immunity 7: 175-178
13. Ceredig R, ten Boekel E, Rolink A, Melchers F, and Andersson J. (1998) Fetal liver organ cultures allow the proliferative expansion of pre-B receptor-expressing pre-B-II cells and the differentiation of immature and mature B cells in vitro. Int Immunol 10: 49-59
14. Owen JJT, Raff MC, and Cooper MD. (1975) Studies on the generation of B lymphocytes in the mouse embryo. Eur J Immunol 5: 468-473
15. Rolink A, Haasner D, Nishikawa SI, and Melchers F. (1993) Changes in frequencies of clonable preB cells during life in different lymphoid organs of mice. Blood 81: 2290-2300
16. Sudo T, Nishikawa S, Ohno N, Akiyama N, Tamakoshi M, Yoshida H, and Nishikawa S. (1993) Expression and function of the interleukin 7 receptor in murine lymphocytes. Proc Natl Acad Sci U S A 90: 9125-9129
17. Köhler G, and Milstein C. (1976) Derivation of specific antibody-producing tissue culture and tumor lines by cell fusion. Eur J Immunol 6: 511-519
18. Andersson J, Melchers F, and Rolink A. (1995) Stimulation by T cell independent antigens can relieve the arrest of differentiation of immature auto-reactive B cells in the bone marrow. Scand J Immunol 42: 21-33
19. Dray S. (1962) Effect of maternal isoantibodies on the quantitative expression of two allelic genes controlling g-globulin allotypic specificities. Nature 195: 677-680

Discussion

John Kearney: Most of the anti-allotype antibodies we have ever used do not see isolated µH-chains, so some conformational change must be occurring with heavy conventional light chain pairing to influence the allotype epitopes [Velardi, A., Kubagawa, H. and Kearney, J.F. (1984) J Immunol 133:2098-2103]. Did you ever try just conventional goat anti-µH antibody?
Jan Andersson: Yes, the result is the same: the anti-µ experiments I showed can be reproduced either by polyclonal goat or rabbit anti-IgM as well as F(ab)2 fragments thereof, or any available monoclonal rat anti-µH-chain antibody. You are absolutely right when it comes to the inability of the available monoclonal anti-IgM allotype antibodies to recognize free µH-chains. The only situation where we can analyze the anti-allotype for its possible interaction with a preB cell receptor, namely a µH-chain associated with λ_5 and V_{preB}, is the IgM^a allotype. None of the available monoclonal anti-IgM^a allotype antibodies react with such a preBCR. We do not have cell lines expressing IgM^b allotype in the absence of conventional light chain. So we do not know how it is with our anti-IgM^b reagents.
Jason Cyster: Have you tried using an Ig transgenic system to see if you can overcome the block at the preB-II stage, given that Ig transgenes are expressed at earlier stages of B cell development?
Jan Andersson: Yes we have, and we cannot arrest differentiation at earlier stages. So we have a transgenic situation which Fritz wanted me to mention, namely an IgM/kappa, called Sp6, which is specific for TNP as well as DNA. When we put this transgene onto a RAG-2 knockout genetic background (RAG-2T), we see the development of a normal preB-II compartment. A number of ligands added, including anti-idiotypic antibodies, free DNA or TNP bound to different thymus-dependent as well as thymus-independent carrier molecules have failed to affect the development of the preB-II compartment in this transgenic model. So we have tried hard to find any possible interaction with a preB cell receptor which would have either positive or negative influences on the developing B cells and we so far have failed.
Fritz Melchers: We have also looked at many heavy chains that are suspected to be auto-reactive by themselves, for instance the heavy chains of Martin Weigert's anti-double-strand DNA-specific antibodies, as a transgene on $RAG^{-/-}$ background. The preB-II compartment always develops normally. Hence you come away with the idea that even that preB cell receptor is not susceptible to any kind of negative influence.
Gary Rathbun: Did you see any difference in RAG expression in your preB-I compartment when you have your reversible block versus your preB-II compartment when you have your irreversible block?
Jan Andersson: No, we did not yet look for RAG expression, but it is obvious that one should. It requires a lot of cell sorting because you get blurred by all the different cell populations present in the FLOC. You have to sort and preferably look at individual cells and we simply have not done that.
Richard Scheuermann: One of the key questions in all this selection business is why some cells respond and get deleted while others do not. Is it the quality or the quantity of the signal? In the case of the preB cells expressing the preB cell receptor, do they express a lot less heavy chain on the cell surface? Could it be related to the quantity of signal that they are getting? Has that ever been addressed?
Jan Andersson: Some Ig transgenics express much higher levels of µH-chain at earlier time points during development.
Richard Scheuermann: You can detect preBCR with antibody?
Jan Andersson: Yes, and there we cannot see any effect either. There are some transgenics (i.e. Sp6) which express the µH-chain already at the preB-I stage and also all attempts to manipulate this compartment with external ligands have failed to show any effect. I do not think it has to do with the quantity. I think it is the quality of the signaling which is different in preB cells and immature B cells.

Jim Kenny: In Fritz's earlier talk he made a point about heavy chains which could associate with the surrogate light chain and that those cells were the ones that in fact went through this expansion during the preB-II phase of development. But you did not see any effect of having put in anti-surrogate light chains?
Jan Andersson: That is correct, we saw the same expansion also in the presence of anti-surrogate light chain antibodies. Now when you use livers from λ_5 knockout mice for FLOC, you find developing B cells which express surface Ig, but they are 20-fold less compared to wild type livers. That deficiency is exactly what you also find in vivo.
Jim Kenny: How does this relate to the idea which Randy Hardy described in a paper in JEM (Wasserman R, Li YS, Shinton SA, Carmack CE, Manser T, Wiest DL, Hayakawa K, and Hardy RR. (1998) A novel mechanism for B cell repertoire maturation based on response by B cell precursors to pre-B receptor assembly. J. Exp. Med. 187: 259-264) suggesting that in the fetal liver, and you are using fetal liver cultures, the heavy chains that could associate with the surrogate light chain were in fact prevented from undergoing expansion, and then at the fetal liver stage it was the ones that did not associate very well with the surrogate light chain that were in fact allowed to go on and develop. How does that fit in?
Jan Andersson: It doesn't fit in. In the paper you are referring to data were obtained by using certain Ig-transgenes, which could be interpreted in the way you just did. The data could, however, also represent a transgenic artefact.
Michael Carroll: Do I understand that you were able to let immature B cells develop in your FLOC system and then treat those with antibodies to IgM, and you saw those cells actually stop developing at that stage? Did you try the same experiment with antibody to CD19, and what was the effect on the immature B cells?
Jan Andersson: Yes we did. Adding it to FLOC initiated from day 14 fetal livers which contain only pre-BI cells, and scoring the cultures after 6 days by FACS analysis for phenotype or function in terms of LPS activation at limiting dilution, these anti-CD19-treated cultures showed no effect. There is only one anti-CD19, the 1D3 clone from Fearon, and titering it into developing FLOC at any time shows no effects.

Negative Selection of Self-reactive B Lymphocytes Involves Complement

M. Carroll
The Center for Blood Research and Department of Pathology, Harvard Medical School, Boston, MA 02115, USA

Introduction

B lymphocytes are regulated at multiple checkpoints during development of the pre-immune and immune repertoire (Goodnow 1996). Encounter of self-antigen within the bone marrow results in deletion, anergy or no effect depending on the strength of signal. In general, membrane self-antigens induce sufficient signal transduction or crosslinking of B cell receptor (BCR) to cause deletion (Nemazee et al. 1989; Hartley et al. 1991). In contrast, soluble antigens such as soluble hen lysozyme (sHEL) induce anergy (Goodnow et al. 1989). B cells expressing an immunoglobulin (Ig) transgene (tg) which bind dsDNA can lead to either deletion in the bone marrow (Chen et al. 1995) or peripheral tolerance (Erikson et al. 1991; Mandik-Nayak et al. 1997) depending on relative binding affinity. Mutations that alter BCR strength of signaling can affect negative selection and these findings support the model. For example, mice bearing targeted disruption of molecules involved in regulation of BCR signaling such as CD22, SHP-1 (Cyster et al. 1995), CD45 (Cyster et al. 1996) or Lyn (Cornall et al. 1998) have altered negative selection of self-reactive B cells in the sHEL/HEL-Ig double tg model. Alternatively, expression of an additional copy of CD19 results in increased sensitivity to BCR signaling and reduction in the number of peripheral tg B cells (Inaoki et al. 1997). The complement system is an important factor in humoral immunity as binding of activated fragments of complement C3 to antigen not only enhances its localization to the lymphoid compartment but induces BCR signal transduction (Fearon et al. 1995; Carroll 1998a) (see review in this issue by M. Carroll). Given the role of complement in B cell activation, we proposed that it might also be involved in B cell tolerance to certain self-antigens such as nuclear proteins and dsDNA.

To examine a role for complement in negative selection of self-reactive B cells, we bred mice bearing targeted deficiencies in complement C4 ^{null}, C3 ^{null} or CD21/CD35 (Cr2^{null}) with mice expressing transgenes encoding HEL-Ig and sHEL. Characterization of the single and double transgenic animals by flow cytometry, immunohistochemistry and functional response to antigen *ex vivo* demonstrated that complement C4 and the receptors CD21/CD35 were critical in maintenance of tolerance in this model of peripheral tolerance.

Deficiency in CD21/CD35 Results in Loss of Anergy in Self-reactive B Cells

Characterization of the sHEL/HEL-Ig double transgenic mice has revealed that self-reactive B cells are not eliminated in the BM but they become anergized and escape into the peripheral lymphoid compartment (Goodnow, et al. 1989). The phenotype of anergic B cells in the sHEL/HEL-Ig model includes a reduction in sIgM, reduction in total number and frequency of mature cells and non-responsiveness to self-antigen *ex vivo*. Further, HEL-specific antibody is not detectable in the blood. The first indication that $Cr2^{+}$ and $Cr2^{null}$ tg B cells were not responding to self-antigen in a similar manner came from analysis of bone marrow (BM) harvested from the two groups of double tg mice. Whereas the relative surface levels of sIgM were reduced on immature (IgD-negative) $Cr2^{+}$ tg B cells, there was a slight increase in sIgM expression on $Cr2^{null}$ tg B cells. Thus, the absence of CD21/CD35 appears to affect the response of immature B cells to self-antigen in the BM (results not shown).

To examine anergy of self-reactive B cells in the $Cr2^{null}$ double tg mice, the frequency of tg cells was analyzed in BM, spleen and lymph nodes (LN) harvested from single and double tg mice. No significant differences were observed among the overall frequency or total numbers of $Cr2^{+}$ $B220^{+}/HEL^{+}$ tg B cells in the BM or spleens of single and double tg mice as expected. However, a modest increase was observed in the total frequency and number of tg B cells in spleens of $Cr2^{null}$ double tg mice. Analysis of mature $B220^{+}$ cells in the LNs revealed a striking decrease in the frequency and number of mature HEL^{+} B cells in $Cr2^{+}$ double tg mice. For example, flow cytometry analysis of mature $CD23^{+}/B220^{+}$ tg B cells demonstrated a 10-fold reduction in the total number ($5.3 \pm 0.9 \times 10^{5}$ versus $0.5 \pm 0.3 \times 10^{5}$, $p < 0.001$). By contrast, only a modest decrease in $CD23^{+}/B220^{+}$ mature B cells was observed in the LNs of $Cr2^{null}$ double tg mice ($3.8 \pm 0.9 \times 10^{5}$ versus $2.0 \pm 1.2 \times 10^{5}$).

The decrease in number of mature HEL^{+} tg B cells in the double tg mice could be explained by a reduced half-life as demonstrated by Fulcher and Basten (Fulcher et al. 1994). Mice were injected with BrdU for seven days to examine the replacement frequency of tg B cells in the single and double tg mice. As expected, approximately 50% of the self-reactive B cells in $Cr2^{+}$ double tg mice were replaced during the labeling period. In contrast, no difference was observed in the turnover of $Cr2^{null}$ self-reactive B cells on comparison of single and double tg animals as approximately 25% of the HEL^{+} cells were labeled over the seven day period (Fig. 1).

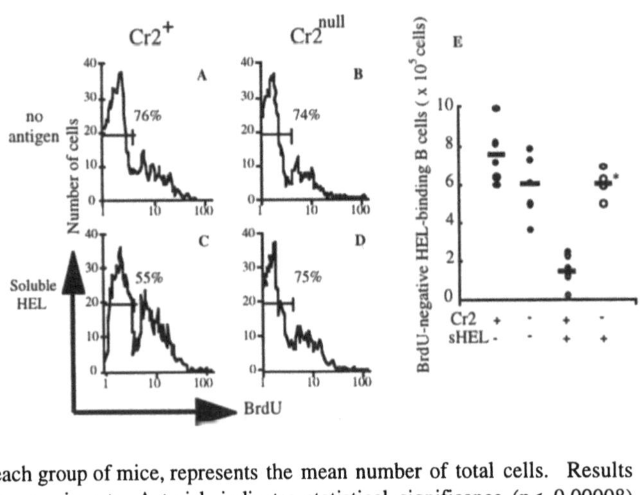

Fig. 1. Life span of $Cr2^{null}$ HEL-binding B cells is not reduced by presence of HEL-self antigen.
(A-D) Representative histograms of relative BrdU fluorescence of HEL-binding B cells of single and double transgenic $Cr2^{+}$ and $Cr2^{null}$ mice.
(E) Scatter plot represents total numbers of BrdU-negative HEL-binding B cells from five lymph nodes per mouse. Horizontal bar for each group of mice, represents the mean number of total cells. Results are from at least 3 separate experiments. Asterisk indicates statistical significance ($p < 0.00008$) comparing number of BrdU-negative HEL-binding B cells harvested from LNs of $Cr2^{+}$ and $Cr2^{null}$ double transgenic mice (from Prodeus et al. 1998).

The hallmark of anergic B cells is impaired response to self-antigen. To characterize the responsiveness of self-reactive B cells to self-antigen *ex vivo*, spleens were harvested from the four groups of tg mice and cultured overnight with an optimal concentration of HEL antigen. $Cr2^{+}$ and $Cr2^{null}$ HEL-Ig B cells were analyzed by three-color flow cytometry for surface expression of HEL, B220 and CD86 (B7-2). CD86 was used as a marker for stimulation as it is expressed on activated B lymphocytes after cross-linking BCR. No difference was observed between the $Cr2^{+}$ and $Cr2^{null}$ HEL-Ig tg B cells harvested from single tg mice as approximately 60% of the tg B cells in both groups expressed CD86 (Fig. 2 A, B, & I). As expected, very few of the $Cr2^{+}$ anergic B cells responded to self-antigen (Fig. 2C). By contrast, the frequency of $CD86^{+}/HEL^{+}$ tg B cells was similar in $Cr2^{null}$ single and double tg mice (Fig. 2 B & D). Thus, $Cr2^{null}$ self-reactive B cells are not rendered nonresponsive in the presence of self- antigen. It is worth noting that self-reactive B cells harvested from both $Cr2^{+}$ and $Cr2^{null}$ tg mice appeared inactivated when analyzed in absence of HEL antigen (Fig. 2E & F). This result is important as it supports the argument that accumulation of $Cr2^{null}$ self-reactive B cells is not likely due to activation *in vivo*.

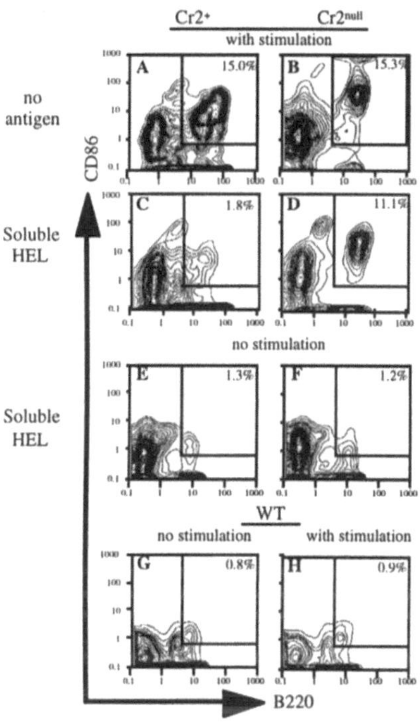

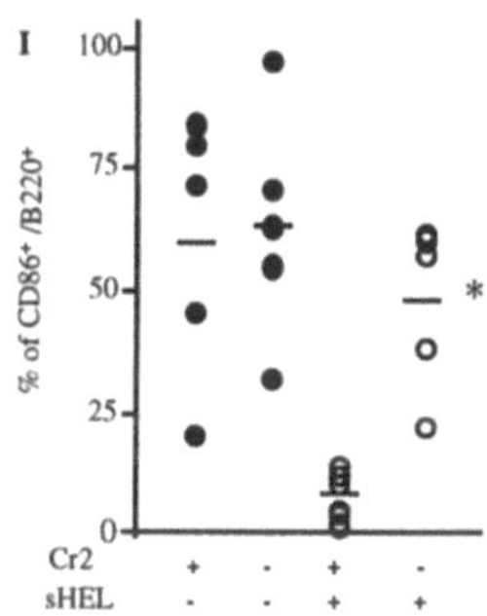

Fig. 2. $Cr2^{null}$ HEL-binding B cells harvested from double transgenic mice are not anergic based on expression of activation marker CD86 in response to antigen stimulation *ex vivo*.
(A-D) Representative flow cytometry results of HEL-binding splenocytes following overnight culture with 100 ng/ml of HEL and then stained with mAb specific for B220 and CD86 (B7-2). HEL^{+}, $B220^{+}$ cells harvested from $Cr2^{+}$ double transgenic mice have an impaired response to HEL-self antigen as expected from previous studies (Cooke et al., 1994). By contrast, only a modest decrease in responsiveness to antigen stimulation was observed in $Cr2^{null}$ cells isolated from double transgenic mice. Number in upper right quadrant represents percent of total lymphocytes gated which are double positive for CD86 and B220. (E,F) Response to culture with antigen was confirmed as specific as very few $B220^{+}$ cells isolated from the two groups of double transgenic mice expressed CD86 *ex vivo* prior to culture with HEL; and (G, H) WT spleen cells express background levels of CD86 *ex vivo* irrespective of culture without or with HEL. (I) Scatter plot summarizing results from three separate experiments demonstrating a significant difference ($p < 0.004$; indicated by asterisk) in the frequency of $CD86^{+}$ $B220^{+}$ cells following overnight culture with HEL isolated from $Cr2^{null}$ compared to $Cr2^{+}$ double transgenic mice. Horizontal bars represent means for each group of mice analyzed. Results represent percent of total $B220^{+}$ cells which were positive for CD86 based on gate settings shown in panels A-D (from Prodeus et al. 1998).

Failure to respond is likely due to a block in BCR signaling. To examine signal transduction via BCR, splenocytes harvested from $Cr2^{+}$ and $Cr2^{null}$ single and double tg B cells were in a calcium ion flux assay in which cells were stained with B220-specific mAb then loaded with a calcium sensitive dye, fluo-3. Cells were cultured briefly with HEL antigen and then analyzed by two color flow-cytometry for release of $Ca^{+2}i$ as an indicator of responsiveness. As reported by Cooke et al. (Cooke et al. 1994), $Cr2^{+}$ $B220^{+}$ self-reactive B cells harvested from double tg mice failed to respond to antigen stimulation. In contrast, $Cr2^{null}$ tg B cells did respond although less than that observed with B cells harvested from single tg mice (results not shown).

Deficiency in Serum Complement C4 Results in Impaired Tolerance

The results obtained with the $Cr2^{null}$ double tg mice demonstrate an unexpected critical role for complement receptors CD21/CD35 in maintenance of tolerance in the sHEL/HEL-Ig model. The major ligands for CD21 and CD35 are activated fragments of C3 and C4. To examine the importance of C3 and C4 in this model, we constructed radiation chimeric mice in which bone marrow harvested from C^{+} HEL-Ig tg mice was engrafted into C^{+}, $C4^{null}$ or $C3^{null}$ sHEL or no antigen recipients. Chimeric mice were prepared rather than germline breeding because the HEL-Ig transgene is located on chromosome 17 near the MHC region (C4 and C3 are encoded on chromosome 17). Therefore, it is difficult to obtain recombinant $C4^{null}$ or $C3^{null}$ Ig tg mice. This approach has been used by others to generate single and double tg mice in the sHEL/HEL-Ig model and the phenotype is similar to that of germline mice (Fulcher and Basten 1994). Single and double tg mice were characterized in a similar manner as $Cr2^{null}$ mice. As expected, self-reactive B cells harvested from the double tg chimeras were anergic based on significant reduction in frequency and total number of $CD23^{+}$ LN cells ($4.1 \pm 1.4 \times 10^{4}$ versus $0.5 \pm 0.3 \times 10^{4}$; $p < 0.0003$). In contrast, a similar number of HEL^{+} cells was observed in single and double tg chimeric mice ($4.3 \pm 1.3 \times 10^{4}$ versus $5.7 \pm 1.8 \times 10^{4}$). Interestingly, dcficicncy in C3 did not significantly alter induction in anergy as an approximately 3-4 reduction in number of $CD23^{+}$ self-reactive B cells was found in the LNs of $C3^{null}$ double tg chimeras ($6.9 \pm 1.8 \times 10^{4}$ versus $2.1 \pm 1.1 \times 10^{4}$; $p<0.0007$). However, it should be noted that BM-derived cells such as monocytes can synthesize C3 (as well as C4) when stimulated and it is possible that low levels of C3 were produced in the lymphoid tissues of the double tg $C3^{null}$ BM chimeras.

To examine further if self-reactive B cells were anergized in the $C4^{null}$ double tg chimeras, splenocytes were harvested from the four groups of chimeras and cultured overnight with optimal concentrations of antigen. Three-color flow cytometry analysis of splenic HEL^{+} tg B cells revealed that self-reactive B cells isolated from the C^{+} or $C3^{null}$ double tg animals failed to express appreciable levels of surface CD86 in response to antigen (Fig. 3 A, C, D, F, J). In contrast, B cells harvested from $C4^{null}$ single and double tg mice responded to a similar degree (Fig. 3 B, E, J). Thus, complement C4 is important in maintenance of B cell anergy in the sHEL/HEL-Ig model.

Fig. 3. HEL-binding B cells harvested from C4^{null} but not C3^{null} chimeric-double transgenic mice respond to antigen *ex vivo* and express the activation marker CD86 (B7-2).

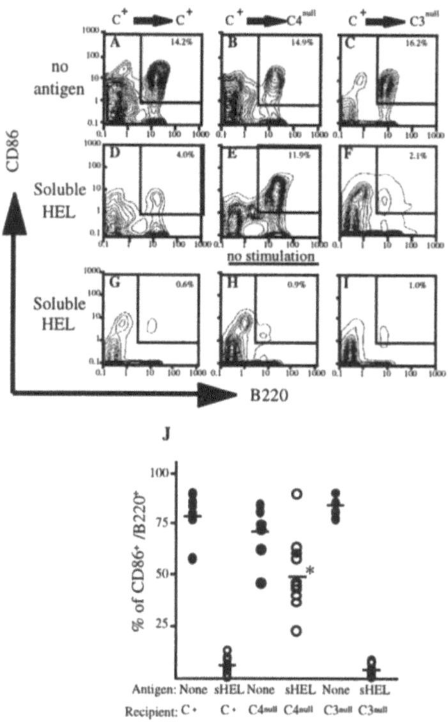

(A-F) Representative flow diagram indicating frequency of B220$^+$ splenocytes harvested from C$^+$, C4^{null} or C3^{null} single and double transgenic mice which express CD86 in response to antigen stimulation *in vitro*. Results reveal that HEL-binding B cells harvested from C4^{null} double transgenic mice are responsive to HEL *in vitro* and therefore do not appear to be anergic. By contrast, HEL-binding B cells harvested from C$^+$ or C3^{null} chimeric double tg mice are anergized. Number in upper right quadrant indicates mean percent of B220/CD86 double positive cells out of total lymphocytes gated. (G-I) Representative flow diagrams of HEL-binding B cells harvested from the three groups of double transgenic mice and analyzed directly without prior stimulation. Results reveal that despite presence of sHEL antigen *in vivo* the B cells do not appear to be activated. (J) Scatter plot summarizing results from three separate experiments comparing frequency of CD86$^+$ cells out of total B220$^+$ splenocytes gated. Horizontal bars indicate mean values. Asterisk indicates statistical significance ($p<0.002$) comparing frequency of CD86$^+$ splenocytes harvested from C$^+$ or C3^{null} with C4^{null} double transgenic mice (from Prodeus et al. 1998).

Discussion

The finding that B cells, like T cells, undergo negative selection suggests that defects in regulation of B cell tolerance could result in autoimmune disease. For example, systemic lupus erythematosus (SLE) is an autoimmune disorder characterized by autoantibodies specific for dsDNA and nuclear proteins. Disease in lupus patients is thought to be mediated by excess immunecomplex formation and in one mouse model, B cell deficiency abrogates disease (Chan et al. 1998). Thus, dysregulation of B cell tolerance might be a major factor in disease susceptibility. Although the cause of SLE in humans is not known, deficiency in early complement components C1q, C4 or C2 (in that order) predisposes to disease. Individuals deficient in C1q or C4 almost always develop lupus (Walport et al. 1991) and disruption of the C1q gene in mice leads to spontaneous autoimmune disease (Botto et al. 1998). It is not clear how complement is involved in SLE; but it has been proposed that its role is in clearance of self-antigens such as apoptotic bodies to prevent activation of self-reactive B cells (Korb et al. 1997; Botto et al. 1998). Our findings with the C4 and Cr2^{null} double tg mice suggest an alternative explanation. We propose that complement is involved in the induction of B cell anergy to soluble self-antigens (Carroll 1998b). This model would not include all soluble antigens but only those in which there are pre-existing natural antibodies. Accordingly, deficiency in C4 or C1q (or complement receptor CD35) would lead to impaired retention of soluble self-antigens such as dsDNA and nuclear proteins within the bone marrow and peripheral lymphoid compartment. (Fig. 4)

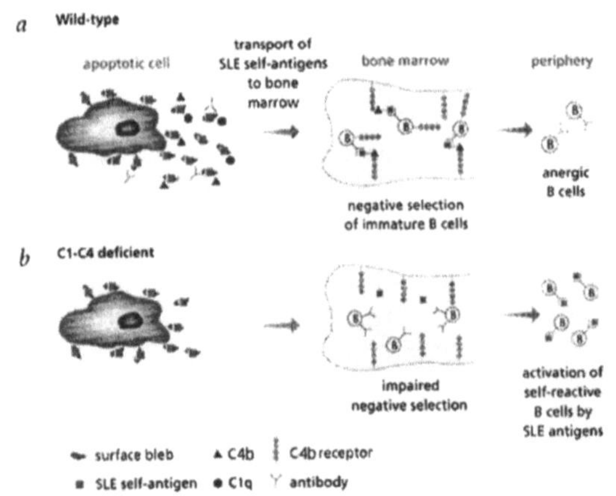

Fig. 4. Role for the complement system in maintenance of B cell tolerance (from Carroll 1998b).

The reduction in efficiency of localization of self-antigens in the BM would result in altered negative selection of self-reactive immature B cells. Thus, in the absence of C1q (which is required for activation of C4) or C4 dsDNA-specific self-reactive B cells would escape into the periphery where they would become available for activation and release of autoantibodies in the presence of T-help. The two different models are not mutually exclusive and it is likely that complement is involved in both stages, i.e. negative selection and antigen clearance.

Further support for a role of complement in lupus disease comes from our findings with C4^{null} or Cr2^{null} *lpr/lpr* mice (Prodeus et al. 1998). Breeding of deficiency in either C4 or CD21/CD35 with the *Fas*-deficient C57BL/6-lpr/lpr strain resulted in an exacerbation of disease. While disease is mild on the B6 background, deficiency in complement C4 or its receptor CD21/CD35 resulted in dramatic increase in anti-dsDNA and nuclear protein antibody levels as well as glomerulonephritis. Our explanation is that in the absence of C4 or CD21/CD35, self-antigens, such as dsDNA were not efficiently retained within the BM and self-reactive B cells were not removed from the repertoire and became activated in the presence of autoreactive T cells.

Acknowledgements

I would like to acknowledge the fellows in my lab who participated in the project, i.e. Andrey Prodeus, Siegfried Goerg, Olga Pozdnyakova, Li-Ming Shen, Elisabeth Alicot, and my colleagues Christopher Goodnow and Garnett Kelsoe for discussions regarding the experiments.

References

Botto M, Dell'Agnola C, Bygrave AE, Thompson EM, Cook HT, Petry F, Loos M, Pandollfi PP, Walport M (1998) Homozygous C1q deficiency causes glomerulonephritis associated with multiple apoptotic bodies. Nature Genet 19: 56-59

Carroll MC (1998a) The role of complement and complement receptors in induction and regulation of immunity. Ann Rev Immunol 16: 545-568
Carroll MC (1998b) The lupus paradox Nature Genet 19: 3-4
Chan O, Shlomchik MJ (1998) A new role for B cells in systemic autoimmunity: B cells promote spontaneous T cell activation in MRL-lpr/lpr mice. J Immunol 160: 51-59
Chen C, Nagy Z, Radic MZ, Hardy RR, Huszar D, Camper SA, Weigert M (1995) The site and stage of anti-DNA B-cell deletion. Nature 373: 252-255
Cooke MP, Heath AW, Shokat KM, Zeng Y, Finkelm A, FD , Linsley PS, Howard M, Goodnow CC (1994) Immunoglobulin signal transduction guides the specificity of B cell-T cell interactions and is blocked in tolerant self-reactive B cells. J Exp Med 179: 425-438
Cornall RJ, Cyster JG, Hibbsd ML, Dunn AR, Otipoby KL, Clark EA, Goodnow CC (1998) Polygenic autoimmune traits: Lyn, CD22, and SHP-1 are limiting elements of a biochemical pathway regulating BCR signaling and selection. Immunity 8: 497-508
Cyster JG, Goodnow CC (1995) Protein tyrosine phosphatase 1C negatively regulates antigen receptor signaling in B lymphocytes and determines the thresholds for negative selection. Immunity 2: 13-24
Cyster JG, Healy JI, Kishihara K, Mak TW, Thomas ML, Goodnow CC (1996) Regulation of B-lymphocyte negative and positive selection by tyrosine phosphatase CD45. Nature 381: 325-328
Erikson J, Radic MZ, Camper SA, Hardy RR, Carmack C, Weigert M (1991) Expression of anti-DNA immunoglobulin transgenes in non-immune mice. Nature 349: 331-334
Fearon DT, Carter RH (1995) The CD19/CR2/TAPA-1 Complex of B Lymphocytes: Linking Natural to Acquired Immunity. Annu Rev Immunol 13: 127-149
Fulcher DA, Basten A (1994) Reduced life span of anergic self-reactive B cells in a double-transgenic model. J Exp Med 179: 125-134
Goodnow CC (1996) Balancing immunity and tolerance: Deleting and tuning lymphocyte repertoires. Proc Natl Acad Sci USA 93: 2264-2271
Goodnow CC, Crosbie J, Jorgensen H, Brink RA, Basten A (1989) Induction of self-tolerance in mature peripheral B lymphocytes. Nature 342: 385-391
Hartley SB, Crosbie J, Brink R, Kantor AB, Basten A, Goodnow CC (1991) Elimination from peripheral lymphoid tissues of self-reactive B lymphocytes recognizing membrane-bound antigens. Nature 353: 765-769
Inaoki M, Sato S, Weintraub BC, Goodnow CC, Tedder TF (1997) CD19 regulated signaling thresholds control peripheral tolerance and autoantibody production in B lymphocytes. J Exp Med 186: 1923-1931
Korb LC, Ahearn JM (1997) C1q binds directly and specifically to surface blebs of apoptotic keratinocytes. J Immunol 158: 4525-4528
Mandik-Nayak L, Bui A, Noorchashm H, Eaton A, Erikson J (1997) Regulation of anti-double stranded DNA B cells in nonautoimmune mice: localization to the T-B interface of the splenic follicle. J Exp Med 186: 1257-1267
Nemazee D, Buerki K (1989) Clonal deletion of autoreactive B lymphocytes in bone marrow chimeras. Proc Natl Acad Sci USA 86: 8039-8043
Prodeus AP, Goerg S, Shen LM, Pozdnykova OO, Chu L, Alicot E, Goodnow CC, Carroll MC (1998) A critical role for complement in maintenance of self-tolerance. 9 721-731
Walport MJ, Morgan BP (1991) Complement deficiency and disease Immunol Today 12: 301-306

Discussion

Fritz Melchers: Do you think that complement affects B cell stimulation in the bone marrow early in B cell development?

Michael Carroll: Yes, we are arguing that there is some effect early on in the bone marrow, but based on what Goodnow has reported I think that this is more of a model of peripheral tolerance; as anergic cells escaping to the periphery where they continue to encounter self-antigen. We are arguing that complement is important for the retention of antigen not only in the bone marrow but also in the periphery.

Jim Kenny: Jason Cyster can correct me, but I was under the impression that in the system of the soluble HEL and anti-HEL the half-life of the B cell in the absence of normal B cells is not greatly different, even though that had been questioned in a paper from Tony Basten, basing it on receptor occupancy.

Jason Cyster: You have 50% survival in one week whereas if you have other cells around none of the HEL-binding cells survive one week.

Jim Kenny: But these animals were not ones in which you should have had, from my understanding of the cross, a lot of endogenous B cells around.

Michael Carroll: When we BrdU labeled for 7 days, we found that there were 50% BrdU positive cells in the $Cr2^+$ double tg animals, whereas in the $Cr2^{null}$ mice, less than 25% of the cells were labeled, demonstrating that half-life is significantly extended in CD21/CD35-deficient B cells. So it may not be days, it may be one week.

Jason Cyster: There seems to be some inconsistency in that observation versus the small numbers of cells that you see. In the spleen and lymph nodes the numbers are down at about a maximum of 50%, whereas in the lymph node you were suggesting the numbers were down a lot.

Michael Carroll: The 10-fold reduction represents total number of $CD23^+$ HEL-binding B cells which is more dramatic than when we gated on total $B220^+$ cells.

Shozo Izui: Have you ever looked at autoantibody production in the $Cr2^{null}$ knockout mice?

Michael Carroll: Yes. Antibody levels were undetectable in the $Cr2^{null}$ double transgenics. We think this is due to absence of T help.

Shozo Izui: How about autoantibodies such as anti-DNA?

Michael Carroll: We have not looked for anti-dsDNA antibody in the complement-deficient mice. However we intend to do this. Mark Walport has reported recently about 25% of mice deficient in C1Q spontaneously make autoantibodies to nuclear antigens at 8 months (Botto et al. 1998, Nat. Genet. 19, 56-59).

Q: In which stage of differentiation of the B cell are complement receptors expressed? Is it only in mature B cells, VpreB or something?

Michael Carroll: CD21/CD35 comes up fairly early, as they are Cr2 expressed at the immature B cell stage.

Q: Which one?

Michael Carroll: We refer to the IgM positive, IgD negative, CD23 negative cells as immature.

Jason Cyster: I thought it came up with IgD.

Michael Carroll: No, we find it on IgD negative cells in the bone marrow.

Jason Cyster: Do you find that IgD negative cells are Cr1 positive?

Michael Carroll: Absolutely.

Fritz Melchers: Ton will talk about a marker that maybe will settle this problem.

Michael Carroll: Mike Holders reported this. I think one problem is that the antibodies used for detecting these receptors bind fairly weakly but with a Cr2 negative control you can readily identify receptor expression. I just want to point out that what I am arguing is not dependent on CD21 expression on the B cell. We are proposing that CD21/CD35 expression on stromal cells in the bone marrow is important for trapping the self-antigen, not coreceptor signaling. The finding that C3-deficient double tgs do not break tolerance supports the idea that costimulation at least via C3d-CD21 is not critical.

Jason Cyster: Why is that? When you need C3 you costimulate?
Fritz Melchers: In the immature stage?
Jason Cyster: To activate Cr1 you need C3 anyway, so how do you separate those two?
Michael Carroll: Well you don't. I have not had a chance to go through the nomenclature but we know that the CR1 (CD35) receptor which is expressed as a coreceptor on a mouse B cell binds also C4b as well as C3d. In fact, C4b is a major ligand for CR1 on human red cells. An important difference between humans and mice is that murine CR1 includes all of the CD21 coding sequence. Therefore, it is possible that CD35 forms a co-receptor with CD19 and can be cross-linked by C4b; although this has not been demonstrated. Anyway we prefer a model in which co-receptor signaling on immature B cells is not critical to negative selection
Frans Kroese: Is there an element of marginal zone B cell development in your system?
Michael Carroll: We have not really looked at that very closely.
Frans Kroese: These tolerant cells do not develop to marginal zone B cells so it seems better in your $Cr2^{null}$ cells.
Michael Carroll: We do observe by immunohistochemistry an increase in the frequency of $Cr2^{null}$ vs. $Cr2^{+}$ HEL-Ig tg B cells within the follicles of double tg mice.

Cross-talk Between CD44 and c-Met in B cells

T.E.I. Taher, R. van der Voort, L. Smit, R.M.J. Keehnen, E.J.M. Schilder-Tol, M. Spaargaren and S.T. Pals.
Department of Pathology, Academic Medical Center, University of Amsterdam, Amsterdam, The Netherlands.

Introduction

Activation of naive B cells in the T cell areas of the secondary lymphoid tissues initiates T cell dependent humoral immune responses. As a consequence of this primary B cell activation, germinal center (GC) cell precursors migrate into B cell follicles where they engage T cells and follicular dendritic cells (FDC), and differentiate into plasma cells or memory B cells. Both the homing of B cells to the GC and their interaction with FDC critically depend on integrin-mediated adhesion. We have recently identified the growth and motility factor, hepatocyte growth factor/scatter factor (HGF/SF) and its receptor, the c-*met*-encoded receptor tyrosine kinase, as a novel paracrine signaling pathway regulating B cell adhesion within the GC microenvironment [22]. The c-Met protein is expressed on B cells localized in the dark zone of the GC (centroblasts) and is induced by combined CD40 and B-cell receptor ligation. Stimulation of c-Met with HGF/SF, which is produced at high levels by tonsillar stromal cells and FDC, leads to enhanced integrin-mediated adhesion of B cells to fibronectin and VCAM-1 [22].

The HGF/SF-c-Met pathway has been shown to regulate growth, motility, and morphogenesis of epithelial, endothelial, and myogenic cells, which requires tightly controlled adhesion. Furthermore, this pathway mediates tumor invasion and metastasis, a process reminiscent of lymphocyte migration [2,24]. HGF/SF is a disulfide-linked heterodimer protein composed of a 69-kDa α-chain and a 34-kDa β-chain that is secreted mainly by mesenchymally derived cells [2]. All known biological effects of HGF/SF are mediated via c-Met. Upon ligand binding, c-Met interacts with different cytoplasmic target proteins resulting in activation of several signaling proteins including Ras and PI3-kinase [2, 14]. In addition to binding c-Met, HGF/SF has a high affinity for heparin, which is present on the cell surface and in the ECM in the form of heparan sulfate proteoglycans (HSPG) [2].

Recent studies indicate that the ability of heparin-binding growth factors to bind to HSPG can add an extra regulatory level to their biological functions *in vivo* [16,17,4,19]. HSPG-binding limits cytokine diffusion, thus allowing the development of chemotactic gradients and the localization of biological activity to the appropriate microenvironment. Furthermore, HSPG can present growth factors, e.g. fibroblast growth factor-2 (FGF-2), to their high-affinity receptors [1,16,17]. CD44 is a multi-functional cell-surface glycoprotein that plays a role in binding to the extracellular matrix, lymphocyte activation and homing, and tumor progression and metastasis [10-13]. The gene encoding the human CD44 protein can be alternatively spliced [1,9,11]. On lymphocytes the short standard form of CD44 (CD44s) predominates, whereas the larger variants are expressed on normal and neoplastic epithelia and on activated lymphocytes and malignant lymphomas [11-13].The principal ligand for CD44 is hyaluronic acid (HA), a major glycosaminoglycan component of the extracellular matrix [11,12,21]. Interestingly, some of the large CD44 variants are cell surface proteoglycans as they carry heparan sulfate (HS) attached to a conserved amino acid motif SGSG encoded by exon v3 [9].

Here we describe and discuss evidence showing that a HSPG form of CD44 on the B-cell surface binds HGF/SF and strongly promotes c-Met signaling in an HS-dependent fashion. Furthermore, we show that binding of the standard isoform of CD44 to HA or anti-CD44 antibodies also promotes signaling through c-Met. These data suggest that distinct routes, i.e. both extracellular and cytoplasmic, account for the promotion of c-Met signaling by different isoforms of CD44. Based on these observations we propose a model to explain the role of CD44 in signaling through c-Met in B cells.

Results and Discussion

A Heparan Sulfate Proteoglycan Isoform of CD44 Binds HGF/SF and Promotes c-Met Signaling.

To study the ability of proteoglycan forms of CD44 to bind HGF/SF, we stably transfected the Burkitt's lymphoma cell line Namalwa with cDNAs encoding either CD44s or CD44v3-10. CD44v3-10 is post-translationally modified by the attachment of an HS chain, whereas the CD44s is not [23]. The binding of HGF/SF to these transfectants was measured by FACS using an anti-HGF/SF antibody. The transfectants which express the HSPG CD44v3-10 bound HGF/SF, whereas the CD44 negative cells and the CD44s transfectant showed weak HGF/SF binding (Fig. 1). The binding of HGF/SF to the cells expressing the CD44v3-10 is HS-dependent, as the binding of HGF/SF to these cells was completely abolished after treatment of the cells with heparitinase, an enzyme which removes the HS side-chain (Fig. 1). Furthermore, an HGF/SF mutant HP1, which lacks the ability to bind HS [7], could not bind CD44v3-10 [23] . These results demonstrate the presence of binding sites for HGF/SF on the HS chain attached to CD44v3-10.

To assess the possible impact of HGF/SF binding to HS-modified CD44 on the activation and signaling through c-Met, we generated double transfectants co-expressing c-Met with either CD44v3-10 or CD44s. Using these cell lines we measured HGF/SF-induced tyrosine phosphorylation of c-Met and other cytoplasmic proteins. In the cells co-expressing CD44v3-10 and c-Met a higher increase in the

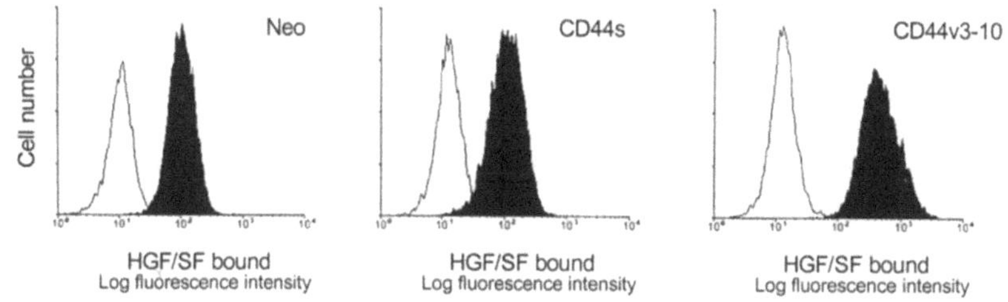

Fig. 1. The HSPG isoform CD44v3-10 binds HGF/SF in an HS-dependent fashion. Namalwa cells, mock-transfected or stably transfected with either CD44s or CD44v3-10 as indicated, were incubated with (*open profile*) or without (*filled profile*) heparitinase (10 U/ml) for 3 hrs and incubated with HGF/SF (18 nM) for the last 1 hr. Binding of HGF/SF was determined by FACS analysis using an anti-HGF/SF antibody.

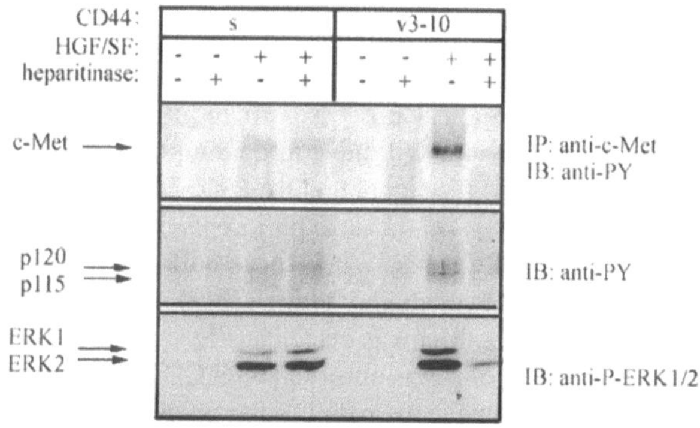

Fig. 2. The HSPG isoform CD44v3-10 promotes c-Met signaling in an HS-dependent fashion. Namalwa cells co-expressing c-Met and either CD44s or CD44v3-10 were treated for 3 hrs with 10 U/ml heparitinase and incubated with HGF/SF (1 nM), as indicated. Subsequently, cells were either directly lysed in sample buffer or cell lysates were immunoprecipitated with anti-c-Met antibody, and immunoblotted using anti-phosphotyrosine antibody or anti-phospho-MAPK antiserum, as indicated.

level of tyrosine phosphorylation of c-Met upon addition of HGF/SF is detected as compared to the cells co-expressing CD44s and c-Met (Fig. 2). Moreover, in the cells co-expressing CD44v3-10 and c-Met, other cytoplasmic proteins were hyperphosphorylated as well, including two major tyrosine phosphorylated proteins with molecular weight of about 115-120 kD (Fig. 2). Two proteins of similar molecular weight have been implicated in c-Met signaling. P120-Cbl, which is highly expressed in B cells, is tyrosine phosphorylated in cells expressing Tpr-Met [6] and is involved in cell adhesion and migration [26]. Furthermore, p115 Grb-2 associated binder (Gab)-1, which was shown to be involved in c-Met-induced morphogenesis [25] as well as B cell receptor signaling [8]. We are currently investigating the identity of the p115 and p120 phosphoproteins in order to study their possible involvement in the c-Met signaling pathways regulating B cell adhesion and migration. Finally, we also observed phosphorylation of the ERK1/2 MAP kinases upon HGF/SF treatment. Again, the phosphorylation of ERK1/2 was stronger in the cells expressing CD44v3-10 as compared to the CD44s expressing cells (Fig. 2).

Using the HGF/SF mutant HP1 [23] and by heparitinase treatment, we provided additional evidence that the striking difference between CD44v3-10 and CD44s in the promotion of c-Met signal transduction is due to the ability of CD44v3-10 to bind HGF/SF by means of its HS moiety. As shown in figure 2, heparitinase treatment strongly reduces the HGF/SF-induced phosphorylation of c-Met on the CD44v3-10 expressing cells. A similar effect of heparitinase treatment was observed with respect to the phosphorylation of p115, p120 and the ERK1/2 MAP kinases (Fig. 2). Taken together, these data clearly demonstrate that the HSPG form of CD44 promotes c-Met activation and downstream signal transduction in an HS-dependent fashion.

CD44-mediated Adhesion Promotes c-Met Signaling

Binding of CD44 to HA, the principal ligand of CD44 and a major component of the extracellular matrix, has been implicated in cell growth and migration, and has been reported to transduce signals to the intracellular compartment leading to activation of different biological processes including cell growth and migration [3,12,13,15]. Since cells *in vivo* will have to deal with more than one ligand at the same time, we assessed how the signaling through c-Met may be affected by CD44-mediated adhesion to HA. For these experiments we used Namalwa cells co-transfected with c-Met and CD44s. When these cells were allowed to adhere to a surface coated with HA and incubated with HGF/SF, a potentiation in the level of tyrosine phosphorylation of c-Met was detected (Fig. 3). We would like to stress that since the potentiating effect of HA is observed with CD44s, the non-HGF/SF-binding isoform, this effect cannot be due to cross-linking or HGF/SF-induced colocalization of c-Met with CD44s. Subsequently, using anti-CD44 antibodies, we investigated whether cross-linking and/or adhesion of CD44 as such, i.e. independent of HA, is sufficient for potentiation of HGF/SF-induced c-Met signaling. Indeed, as shown in figure 3, a similar potentiating effect on c-Met signaling can be induced by cross-linking and/or adhesion of CD44 by means of the anti-CD44 antibody Hermes-3 in an HA-independent fashion. These results suggest that the cytoplasmic domain of CD44 may be involved in an outside-in signaling mechanism by which CD44-mediated adhesion can promote signaling through c-Met.

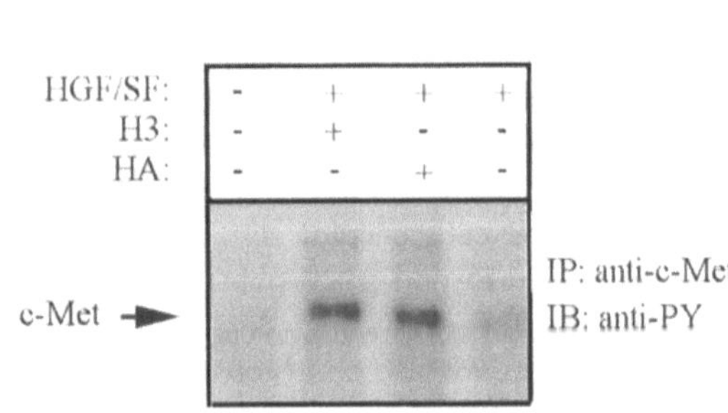

Fig. 3. The CD44s isoform promotes c-Met signaling in an adhesion-dependent fashion. Namalwa cells co-expressing c-Met and CD44s were allowed to adhere for 10 min, either in the presence or absence of HGF/SF (1 nM), to a surface which, before being blocked with 1% BSA, had been coated with either 50 μg/ml hyaluronic acid (*HA*), 10 μg/ml Hermes-3 (*H3*) or nothing, as indicated. After cell lysis, c-Met was immunoprecipitated with anti-c-Met antibody and immunoblotted with anti-phosphotyrosine antibody.

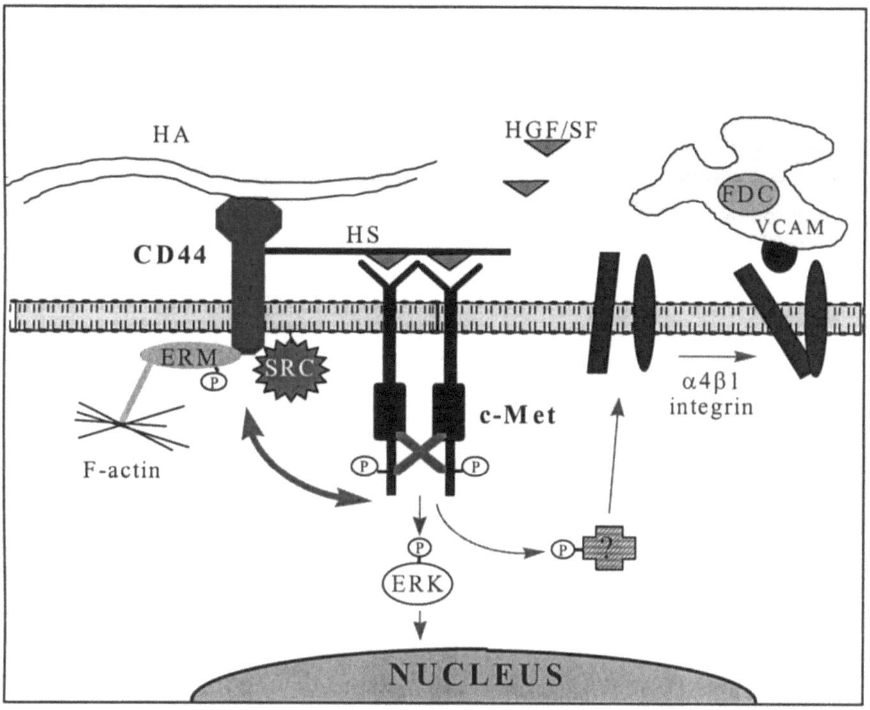

Fig. 4. Different isoforms of CD44 can promote c-Met signaling by distinct mechanisms. CD44v3-10 promotes c-Met signaling by heparan sulfate-mediated presentation of HGF/SF to c-Met, whereas CD44 can also promote c-Met signaling as a consequence of adhesion to HA. See text for further details.

Functional Cross-talk Between CD44 and c-Met: a Model

In summary, our results show that an HSPG form of CD44 can act as a low affinity receptor for HGF/SF and can promote signaling through c-Met in an HS-dependent fashion. Furthermore, binding of the standard form of CD44 to HA can also promote c-Met activation by HGF/SF. We propose the following model to explain the possible role for CD44 in the signaling through c-Met (Fig. 4).

The promotion of HGF/SF-induced c-Met signaling in the cells expressing the HSPG form of CD44 may be due to an increased effective concentration of HGF/SF on the plasma membrane, thereby increasing the binding of HGF/SF to c-Met. Similar mechanisms were proposed for signaling through the FGF-receptor [16,17]. In addition, the binding of several HGF/SF molecules to the HSPG form of CD44 may promote di-/oligomerization of c-Met, leading to enhanced receptor activation. Furthermore, the potentiation of c-Met activation may be partially explained by HGF/SF-mediated co-localization of HS-modified CD44 and c-Met, which may bring relevant intracellular signaling molecules in the proximity of each other. The results showing that binding to HA (or anti-CD44 antibody) of the CD44s isoform, which is unable to bind HGF/SF, promotes HGF/SF-induced c-Met activation, provide further support for the existence of intracellular cross-talk between CD44 and c-Met. This intracellular cross-talk may be the consequence of outside-in signaling by CD44 due to either ligand binding, cross-linking or substrate adhesion. Indeed, the intracellular domain of CD44 may affect signaling through c-Met, as we have previously shown that CD44 physically and functionally interacts with the Src-family protein tyrosine kinase Lck in T lymphocytes [18], and it has been shown that Src kinases are involved in c-Met signaling [14]. Besides the Src family tyrosine kinases, also ERM family members (e.g. ezrin) may be involved in intracellular cross-talk between CD44 and c-Met. Ezrin binds directly to the cytoplasmic domain of CD44 and to the actin cytoskeleton [3, 20]. Furthermore, ezrin is a substrate for c-Met shown to be involved in HGF/SF-induced cell migration [5]. Since the interaction of ezrin with the cytoskeleton and plasma membrane receptors is crucial for induction of cell migration [5], it is tempting to speculate that tyrosine phosphorylation of ezrin by c-Met may increase its binding to the cytoskeleton and CD44, thereby regulating cell adhesion and migration. In conclusion, we have obtained evidence that HSPG isoforms of CD44 can promote c-Met signaling in an HGF/SF-dependent manner by an extracellular mechanism, whereas the standard isoform of CD44 may promote c-Met signaling in an adhesion-dependent manner by an intracellular mechanism. Thus, by means of distinct mechanisms different isoforms of CD44 are able to promote signaling by c-Met, thereby regulating B cell adhesion and migration.

Currently, we are further unravelling the possible mechanisms of extracellular and intracellular cross-talk between CD44 and c-Met, as well as the signaling pathways involved in the regulation of B cell adhesion and migration. Obviously, the proposed model brings enormous flexibility and power to the mechanism of modulation of receptor tyrosine kinase signaling by HSPG and thereby to the regulation of processes like lymphocyte homing and the immune response, as well as tumor progression and metastasis.

Acknowledgment- This work was supported by grant no. 98-267 from the AICR

References

1. Bennett KL, Jackson DG, Simon JC, Tanczos E, Peach R, Modrell B, Stamenkovic I, Plowman G, and Aruffo A (1995) CD44 isoforms containing exon V3 are responsible for the presentation of heparin-binding growth factor. J Cell Biol 128:687-698.
2. Birchmeier C, and Gherardi E (1998) Developmental roles of HGF/SF and its receptor, the c-Met tyrosine kinase. Trends Cell Biol 8:404-410.
3. Bourguignon LYW, Zhu D, and Zhu H (1998) CD44 isoform-cytoskeleton interaction in oncogenic signaling and tumor progression. Front Biosci 3:D637-649.
4. Carey DJ (1997. Syndecans: multifunctional cell-surface co-receptors. Biochem J 327:1-16.
5. Crepaldi T, Gautreau A, Comoglio PM, Louvard D, and Arpin M (1997) Ezrin is an effector of hepatocyte growth factor-mediated migration and morphogenesis in epithelial cells. J Cell Biol 138:423-434.
6. Fixman ED, Naujokas MA, Rodrigues GA, Moran MF, and Park M (1995) Efficient cell transformation by the Tpr-Met oncoprotein is dependent upon tyrosine 489 in the carboxy-terminus. Oncogene 10:237-249.
7. Hartmann G, Prospero T, Brinkmann V, Ozcelik O, Winter G, Hepple J, Batley S, Bladt F, Sachs M, Birchmeier C, Birchmeier W, and Gherardi E (1998) Engineered mutants of

HGF/SF with reduced binding to heparan sulfate proteoglycans, decreased clearance and enhanced activity in vivo. Curr Biol 8:125-134.

8. Ingham RJ, Holgado-Madruga M, Siu C, Wong AJ, and Gold MR (1998) The Gab1 protein is a docking site for multiple proteins involved in signaling by the B cell antigen receptor. J Biol Chem 273:30630-30637.
9. Jackson DG, Bell JI, Dickinson R, Timans J, Shields J, and Whittle N (1995) Proteoglycan forms of the lymphocyte homing receptor CD44 are alternatively spliced variants containing the v3 exon. J Cell Biol 128:673-685.
10. Koopman G, van Kooyk Y, de Graaff M, Meyer CJ, Figdor CG, and Pals ST (1990) Triggering of the CD44 antigen on T lymphocytes promotes T cell adhesion through the LFA-1 pathway. J Immunol 145:3589-3593.
11. Lesley J, Hyman R, and Kincade PW (1993) CD44 and its interaction with extracellular matrix. Adv Immunol 54:271-335.
12. Lesley J, and Hyman R (1998) CD44 structure and function. Front Biosci 3:D616-630.
13. Ponta H, and Herrlich P (1998) The CD44 protein family: roles in embryogenesis and tumor progression. Front Biosci 3:d650-656.
14. Ponzetto C, Bardelli A, Zhen Z, Maina F, dalla Zonca P, Giordano S, Graziani A, Panayotou G, and Comoglio PM (1994) A multifunctional docking site mediates signaling and transformation by the hepatocyte growth factor/scatter factor receptor family. Cell 77:261-271.
15. Rafi A, Nagarkatti M, and Nagarkatti PS (1997) Hyaluronate-CD44 interactions can induce murine B-cell activation. Blood 89:2901-2908.
16. Spivak-Kroizman T, Lemmon MA, Dikic I, Ladbury JE, Pinchasi D, Huang J, Jaye M, Crumley G, Schlessinger J, and Lax I (1994) Heparin-induced oligomerization of FGF molecules is responsible for FGF receptor dimerization, activation, and cell proliferation. Cell 79:1015-1024.
17. Steinfeld R, Van Den Berghe H, and David G (1996) Stimulation of fibroblast growth factor receptor-1 occupancy and signaling by cell surface-associated syndecans and glypican. J Cell Biol 133:405-416.
18. Taher TE, Smit L, Griffioen AW, Schilder-Tol EJ, Borst J, and Pals ST (1996) Signaling through CD44 is mediated by tyrosine kinases. Association with p56lck in T lymphocytes. J Biol Chem 271:2863-2867.
19. Tanaka Y, Kimata K, Adams DH, and Eto S (1998) Modulation of cytokine function by heparan sulfate proteoglycans: sophisticated models for the regulation of cellular responses to cytokines. Proc Assoc Am Physicians 110:118-125.
20. Tsukita S, Oishi K, Sato N, Sagara J, and Kawai A (1994) ERM family members as molecular linkers between the cell surface glycoprotein CD44 and actin-based cytoskeletons. J Cell Biol 126:391-401.
21. van der Voort R, Manten-Horst E, Smit L, Ostermann E, van den Berg F, and Pals ST (1995) Binding of cell-surface expressed CD44 to hyaluronate is dependent on splicing and cell type. Biochem Biophys Res Commun 214:137-144.
22. van der Voort R, Taher TE, Keehnen RM, Smit L, Groenink M, and Pals ST (1997) Paracrine regulation of germinal center B cell adhesion through the c- Met-hepatocyte growth factor/scatter factor pathway. J Exp Med 185:2121-2131.
23. van der Voort R, Taher TE, Wielenga VJM, Spaargaren M, Prevo R, Smit L, David G, Hartmann G, Gherardi E, and Pals ST. Heparan sulfate-modified CD44 promotes hepatocyte growth factor/scatter factor-induced signal transduction through the receptor tyrosine kinase c-Met. J Biol Chem, in press.
24. Weidner KM, Sachs M, and Birchmeier W (1993) The Met receptor tyrosine kinase transduces motility, proliferation, and morphogenic signals of scatter factor/hepatocyte growth factor in epithelial cells. J Cell Biol 121:145-154.
25. Weidner KM, Di Cesare S, Sachs M, Brinkmann V, Behrens J, and Birchmeier W (1996) Interaction between Gab1 and the c-Met receptor tyrosine kinase is responsible for epithelial morphogenesis. Nature 384:173-176.
26. Zell T, Warden CS, Chan AS, Cook ME, Dell CL, Hunt SW, 3rd, and Shimizu Y (1998) Regulation of beta 1-integrin-mediated cell adhesion by the Cbl adaptor protein. Curr Biol 8:814-822.

Discussion

Kenneth Nilsson: At what stage of B cell differentiation do you find c-Met expressed?
Steven Pals: We have not looked at any precursor B cells so far. We will do that in collaboration with Ton Rolink. We have only looked in tonsillar or mature B cells and we find expression in IgD CD38 double-positive cells, which are presumably germinal center precursors, and in CD38 positive cells which are IgD negative, and then most prominently in the cells which are CD77 positive, so in the centroblasts.
Kenneth Nilsson: Have you looked at myeloma?
Steven Pals: We have not looked in myeloma but we also see expression in plasma cells; there are two reports that c-Met is expressed in myeloma.
George Klein: How good is the correlation between c-Met and CD77 expression in a collection of Burkitt lines? Do all Burkitt lines express it? How about the lymphoblastic cell lines, do they not express it?
Steven Pals: I cannot answer the question as we did not go into this in detail in the Burkitt lines. We know that some Burkitt lines express it and others do not. Also, some primary, spontaneous Burkitt lymphomas express c-Met and others do not. But we did not correlate this so far with expression of CD77; this correlation has only been examined for the normal B cells.
Georg Bornkamm: Did you correlate with CD38 expression?
Steven Pals: No, we did not correlate it with the CD38. We have only taken a panel of known Burkitt lymphoma cell lines and looked if they had c-Met expression – some have and others do not. But we have not correlated it.
Isaac Witz: Could you induce c-Met expression by antigen or anti-IgM plus anti-CD40? Does the hepatocyte growth factor bind to plasminogen activator? In other words, can it be hooked up to the plasminogen activator receptor cascade?
Steven Pals: What was the first question?
Isaac Witz: Can you induce c-Met by anti-IgM?
Steven Pals: No, if you crosslink the B cell receptor alone, you see virtually no effect on c-Met expression. CD40 ligation, plus anti-IgM, induces strong c-Met expression.
Isaac Witz: What would be the physiological stage?
Steven Pals: We believe that right in the primary response, the B cells probably get the signal to upregulate c-Met and then go to the germinal center.
Garnett Kelsoe: The CD77 population, the dividing centroblasts, has the least contact with the FDC, not the most. I assumed your model would have predicted that the light zone would have the highest expression of c-Met and the dark zone the lowest, but that is the opposite, is it not?
Steven Pals: You are right, CD77 positive cells are the most strongly positive, the others have less expression. But of course we do not know how long the integrin remains active after the stimulation.
Frans Kroese: Do B-1 cells express c-Met, CD5 positive cells or CLLs? Might they be expressed first in germinal centers?
Steven Pals: I cannot answer this for the normal B-1 compartment, and I believe CLLs are not positive.
George Klein: Are follicular lymphomas positive?
Steven Pals: Yes, some of them are positive.

The Transition from Immature to Mature B Cells

A. G. Rolink, F. Melchers and J. Andersson
Basel Institute for Immunology, Postfach, 4005 Basel, Switzerland

Introduction

The small pre-B II cells, such as those that can be found in the bone marrow, form the direct precursor pool of immature B cells that first express IgM at their surface. Experiments by Osmond and his colleagues have shown that mice produce about 2 x 10^7 of these immature B cells per day [1]. Some of them are thought to exit bone marrow [2] and home to extrafollicular areas of the spleen [3]. At these sites in the spleen, B cells are still immature and can be distinguished from their mature counterparts by their half-life (3-4 days versus 6 weeks), their lower B220 and sIgD and their higher HSA and sIgM expression levels [4; 5]. Experiments by a number of investigators have shown that only 5-10% of the newly generated immature B cells are selected into the pool of long-lived mature B cells [1; 3; 4; 6; 7]. Why and how only such a small proportion of immature B cells is selected is largely unknown.

Results and Discussion

We recently described [8] a new mAb, called 493, that allows us to distinguish immature from mature B cells found in bone marrow and in spleen of all mouse strains tested so far. In Fig. 1A, we present 493/B220 double staining analysis of spleen cells derived from a 6-week-old C57Bl/6 mouse. Thus 30% of all the splenic B cells in this mouse express the 493 marker and are immature B cells, just as we also verified previously by short term BrdU labeling. These immature splenic B cells have a life span of about 4 days. Based on the total number of immature B cells in the spleen, which is about 8 x 10^6, and their short half-life time, only 10-20% of the immature B cells made in the bone marrow reach the spleen. Long term BrdU labeling and chase experiments revealed that the majority of immature splenic B cells enter the pool of mature B cells ($B220^+$ 493^-) and become long-living cells (15-20 weeks). With respect to LPS reactivity, immature and mature B cells are indistinguishable, in contrast to the stimulatory action of anti-CD40 which is stronger on mature than on immature splenic B cells. The behavior of immature and mature B cells upon cross-linking of the Ig receptor by anti-IgM antibodies is, on the other hand, completely different. Mature B cells go into proliferation upon Ig cross-linking, as opposed to immature B cells which die by

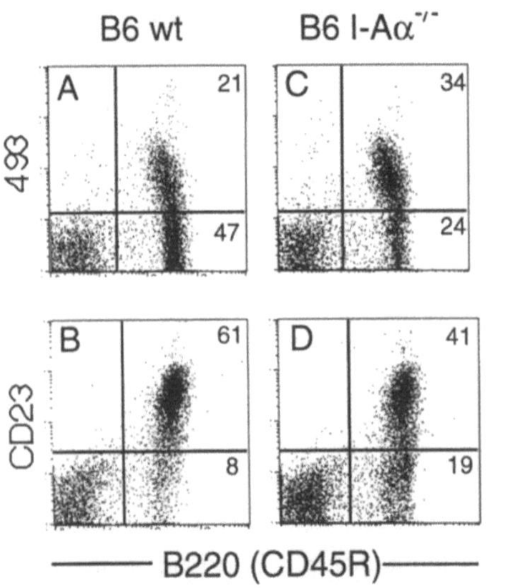

Fig. 1 Double staining of spleen from 6 week old B6 and B6 I-Aα$^{-/-}$ mice using biotinylated mAb 493 or anti-CD23 together with FITC-labelled anti-B220.

apoptosis. Therefore, immature splenic B cells are still sensitive to negative selection. *In vitro* this negative selection can be overcome by co-stimulation with anti-CD40 or by transgenic Bcl-2 expression.

Previously, the differential expression of B220, IgM, IgD and HSA has been used to distinguish immature from mature B cells [5] Thus, immature B cells are B220^{intermediate}, IgM^{high}, IgD^{low} and HSA^{high}, while mature B cells are B220^{high}, IgM^{low}, IgD^{high} and HSA^{low} [2; 5]. Furthermore, CD23 has often been considered as a marker for mature B cells [5]. However, as shown in Fig. 1A and B, at least a considerable number of immature B cells also express CD23. B-I type of B cells are B220^{intermediate}, IgM^{high}, IgD^{low} and HSA^{high}, i.e. appear as if they belong to the immature B cell compartment [9]. In contrast, mAb 493 does not stain peritoneal B cells, which are enriched for B-1 B cells (Fig. 2A and B). So, from this we determine that the mAb 493 is a nice, simple tool with which we can distinguish immature from mature B cells.

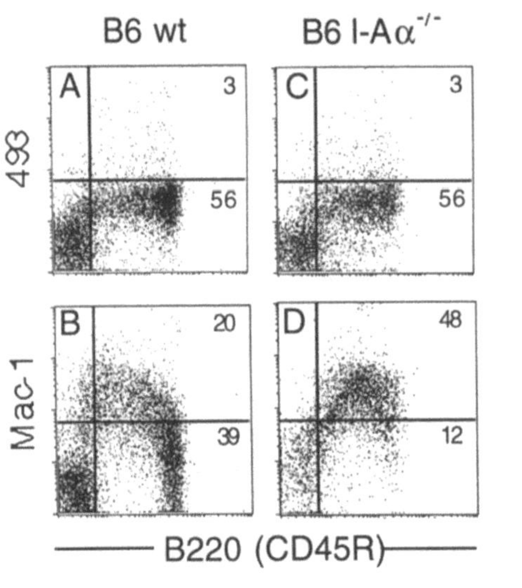

Fig. 2 Double staining of peritoneal cells from the same animals as in Fig. 1. Using biotinylated mAb 493 or anti-Mac-1 together with FITC-labelled anti-B220.

We have been using this mAb currently to analyze mutant mice for defects in immature and mature B cell compartments. By doing so, we found that MHC class II deficient C57Bl6 I-Aα$^{-/-}$ mouse strain [10] has a severely reduced mature B cell compartment (Fig. 1C). In fact, the absolute number of mature B cells in these mice is cut 4 fold lower than in WT control animals. The immature splenic B cell compartment of I-Aα$^{-/-}$ mice is comparable in size to that found in WT mice. In addition, many of these immature B cells express CD23 (Fig. 1.C and D), showing yet again that CD23 cannot be regarded as a mature B cell marker.

B cell development in the bone marrow of B6 I-Aα$^{-/-}$ mice is normal. Moreover, normal numbers of B 1 cells can be found in the peritoneal cavity of B6 I-$A\alpha^{-/-}$ mice (Fig. 2.C), while, as in other peripheral lymphoid organs, conventional mature B cells are also severely reduced (Fig. 2B and C).

BrdU labeling and chase kinetics revealed that the mature B cells in B6 I-$A\alpha^{-/-}$ mice have a half-life time of about 4 weeks. Since the life span of mature B cells in WT mice is 15-20 weeks, the reduced mature B cell compartment in B6 I-$A\alpha^{-/-}$ mice is very likely due to the reduced half-life time of the mature B cells in these mice.

In order to test whether an $E\alpha^d$ transgene can rescue the B cell defect in B6 I-$A\alpha^{-/-}$ mice, two different $E\alpha^d$ transgenes were introduced by back-crossing [11; 12] The $E\alpha^d$ transgene which gives rise to MHC class II expression on precursor and immature B cells could rescue B cell maturation in B6 I-$A\alpha^{-/-}$ mice. Conversely, the $E\alpha^d$ transgene which is expressed only on mature B cells could not. This makes us favor the idea that MHC class II expression on precursors and/or immature B cells is required for optimal B cell maturation. However, these experiments do not yet completely rule out the possibility that MHC class II on non-hematopoietic and/or hematopoietic cells other than B cells could also be involved. Therefore, 950 rad irradiated normal B6 mice were reconstituted with a one in one mixture of B6 I-$A\alpha^{-/-}$ $Ly5.2^+$ and B6 WT $Ly5.1^+$ bone marrow cells. Six weeks after reconstitution, the mice were analyzed. The different stages of B cell development found in the bone marrow were derived equally from the B6 I-$A\alpha^{-/-}$ and the B6 $Ly5.1^+$ donor cells. As shown in Fig. 3, in the spleens of these chimeras, 40% of the cells are derived from the B6 I-$A\alpha^{-/-}$ $Ly5.2^+$ donor and 60% from the B6 $Ly5.1^+$ donor. With respect to the immature B cell compartment in the spleen, both donors contributed equally (Fig. 3). On the other hand, 70-80% of the mature B cells found in these chimeras is derived

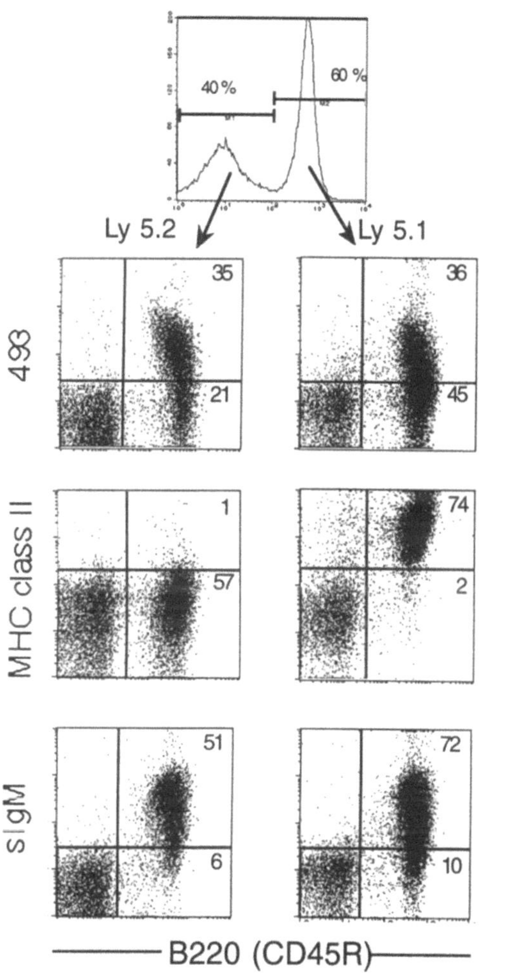

Fig. 3 Phenotypic analyses by FACS of spleen cells from mixed chimeras 6 weeks after adoptive transfer of bone marrow cells from normal B6 (Ly5.1) and from B6 I-$A\alpha^{-/-}$ (Ly5.2) mice.

from the normal B6 WT Ly5.1$^+$ donor (Fig. 3). Thus, in a normal MHC class II expressing environment, the B6 I-A$\alpha^{-/-}$ B cell maturation defect is also obvious. Consequently, this defect is most likely an intrinsic feature of the B cells. Further, MHC class II expression, or at least I-Aα during early stages of B cell development, is required for the formation of a proper long-lived mature B cell compartment.

Others have also reported the involvement of MHC class II on B cell maturation. Shachar and Flavell [13] reported that mice lacking the invariant chain (Ii) associated with MHC class II molecules have an impaired B cell maturation. Similar findings were made by analyzing mice lacking DM [14]. Surprisingly, no B cell maturation defect is observed in B6 I-A$\beta^{-/-}$ mice [15; 16]. If MHC class II expression is required for proper B cell maturation, how do B6 I-A$\beta^{-/-}$ mice manage? Ruberti et al., described heterodimers of Aβ^d Eα^d which play an important role in the immune response against a peptide from sperm whale myoglobin [17] Several laboratories have also shown that AβEα heterodimers can be formed by *in vitro* transfection experiments [18-21]. Hence, the B6 I-A$\beta^{-/-}$ mice might be able to form heterodimers between Aα and Eβ, and the expression of these heterodimers might be the reason for the normal B cell development. However, it must be noted that the existence of AαEβ heterodimers has never been documented experimentally. Alternatively, it might be hypothesized from the experiments presented here, that Aα can associate with other molecules to form a complex involved in B cell maturation either directly, i.e. in contact with a ligand in the environment of bone marrow, or indirectly, i.e. by providing structures for such a contact.

The mechanism by which MHC class II participates in B cell maturation is unknown. The three molecules known to interact with MHC class II, namely the TCR-CD3 complex, CD4, and LAG3 do not appear to be involved (Data not shown). So, another, yet unknown molecule capable of interacting with MHC class II might be involved, and this molecule might be expressed either on immature B cells or on cooperating cells which are not the classical CD4$^+$ helper T cells.

Acknowledgements

The Basel Institute for Immunology was founded and is supported by F. Hoffmann-La Roche Ltd, Basel, Switzerland.

References

1. Osmond DG. (1991) Proliferation kinetics and the lifespan of B cells in central and peripheral lymphoid organs. Curr Opin Immunol 3: 179-185
2. Allman DM, Ferguson SE, Lentz VM, and Cancro MP. (1993) Peripheral B cell maturation. II. Heat-stable antigen^{hi} splenic B cells are an immature developmental intermediate in the production of long lived marrow-derived B cells. J Immunol 151: 4431-4444
3. MacLennan I, and Chan E. (1993) The dynamic relationship between B-cell populations in adults. Immunol Today 14: 29-34

4. Förster I, and Rajewsky K. (1990) The bulk of the peripheral B-cell pool in mice is stable and not rapidly renewed from the bone marrow. Proc Natl Acad Sci USA 87: 4781-4784
5. Hardy RR, Carmack CE, Shinton SA, Kemp JD, and Hayakawa K. (1991) Resolution and characterization of proB and pre-pro B cell stages in normal mouse bone marrow. J Exp Med 173: 1213-1225
6. Thomas-Vaslin V, and Freitas AA. (1989) Lymphocyte population kinetics during the development of the immune system. B cell persistence and life-span can be determined by the host environment. Int Immunol 1: 237-246
7. Sprent J. (1993) Lifespans of naive, memory and effector lymphocytes. Curr Opin Immunol 5: 433-438
8. Rolink AG, Melchers F, and Andersson J. (1998) Characterization of immature B cells by a novel monoclonal antibody, by turnover and by mitogen reactivity. Eur J Immunol 28: 3738-3748
9. Hardy RR, and Hayakawa K. (1991) A developmental switch in B lymphopoiesis. Proc Natl Acad Sci USA 88: 11550-11554
10. Kontgen F, Suss G, Stewart C, Steinmetz M, and Bluethmann H. (1993) Targeted disruption of the MHC class II Aα gene in C57BL/6 mice. Int Immunol 5: 957-964
11. Widera G, Burkly LC, Pinkert CA, Bottger EC, Cowing C, Palmiter RD, Brinster RL, and Flavell RA. (1987) Transgenic mice selectively lacking MHC class II (I-E) antigen expression on B cells: an in vivo approach to investigate Ia gene function. Cell 51: 175-187
12. Yamamura K, Kikutani H, Folsom V, Clayton LK, Kimoto M, Akira S, Kashiwamura S, Tonegawa S, and Kishimoto T. (1985) Functional expression of a microinjected Ed alpha gene in C57BL/6 transgenic mice. Nature 316: 67-69
13. Shachar I, and Flavell RA. (1996) Requirement for invariant chain in B cell maturation and function. Science 274: 106-108
14. Kenty G, Martin WD, Van Kaer L, and Bikoff EK. (1998) MHC class II expression in double mutant mice lacking invariant chain and DM functions. J Immunol 160: 606-614
15. Cosgrove D, Gray D, Dierich A, Kaufman J, Lemeur M, Benoist C, and Mathis D. (1991) Mice lacking MHC class II molecules. Cell 66: 1051-1066
16. Markowitz JS, Rogers PR, Grusby MJ, Parker DC, and Glimcher LH. (1993) B lymphocyte development and activation independent of MHC class II expression. J Immunol 150: 1223-1233
17. Ruberti G, Paragas V, Kim D, and Fathman CG. (1993) Selection for amino acid sequence and J beta element usage in the beta chain of DBA/2V beta b- and DBA/2V beta a-derived myoglobin-specific T cell clones. J Immunol 151: 6185-6194
18. Anderson GD, Banerjee S, and David CS. (1989) MHC class II A alpha and E alpha molecules determine the clonal deletion of V beta 6^+ T cells. Studies with recombinant and transgenic mice. J Immunol 143: 3757-3761
19. Anderson GD, and David CS. (1989) In vivo expression and function of hybrid Ia dimers (E alpha A beta) in recombinant and transgenic mice. J Exp Med 170: 1003-1008
20. Matsunaga M, Seki K, Mineta T, and Kimoto M. (1990) Antigen-reactive T cell clones restricted by mixed isotype A beta d/E alpha d class II molecules. J Exp Med 171: 577-582
21. Mineta T, Seki K, Matsunaga M, and Kimoto M. (1990) Existence of mixed isotype A beta E alpha class II molecules in Ed alpha gene-introduced C57BL/6 transgenic mice. Immunology 69: 385-390

Discussion

Gary Rathbun: Have you used your antibody for any histochemistry?
Ton Rolink: We have tried but it does not work.
Frans Kroese: I would like to make a comment. We got exactly the same data as you in rats, which we published a while ago, using Thy-1 as a marker (Deenen GJ and Kroese FGM [1993] Int Immunol 5:735-741; Kroese FGM et al. [1995] Cell Immunol 162:185-193). Thy-1 is a beautiful marker in rats for distinguishing immature from mature B cells, and we can subdivide the immature compartment into two subpopulations – one that is IgD low and the other IgD high. So we consider the IgD low ones real uniform B cells, and called that population uniform B cells, and the other ones are IgD high and we called those cells early recirculating follicular B cells, as the most immature cells that entered the mature compartment. So my question is: do you have data similar to ours whereby using IgD as a marker you can distinguish between the two subsets, and what is the nomenclature of the cells? I would like that you use the same nomenclature.
Ton Rolink: We have done the correlation but I did not show the data. Immature B cells in a mouse were in before characterized as being $IgD^{-/low}$, HSA^{high}, IgM^{high}. Now doing four-color staining with our marker, it correlates. One problem in the mouse with these old markers, is that one cannot distinguish immature B cells from mature B-1 cells
Frans Kroese: Well, we do have problems in rats because we cannot find B-1 cells.
Ton Rolink: The B-1 as well as the marginal zone B cells in the mouse are 493 negative.
Frans Kroese: But can you find a subset of IgD bright cells in that population that expresses your marker?
Ton Rolink: Yes, but the IgD staining is not very homogeneous anyhow, so based on IgD expression levels I would not subdivide my cells again.
Garnett Kelsoe: What is the relation of your marker to CD23 and CD21 expression?
Ton Rolink: CD23 is expressed on a large number of 493 positive immature B cells, while CD21 is not.
Andreas Radbruch: With respect to the class II-deficient mice, is the half-life of mature B cells affected in T cell-deficient mice?
Ton Rolink: No, we have looked in CD3 knockouts as well as beta/delta TCR knockouts and there the B cells are normal, so it is not the normal interaction with the TCR that gives the long lifespan.
Fritz Melchers: And it is only that one chain.
Michael Carroll: Did you show that CD40 deficiency also had an effect?
Ton Rolink: CD40 deficiency alone has no effect. Only when you cross it onto a BTK mutation do you get an accumulation of the defect.
Jason Cyster: Ian MacLennan and others have shown that when you deplete the mature B cell repertoire it refills within a week, which would not fit with these numbers. Do you have data to indicate that the numbers that come out are enlarged when there is less in the periphery?
Ton Rolink: All the data I showed you came from adult mice. Thus far we have not yet carefully analyzed young mice or chimeras where the situation indeed could be different.
Shozo Izui: In the experiments on the I-A beta knockout mouse, have you looked for expression of the alpha chain? Might the alpha chain combine with another chain?
Ton Rolink: We have looked for it but have not found expression on the surface of cells

CD21^{high} IgM^{high} Splenic B Cells Enriched in the Marginal Zone: Distinct Phenotypes and Functions

F. Martin and J. F. Kearney
Department of Microbiology, Division of Developmental and Clinical Immunology, University of Alabama at Birmingham, Birmingham, AL 35294-3300, USA

Splenic B Cell Subpopulations

Upon generation in the fetal liver and adult bone marrow, B lymphocytes are selected into a long-lived pool that participates in the immune response against exogenous antigens. Processes leading to the generation of long-lived naive B cells are still poorly understood, but it is clear that they include the selection of particular clones over others depending on receptor specificity and individual micro-environmental experiences.

Adult spleen contains follicular and marginal zone long-lived B cells that differ in their topographical location, phenotype and functional capabilities (Gray et al., 1982; Oliver et al., 1997). Although there is not a perfect overlap between phenotype and topography, it is clear that IgM^{hi}/IgD^{lo}/CD21^{hi}/CD23^{lo} B lymphocytes predominate in the marginal zone (MZ) while IgM^{lo}/IgD^{hi}/CD21^{int}/CD23^{hi} represent recirculating follicular (FO) cells (Grey et al., 1984; Waldschmidt, 1991; Oliver et al., 1997). Bacteria and other particulate antigens reaching the blood are retained with high efficiency in the marginal zone of the spleen (Kraal, 1992; FM and JFK, unpublished observations) by specialized macrophages bearing a variety of scavenger receptors. In addition to dendritic cells, B cells located in the marginal zone will also be exposed early in the immune response to capsular and cell wall antigens not requiring a special pathway for processing.

Recent work has shown that in the T cell compartment there are subsets of cells that respond rapidly to nonprotein antigens. These include NK T cells activated by glycolipids and some γδ T cells compartmentalized at mucosal surfaces that recognize unprocessed protein and nonprotein antigens (Fig. 1). As a result of an evolutionary selection these cells have restricted TCR genes: Vα24 paired mostly with Vβ8 for NK T cells and Vγ5 or Vγ6 for γδ T cells in the skin and reproductive tract respectively. Although no such extreme restriction has been described so far in the B cell compartment (with the exception of some clones selected in the B1 peritoneal cavity population), the data presented here suggest that MZ B cells contain such selected clones and that they represent potent effector B cell progenitors.

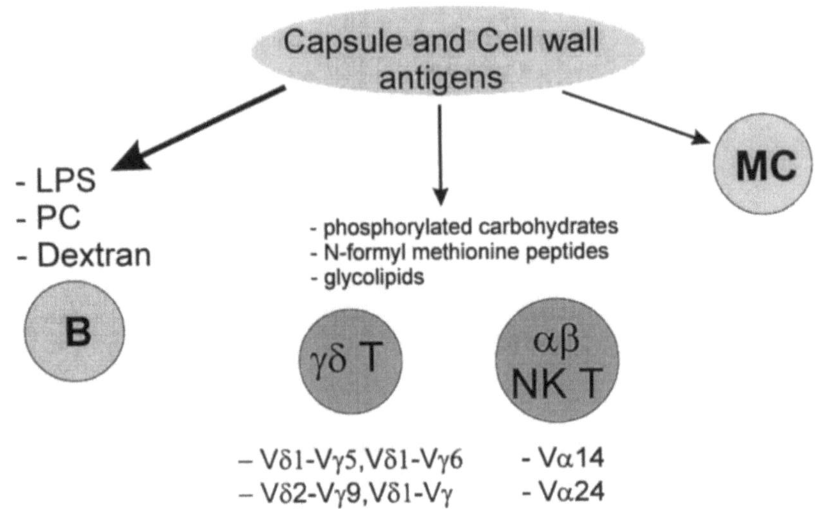

Fig. 1. The first line of response against bacterial antigens involves capsule and cell wall determinants that act on mast cells (MC) and very specialized lymphoid T and possible B cell subpopulations.

Marginal Zone B Cells are Strongly Selected and Show Signs of Previous Antigenic Experience

The marginal zone (MZ) was initially described as the major B cell compartment in the rat spleen that develops independently of T cells (Gray et al., 1982). Recently we have shown that several immunoglobulin heavy chain transgenic mice (HC tg) have an enlarged MZ compartment which facilitates the isolation and detailed characterization of these cells (Oliver et al., in press). All of these models: 81x tg (Chen et al., 1997; Martin et al., 1997) MD2 tg (Goodnow et al., 1988), 81x $TCR^{-/-}$ (Oliver et al., in press) have a proportionally larger marginal zone than their littermates (C57Bl/6 or $TCR^{-/-}$ C57Bl/6) and show that indeed generation of this compartment is largely T cell independent. A detailed phenotypic study shows that MZ B cells are slightly larger and express some markers indicative of previous stimulation (lower levels of CD62L, higher levels of the B7 co-activation molecules) (Fig. 2, Oliver et al., in press). In addition, by following the generation and selection of a particular B cell clone in the 81x tg mice (VH81x-Vκ1C-Jκ5), we showed the extreme enrichment of this clone in the MZ repertoire (F. Martin and J. F.Kearney, in press). VH81X-Vκ1C idiotype positive B cells

(Id+) represent ~5% of the newly emerging B cells in both fetal liver and adult bone marrow. Identical, independently derived clones acquire maturation markers, are enriched to 10-20% of B cells in the transitional compartments of the spleen and finally dominate in the MZ repertoire where they represent ~50% of the B cells. Pulse-chase experiments using BrdU show that the accumulation of Id+ cells is the result of a preferential generation of clones with this receptor and not the result of a selective longer survival. The receptor found on these B cells binds to intracellular self antigens as well as to bacterial phosphorylcholine, both of which might play a role in the peripheral selection of these B cell populations. A similar mechanism of enrichment in the MZ compartment was seen in the case of a VH1-Vκ24 B cell clone in M167 transgenic mice suggesting that a similar mechanism operates in the general selection of the normal MZ B cell repertoire.

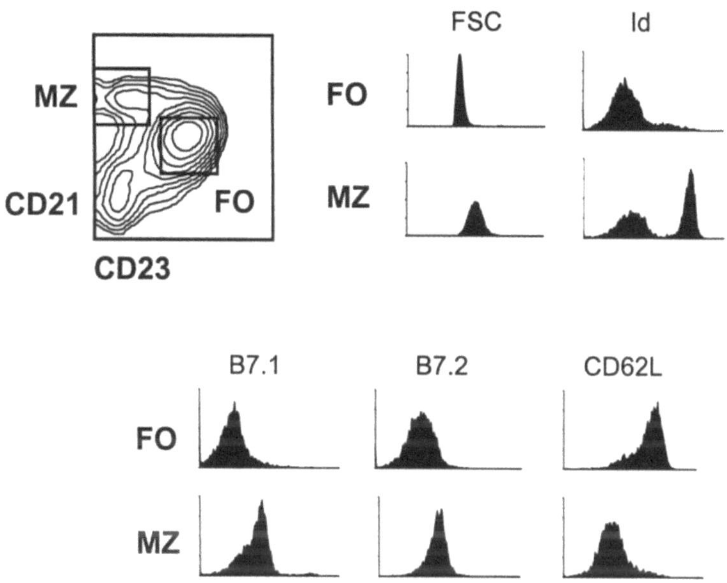

Fig. 2. Mature B lymphocyte subpopulations in the spleen of the VH81x transgenic mice. Idiotype (Id) B cells are enriched in the "natural" activated B cells predominant in the marginal zone (MZ).

CD21^{hi} IgM^{lo} B Cells Respond Rapidly in the Immune System to Present Antigens and Produce Antibodies

From transgenic mice sufficient numbers of purified MZ B cells can be isolated to facilitate the analysis of their functional potential in early stages of *in vitro* and *in vivo* activation. As reported previously (Oliver et al., 1997), MZ B cells proliferate in response to LPS and anti-CD40 (Fig. 3A) and more poorly to anti-IgM stimulation than follicular B cells. MZ B cells also generated higher calcium influxes after crosslinking of their surface IgM receptors. The kinetics of

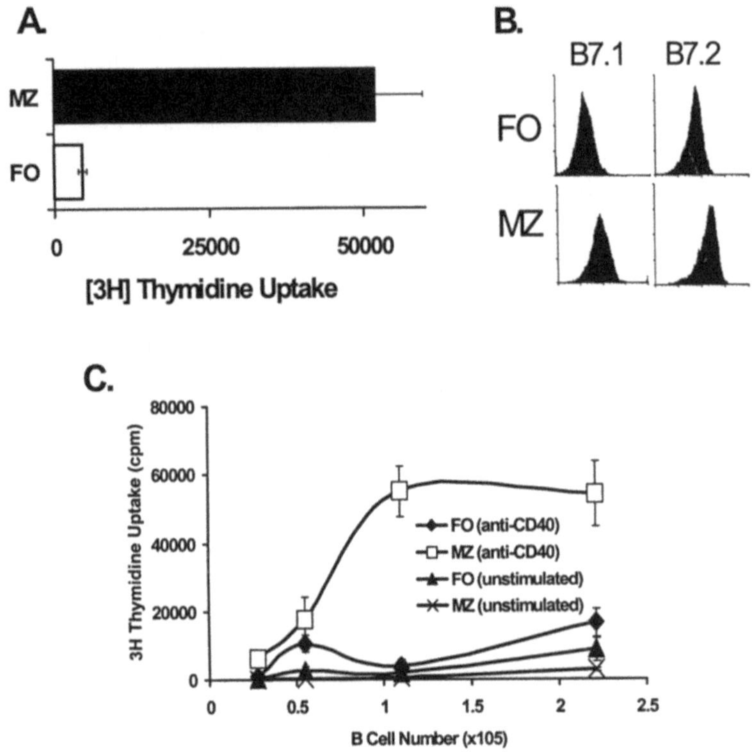

Fig. 3. Marginal zone B cells respond cells to anti-CD40 stimulation better than follicular B by rapidly entering the cell cycle (A), upregulating B7 costimulatory molecules after only 6 hours of activation (B) and by presenting antigen to alloreactive T cells (C).

upregulation for T cell costimulatory molecules B7.1 and B7.2 is also faster on MZ cells (Oliver et al., in press). These findings taken together support the possibility that MZ B cells could function as antigen presenting cells (APC) for T cells. As seen in Fig. 3B, after a very brief (6 hours) activation with anti-CD40 B7.2, although present on unstimulated MZ B cells at a higher level than FO B cells, is upregulated to even higher levels. In parallel the antigen-presenting capacity of MZ B cells is also dramatically increased compared to their follicular counterparts (Fig. 3C).

Summary and Conclusions

Collectively, these findings suggest that MZ B cells have unique signaling and subsequent differentiative capabilities that permit them to react much more vigorously than the majority of splenic B cells (FO) in the earliest stages of an *in vivo* immune response. This is particularly evident with limiting T cell help, low concentration of thymus-independent mitogens or low amounts of particulate blood-borne antigen in the spleen (Fig. 4). They are uniquely situated adjacent to the marginal sinuses and a rich array of antigen trapping macrophages. Because of this location the MZ B cells are ideally positioned for immediate exposure to blood-borne antigens. In contrast, the FO B cells are in juxtaposition to the PALS which may expedite the interactions of FO B cells with T cells and antigen presenting cells. Collectively these properties point to a role for FO B cells in antibody responses to T dependent antigens generated in germinal centers. These responses occur temporally later in immune responses and may be involved principally in the response to protein antigens.

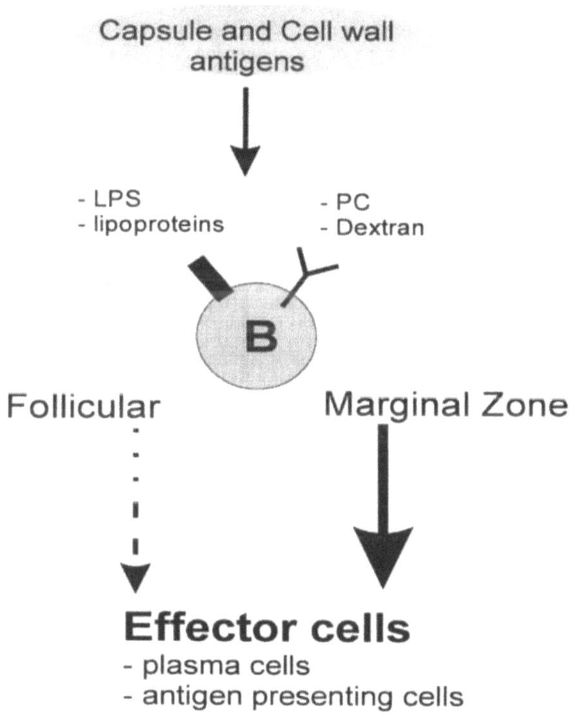

Fig. 4. "Natural" activated B cells enriched in the marginal zone of the spleen (MZ) generate effector cells faster than the bulk of mature recirculating follicular B cells.

Acknowledgements

We gratefully acknowledge the following for transgene constructs, mouse lines, monoclonal antibodies and critical discussions: C. Goodnow, J. Kenny, G. Kraal, P. Burrows, J. Cyster, and Tom Waldschmidt. This work was supported by NIH grants AI 14782 and CA13148.

References

Chen, C., F. Martin, K.A. Forbush, R.M. Perlmutter, and J.F. Kearney. 1997. Evidence for selection of a population of multi-reactive B cells into the splenic marginal zone. *Int. Immunol.* **9**:27-41.

Gray, D., I.C.M. MacLennan, H. Bazin, and M. Khan. 1982. Migrant $\mu^{+}\delta^{+}$ and static $\mu^{+}\delta^{-}$ B lymphocyte subsets. *Eur. J. Immunol.* **12**:564-569.

Gray, D., I. Mcconnell, D.S. Kumararatne, J.H. Humphrey, and H. Bazin. 1984. Marginal zone B cells express CR1 and CR2 receptors. *Eur. J. Immunol.* **14**:47-52.

Goodnow, C.C., J. Crosbie, S. Adelstein, T.B. Lavoie, S.J. Smithgill, R.A. Brink, H. Pritchard-Briscoe, J.S. Wotherspoon, R.H. Loblay, K. Raphael, R.J. Trent, and A. Basten. 1988. Altered immunoglobulin expression and funcitonal silencing of self-reactive B lymphocytes in transgenic mice. *Nature* **334**:676-679.

Kraal, G. 1992. Cells in the marginal zone of the spleen. *Int. Rev . Cytol.* **132**:31-74.

Martin, F., X. Chen and J.F. Kearney. 1997. Development of VH81X transgene-bearing B cells in fetus and adult: sites for expansion and deletion in conventional and CD5/B1 cells. *Int. Immunol.* **9**:493-505.

Oliver, A.M., F. Martin, G.L. Gartland, R.H. Carter, and J.F. Kearney. 1997. Marginal zone B cells exhibit unique activation, proliferative and immunoglobulin secretory responses. *Eur. J. Immunol.* **27**:2366-2374.

Oliver, A.M., F. Martin, and J.F. Kearney. 1999. $IgM^{high}CD21^{high}$ lymphocytes enriched in the splenic marginal zone generate effector cells more rapidly than the bulk of follicular B cells. *J. Immunol. In press.*

Waldschmidt, T.J., F.G.M. Kroese, L.T. Tygrett, D.H. Conrad, and R.G. Lynch. 1991. The expression of B cell surface receptors. III. The murine low-affinity IgE Fc receptor is not express on Ly1 or 'Ly1-like' B cells. *Int. Immunol.* **3**:305-315.

Discussion

Frans Kroese: You have put a question mark between follicular cells and marginal zone B cells. We have some evidence in rats that the most mature Thy-1 negative recirculating follicular B cells can give rise to marginal zone B cells. Do you have some additional evidence for that?
John Kearney: We have done multiple transfer experiments: if you separate follicular and marginal zone cells and inject them, within the first 24 or 48 hrs, each population homes to the correct sites from which they were sorted. Later on we found some follicular cells beginning to appear in the marginal zone. That would agree (in essence) with what you found.
Frans Kroese: Are you saying that when you inject marginal B cells they go back to the marginal zones?
John Kearney: Yes.
Frans Kroese: That is surprising because I thought that marginal zone B cells are being trapped by liver when you inject them.
John Kearney: No, not in our hands. Maybe it has something to do with the antibody you use to sort them. Marginal zone cells clearly home into the marginal zone areas when you sort them with the CD21 reagent.
Fritz Melchers: Did you show that anti-IgM does not stimulate them?
John Kearney: Marginal zone B cells, similar to B-1 cells, are highly susceptible to cross-linking of the BcR by anti-μ antibodies and undergo apoptosis.
Fritz Melchers: The immature B cells? The 493 positive cells?
John Kearney: Antibody 493 is negative for the marginal zone.
Fritz Melchers: Yes I know, but 493 positive cells of the spleen and the bone marrow drop dead, as you say.
Michael Carroll: John, you focused on B cells that respond to bacterial-type antigens. Do you think those cells were selected there because marginal zone macrophages are binding carbohydrate antigens?
John Kearney: I think there is a lot of evidence that memory B cells specific for haptens such as dinitrophenol locate in the marginal zone, but we also think that the marginal zone is also a repository for cells with evolutionary memory. This may include B cells with germline-encoded specificities to phosphorylcholine and other multi-specific B cells which may locate there. This would make sense if you wanted to have B cells bearing polyreactive receptors which may help them present antigen when they migrate into follicular areas.
Kenneth Nilsson: You said that the plasma cells derived from marginal cells were short lived, did you actually prove that or could it be that they home back to the bone marrow?
John Kearney: No, they do not home back to the bone marrow. That is one question that we can answer definitively. We have used idiotypic markers in several Ig transgenic mice and looked at different times after exposure to this antigen, and you do not see them appearing in the bone marrow. This is an interesting finding compared to what others have published, including Andreas Radbruch, with respect to long-lived plasma cells: the plasma cells that I have talked on today are short lived and are not part of the T-dependent response.
Kenneth Nilsson: Are there any other differences between those cells and the long-lived plasma cells?
John Kearney: I don't know. After reaching a peak frequency in the spleen, at about 3 days after immunization they disappear on spleen sections, and they appear to be disintegrating.
Carel van Noesel: According to your scheme there are two populations of plasma cells that can be formed in a T-independent fashion. One population is marginal zone B cells and another one is out of the follicular cells.
John Kearney: The follicular-derived plasma cells appear later in our scheme, and Garnett Kelsoe has a lot of evidence relating to those cells: they take longer to develop after antigen exposure and they are not morphologically similar to those that we are discussing. We have not identified where these cells are in relation to the early appearing IgM-producing plasma cells.

Andreas Radbruch: In the beginning you said that the marginal zone B cells present antigen to T cells but then later in your model the T cell-B cell interaction does not play a role for marginal zone B cells. Are they reactivated by the T cells later and where do they present the antigen to the T cells?

John Kearney: We hypothesize that they can do either depending on the kind of antigen they are exposed to. We've looked at idiotype-bearing antibodies in a variety of transgenic mice and 3 days after immunization, you see that a lot of antibody appears to coat a variety of cells in the follicle. We don't know yet what controls whether a marginal zone B cell migrates into the follicle versus the red pulp but the potential is there and it may depend on the kind of antigen.

Isaac Witz: What is the mechanism for the LPS response? Is it a high concentration or a high affinity of the CD14? Do B-1 cells respond better to LPS than B2 cells?

Fritz Melchers: The answer to the latter question is no: CD14 is not implied as an LPS receptor.

Sandy Morse: The marginal zone cells also express very high levels of CD1. Do you relate that in any way to their possible stimulation by specific T cell subsets?

John Kearney: No, but it is another interesting finding that CD1 is expressed in very high levels on these cells and it fits with the more innate kind of immune response produced by marginal zone B cells.

Jim Kenny: You showed two examples of these marginal zone cells, one was your 81X transgenic animal, and the other one was the phosphorylcholine with the M167 Vkappa 24, and both of those specificities are heavy-light chain specificities which appear to have low affinity autoreactivity for self-antigens. Is there a possibility that this whole population that survives out there is cells that are already pre-activated?

John Kearney: That may be true, but also the MD2 mice have a large marginal zone population. I think it is characteristic that in the absence of competition a certain population of B cells preferentially localizes in this site, which may have been selected by unknown autoantigens.

Jim Kenny: So are there any specificities in the marginal zone that are not potentially autoreactive?

John Kearney: That will take a lot of sorting out. We do not know.

Fritz Melchers: Bacteria, you stimulated them.

Jim Kenny: That is just cross-reactivity.

Martin Bachmann: What do you think is the role of these marginal zone B cells for neutralizing anti-viral B cell responses?

John Kearney: I thought your group in Zurich proposed that there is a lot of IgM antibody that is involved in reactivity and protection against certain viruses, which also appear after immunization to localize in the marginal zone.

Martin Bachmann: Many viruses induce T cell-independent B cell responses by efficiently cross-linking the B cell receptor. Thus, receptor cross-linking on marginal zone B cells would be important for these responses, but now you say these marginal zone B cells drop dead if you cross-link the IgM.

John Kearney: But they can also present antigen very quickly too.

Jason Cyster: Could it be strength of signal? An anti-IgM polyclonal is too strong a signal perhaps? You need to titrate these things.

John Kearney: I agree.

Siegfried Janz: I wonder whether the plasmacytic differentiation of marginal zone B cells is a one-way street. Do all plasma cells derived from marginal zone B cells die, or is there a possibility that at least some of the marginal zone-derived plasma cells or plasmablast-like cells return to the marginal zone? If able to return, could the cells go through this pathway of recirculation and reactivation several times?

John Kearney: Like retired antibody-forming cells? We do not have any evidence for or against that possibility at the moment.

Do Germinal Centers Have a Role in the Generation of Lymphomas?

K. Yang, M. Davila, and G. Kelsoe
Department of Immunology, Duke University Medical Center, Durham, North Carolina 27710, USA.

In the spirit of this meeting I brought only a few slides but I was just told that Ian MacLennan, the real expert on germinal centers, couldn't come and that I should give a bit of an introduction to germinal centers and the germinal center reaction. I can't do that as well as Ian but I would like to talk about three things that I hope you will find interesting and relevant to tumorigenesis.

Figure 1 illustrates a germinal center 16 days after primary immunization with my favorite antigen, the K`ln antigen: nitrophenyl(acetyl) coupled to chicken γ-globulin (NP-CG). The cell nuclei have been labeled with a 3 hour pulse of 2-deoxybromouridine (BrdU) and the blue is staining for the RAG1 protein of the V(D)J recombinase. There are two zones in germinal centers, a , so-called dark zone which is the proliferating zone of the germinal center. B cells enter the DZ, downregulate membrane Ig (mIg), and proliferate as centroblasts. The number of mitotic rounds that centroblasts enter is not known but on average it can not be many because after very brief pulses of BrdU, one can follow migration of labeled cells into the germinal center light zone (LZ). By 6 hours after a pulse of BrdU, virtually all the labeled GC cells will, as Ian MacLennan has shown, have entered the GC LZ (MacLennan, 1994). The LZ is the region of GCs where relatively little proliferation takes place and the site of cell-to-cells interaction between T- and B lymphocytes – here called centrocytes – and follicular dendritic cells. Centrocytes are derived from centroblasts but unlike them, express mIg and do not divide. It is in the LZ that antigen-dependent selection is believed to occur. Following selection in the LZ, centrocytes are thought to either leave the germinal center as memory cells or to return to the DZ and enter another round of division as centroblasts. By reiterating rounds of mutation, proliferation and selection, GC B cells can achieve extraordinary levels of non-debilitating mutations and form extensive genealogies of common descent.

Note that much of the RAG1 staining is present in the cytoplasm of these cells and distinct from the nuclei that are defined by BrdU-labeling (Fig. 1). We have been worried about this staining pattern for we are quite sure that RAG1 is confined to the nucleus of thymocytes and believe that pro- and pre-B cells have only nuclear RAG as well. This histology reveals an interesting difference which may or may not be real but is being pursued by Kaiyong Yang in my laboratory. In his studies, Kaiyong has used the pre-B cell line of Naomi Rosenberg, 103/bcl-2 (Chen et al., 1994), to follow RAG expression and its translocation to the nucleus. This cell line is transformed by a temperature-sensitive Abelson leukemia virus that drives cellular proliferation at 34°C but carries a mutant *v-abl* gene whose product is unstable at 39°C. Thus, when cultured 103/bcl-2 cells are shifted to the higher temperature, they leave cycle and promptly upregulate recombinase activity. In contrast to the original description of temperature-induced production of RAG1 and RAG2, we find RAG1 protein present at all times in these cells with only modest increases in amount following temperature-shift. RAG2, on the other hand, clearly increases after the transition to higher temperature. We presume that this increase reflects the

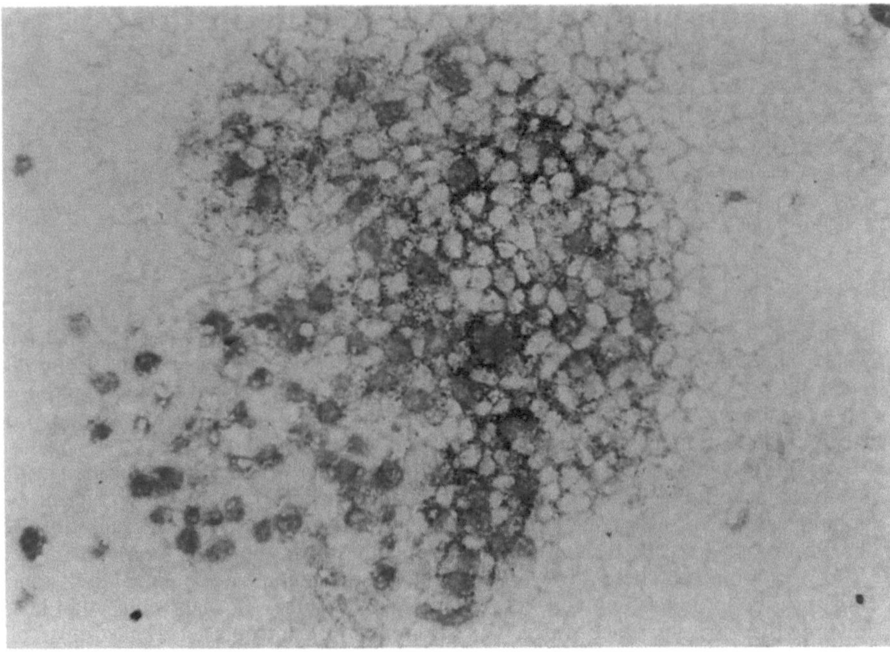

Fig. 1. A primary germinal center illustrating cytoplasmic distribution of RAG1 protein. Sixteen days after a primary immunization with NP-CG, mice were injected i.p. with BrdU and killed 3 h later. Spleens were prepared for immunohistology (Zheng et al., 1996; Han et al., 1996) to reveal BrdU (red) and RAG1 (blue). Note that RAG1 is observed only in the germinal center LZ and is present in the cytoplasm of non-dividing centrocytes (blue cytoplasm/unlabeled nucleus) and centroblasts that have recently left the DZ (blue cytoplasm/red nucleus). Cytoplasmic RAG1 is not observed in thymocytes.

inhibition of RAG2 degradation by cyclin-dependent phosphorylation. Where is the RAG1 protein in 103/bcl-2 cells before and after temperature shift? Kaiyong has addressed this by fractionating the nuclear and cytoplasmic/membrane components of the cells and precipitating each for western blots. Here (Fig. 2) we see that RAG1 is present only in the nuclear fraction both before and 24 hours after cultures are shifted to 39°C. RAG2 also seems only to be found in the nuclear fraction of 103 cells and only after temperature-shift. Does this mean that our histological demonstration of cytoplasmic RAG1 is only an artifact? Perhaps, but Kaiyong has also shown that transfection of fibroblasts with a shuttle vector encoding the complete RAG1 protein results either in RAG1 protein present in the cytoplasm only or in a roughly equal distribution between the cytoplasmic and nuclear compartments (Fig. 3). It may be that the efficient translocation of RAG1 to the nucleus depends on the presence of RAG2 (although this seems unlikely given the presence of nuclear RAG1 in 103 cells held at permissive temperatures), or on transport factors present only in lymphoid cells, or perhaps on factors that are stage-specific in lymphoid development.

This last possibility is especially intriguing given the recent reports from the laboratories of David Schatz (Agrawal et al., 1998) and Martin Gellert (Hiom et al., 1998) on the ability of RAG1 and RAG2 to function as a transposase. Could it be that RAG activity is uniquely suited to the invasion of other gene loci in germinal

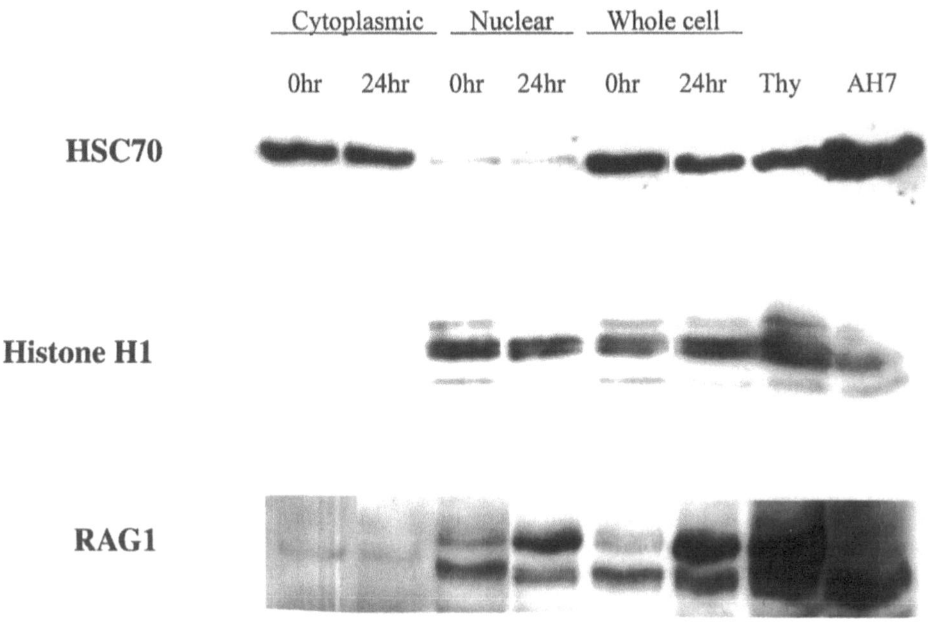

Fig. 2. Subcellular localization of RAG1 protein in 103/bcl-2 cells. 103/bcl-2 cells were fractionated as described by Spanopoulou et al (1995). Cell extracts were separated by SDS-PAGE and proteins were transferred to membrane and blotted with anti-HSC70, anti-histone H1 and anti-RAG1 antibody respectively. Lanes 1-6 are cell extractions from 103/bcl-2 cells before and after temperature induction. Cytoplasmic, Nuclear, and Whole cell refer to each extraction. Thy refers to whole cell extractions of thymocytes and AH7 is a whole cell extract of a $RAG1^{-/-}$ pre-B cell line. For 103/bcl-2 cells, all lanes are equivalent to 5×10^5 cells. For thymocytes and AH-7, both lanes are equivalent to 5×10^6 cells. 0hr indicates 103/bcl-2 cells cultured at the permissive temperature (34°). 24hr indicates 103/bcl-2 cells cultured at the non-permissive temperature (39°) for 24 hours.

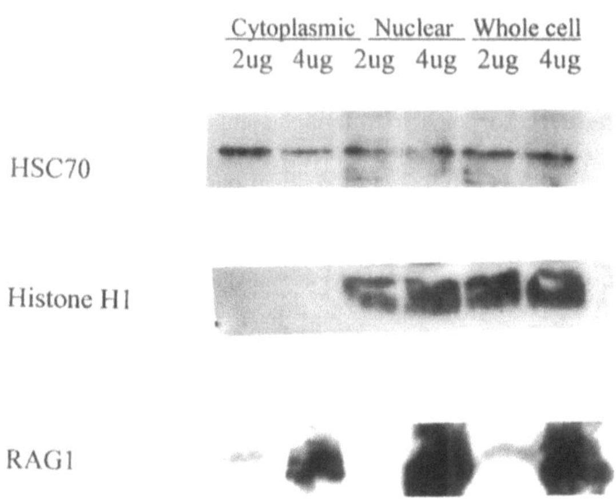

Fig. 3. Subcellular localization of RAG1 protein in 293T transfectants. 2 μg, 4μg and 10 μg RAG1 plasmid were transfected into 293T fibroblast cells. 48-72 hours later, transfected cells were harvested and fractionated as described for figure 2 . All subcellular fractions were run on SDS-PAGE and blotted with anti-HSC70, anti-histone H1 and anti-RAG1 antibodies.

center cells as opposed to other stages in B cell development where RAG and V(D)J recombination may be better regulated? This is only speculation but it is remarkable that the majority of lymphomas and leukemias that carry chromosomal translocations that appear RAG-dependent have cellular phenotypes consistent with mature- rather than developing B cell origins. Certainly recombinase activity in germinal center B cells is substantial. Recombination in germinal center B cells is largely confined to a $B220^{low}$ population leading to the possibility that these cells may not represent mature B cells. However these $B220^{low}$ cells carry rearranged and mutated heavy- and light chain genes, express mIg capable of transducing activation signals, and are antigen-reactive (Han et al., 1997; Meffre et al., 1998; Hertz et al., 1998). Nonetheless, I believe that the jury is still out with regard to whether these cells represent some intermediate stage of cellular maturity or mature cells that have acquired immature characters.

Several groups, including my own and those of David Nemazee (Hertz et al., 1998) and Michel Nussenzweig (Meffre et al., 1998), have shown that germinal center B cells actively engage in the rearrangement of *Ig* genes and revision of mIg. Significantly, this activity does not exhibit allelic exclusion, even at the heavy chain loci. Pam Fink has just reported that secondary rearrangements may also take place in the TCR β and -α loci of germinal center T cells (McMahan and Fink, 1998). The absence of allelic exclusion in V(D)J recombination in germinal centers is very different from that occurring in the bone marrow and thymus and it may be profitable to go after other recombinase activities in peripheral lymphocytes. One possibility is that RAG activity in germinal center lymphocytes catalyzes chromosomal translocations and drives the formation of leukemias and lymphomas. Marco Davila in my laboratory has begun to lay the ground work for determining the frequency of RAG-translocations by studying 103/bcl-2 cells that have been held at non-permissive temperatures for periods as long as 72 hours. You will recall that 103 cells leave cycle at 39°C, upregulate RAG1 and RAG2, and initiate V-to-J rearrangements in the *Igκ* loci on chromosome 6 (Chen et al., 1994). Marco has shown that even after 72 hours of growth arrest and recombinase activity, a low frequency of 103 cells may be rescued by a return to culture at 34°C (Fig. 4). These cells can then be subcloned to study the effects of extended recombinase activity. Although subcloned 103/bcl-2 cells retain good cloning efficiencies after 24 hours at the nonpermissive temperature, additional time at 39°C results in a sharp decline in the clonability of viable cells (Fig. 4). This decline is correlated with the appearance of secondary rearrangements in the κ locus and we speculate that some RAG-dependent events might permit viability but impede mitosis; aberrant chromosome structure is a candidate for this effect. To screen for translocations generally, Marco has adopted a strategy of chromosome painting and focussed on chromosome 6, a known site of recombinase activity in the 103/bcl-2 cells. Chromosome painting is a valuable technique for the identification of mouse chromosomes because all mouse chromosomes are acrocentric and similar in size. Figure 5 illustrates the standard karyotype of 103 cells with chromosomes labeled by DAPI (blue) and a paint probe specific for chromosome 6 (red). The simplicity of this pattern means that translocations involving chromosome 6 should be readily detectable as a novel red/blue chromosome and need not be transforming. Screening for this kind of event is easy and we estimate that events with frequencies as low as 5×10^{-4} can be recovered with no special efforts. Any success with this *in vitro* model would lead us in the direction of similar screens of cells recovered from the germinal centers of mice.

The germinal center reaction to non-replicating antigens is over relatively quickly. By about 4-5 weeks after primary immunization, the frequency of splenic B cells with the germinal center phenotype returns to levels present in naïve mice. Yoshimasa Takahashi has made the interesting observation that affinity maturation

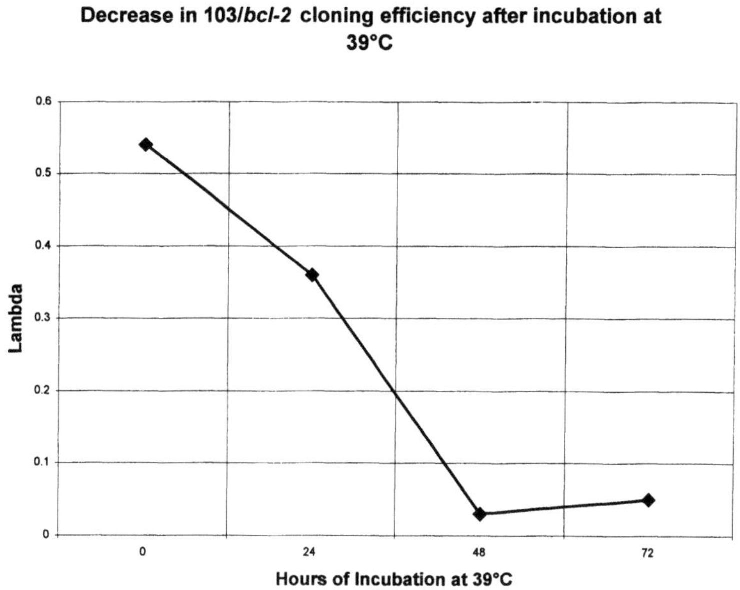

Fig. 4. 103/bcl-2 cells were incubated at 39° for 0, 24, 48, and 72 hours. After returning the cells to 34° for 12 hours, viable cells were recovered by centrifugation through Lympholyte-M and then subcloned at 1 cell/well in 96-well plates. After 7 days at 34°C the number of positive (wells containing proliferating cells) and negative wells were recorded and the Poisson distribution was used to analyze the results. Using the observed frequencies of negative wells, we calculated the cloning efficiency (λ) for the plated cells. λ values < that determined for cells held at permissive temperatures indicate that the ability to transit the cell cycle has been impaired by incubation at the non-permissive temperature.

of the serum antibody continues well after the end of the germinal center reaction (Takahashi et al., 1998). Thus while the germinal center has been touted as the immune response's Darwinian microcosm, much affinity maturation occurs after germinal centers are no longer present. Where does this maturation take place and what controls it? In collaboration with the laboratory of Tim Behrens, Yoshi studied the role of Bcl-2 and Bcl-x_L in germinal center B cells and in the early and late phases of affinity maturation. Yoshi found that germinal center B cells are similar to pre-B cells in that they express little or no Bcl-2 but contain substantial amounts of Bcl-x_L. Craig Thompson and his colleagues have also observed this pattern of expression in human germinal center cells (Tuscano et al., 1996). Yoshi also noted diminished apoptosis in germinal centers of the transgenics, retention of uncharacteristic VDJ rearrangements late into the primary response, and poor affinity maturation in the serum antibody. He also followed the somatic genetics of the long-lived plasmacytes that maintain serum antibody. These antibody-forming cells (AFCs) were purified from the bone marrow by flow cytometry; recovered cells were used in ELISPOT assays to measure antibody affinity or subjected to RT-PCR assays to identify the VDJ rearrangements present in the population. Like the germinal centers, the bone marrow AFC compartment in transgenic mice showed evidence for relaxed negative selection: the fraction of AFC that secreted low affinity, IgG_1 antibody specific for NP was significantly increased as was the

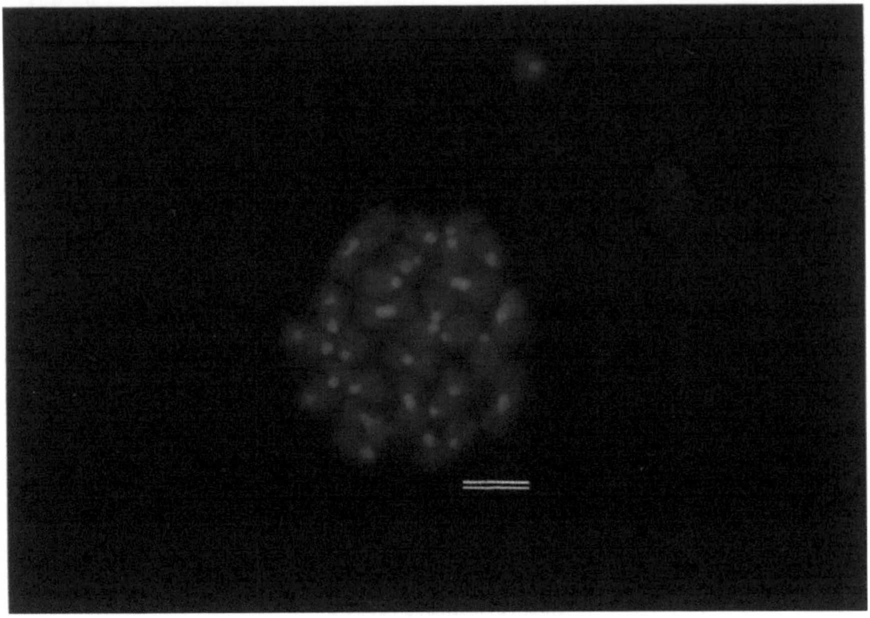

Fig. 5. Identification of chromosome 6 in 103/bcl-2 cells. A chromosome-specific paint probe was used to identify chromosome 6 in dividing 103/bcl-2 cells according to a protocol supplied by the manufacturer (ONCOR, Gaithersburg, MD). Briefly, slides of metaphase chromosomes were prepared and incubated with digoxigenin-labeled chromosome 6 probe. Bound probe was detected with rhodamine-labeled sheep anti-digoxigenin antibody; other chromosomes were counterstained with DAPI (4',6-diamidino-2-phenylindole), and photographed with a Olympus BX60/PM20 microscope at 250x magnification. Chromosome 6 is stained red and all other chromosomes are stained blue. Bar equals 10 μm.

frequency of VDJ rearrangements that used V_H gene segments other than V186.2. Indeed, about 90% of the VDJ rearrangements amplified from the bone marrow AFC of control mice contained the canonical V186.2 segment versus less than 50% in transgenics. The persistence of non-canonical, low affinity AFCs in transgenic but not normal mice suggests that Bcl-x_L may spare cells in both compartments from apoptosis.

These observations would not be surprising if it were not for prior work from the laboratory of David Tarlinton (Smith et al., 1994) on the role of a *bcl-2* transgene in affinity maturation. In brief, transgenic Bcl-2 did not measurably alter affinity maturation in these mice despite its demonstrated presence in germinal center cells. In addition, Bcl-2 clearly prolongs the lifetime of splenic AFCs whereas Yoshi found that the *bcl-x_L* transgene did not. This is a bit of a conundrum and raises the possibility that Bcl-2 and Bcl-x_L may not serve identical roles in B lymphocytes.

My final point on Yoshi's work is that all of us who study germinal centers are bird watchers, natural historians, at heart. We believe that the germinal center is a sort of laboratory of evolution, an island with finches, and that we follow the result of clonal competition and the exhaustion of antigen. This view does not fit well with our studies on the *bcl-x_L* transgenic mice. Even if programmed death is reduced in the germinal center, the selective proliferation of higher affinity clones under conditions of limiting antigen should drive affinity maturation by the overgrowth of cells with avid receptors. This "affinity maturation by neglect" should be evident at late times after immunization when residual antigen concentrations fall. However, Yoshi did not see any evidence for selective proliferation; the ratio of canonical to non-canonical VDJ rearrangements present in germinal center B cells at day 12 of the response was almost that present in the bone marrow AFCs 108 days later. Thus, antigen as a limiting growth resource for competing cells may not solely define the outcome of clonal selection in immune responses. Physiologic regulators, *e.g.* coreceptor activity, BCR signal enhancement by complement, *etc.*, may have substantial roles in determining the winners and losers of immune responses.

To find out more about the role of receptor affinity in recruiting B cells into the early AFC- and germinal center populations, Joe Dal Porto in my laboratory collaborated with Mark Shlomchik to measure the affinities of B cells actively participating in primary responses to NP-CG. Joe's "experiment" was a remarkable bit of natural history. He used microdissection to recover AFCs and germinal center cells from frozen sections of immune spleen, used a PCR to amplify VDJ rearrangements present in these cells, and transfected these rearrangements into a plasmacytoma line. The end result was recreation of the antibody molecules that directed clonal recruitment. This work has been published (Dal Porto et al., 1988) and so I shall not detail Joe's results except to note that he observed a wide range of affinities in these unmutated receptors; K_a s varied from 6-8 x 10^4 to 1-2 x 10^6 M^{-1}. The lower values are roughly that of a bad T cell antigen receptor and what most immunochemists would dismiss as junk.

Can very low affinity antigen receptors provide a full range of activating signals? Joe and Mark took these VDJ rearrangements that encoded very low affinity antibodies and made heavy chain transgenic mice. These animals exhibited excellent allelic exclusion and the transgenic heavy chain paired in the expected proportions with endogenous κ- and λ light chains. Importantly, the density of mIg on the splenic B cells of transgenic animals was not different from that of control mice. The transgenic heavy chains made anti-NP antibodies only when paired with the λ1 light chain; this meant that no more than 2% of peripheral B cells could respond to NP immunization. To make this too long story shorter, Joe found that the transgenic mice did respond to immunization with NP-CG and that antibody affinities of ≈1 x 10^5 M^{-1} to 5 x 10^4 M^{-1} were sufficient to drive antibody production and the formation of germinal centers. At this point the responses of the lower affinity mice diverged from that of normal animals and transgenic mice with K_a s ≥1 x 10^5 M^{-1}. To our astonishment, the lower affinity germinal center cells were transformed *en mass* by the reactivation of RAG1 and RAG2 and rearrangement of the endogenous heavy chain genes. This occurred in the absence of hypermutation and was driven, we think, by the low affinity of the transgenic mIg. Many, perhaps most, low affinity B cells that become activated by antigen travel to the germinal center and initiate secondary V(D)J recombination.

The role of such cells – if any – in the antibody response is not known. These cells may provide new gene associations capable of forming better antibodies than could be achieved by mutation alone. These cells may simply die as bystanders in a race to protective immunity. I do not know. However, these low affinity cells do offer the possibility that some fraction of them may undergo chromosomal translocations that are oncogenic. The germinal center may be not only a cradle of protective immunity but also of malignancy.

Acknowledgements

We wish to thank Dr. B. Zheng for providing us with Figure 1 and M. Gendelman for her assistance in the projects described. Drs. T. Behrens and M.J. Shlomchik have collaborated in our studies of apoptosis and selection in germinal centers and plasmacytes. This work was supported in part by USPHS grants AI 24335, AG 13789, and AG 10207.

References

Agrawal, A, Eastman, QM, Schatz, DG (1998) Transposition mediated by RAG1 and RAG2 and its implications for the evolution of the immune system. Nature 394, 744-751

Chen, Y, Wang, LC, Huang, MS, Rosenberg N (1994) An active v-*abl* protein tyrosine kinase blocks immunoglobulin light-chain gene rearrangement. Genes & Development 8, 688-697

Dal Porto, J, Haberman, AM, Shlomchik, MJ, Kelsoe, G (1998) Antigen drives very low affinity B cells to become plasmacytes and enter germinal centers. J Immunol 161, 5373-5381

Han, S, Zheng, B, Schatz, DG, Spanopoulou, E, Kelsoe G (1996) Neoteny in lymphocytes: Rag1 and Rag2 expression in germinal center B cells. Science, 274, 2094-2097

Han, S, Dillon, SR, Zheng, B, Shimoda, M, Schilesse, MS, Kelsoe, G (1997) V(D)J recombinase activity in a subset of germinal center B lymphocytes. Science, 278, 301-305

Hertz, M, Kouskoff, V, Nakamura, T, Nemazee, D(1998) V(D)J recombinase induction in splenic B lymphocytes is inhibited by antigen-receptor signaling. Nature 394, 292-295

Hiom, K, Melek, M, Gellert, M (1998) DNA transposition by the RAG1 and RAG2 proteins: A possible source of oncogenic translocations. Cell 94, 463-470

MacLennan, ICM, (1994)Germinal centers. Annu. Rev. Immunol 12, 117-139

McMahan, CJ, Fink, PJ (1998) RAG reexpression and DNA recombination at T cell receptor loci in peripheral CD4+ T cells. Immunity 9, 1-20

Meffre, E, Papavasiliou, F, Cohen, P, de Bouteiller, O, Bell, D, Karasuyama, H, Schiff, C, Banchereau, J, Liu, YJ, Nussenzweig, MC (1998) Antigen receptor engagement turns off the V(D)J recombination machinery in human tonsil B cells. J.Exp Med188, 765-772

Smith, KG, Weiss, U, Rajewsky, K, Nossal, GJ, Tarlinton, DM (1994) Bcl-2 increases memory B cell recruitment but does not perturb selection in germinal centers. Immunity 1, 803-813

Spanopoulou, E, Cortes, P, Shih, C, Huang, CM, Silver, DP, Svec, P, Baltimore, D, (1995) Localization, interaction, and RNA binding properties of the V(D)J recombination activating proteins RAG1 and RAG2. Immunity 3, 715-726

Takahashi, Y, Dutta, PR, Cerasoli, DM, Kelsoe, G (1998)In situ studies of the primary immune response to (4-hydroxy-3-nitrophenyl)acetyl. V. Affinity maturation develops in two stages of clonal selection. J Exp Med 187, 885-895

Tuscano, JM, Druet, KM, Riva, A, Pena, J Thompson, CB, Kehrl, JH (1996) Bcl-x rather than Bcl-2 mediates CD40-dependent centrocyte survival in the germinal center. Blood 88, 1359-1364

Zheng, B, Han, S, Zhu, Q, Goldsby, R, Kelsoe G (1996) Alternative pathways for the selection of antigen-specific peripheral T cells. Nature 384, 263-266

Discussion

Jim Kenny: Do the transgenics that you made with the heavy chains, from what I understand, all associate with λ1 to recognize NP?
Garnett Kelsoe: Yes.
Jim Kenny: Then if you take equal numbers of those two cells and put them into an animal and immunize with NP, the prediction of that experiment would be that the cells of the lowest affinity, when you looked in the germinal centers, would be the ones that would be dying and lost, and the ones which started out with the higher affinity would be those that were selected and undergo further affinity maturation. Was that the case?
Garnett Kelsoe: Yes, I think that would be the outcome but not as an individual event. If you rearrange the endogenous Ig locus, however unlikely it may be, you may be lucky and find a rearrangement that encodes good antibody. Lucky chances are why lotteries are so popular in the United States and Europe. Winning may be rare but you can reap tremendous benefit. On the other hand virtually everyone else in the population loses. Thus on the scale of the whole population, what you predict is likely to be true, but I have not done the experiment.
Gary Rathbun: I am interested in the RAG expression patterns you described. Have you looked at those cells that express RAG and presumably translocate to the nucleus, over a period of time? Have you looked at it with a tunel assay to look for apoptosis? Do these cells actually persist or do they die?
Garnett Kelsoe: Watching nuclear translocation has been done only in the 103 bcl-2 line and fibroblasts. 103/bcl-2 cells have high constitutive bcl-2 but they die during non-permissive culture. I have not correlated apoptosis and RAG translocation *in vivo* and therefore I cannot answer your question.
Richard Scheuermann: In that same experiment you seem to see an inverse correlation between RAG activity or expression and proliferation. Have you looked into that in any more detail in some of your other systems?
Garnett Kelsoe: In what sense?
Richard Scheuermann: Proliferation would be the signal that you are getting a good response to an antigen and might not need to edit your receptor, whereas if you are not proliferating you are not responding, and that is what gives the signal to upregulate RAG?
Garnett Kelsoe: Sure, we know that at the message level this is not true, but, trivially, since RAG-2 protein is phosphorylated on threonine 490, any cell in cycle will not be capable of undergoing VDJ recombination or transposition. We do know that you can get non-dividing centrocytes that have no RAG message or protein. So while there are many ways of regulating RAG activity in germinal center cells, I do not know what actually occurs *in vivo*. I have only correlative data that restricts RAG protein to the centrocyte compartment.
Mike Potter: Hearing you talk now and that seminar you gave us before, and reading Andreas Radbruch's paper on long-lived plasma cells, do you predict that the bone marrow long-lived plasma cell has any capacity whatsoever to synthesize DNA and replicate?
Garnett Kelsoe: It clearly has limited capacity because in Andreas Radbruch's experiments with very long-term bromodeoxuridine labeling a small percent of cells, about 15%, label over a 30-day period.
Mike Potter: 15% for the whole lot.
Garnett Kelsoe: That's true, I think.
Andreas Radbruch: I would say that these plasma cells do not react to antigen at all.
Mike Potter: But that's not the issue.
Fritz Melchers: The question is the half-life.
Andreas Radbruch: From about six weeks after their generation, we find no DNA synthesis in long-lived plasma cells.
Mike Potter: This is crucial for the understanding of multiple myeloma. Is something going on proliferatively in your plasma cell population in the bone marrow?
Garnett Kelsoe: We have not done that experiment; indirectly, if we are right, if that's the population that undergoes selection, there must be some proliferation and turnover. Although the population size remains constant, unequivocally the gene frequencies of the optimal antibody type increase over time. I know that to be a fact.
Andreas Radbruch: I have a question specific to this experiment: did you use one particular antigen concentration or did you increase the antigen concentration? You could speculate that if there is enough serum antibody generated in previous immunizations, the antigen at a certain

timepoint will be neutralized, there will be no new memory cells recruited or plasma cells generated, and the affinity will not increase. But if you then would immunize with higher amounts of antigen, you would again reactivate the memory B cell pool and get new higher affinity antibodies.
Garnett Kelsoe: We only immunize with a single standard dose which was 50μg in this experiment.
Siegfried Janz: Your model on the re-activation or re-expression of RAG in B cells suggests that this reactivation is dependent on the affinity to antigen of the surface immunoglobulin expressed by the B cells. Does this mean that the germinal center B cells with the low affinity immunoglobulin are at increased risk to undergo re-expression of RAG and become subjected to its transferase activity?
Garnett Kelsoe: Yes, we provided indirect evidence for this in our paper (Han et al [1997] Science 27B:301-305) and David Nemazee's more recent paper (Hertz et al [1998] Nature 394:292-295) showed directly that the higher affinity interaction on the surface Ig strongly suppressed RAG activity, whereas low or no interaction promoted RAG activity. The other interesting point is that you can be a pretty bad B cell in terms of affinity and enter a germinal center reaction, so it's quite a large population which enters and is lost either by apoptotic death or by receptor revision.
Siegfried Janz: Can a B-1 cell with low affinity Ig participate in the germinal center reaction?
Garnett Kelsoe: People say not, but there are phosphocholine-specific germinal centers that in BALB/c mice (my colleague Jan Cerny has shown this) carry the classical VDJ gene rearrangements that are associated with the B-1 population.
Paolo Ghia: Is there the possibility that these RAG-1 expressing cells may be from different stages of development? In the past we analyzed human tonsils and human B cell sub-populations and the presence of RAG expression correlated with the presence of VpreB or λ5 expression. Do you have similar data?
Garnett Kelsoe: About four years ago, we showed that λ5 transcripts were also up in this population, which made everyone worry that these were in some way immature or even preB cells that were caught in this environment. I think the best work that describes this is a JEM paper by Michael Nussenzweig who shows that λ5 is coexpressed with Ig light chain. Certainly the Nemazee work in the mouse indicates that there is a true BCR complex that transmits an antigen-specific signal, so at least in that case these cells may not be mature but they are certainly not preB cells.
Michael Carroll: When you introduced the *bcl-xL* transgene, you found that the low affinity cells that formerly were knocked-off survived, and that affected affinity maturation. How would you explain that?
Garnett Kelsoe: Over a long period, and our experiment went over 70 days, one would have guessed that even if the low affinity cells did not easily die, eventually their weak affinity receptors would no longer recognize the tiny amounts of retained antigen. But that did not seem to be the case. That is as much of a conundrum for me as it is for anyone else. The only way I can interpret this observation now is that once you survive the germinal center reaction and enter the long-lived AFC compartment, BCR affinity is not nearly as important as (costimulatory?) signals that provide some anti-apoptotic cell cushion.
Fritz Melchers: Unless there is a homeostatic effect. If a B cell compartment has a given size, if you put in a lot of long-lived cells the good ones which die rapidly have a harder time to expand.
Mike Potter: Human myeloma cells, if I understand correctly, express lots of bcl-2, and since they are bone marrow cells, would that be what you predict?
Garnett Kelsoe: No, there is this interesting difference. Bcl-2 mouse transgenics, which are all I know about, have this incredible long-lived splenic AFC population, and the Australian group of Cory, Adams and Strasser has shown this very nicely. I think a lot of these mice actually die from kidney disease because once formed, they have plasmacytes forever. The consequent high antibody titers and immune complexes damage the glomeruli. The *bcl-xL* transgenic mice do not have accumulations of splenic plasmacytes and the transient AFC population is perfectly normal; AFC numbers are a little higher but the kinetics of loss is identical to controls. So the working hypothesis for us is that the short-lived plasmacytes are regulated by Bcl-2, and the bone marrow long-lived plasmacytes are regulated by Bcl-xL.
Mike Potter: That has to be straightened out for myeloma.
Kenneth Nilsson: I think this points to the difference that one sees from myeloma and plasmacytoma also where in the mouse the *bcl-2* gene might not be used to protect against apoptosis. Maybe we are faced with a species difference where the usage of Bcl-2 family proteins, or some other genes involved in survival, differs from species to species. Otherwise this is strange.

Role of Complement Receptors CD21/CD35 in B Lymphocyte Activation and Survival

M. Carroll
The Center for Blood Research and Department of Pathology, Harvard Medical School, Boston, MA 02115, USA

Introduction

Over the past two decades, evidence has accumulated that strongly supports a role for the serum complement system in enhancement of the humoral response to thymus-dependent antigens (Pepys 1972; Humphrey et al. 1984; Bottger et al. 1986; Bitter-Suermann et al. 1989). More recent biochemical (Fearon et al. 1995) and *in vivo* studies in knock out mice have revealed that the complement effect is mediated via complement receptors CD21/CD35 (Carroll 1998). The classical pathway of complement is activated by recognition proteins such as mannan binding protein (Epstein et al. 1996), C-reactive protein (Szalai et al. 1997) or complement (Ebenbichler et al. 1991) of innate immunity which bear carbohydrate recognition domains encoded in the germline (Fearon et al. 1996). Natural IgM (encoded in the germline) although a component of adaptive immunity is also an important activator of classical pathway complement and is particularly important in recognition of protein antigens in addition to carbohydrate. For the purposes of this review, the enhancing effect of complement is most probably mediated by natural IgM, as deficiency in secretory IgM results in an impaired B cell response to suboptimal doses of T-dependent antigens (Boes et al. 1998). Recognition of foreign antigens by natural antibody results in activation of classical pathway complement leading to covalent attachment of the third component, C3b, via a transacylation reaction to the antigen (Law et al. 1980).

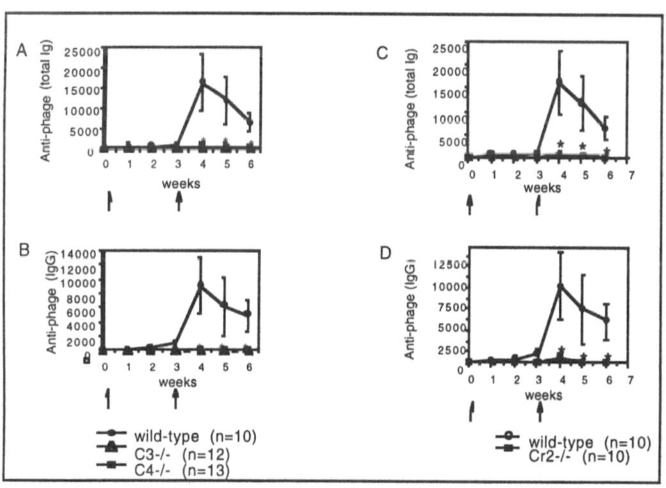

Fig. 1. Mice deficient in complement C4, C3 or CD21/CD35 have an impaired humoral response to thymus-dependent antigens. Total anti-phage response (vertical axis, panels A & C) or IgG anti-phage response (vertical axis, panels B & D) were determined by bacteriophage neutralization assay following immunizations at day 0 and week 3 (horizontal axis, panels A-D) with 2 X 10^7 PFU of OX174.

This event is critical as it alters the fate of the antigen. The importance of classical pathway complement in the humoral response to T-dependent antigens was confirmed and extended by analysis of mice bearing a targeted deficiency in either complement proteins C4 or C3 (Fig. 1 A,B).

The deficient mice were equally impaired in their primary and secondary responses to the classic bacteriophage antigen (Fischer et al. 1996). The defect was localized to the B cell level as T-cells were primed as shown by adoptive transfer experiments (Fischer et al. 1996). The attachment of activated C3b, which is rapidly converted to C3d, to antigen provides a ligand for complement receptors CD21/CD35 expressed on the surface of B cells and follicular dendritic cells (FDC) (Fig. 2).

Binding of C3d-antigen adducts by CD21/CD35 alters the B cell response in at least two ways. First, trapping of antigen by FDCs via CD21/CD35 provides a source of antigen for presentation to naive B cells and for maintenance of memory (Fang et al. 1998). Equally important, binding of C3d-adducts by the CD21/CD19/Tapa-1 coreceptor on antigen-specific B cells enhances BCR signaling (Fearon and Carter 1995). The importance of expression of CD21/CD35 was demonstrated recently by examination of the humoral response of mice totally deficient in the complement receptors (Ahearn et al. 1996; Molina et al. 1996) (Fig 1 C,D). The B cell response to T-dependent antigens was impaired in the deficient mice and depending on the antigen, the response was characterized by a reduced number and size of germinal centers. The impaired response could be restored in part by transfer of bone marrow (BM) from wild type (WT) into irradiated deficient animals (Ahearn et al. 1996). Thus, the short term memory and GC responses were reconstituted with CD21/CD35-positive BM. These results support the importance of B cell expression of the CD21/CD19/Tapa-1 coreceptor as the chimeric mice remained deficient in complement receptor expression by radio-resistant FDCs. It was noted in the immunized chimeric animals that the secondary antibody response dropped-off markedly following antigen challenge suggesting that in the absence of efficient retention of antigen on FDC memory was only transient (Ahearn et al. 1996). A similar observation was made in chimeric animals using a different T-dependent antigen (Fang et al. 1998).

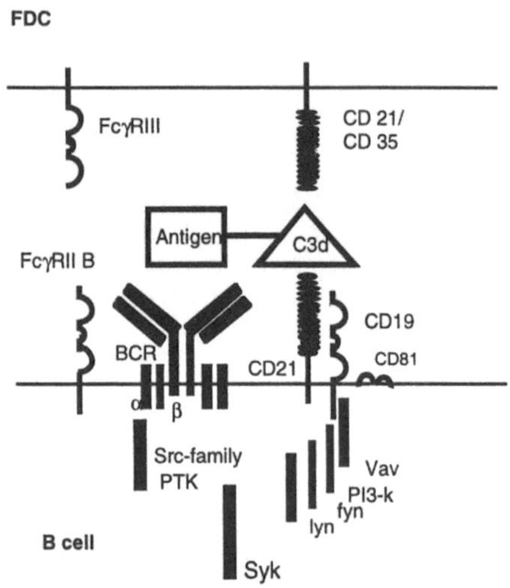

Fig 2. CD21 and CD35 are coexpressed on B cells and follicular dendritic cells.

Importance of Coreceptor Expression in B Cell Survival

To examine the importance of B cell expression of the CD21/CD19/Tapa-1 coreceptor in the presence of normal FDCs and primed T cells, we used the adoptive transfer system of Shokat and Goodnow (Shokat et al. 1995). In this model, splenocytes harvested from $Cr2^{+}$ or $Cr2^{null}$ HEL/ immunoglobulin (Ig) transgenic (tg) mice were transferred into WT mice immunized 7 days previously with 50ugs of lysozyme. The HEL-Ig tg was constructed from the well known HEL-10 hybridoma (Hy-HEL 10) which binds lysozyme from different species at varying relative affinities (Lavoie et al. 1992). For example, Hy-HEL 10 binds turkey lysozyme (TEL) at an unusually high affinity of 2×10^{10} M^{-}. In contrast, duck lysozyme (DEL) binds approximately 1000-fold less affinity (2×10^{7} M^{-}). By using these two different antigens for immunization, we were able to compare the importance of coreceptor signaling to intermediate and very high affinity antigens, respectively.

In the first series of experiments, spleens were harvested at days 1, 3 and 5 following adoptive transfer of $Cr2^{+}$ or $Cr2^{null}$ tg B cells into DEL-immunized recipients. Two-color immunohistochemical analysis of the two groups of recipients demonstrated no difference in the number of tg cells within the follicles within 24 hours of transfer. However by day 5, forty-fold fewer $Cr2^{null}$ than $Cr2^{+}$ tg B cells were identified within the follicular region (Fischer et al. 1998). It was proposed that the dramatic reduction in $Cr2^{null}$ tg B cells was due to an active process such as elimination or migration because no difference in the number of tg B cells was observed 5 days after transfer into non-immune recipients (Fig. 3a).

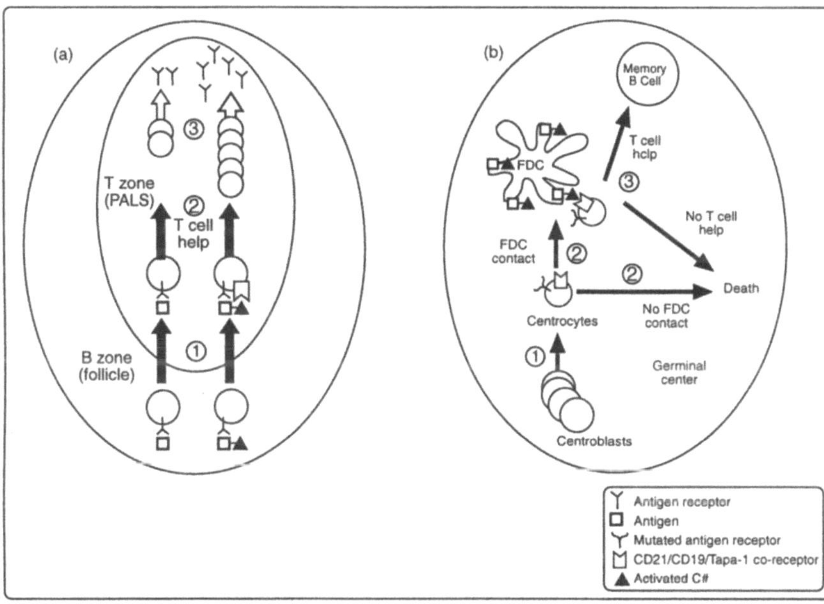

Fig. 3 (a,b). Expression of CD21 on B cells is critical for at least two stages of B cell survival.

One mechanism for regulation of activated lymphocytes is by CD95 (Fas). For example, B cells upregulate CD95 on CD40L signaling from cognate T cells. Fas ligand expressed on the surface of the activated $CD4^{+}$ T cell crosslinks CD95 resulting in a death signal unless countered by a threshold signal via the BCR (Rothstein et al. 1994). The CD95 gene maps to the *lpr* locus in mice (Watanabe et al. 1992). To examine if the loss of $Cr2^{null}$ B cells was due to Fas-mediated elimination, a similar experiment was performed in lpr mice. Interestingly, in contrast to that observed in WT mice, no difference was found in the survival of Cr2$^+$ and Cr2^{null} Fas-deficient tg B cells in the DEL-immune B6.lpr/lpr mice at day 5 after transfer (Table 1). Thus, in the absence of Fas regulation, Cr2^{null} tg B cells were equally competitive with Cr2$^+$ tg B cells in follicular survival. Our interpretation is that Cr2^{null} tg B cells receive a sub-threshold signal relative to Cr2-sufficient B cells and in the presence of HEL-specific CD4$^+$ T cells are eliminated by a Fas-dependent mechanism. Interestingly, the requirement for coreceptor signaling is apparently overridden when the antigen binds at very high affinity such as TEL as described below.

Table 1

Strain	No. of Follicles[1]	No. of HEL$^+$ Follicles[2]	% HEL$^+$ Follicles	No. of GC[3]	No. of HEL$^+$ GC[4]	%HEL$^+$ GC
Cr2$^+$ /HEL Ig tg (n = 12)	32.8 ± 3.9	28.2 ± 5	86. 1	28.7 ± 5.9	1.1 ± 0.4	3.8
Cr2^{null} /HEL Ig tg (n = 16)	31.1 ±4.7	2.9 ± 2.9	9. 5	21.9 ± 9.4	0.1 ± 0.1	0.6
Cr2$^+$ /HEL Ig tg *lpr* (n = 8)	24.3 ± 11.3	15.0 ± 10.9	61. 5	11.6 ± 6.0	0.2 ± 0.2	1.4
Cr2^{null} /HEL Ig tg *lpr* (n = 11)	29.8 ± 6.5	15.7 ± 6.1	52. 6	17.6 ± 7.7	0.3 ± 0.3	1.7

1. mean + (SD) number of follicles per-section counted
2. mean + (SD) number of follicles per-section counted with ≥ 10 HEL Ig tg B cells
3. mean + (SD) number of germinal centers per-section counted
4. mean + (SD) number of germinal centers per-section counted with ≥ 10 HEL Ig tg B cells
5. total number of mice

The threshold hypothesis predicts that naive B cells require CD21/CD19/ Tapa-1 coreceptor signaling to overcome a threshold for activation by low affinity antigens (Fearon and Carter 1995). To examine if coreceptor signaling is required also by B cells binding very high affinity antigen, we adoptively transferred Cr2$^+$ or Cr2^{null} tg B cells into WT mice immunized with TEL.

As discussed above, HEL-Ig tg B cells bind TEL with a 1000 fold higher affinity than DEL. At this unusually high affinity, it was predicted that coreceptor signal was not required for survival. To test this hypothesis, Cr2$^+$ and Cr2^{null} tg B cells were adoptively transferred into WT mice previously immunized with TEL antigen. Two-color immunohistochemical (PNA and HEL-ligand) characterization of cryosections of spleens harvested from the recipients revealed a similar number of tg B cells within the splenic follicles five days after transfer (Fischer et al. 1998). Thus, Cr2^{null} tg B cells received sufficient signal via high affinity antigen binding to block Fas-killing and survive within the follicles. By contrast, examination of germinal center (GC) B cells identified six-fold fewer GCs with Cr2^{null} than Cr2$^+$ B cells, i.e. 6.3± 2.2 % versus 53.3 ± 3.6 %; P< 3 X 10^{-5} (Fischer et al. 1998). Thus, despite the presence of unusually high affinity antigen, Cr2^{null} tg B cells did not survive within the GCs relative to Cr2$^+$. These findings were not predicted and suggest a novel role for coreceptor signaling in GC B cell survival. The low number of Cr2^{null} B cells within the GC explains the findings that GCs in C3^{null}, C4^{null} or Cr2^{null} mice immunized with T-dependent antigens are approximately 10-fold smaller than in WT controls (Ahearn et al. 1996; Fischer et al. 1996).

The GC represents a specialized microenvironment within the secondary follicles where B cells undergo somatic hypermutation and clonal selection. Mutated GC B cells compete for antigen binding and T cell help within the distal region (light zone) of the GC (MacLennan 1994; Kelsoe 1995) (see review by Kelsoe). Antigen is retained in the GC on the surface of FDC primarily by binding to CD21/CD35 receptors via C3b/C3d ligands. We propose that B cell survival in the GC requires signaling between B cell coreceptor and C3d ligand bound to FDC surface. Thus, C3d ligand serves both to anchor antigen to the FDC surface and to provide a signal to the B cell via the CD21/CD19/Tapa-1 coreceptor (Fig. 3b). As a further test of this hypothesis, we treated TEL-immune WT mice at optimal germinal center period (day 8, 9 and 10 following immunization) with 200ugs of soluble CD21 ($[CR2]_2$-IgG1) i.v. (Hebell et al. 1991). Examination of splenic cryosections 48hours later revealed 87% reduction in GC area in treated spleens compared to controls injected with IgG1 (Fischer et al. 1998). Thus, blocking of contact between CD21/CD35/Tapa-1 coreceptor on the GC B cell and C3d on the FDC results in loss of B cells from the GC. It will be important to determine if the B cells migrated out or became apoptotic in the absence of coreceptor signaling. A similar phenomenon occurs when GCs are flooded with specific antigen, i.e. GC B cells are eliminated or migrate out of the GC within a few hours (Han et al. 1995; Pulendran et al. 1995; Shokat and Goodnow 1995). One explanation is that soluble antigen in the absence of C3d ligand blocks contact between the B cell and FDC. This model is supported further by *in vitro* studies by Tew and colleagues who reported that coculture of FDCs (bearing specific antigen) with activated B and T cells promotes survival of the B cell and the effect is dependent on CD21 expression on the B cell and C3d bound to FDC (Qin et al. 1998).

Summary

In summary, the complement system has evolved an important function in regulation of humoral immunity to T-dependent antigens. Covalent attachment of activated C3 to antigen alters its fate by enhancing uptake on the surface of FDC via CD21/CD35; and by enhancing signal transduction via the B cell coreceptor CD21/CD19/Tapa-1. In the absence of complement receptors CD21/CD35 or C3 ligand, naive B cells bearing low affinity BCR fail to effectively survive within the lymphoid follicle following contact with antigen and death is mediated by a Fas-dependent mechanism. Alternatively, B cells sufficiently activated to initiate a GC reaction fail to survive in the absence of CD21-CD21L interaction.

References

Ahearn J, Fischer M, Croix D, Goerg S, Ma M, Xia J, Zhou X, Howard R, Rothstein T, Carroll M (1996) Disruption of the Cr2 locus results in a reduction in B-1a cells and in an impaired B cell response to T-dependent antigen. Immunity 4: 251-262

Bitter-Suermann D, Burger R (1989) C3 Deficiencies. Current Topics in Microbiology and Immunology 153: 223-233

Boes M, Esau C, Fischer MB, Schmidt T, Carroll MC, Chen J (1998) Enhanced B-1 cell development, but impaired IgG antibody responses in mice deficient in secreted IgM. J Immunol 160: 4776-4787

Bottger EC, Metzger S, Bitter-Suermann D, Stevenson G, Kleindienst S, Burger R (1986) Impaired humoral immune response in complement C3-deficient guinea pigs: absence of secondary antibody response. Eur J Immunol 16: 1231-1235

Carroll MC (1998) The role of complement and complement receptors in induction and regulation of immunity. Ann Rev Immunol 16: 545-568

Ebenbichler CF, Thielens NM, Vomhagen R, Marschang P, Arlaud GJ, Dierich UT (1991) Human immunodeficiency virus type I activates the classical pathway of complement by direct C1 binding through specific sites in transmembrane glycoprotein gp41. J Exp Med 174: 1417-1424

Epstein J, Eichbaum QE, Sheriff S, Ezekowitz RAB (1996) The collectins in innate immunity. Curr Opin Immunol 8: 29-35

Fang Y, Xu C, Fu Y, Holers VM, Molina H (1998) Expression of complement receptors 1 and 2 on follicular dendritic cells is necessary for the generation of a strong antigen-specific IgG response. J Immunol 160: 5273-5279

Fearon DT, Carter RH (1995) The CD19/CR2/TAPA-1 Complex of B Lymphocytes: Linking Natural to Acquired Immunity. Annu Rev Immunol 13: 127-149

Fearon DT, Locksley RM (1996) The instructive role of innate immunity in the acquired immune response. Science 272: 50-54

Fischer M, Ma M, Goerg S, Zhou X, Xia J, Finco O, Han S, Kelsoe G, Howard R, Rothstein T, et al. (1996) Regulation of the B cell response to T-dependent antigens by classical pathway complement J Immunol 157: 549-556

Fischer MB, Goerg S, Shen LM, Prodeus AP, Goodnow CC, Kelsoe G, Carroll MC (1998) Dependence of germinal center B cells on expression of CD21/CD35 for survival. Science 280: 582-585

Han S, Zheng B, Dal Porto J, Kelsoe G (1995) In situ studies of the primary immune response to (4-hydroxy-3-nitrophenyl)acetyl. IV. Affinity-dependent, antigen-driven B cell apoptosis in germinal centers as a mechanism for maintainingh self-tolerance. J Exp Med 182: 1635-1644

Hebell T, Ahearn JM, Fearon DT (1991) Supression of the immune response by a soluble complement receptor of B lymphocytes Science 254: 102-105

Humphrey JH, Grennan D, Sundaram V (1984) The origin of follicular dendritic cells in the mouse and the mechanism of trapping of immune complexes on them. Eur J Immunol 14: 859-864

Kelsoe G (1995) The germinal center reaction. Immunology Today 16: 324-326

Lavoie T, Drohan W, Smith-Gill S (1992) Experimental analysis by site-directed mutagenesis of somatic mutation effects on affinity and fine specificity in antibodies specific for lysozyme. J Immunol 148: 503-513

Law SK, Lichtenberg NA, Levine RP (1980) Covalent binding and hemolytic activity of complement proteins. Proc Natl Acad Sci USA 77: 7194-7198

MacLennan I (1994) Germinal Centers. Annu Rev Immunol 12: 117-139

Molina H, Holers V, Li B, Fung Y, Mariathasan S, Goellner J, Strauss-Schoenberger J, Karr R, Chaplin D (1996) Markedly impaired humoral immune response in mice deficient in complement receptors 1 and 2. Proc Natl Acad Sci USA 93: 3357-3361

Pepys MB (1972) Role of complement in induction of the allergic response. Nature:New Biology 237: 157-159

Pulendran B, Kannourakis G, Nouri S, Smith KGC, Nossal GJV (1995) Soluble antigen can cause enhanced apoptosis of germinal center B cells. Nature 375: 331-333

Qin D, Wu J, Carroll MC, Burton GF, Szakal AK, Tew JG (1998) Antibody production and B cell-FDC communication via CD21-CD21 ligand. J Immunol 161: 4549-4554

Rothstein TL, Wang JKM, Panka DJ, Foote LC, Wang Z, Stanger B, Cui H, Ju ST, Marshak-Rothstein A (1994) Protection against Th1-mediated apoptosis by antigen receptor engagement in B cells. Nature 374: 163-165

Shokat K, Goodnow C (1995) Antigen-induced B-cell death and elimination during germinal centre immune response. Nature 375: 334-338

Szalai AJ, Agrawal A, Greenhough TJ, Volanakis JE (1997) C-reactive protein: structural biology, gene expression, and host defense. Immunol Res 16: 127-36

Watanabe FR, Brannan CI, Copeland NG, Jenkins NA, Nagata S (1992) Lymphoproliferation disorder in mice explained by defects in FAS antigen that mediates apoptosis. Nature 356: 314

Discussion

Jim Kenny: When you have your complement receptor knockout, in fact when you put either one of these antigens in, what is the evidence that you have effectively engaged the same number of immunoglobulin receptors?

Michael Carroll: In this case we are doing adoptive transfer experiments: we are immunizing wild-type mice and transferring in either $Cr2^{+}$ or $Cr2^{null}$ transgenic cells, and we assume the recipient has a normal endogenous antibody response in both cases. So we think that competition from the endogenous background is the same whether we are getting $Cr2^{+}$ or $Cr2^{null}$ cells. Is that your question?

Jim Kenny: No. The question is that at some point it would seem to be necessary to demonstrate that in the knocked out the complement receptor does not alter the number of immunoglobulin receptors effectively.

Michael Carroll: We have performed the appropriate *in vitro* controls in which we culture $Cr2^{+}$ or $Cr2^{null}$ HEL Ig transgenic cells with increasing concentrations of HEL antigen and assay for B7.2 (CD86) expression or mitogenic proliferation. In these types of functional comparisons in which complement ligand is not involved, we fail to find a difference. So my interpretation is that the absence of CD21/CD35 does not affect functional levels of the B cell receptor.

Jim Kenny: But does it change the interaction with antigen in terms of being able to form stable complexes? If your antigen has to engage the immunoglobulin receptor and form stable receptor signaling complexes, is there any evidence that if you take your duck lysozymes, you encounter this cell, and you form the same number of ligated receptors?

Michael Carroll: We have addressed that issue at least in terms of functional response of the B cell, independent of complement. If you take complement out of the system, do the experiment *in vitro*, with just varying concentrations of duck or turkey lysozyme antigen, we find that the expression is similar whether you use $Cr2^{null}$ or $Cr2^{+}$ transgenic cells. However, we have not directly addressed your question, as I understand it, if co-receptor crosslinking enhances overall avidity of antigen binding to the BCR.

Katherine Siminovitch: Do you think that CD21 or Cr2 directly affects the threshold for signaling in a positive way or that the receptor provides a mechanism for impeding fas-mediated signaling?

Michael Carroll: It could just be a threshold for regulating fas (CD95), or the combined effect of the coreceptor and the B cell receptor. Biochemical studies by Doug Fearon and colleagues have demonstrated coligation of the coreceptor with the B cell receptor lowers the threshold for the amount of antigen required for optimal stimulation by 10-100 fold. So you could account for it that way, or there may be a separate more direct interaction between the coreceptor and regulation of fas, and we are trying to test that by several procedures.

Garnett Kelsoe: Tom Tedder and I have done a study with CD19 transgenic mice which works from the opposite direction of your experiment. These are mice hyper-responsive because CD19 density is higher. Coreceptor, or CD19, density is 3-fold above wildtypes but in anti-NP responses you recruit cells that have at least a 100-fold lower, perhaps even 1000-fold, lower affinity than the B cells normally present in the response. It is really impressive that the co-receptor makes such an important difference: small changes in the coreceptor more than compensate for huge affinity changes, and I think that is a point that we should remember. My other point is that germinal center people are the most morbid of all B cell biologists. We always presume that if something is not there it is dead. In fact, disappearing cells, especially if you use antigen-binding system to recognize them, can also leave the germinal center or revise their receptors to a lower affinity form. In both cases, the cells will not be detected and declared dead, not missing. We may overplay the role of death in germinal centers.

Fritz Melchers: As long as we weren't used to your unorthodox thinking!

Michael Carroll: I will describe one other control that might get at your question. We found that injection of soluble CR2 (CD21) into immunized WT mice at optimal GC period results in elimination of the majority of GC B cells. Our interpretation is that soluble CD21 competes for C3d on the surface of the FDC and blocks delivery of a survival signal. Thus, the GC B cells either die or leave the GC. We have not tested which of these two possibilities is correct.

Long-lived Plasma Cells Survive Independent of Antigen

R. A. Manz, G. Cassese, A. Thiel and A. Radbruch
Deutsches Rheuma-Forschungszentrum Berlin (DRFZ), Hannoversche Strasse 27, D-10115 Berlin, Germany

I here address the old question of whether the humoral memory is based on the continuous generation of plasma cells from memory cells or whether there are long-lived plasma cells which are the cellular correlates of humoral memory.

To show that the memory cells might not really be essential for the maintenance of humoral memory, we have compared the serum titer of phospholipaseA2-specific IgG to the frequency of phospholipaseA2-specific IgG^+ B cells in the blood of individual donors. There is no correlation. In general, the number of memory B cells does not correlate to the serum titer in response to particular antigens. Apart from phospholipase A2 we also tested tetanus toxin, with the same result. However, to really demonstrate that humoral memory is independent of the memory B cell pool, we have directly addressed the question of how long-lived plasma cells are?

To this end we have used a new technique, developed by us earlier, the cellular affinity matrix technology. It makes secreted proteins, and any other cell product which is secreted, accessible to flow cytometric analysis and cell sorting. The idea is based on a concept that Georges Köhler developed decades ago, i.e. coating the cell surface with an affinity matrix for the secreted product. We take antibodies that are specific for our product of interest, allow the cells to secrete whatever they want to secrete, in vitro. The secreted product of interest is caught by the affinity matrix and converted in a cell surface marker. We then need a second reagent that detects a distinct cpitope of the secreted product, and that labels the cell by fluorescence or magnetically. Essentially, to use the approach, a pair of antibodies is required, as for an ELISA.

To mark cells without affecting their viability, our first approach has been to use palmitylic acid as hydrophobic anchor, with a dextran backbone conjugated to it, and biotins conjugated to that backbone. Avidin-antibody conjugates would bind to this biotin-matrix and thus form an affinity matrix with the specificity of the antibody. This original approach is quite laborious and we soon replaced it with direct biotinylation of the cell surface, i.e. arbitrary proteins on the cell surface were labeled with biotin and then used to anchor our avidin antibody conjugates. At present we are developing bi-specific antibodies that are anchored on the cell surface by antibody with the other one forming the specific affinity matrix. We have used the cellular affinity matrix technology in two major lines of research. One is the analysis of cytokine-secreting cells and the other, which I will talk about today, is antibody-secreting cells.

To analyse lifetime and differentiation of plasma cells, we have used a murine model system. We have primed and boosted mice with ovalbumin, and then used the technology I just outlined to label the cells for secreted IgG1. Simultaneously, the cells were labelled for surface Ig. The cells were analysed by flow cytometry, gated according to light scatter and propidium iodide. Only a few cells express low or no surface Ig and are marked clearly for secreted IgG1. If those cells are sorted out, they secrete nearly all the secreted ovalbumin(ova)-specific antibody if kept in culture for one more day. According to this experiment, we have identified and isolated the cells secreting ova-specific IgG1.

We have then shown that those cells that are stained for secreted IgG1 can be labeled exclusively with antigen intracellularly. We used fluoresceinated ova for intracellular staining. This gives us an easy way to cytometrically track cells that secrete ovalbumin-specific antibodies, by intracellular staining with the antigen. Among spleen cells of an immunized mouse at about 1 week after boost, ova-specific plasma cells make up a considerable fraction of the IgG1 secreting cells.

In a systematic approach, we have then enumerated the ova-specific antibody-secreting cells in the spleen and in the bone marrow over a time course of about 100 days. Within two weeks, their cell number in the spleen peaks at 150,000 cells in total, then the numbers go down rapidly. After about three weeks, there are only 10,000 ova-specific plasma cells left in the spleen. At the same time, the number of cells in the bone marrow increases to about 60,000 per animal, and then remains at that level over the period of observation.

In the next experiment we tried to determine whether the ova-specific antibody secreting cells are continuously generated *de novo*, e.g. by residual antigen from memory B cells, or whether they are generated in the initial phase of the secondary immune response, and then survive in the bone marrow for long time periods. We used BrdU-incorporation to determine the frequencies of cells undergoing DNA-synthesis and cell division. We made up two complementary BrdU incorporation groups. One group of mice were fed BrdU for about 3 weeks, after boosting, and then left without BrdU until analysis of BrdU labelling after up to 150 days. In the other group we did not label the cells in the first 3 weeks and then fed BrdU for the rest of the time, until day 150. So all the cells generated by cell division from three weeks after boosting onwards, would be labeled in this group, and would not be labeled in the first group.

After the initial 19 days, the number of new plasma cells increases to about 30% of all plasma cells in the bone marrow within another 4 to 6 weeks. Later and until the end of the observation period few if any new plasma cells enter the pool of specific bone marrow plasma cells. In other words, most of the ova-specific plasma cells have been generated in the initial phase of the secondary immune reaction and then have survived for the rest of the observation period.

Are there any surrogate markers that distinguish the old from the new plasma cells? The most interesting one is probably MHC class II expression: 6 days after the boost most of the plasma cells in the bone marrow express elevated levels of MHC class II on the cell surface, compared to resting B lymphocytes. Later after the boost, most of the plasma cells return to expression of low levels of MHC class II.

The same is true in the spleen. Compared to the bone marrow, there are not so many plasma cells in total, only about 10,000 per mouse. Splenic plasma cells initially show upregulated MHC II expression at day 3, a fraction of them still shows it on day 12, while the few plasma cells remaining in the spleen after 40 days are MHC class II^-. In other words they have, according to this marker, the characteristics of "old" plasma cells.

Are there any other markers that characterize or discriminate young and old plasma cells? I do not want to mention syndecan (CD138), but about B220, or CD45, which we used for separation of the plasma cells from other lymphoid cells, esp. memory B cells, to determine by transfer experiments the relative contribution of memory B and plasma cells to humoral memory and their dependency on antigen. Plasma cells are negative for B220, and we used that marker to separate them from memory B cells in the bone marrow, as a strategy not to touch the plasma cells. B220 positive and negative cells could be separated by magnetic cell sorting to rather high purity and in large numbers for cell transfer experiments.

We then transferred those sorted cells into irradiated Ig^- allotype mismatched hosts and monitored the ova-specific serum titers of the transferred allotype. The humoral immunity, i.e. the serum titer is conferred with the $B220^-$ cells, the cell fraction including the plasma cells, but not so with the fraction of $B220^+$ cells, including the memory B cells.

Next we asked whether antigen matters for the survival of the plasma cells. To this end, the cells were transferred with and without antigen. The $B220^-$ cells do not react to the antigen; no matter whether transferred with or without antigen, they provide the same, stable serum titer. The serum does not go up but also not down, although the cells still may be able to see the antigen, at least they appear to have still a little surface Ig. In contrast, there is a drastic increase in the secreted antibodies derived from $B220^+$ cells, pointing to the rapid generation of plasma blasts and cells from memory B cells.

In conclusion, our data challenge some views that some people may currently have. From our work it is not clear whether primary activation of B cells does generate long-lived plasma cells, but secondary activation does, as we have shown unequivocally. One possibility could be that long-lived plasma cells can only be generated from long-lived memory B cells. This would make sense for the immune system because the antibodies selected in the first line of defense often may not be so specific for a particular antigen. In secondary responses they would have already matured a little. The plasma cells secreting them will then go to the bone marrow and reside there as long-lived plasma cells. They will not divide, continue to secrete their antibody, will not react to new antigen that enters the system, and provide a protective serum antibody titer that can fence off a certain amount of antigen, in a way that memory B cells are not activated. If the immune system would be confronted with more antigen than the serum antibodies could handle, new, long-lived plasma cells would be generated from memory B cells, which are activated by the surplus antigen. The antibodies of the new plasma cells may even have been more matured and have adjusted fine specificities. As a result, the serum antibody titer for that particular antigen is adjusted to the maximum antigen concentration of the environment the immune system lives in.

Rudolf Manz was the primary investigator in this study.

References

1. RA Manz, Thiel, A. and Radbruch, A. (1997) Lifetime of plasma cells in the bone marrow. Nature 388:133-134.
2. RA Manz, Löhning M, Cassese G, Thiel A and Radbruch A (1998) Survival of long-lived plasma cells is independent of antigenInt. Immunology 10:1703-1711

Discussion

Fritz Melchers: Do the long-lived memory cells express CD40? Would they be sensitive to antigen stimulation in a T-dependent way although they don't express class II molecules?
Andreas Radbruch: We didn't do CD40.
Mike Potter: It would be important to do CD40 because myeloma cells express CD40. It was not clear to me about the DNA synthesis: is there a very small amount in the bone marrow plasma cells?
Andreas Radbruch: There is always a limit of sensitivity to the technology. We are working on the borderline, so I cannot exclude that there is not any DNA synthesis. But I think it makes no difference for the concept. All these cells are lying in the bone marrow as time-bombs. The only thing they lack is proliferation, so if they would just switch that on...
Bernhard Klein: Just as a comment, the myeloma CD40 is not functional.
Mike Potter: Not functional in myeloma cells?
Bernhard Klein: No.
Jason Cyster: A nice system for tracking the plasma cells. Have you done anything to see if the enumeration of what you've got in suspension amounts to what you have got *in situ*, so that you know whether or not you've isolated all the plasma cells?
Andreas Radbruch: By ELISA spot?
Jason Cyster: No, by extracting them out of the tissue. Is it clear that they are all extractable?
Andreas Radbruch: Yes, they are cells that we extracted according to antibody secretion.
Jason Cyster: No, but have you compared it towards what is *in situ*?
Andreas Radbruch: No, not by histology, not yet.
Kenneth Nilsson: It was not clear to me why you wanted the memory B cell response to be the sort of backup protective system, and not the first line of defense. If you go from normal B cells, you would go through a wave of proliferation to expand the clone to derive the plasma cells. This would take time, while B cells would be able to go into plasma cells in just a few hours, as we heard before.
Andreas Radbruch: The concept would be that in the initial response you would not generate long-lived plasma cells because these antibodies are not worth much. But they mature then and if the antigen comes around a second time, you would want to generate long-lived plasma cells because they are continuously providing secreted antibody. I think that this is the fastest way: presence of the protective antibody when the antigen enters the system. It somehow covers a

certain amount of antigen; the idea being that the memory cells are only required if the amount of antigen is more than what can be covered by the already existing humoral antibody. In that case you would generate new plasma cells and these plasma cells would be derived from memory cells of course, and that would be fast.

Kenneth Nilsson: But why not have long-lived plasma cells in the bone marrow from both cell types? Why distinguish between...?

Andreas Radbruch: From primary responses?

Kenneth Nilsson: How do you know this?

Andreas Radbruch: I don't know it. This is completely hypothetical. We were not able to determine the longevity of plasma cells that were generated in primary immune responses because their numbers are too low. As I said, we are working on the borderline of sensitivity: the spleen with 10,000 plasma cells per organ, that is what we can do, and that is the maximum generated in this kind of response in primary activation.

John Kearney: I can't let you get away with saying that the antibody made by the early plasma cells "is not worth much"! It might be with a specificity of albumin!! But early IgM antibody towards *S. pneumoniae* (as an example) will protect mice from death, so I think you need to make a distinction between the functional aspects of antibody from early appearing short-lived plasma cells compared to long-lived plasma cells in the bone marrow.

Andreas Radbruch: It depends on which angle you look at it. It could also be autoreactive.

Charles Rabkin: Do you have any data showing that the number of plasma cells correlated with the serum antibody titer?

Andreas Radbruch: No.

Charles Rabkin: Would your methods not be sensitive enough for that?

Andreas Radbruch: Yes.

Frans Kroese: Could you speculate why they migrate to the bone marrow?

Andreas Radbruch: We *are* just speculating! That is a subject for the next meeting, which kind of chemokine receptors and chemokines are expressed, and maybe bone marrow-specific. I don't have a clue.

Ivan Lefkovits: There are some old experiments of Robbert Benner, and other ones of Claudia Henry and Humberto Cosenza, in which they show that all this depends on the kind of antigen one uses. The fate of the plasma cells depends on whether it is a thymus-dependent or a thymus-independent antigen, and of course KLH-hapten differs from ovalbumin-hapten, and there are a number of differences in the lifespan of plasma cells just because of these variables.

Andreas Radbruch: It is very clear that there are short-lived plasma cells and I am not saying that all plasma cells are long-lived. That's why we chose this T-dependent antigen ovalbumin because we knew that the titers would be stable for a long time and that ovalbumin is not a very persisting antigen, unlike viral antigen, and that we could hope that with this system we would find out how long-lived the plasma cells really are.

Ivan Lefkovits: It is important to realize that what you are describing is not a general phenomenon, because if it were, you would not expect a very sharp peak in response to many antigens. The simple fact that antibody-forming cells might totally disappear within a few days and that the response sharply declines means that the plasma cells are gone.

Bart Barlogie: The homing to the marrow may somehow be related to an activated bone marrow microenvironment, at least when you look at data from the human myeloma system.

II

Chemokines and Chemokine Receptors

Regulation of Expression of Chemokine Receptor BLR1/CXCR5 during B Cell Maturation

V. Pevzner, I. Wolf, R. Burgstahler, R. Förster and M. Lipp
Max-Delbrück-Center for Molecular Medicine, Department of Tumor- and Immunogenetics, Robert-Rössle-Straße 10, 13092 Berlin, Germany

Introduction

Functional interactions of chemokines and their receptors, which belong to the family of seven-transmembrane-domain proteins, signaling through heterotrimeric G proteins, have been shown to be primarily implicated in pathophysiological inflammatory processes [1]. Leukocytes are recruited from blood by locally produced chemokines towards sites of inflammation, arising from infections, injury, allergic reactions, arthritis and artherosclerosis. Several lines of evidence suggest that members of the chemokine receptor family may also be involved in lymphocyte migration to distinct lymphoid organs. Mature B and T lymphocytes continuously recirculate between blood and lymphatics to mediate immune surveillance. In this process they have to interact and to pass specialized endothelia: postcapillary venules in non-lymphoid organs and high endothelial venules in lymph nodes. Migration of B and T cells into secondary lymphatic organs is a prerequisite for the development of an antigen-specific immune response. The recent finding, that the chemokine receptor BLR1 is needed for B cell migration into lymphoid follicles [2], supports the view that chemokine receptors play an essential role as conductors of an orchestra of adhesion molecules, which allow lymphocyte subsets to navigate to different anatomical locations and are involved in the functional compartmentalization of lymphoid organs.

Interestingly, the properties of chemokine receptors are widely used by several human viruses. Fusin/CXCR4 is utilized by T-tropic isolates of HIV as a co-receptor for entry into T cells [3], and the chemokine receptor CCR5 fulfills a similar function for M-tropic HIV strains [4]. EBV strongly upregulates expression of BLR2/CCR7 in B cells [5], and moreover several human lymphotropic herpes viruses encode chemokine receptor-like molecules [6, 7].

Below we will concentrate on the expression patterns of three members of the chemokine receptors' family, as well as discuss the mechanisms of transcriptional control which allow restricted expression of one of them in specific lymphoid subpopulations. One of these receptors, initially termed BLR1 and now assigned the name CXCR5 according to the chemokine receptor nomenclature, was isolated from a Burkitt's lymphoma line [8]. The other – BLR2/EBI1/ – was detected

Table 1. Differential expression of CXCR5, CCR7 and CXCR4 on peripheral blood cells

	Ligand	Neutro-phils	Mono-cytes	B cells	CD4+		CD8+	
					naïve	memory	naïve	memory
CXCR5/BLR1	BLC	-	-	++	-	+	-	-
CCR7 /BLR2	ELC,SLC	-	+/-	+	+	+/-	+	+/-
CXCR4/Fusin	SDF-1	+	+	+	+	+/-	+	+/-

in activated peripheral blood lymphocytes [5, 9]. The ligands of both these receptors have been identified recently. BLC/BCA-1, a strong B cell chemoattractant produced in lymphoid follicles binds BLR1 [10, 11], and ELC is a ligand for BLR2 [12]. Finally, the third of the receptors, discussed below – fusin/CXCR4 – was isolated by several groups and attracted widespread attention as the first identified coreceptor of HIV entry (see above). The corresponding ligand was shown to be the stroma-derived factor SDF-1 [13].

Results and Discussion

Differential Expression of Chemokine Receptors on Lymphocyte Subsets

To gain insight into the physiological functions of BLR1, BLR2 and CXCR4 a panel of rat monoclonal antibodies was generated, and peripheral blood cells from healthy volunteers were analyzed by means of three-colour flow cytometry [14, 15]. The analysis demonstrated that these receptors are expressed differentially within the hematopoietic lineage (Table 1).

Expression of BLR1 is restricted to mature $CD19^+$ B cells and to a subpopulation of $CD4^+$ T-helper cells. This subpopulation, which makes up approximately 15% of all recirculating $CD4^+$ cells, is characterized by low levels of L-selectin, high levels of CD44, and expression of CD45RO. This defines the BLR1 expressing T cell subset as resting memory cells. Whereas BLR2 shows a relatively unrestricted pattern of expression on various lymphocyte subsets, but is only weakly expressed on monocytes and can not be detected on neutrophils, CXCR4 is widely expressed on various peripheral blood cell subsets, including monocytes and neutrophils. Of particular interest is the fact that within the T cells, expression of both BLR2 and CXCR4 is primarily restricted to naive antigen-inexperienced T cells, as defined by coexpression of high levels of L-selectin and CD45RA. As T cell expression of most of the known chemokine receptors is usually restricted to activated and memory T cells, BLR2 and CXCR4 are the first identified chemokine receptors showing preferential expression on naive T cells.

Expression of BLR1 in murine tissues tightly follows the expression pattern of BLR1 in humans, and thus is highly conserved in both species [2]. To follow the expression of BLR1 at different stages during B cell development we analyzed

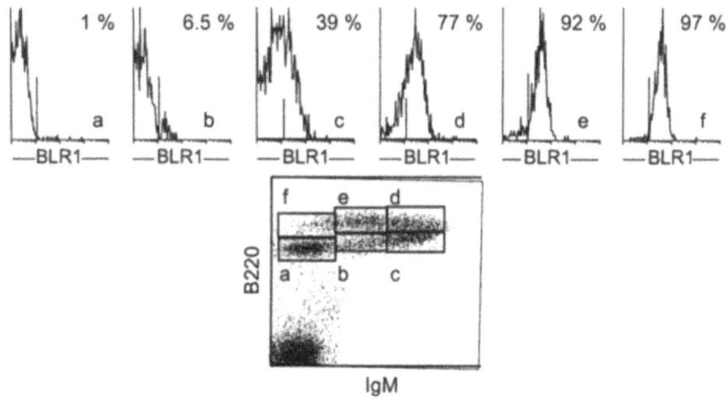

Fig. 1 Expression of BLR1 during the process of B cell maturation in the bone marrow. Bone marrow cells were triple-stained with anti-IgM, anti-B220 and anti-BLR1. The expression levels of BLR1 were determined on various B cell populations (indicated a - f), which were chosen based on the expression of IgM and B220. For detailed description of each population see the text.

murine bone marrow cells with a panel of B cell differentiation markers together with the monoclonal antibody against murine BLR1. Below 1% of cells at pro-B- and early pre-B-stages ($B220^{low}IgM^{-}$, Fig 1a) express BLR1. As the cell progresses from the pre-B- to the immature-B-stage, which is reflected by the elevation of IgM levels on the cell surface, the detected levels of BLR1 also gradually increase (from 6.5% at the stage $B220^{low}IgM^{low}$ to 39% at the stage $B220^{low}IgM^{high}$, Fig. 1b-c). At the end of the B cell maturation process the expression of BLR1 reaches its maximum and can be detected on 77-97% of all $B220^{+}IgM^{+}$ cells (Fig. 1d-f).

Cell-type Restricted Pattern of BLR1 Expression is Regulated by the Combinatorial Action of Oct-2, Bob1 and NF-κB

Comparison of the promoters of human and murine *BLR1* genes reflects the conservative mode of receptor expression in both species. Both promoter nucleotide sequences show high degree of overall homology, and the sequences and positioning of the identified consensus binding sites of transcription factors are almost identical in both promoters [16]. In both cases the classical transcriptional initiator sequences like the TATA-box are absent. However, we could detect protein binding to a single site located in close proximity (-36) to the start of transcription. Although the bound proteins remained unidentified, the location of this promoter element as well as its functional significance, revealed in the mutational analysis of this site, testify for the presumable role of a substitute for initiator sequence. Therefore this element was termed a functional promoter region (FPR).

The sequence of the human *BLR1* promoter spans over the genomic region of over 1.2 kb and encompasses the transcriptional start site. Deletional analysis of this region revealed that the elements critical for the promoter function are located in the core region, positioned between nucleotides –78/+215 respective to the start site. In addition to the above mentioned FPR, this region contains a noncanonical

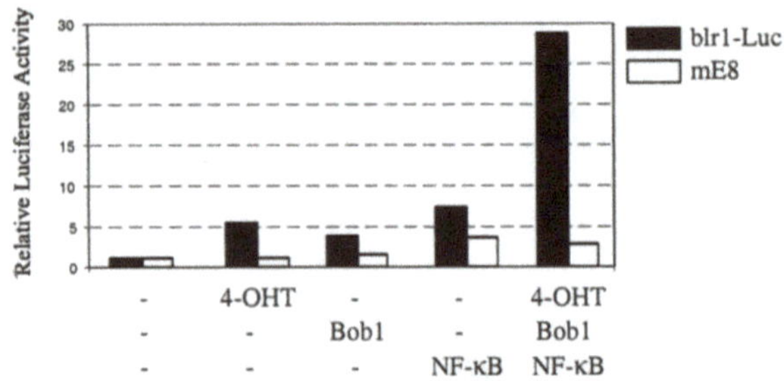

Fig. 2 Oct-2, NF-κB, and Bob1 dependent activation of the murine *blr1* promoter. 20μg of blr-Luc plasmid or mE8 construct were transfected or cotransfected with NF-κB p50/p65 (5μg each) and Bob1 (10 μg) in Abl/Oct2-ER cells. Each transfection was split in half and 4-hydroxytamoxifen (4-OHT) was added to one part to the final concentration of 1 μM where indicated. Luciferase activity of mblr1-Luc or m-E8 alone was set to 1 in all experiments and the other bars present data of at least 3 experiments as fold activation of luciferase activity above that.

octamer sequence, an NF-κB binding site and an E-box. These sites attracted our particular attention, as they are known to be bound by transcription factors involved in regulation of many other B cell-specific genes. In particular, the classical octamer site 5'-ATGCAAAT-3', which is essential for regulation of Ig genes, is recognized by the ubiquitously expressed Oct-1 and the B cell-restricted Oct-2 factors and their coactivator Bob1. Also, an NF-κB-site is frequently found in promoters of many genes induced in early stages of inflammatory and immune response and mediates their rapid activation. At the same time several potentially interesting sites (AP-1, LEF-1, and two additional NF-κB sites) remain outside of the identified core region and seem not to influence the functioning of the *BLR1* promoter under tested conditions. However, it is likely that they are involved in the fine-tuning of BLR1 expression in T cells or under certain specific conditions.

To analyse the functional role of octamer and NF-κB sites in the core region of the *BLR1* promoter, we placed a firefly luciferase reporter gene under the control of the murine promoter region. The resulting construct (blr1-Luc) as well as the construct with the mutated octamer sequence (mE8) were transfected into Abl/Oct2-ER cells. This B cell line allows the differentiation of the input of Oct-1 and Oct-2 into the regulation of the analysed promoter. The cells express Oct-1 but Oct-2 is normally not expressed and can be functionally activated by treatment with estrogen derivatives like 4-OHT [17]. In this line transfected with blr1-Luc alone only minimal reporter activity could be detected, suggesting that Oct-1 is unable to provide a significant level of promoter function. Addition of either 4-OHT, Bob1, or NF-κB to the transfected cells resulted in 4 to 7-fold activation of the *blr1* promoter (Fig. 2), but combinatorial action of Bob1 and NF-κB complemented with the induction of Oct-2 by 4-OHT resulted in strong activation of the promoter (~30-fold). In contrast, the mutated construct mE8 showed only weak response to NF-κB, thus reflecting the primary significance of the functional octamer site for the activity of the *BLR1* promoter. In accordance with this result the expression of BLR1 in spleen lymphocytes from newborn progeny of Oct-$2^{-/-}$

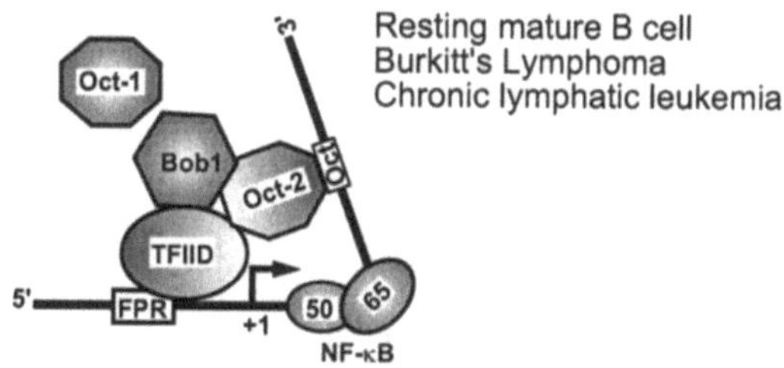

Fig. 3 Proposed model of cooperative action of Oct-2, Bob1, and NF-κB on the *BLR1* promoter.

mice was only barely detectable, whereas cells isolated from wild-type littermates expressed levels of BLR1 usually observed in newborns [16]. Furthermore, also in mice defective for Bob1 or NF-κB factors, the expression of BLR1 was markedly affected. It was more than 50% reduced in B220+ cells derived from lymph nodes or spleen of Bob1 null mutant mice and was virtually absent in mice lacking both p50 and p52 NF-κB subunits [16].

BLR1 is not expressed on continuously activated B cells and plasma cells, and obviously mechanisms of downregulation of its expression on mature B lymphocytes exist. An interesting candidate site for mediating this downregulation could be the E-box located downstream of the octamer site. The E-box is a recognition site of the factors belonging to the basic helix-loop-helix (bHLH) proteins' class. Recently a novel bHLH factor, ABF-1, with the function of transcriptional repressor was identified in activated B cells [18]. To test if ABF-1 represses the activity of the *BLR1* promoter, we cotransfected a blr1-Luc construct with an ABF-1 expression vector in Raji cells. The promoter is fully active in these cells and the level of reporter expression was unaffected by ABF-1, thus showing that this factor is not mediating BLR1 downregulation in activated B cells.

Taken together the reported results suggest a hypothetical model of *BLR1* promoter regulation (Fig. 3). The binding of NF-κB p50/p65 subunits to DNA causes a bend in the DNA molecule and brings FPR and the octamer element into close proximity to each other. The resulting interaction of octamer-bound factors with the protein(s) bound to FPR seems to be critical for the formation of the preinitiation complex.

References

1. Rollins BJ (1997) Chemokines. Blood 90: 909-928

2. Förster R, Mattis AE, Kremmer E, Wolf E, Brem G, Lipp M (1996) A putative chemokine receptor, BLR1, directs B cell migration to defined lymphoid organs and specific anatomic compartments of the spleen. Cell 87: 1037 – 1047
3. Feng Y, Broder CC, Kennedy PE, Berger EA (1996) HIV-1 entry cofactor: functional cDNA cloning of a seven-transmembrane, G protein-coupled receptor. Science 272: 872-877
4. Moore JP, Trkola A, Dragic T (1997) Co-receptors for HIV-1 entry. Curr Opin Immunol 9: 551-562
5. Burgstahler R, Kempkes B, Steube K, Lipp M (1995) Expression of the chemokine receptor BLR2/EBI1 is specifically transactivated by Epstein-Barr virus nuclear antigen 2. Biochem Biophys Res Commun 215: 737-743
6. Ahuja SK, Murphy PM (1994) Molecular piracy of mammalian interleukin-8 receptor type B by herpesvirus saimiri. J Biol Chem 268: 20691 – 20694
7. Arvanitakis L, Geras-Raaka E, Varma A, Gershengorn MC, Cesarman E (1997) Human herpesvirus KSHV encodes a constitutively active G-protein-coupled receptor linked to cell proliferation. Nature 385: 347 – 350
8. Dobner T, Wolf I, Emrich T, Lipp M (1992) Differentiation-specific expression of a novel G protein-coupled receptor from Burkitt's lymphoma. Eur J Immunol 22: 2795 – 2799
9. Birkenbach M, Josefsen K, Yalamanchili R, Lenoir G, Kieff E (1993) Epstein-Barr virus-induced genes: first lymphocyte-specific G protein-coupled peptide receptor. J Virol 67: 2209 – 2220
10. Gunn MD, Ngo VN, Ansel KM, Ekland EH, Cyster JG, William LT (1998) A B-cell-homing chemokine made in lymphoid follicles activates Burkitt's lymphoma receptor-1. Nature 391: 799 – 803
11. Legler DF, Loetscher M, Roos RS, Clark-Lewis J, Baggiolini M, Moser B (1998) B cell-attracting chemokine 1, a human CXC chemokine expressed in lymphoid tissues, selectively attracts B lymphocytes via BLR1/CXCR5. J Exp Med 187: 655 – 660
12. Yoshida R, Imai T, Hieshima K, Kusuda J, Baba M, Kitaura M, Nishimura M, Kakizaki M, Nomiyama H, Yoshie O (1997) Molecular cloning of a novel human CC chemokine EBI1-ligand chemokine that is a specific functional ligand for EBI1, CCR7. J Biol Chem 272: 13803 – 13809
13. Bleul CC, Farzan M, Choe H, Parolin C, Clark-Lewis I, Sodroski J, Springer TA (1996) The lymphocyte chemoattractant SDF-1 is a ligand for LESTR/fusin and blocks HIV-1 entry. Nature 382: 829 – 833
14. Förster R, Emrich T, Kremmer E, Lipp M (1994) Expression of the G-protein-coupled receptor BLR1 defines mature, recirculating B cells and a subset of T-helper memory cells. Blood 84: 830 – 840
15. Förster R, Kremmer E, Schubel A, Breitfeld D, Kleinschmidt A, Nerl C, Bernhardt G, Lipp M 1998) Intracellular and surface expression of the HIV-1 coreceptor CXCR4/fusin on various leukocyte subsets: rapid internalization and recycling upon activation. J Immunol 160: 1522 – 1531
16. Wolf I, Pevzner V, Kaiser E, Bernhardt G, Claudio E, Siebenlist U, Förster R, Lipp M (1998) Downstream activation of a TATA-less promoter by Oct-2, Bob1, and NF-κB directs expression of the homing receptor BLR1 to mature B cells. J Biol Chem 273: 28831 – 28836
17. König H, Pfisterer P, Corcoran LM, Wirth T (1995) Identification of *CD36* as the first gene dependent on the B-cell differentiation factor Oct-2. Genes and Dev 9: 1598-1607
18. Massari ME, Rivera RR, Voland JR, Quoung MW, Breit TM, van Dongen J, de Smit O, Murre C (1998) Characterization of ABF-1, a novel basic helix-loop-helix transcription factor expressed in activated B lymphocytes Mol Cell Biol 18: 3130 - 3139

Acknowledgements

The authors are grateful to Thomas Wirth for providing Abl/Oct2-ER cell line, to Walter Schaffner for Bob1 expression vector and to Mark Eben Massari for ABF-1 expression vector. This study was supported by the Deutsche Forschungsgemeinschaft grants Li 374/8-1. V.P. is supported by a fellowship from Boehringer Ingelheim Fonds.

Discussion

Richard Scheuermann: How do these chemokines affect expression of adhesion molecules?
Martin Lipp: It has been postulated that chemokine receptors, which couple to heterotrimeric G proteins, activate adhesion molecules like the integrins by inducing a conformational alteration, which in turn allows firm interaction with the counter receptor of the Ig superfamily on endothelial cells. It is also well established that small G proteins like rho and rac are involved. However, the complete signaling cascade leading finally to integrin activation is still not resolved at the molecular level.
Ton Rolink: How is CXCR5 expression regulated during B cell development? I am asking this because you showed involvement of Bob1, also known as OBF-1. We showed that OBF-1 knockout mice have a very dramatic problem in transporting B cells from the bone marrow into the spleen.
Martin Lipp: As I said, in Bob1-deficient mice expression of CXCR5 was reduced significantly in $B220^{+}$ splenocytes.
Ton Rolink: So CXCR5 could be involved in the transition from bone marrow to the spleen?
Martin Lipp: Yes, because all B cells in the spleen express CXCR5, including those which are immature in your definition.
Martin Bachmann: TNFα and lymphotoxin are very important for the organogenesis of lymph nodes and for the formation of germinal centers. Do you know whether they regulate expression of CXCR5?
Martin Lipp: This is a good question. There are probably some connections to the chemokine system, but we have no indication that CXCR5 is directly regulated by lymphotoxins.
Siegfried Janz: Is CXCR5 a target gene for c-myc?
Martin Lipp: No. The c-myc binding sequence is only present in the human promoter. Ectopically expressed MYC did not influence the activity of the promoter.

Chemokines and B-cell Homing to Follicles

J.G. Cyster, V.N. Ngo, E.H. Ekland, M.D. Gunn[†], J.D. Sedgwick[§] & K.M. Ansel

Department of Microbiology and Immunology, and [†]Cardiovascular Research Institute, University of California at San Francisco, San Francisco, California 94143, USA; [§]Centenary Institute of Cancer Medicine, and Cell Biology, Sydney, NSW, Australia 2050

B cells that bind autoantigen in the periphery may be excluded from lymphoid follicles and rapidly eliminated (Cyster, 1997). To understand the basis for follicular exclusion we considered whether Gi coupled chemokine receptors might play a role by testing the effect of treatment with pertussis toxin (PTX), an inhibitor of Gi signaling, on B cell migration into splenic follicles. Strikingly, PTX treated B cells were unable to migrate into follicles or the white pulp cords of the spleen, whereas cells treated with buffer alone or with the oligomer B subunit of PTX could migrate into follicles normally (Cyster and Goodnow 1995). These observations led us to consider which chemokine receptors and chemokines might have a role in B cell positioning within lymphoid organs. We focused on two orphan receptors, BLR1 and EBI1, because these had been shown to be constitutively expressed by B cells in humans (Birkenbach et al. 1993; Dobner et al. 1992). To track expression of the mouse receptors, the amino-terminal ectodomains were expressed as GST fusion proteins and used to immunize rabbits. An antiserum against BLR1 was isolated and affinity purified using the same BLR1 fragment expressed as a fusion protein with mannose-binding protein. Flow cytometric analysis of mouse lymphoid tissues showed BLR1 expression on all mature B cells (Schmidt et al. 1998) with slightly higher surface expression on B cells with a $CD21^{hi}IgD^{lo}$ marginal zone phenotype (Fig. 1). BLR1 expression was also observed on $B220^{+}CD5^{+}$ peritoneal B-1 cells (Fig. 1). In B cell development, there was little or no BLR1 detectable on $B220^{+}IgM^{-}$ pro/pre-B cells, whereas $B220^{+}IgM^{+}$ immature B cells showed weak expression (Fig. 1; note that as BLR1 is detected with a polyclonal antiserum it is necessary to be cautious in interpreting the significance of weak signals such as seen on many of the cells in bone marrow gate G4). BLR1 expression became strongly upregulated on immature B cells at about the same time as surface IgD and CD21 (Fig. 1). The low expression by immature B cells is consistent with findings that immature B cells are inefficient at entering follicles (Cyster 1997) and suggests that BLR1 upregulation may be an important part of the immature to mature B cell transition.

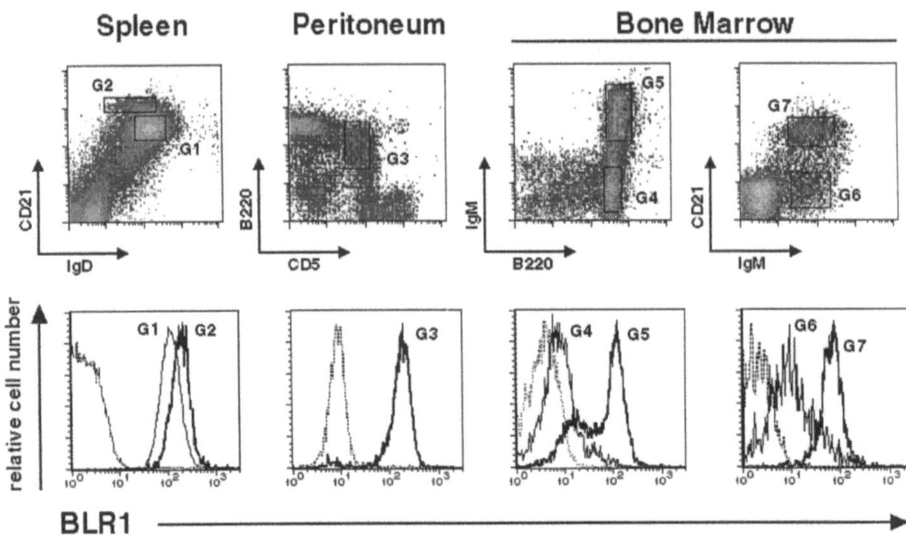

Fig. 1. Surface BLR1 expression by murine B lymphocytes. Cell suspensions prepared from the indicated tissues of C57BL/6 mice were stained with the antibodies shown in the upper panel and with rabbit anti-BLR1. BLR1 expression on cells within the gated regions in the upper panels is plotted in the lower panels. The gates correspond approximately to the following cell populations: G1, mature recirculating B cells; G2, marginal zone B cells; G3, peritoneal B-1 B cells; G4, pro/pre-B cells; G5, immature and mature bone marrow B cells; G6, immature bone marrow B cells; G7, mature recirculating bone marrow B cells. In the left and right-most panels, rabbit anti-BLR1 was detected with anti-rabbit-PE and in the center panels with anti-rabbit-FITC. The leftmost profiles in each histogram plot are samples stained without anti-BLR1 primary antibody as a control.

To allow identification and characterization of BLR1 ligands, BLR1 transfected 293 cells, Jurkat cells and E300-19 pre-B cells were generated. In situ hybridization experiments using novel expressed sequence tags (ESTs) related to chemokines as probes led to identification of one EST that hybridized to follicles in spleen, lymph nodes and Peyer's patches (Gunn et al. 1998). A recombinant form of the CXC chemokine encoded by this EST promoted calcium flux and chemotaxis responses in BLR1 transfected but not control cells, providing evidence that it was a ligand for BLR1 (Gunn et al. 1998). Chemotaxis assays with freshly isolated cells showed that the mouse chemokine was an efficacious attractant of B cells, but attracted only small numbers of CD4 T cells and few or no macrophages or granulocytes (Gunn et al. 1998). These findings lead us to call the mouse chemokine and its human homolog, BLC for B-lymphocyte chemoattractant. In independent studies Legler et al., isolated the same molecule, termed it B-cell attracting chemokine (BCA)-1, and showed it was an efficacious attractant of human B cells (Legler et al. 1998). Based on these functional studies it has been concluded that BLC is a ligand for BLR1, leading to the renaming of BLR1 as CXCR5. Interactions between G-protein coupled receptors and their ligands frequently lead to modulation of surface receptor expression (Samanta et al. 1990; von Zastrow and Kobilka 1992). To further test the specificity of the BLR1/BLC interaction, splenic B cells were incubated in the presence of BLC or, as a control, IL-8, for 30 minutes at 37°C and then washed and stained for surface BLR1. Incubation with BLC, but not IL-8, lead to a two-fold modulation in surface BLR1 expression (Fig. 2). Kinetic analysis showed that BLR1 was modulated within 10 minutes of adding BLC. These results provide further evidence for the specificity of the BLC/BLR1 interaction and suggest that surface modulation may play a role in ligand mediated desensitization of this receptor.

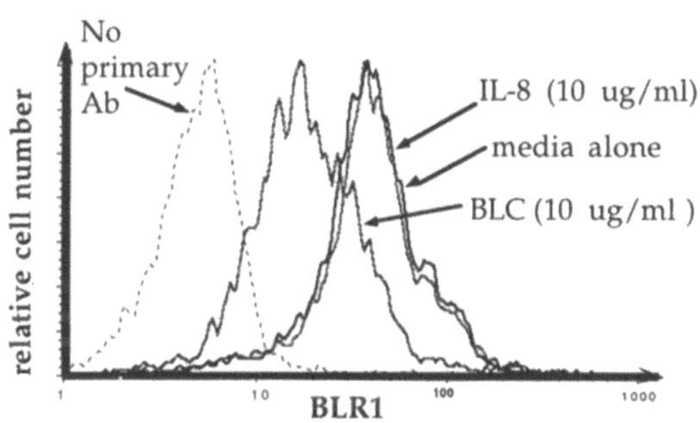

Fig. 2. Incubation with BLC induces internalization of BLR1. B cells were incubated in the absence or presence of chemokine as indicated for 30 minutes at 37°C and then stained on ice for BLR1.

In situ hybridization analysis demonstrated that BLC was highly expressed by cells with dendritic morphology in follicles (Fig. 3). Although BLC was not detected in resting lymphocytes, lymphocyte deficient RAG1-knockout mice expressed 10-fold less BLC than wildtype controls (Fig. 3 and Gunn et al. 1998). Analysis of B and T cell deficient mice established that B cells but not T cells are needed for normal basal expression of BLC (Fig. 3 and Ngo et al. 1999). These findings are consistent with BLC being made by follicular dendritic cells, because maturation of these cells is B lymphocyte dependent (Yoshida et al. 1994). However, the expression pattern of BLC does not fully overlap with that of the FDC marker

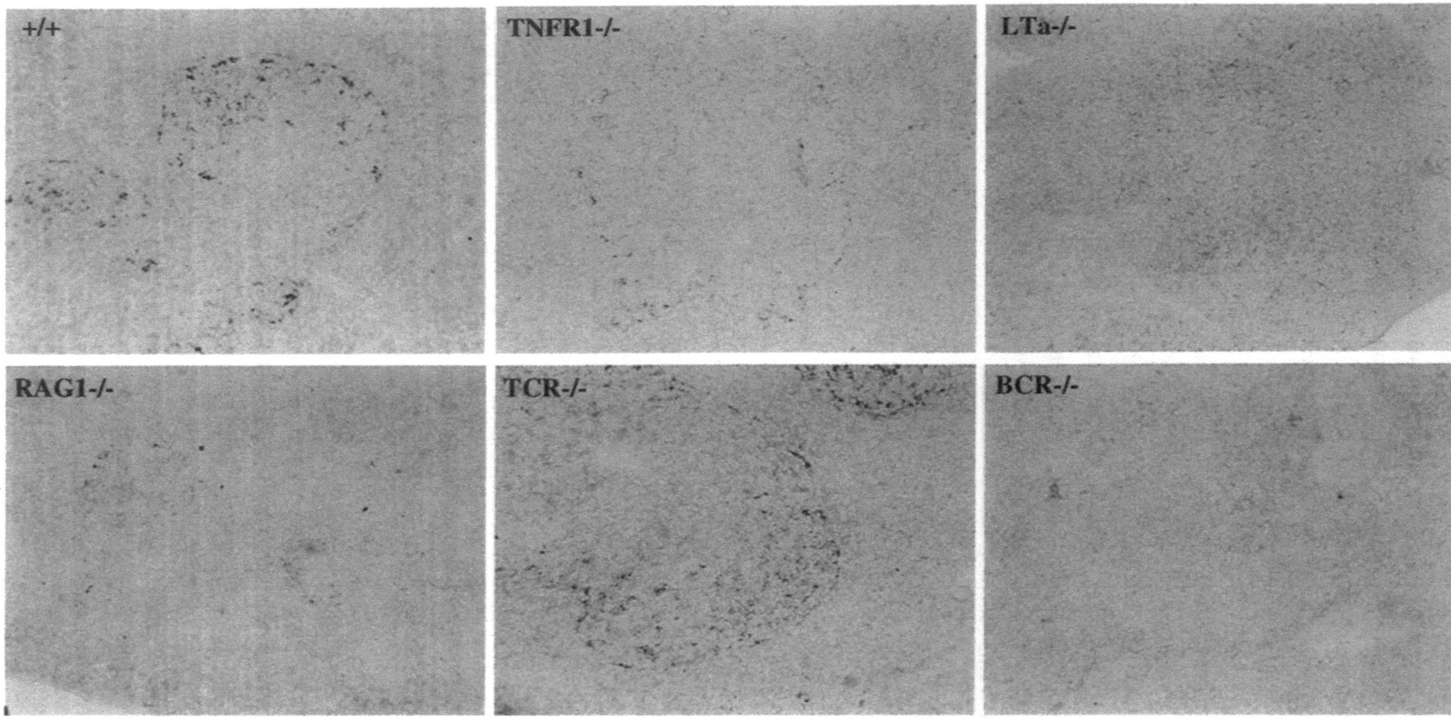

Fig. 3. In situ hybridization analysis of BLC expression in mouse spleen tissue from wildtype (+/+), TNFR1-/-, LTα-/-, RAG1-/-. TCRβ-/-δ-/- (TCR-/-), and μMT (BCR-/-) mice. Hybridization with the anti-sense BLC probe is seen as black staining. No signal was seen with a sense probe. Original magnification, 10x. In situ analysis was performed as described in Ngo et al., 1999.

CD35. Pending further analysis on isolated cells, we refer to BLC producing cells as stromal cells since this designation encompasses FDC and other reticular cell types present in follicles. To further investigate the requirements for BLC expression by follicular stromal cells we studied mice deficient in TNF and lymphotoxin (LT) α/β. Mice deficient in TNF, LTα or LTβ lack organized follicles in the spleen (Matsumoto et al. 1997). The strikingly similar disruption of follicles in TNF-deficient mice and BLR1-deficient mice (Forster et al. 1996), suggested a genetic relationship between TNF and BLR1 (Goodnow and Cyster 1997). Analysis of BLR1 expression in TNF deficient mice and LTα deficient mice showed that BLR1 expression was not reduced but instead was slightly elevated (Cook et al. 1998). However, striking deficits were observed in expression of the BLR1 ligand, BLC, in these animals (Ngo et al. 1999). These reductions were readily apparent by in situ hybridization analysis (Fig. 3). When quantitated by Northern blot of total spleen RNA, an approximately three-fold reduction was detected in TNF-deficient animals and a 20-fold decrease in mice lacking LTα/β (Ngo et al. 1999). Expression of stromal cell derived factor 1 (SDF1) was not depressed in the mutant animals, providing some evidence for selectivity in the effect on BLC expression. Since BLR1 is required for normal organization of B cells in splenic follicles and since BLC is currently the only known ligand for BLR1, it is reasonable to propose that TNF and LTα/β promote lymphocyte compartmentalization in follicles by promoting BLC expression. Future studies must address whether TNF and LTα/β induce BLC expression directly or whether their role is indirect, promoting maturation of BLC expressing stromal cells.

Acknowledgements

EHE and KMA are supported by HHMI predoctoral fellowships and JGC is a Pew Scholar. This work was supported in part by NIH grant AI-40098.

References

Birkenbach M, Josefsen K, Yalmanchili R, Lenoir G, Kieff, E (1993) Epstein-Barr virus induced genes: first lymphocyte-specific G-protein coupled peptide receptors. J Virol 67: 2209-2220

Cook MC, Korner H, Riminton DS, Lemckert FA, Hasbold J, Amesbury M, Hodgkin PD, Cyster JG, Sedgwick JD, Basten, A (1998) Generation of splenic follicle structure and B cell movement in tumor necrosis factor-deficient mice. J Exp Med 188:1503-1510

Cyster JG (1997) Signaling thresholds and interclonal competition in preimmune B-cell selection. Immunol Rev 156: 87-101

Cyster JG, Goodnow CC (1995) Pertussis toxin inhibits migration of B and T lymphocytes into splenic white pulp cords. J Exp Med 182: 581-586

Dobner T, Wolf I, Emrich T, Lipp M (1992) Differentiation-specific expression of a novel G protein-coupled receptor from Burkitt's lymphoma. Eur J Immunol 22: 2795-2799

Forster R, Mattis AE, Kremmer E, Wolf E, Brem G, Lipp, M (1996) A putative chemokine receptor, BLR1, directs B cell migration to defined lymphoid organs and specific anatomic compartments of the spleen. Cell 87: 1037-47

Goodnow CC, Cyster JG (1997) Lymphocyte homing: the scent of a follicle. Curr Biol 7: R219-22

Gunn MD, Ngo VN, Ansel KM, Ekland EH, Cyster JG, Williams LT (1998) A B-cell-homing chemokine made in lymphoid follicles activates Burkitt's lymphoma receptor-1. Nature 391: 799-803

Legler DF, Loetscher M, Roos RS, Clark-Lewis I, Baggiolini M, Moser, B (1998) B cell-attracting chemokine 1, a human CXC chemokine expressed in lymphoid tissues, selectively attracts B lymphocytes via BLR1/CXCR5. J Exp Med 187: 655-60

Matsumoto M, Fu YX, Molina H, Chaplin DD (1997) Lymphotoxin-alpha-deficient and TNF receptor-I-deficient mice define developmental and functional characteristics of germinal centers. Immunological Reviews 156: 137-44

Ngo VN, Korner H, Gunn MD, Schmidt KN, Riminton DS, Cooper MD, Browning JL, Sedgwick JD, Cyster JG (1999) Lymphotoxin-α/β and tumor necrosis factor are required for stromal cell expression of homing chemokines in B and T cell areas of the spleen. J Exp Med 189(2): in press

Samanta AK, Oppenheim JJ, Matsushima K (1990) Interleukin 8 (monocyte-derived neutrophil chemotactic factor) dynamically regulates its own receptor expression on human neutrophils. J Biol Chem 265: 183-9

Schmidt KN, Hsu CW, Griffin CT, Goodnow CC, Cyster, JG (1998) Spontaneous follicular exclusion of SHP1-deficient B cells is conditional on the presence of competitor wild-type B cells. J Exp Med 187: 929-37

von Zastrow M, Kobilka BK (1992) Ligand-regulated internalization and recycling of human beta 2-adrenergic receptors between the plasma membrane and endosomes containing transferrin receptors. J Biol Chem 267: 3530-8

Yoshida K, van den Berg TK, Dijkstra CD (1994) The functional state of follicular dendritic cells in severe combined immunodeficient (SCID) mice: role of the lymphocytes. Eur J Immunol. 24: 464-468

Discussion

Paolo Ghia: As the TNF alpha and beta have been shown to be growth factors for the follicular dendritic cells, don't you think it is just a matter of quantity in the sense that you have fewer follicular dendritic cells in the lymph nodes, so you also have less BLC?
Jason Cyster: Yes, that is certainly a reasonable possibility of how direct it is, but I think the experiments indicate that you need these cytokines for normal expression of BLC. We cannot say whether the cytokines are acting to lead to the maturation of a follicular stromal cell population which then produces the chemokine.
Paolo Ghia: Did you try to correlate the BLC expression with another FDC-specific marker?
Jason Cyster: Yes, kinetically the FDC markers disappear as fast, if not faster than the chemokine, so we cannot disagree with what you are saying.
Garnett Kelsoe: In some of the knockout systems which have been examined, there seems to be a difference between the FDC that is recognized by FDC M1 and M2. Do you have any data on their ability to express BLC?
Jason Cyster: No. I can say that in the spleen we see very weak or no expression of BLC in germinal centers.
Frans Kroese: When you look at BLC expression during ontogeny, you do get a similar kind of morphology, where B cells surround the T cell area, so you expect no BLC expression?
Jason Cyster: We should not say no BLC expression. All of these mice ($TNF^{-/-}$, $LT\alpha^{-/-}$) still have some.
Isaac Witz: What happens to BLC in situations where TNF is upregulated, i.e. in septic shock or in similar situations?
Jason Cyster: That is a good question. We are looking at non-lymphoid sites for some of those things at the moment. However, as regards in the lymphoid tissue itself, we have not looked in such situations.
Kenneth Nilsson: Is BLC present in the bone marrow?
Jason Cyster: We could not see it at a Northern blot level of detection.
Katherine Siminovitch: Have you ever determined whether BLC expression is upregulated by TNF in an *in vitro* system?
Jason Cyster: We have attempted to do that and we are still trying.
Paolo Ghia: My experience is with human cells, so I would like to know if you have tried to sort mouse FDCs and checked if they express the chemokine BLC?
Jason Cyster: Yes, that is a project that I am expecting a student in the lab to take several years to do, but he has started.
Paolo Ghia: We actually tried and we were never able to show it.
Jason Cyster: It drops very quickly *in vivo* when you block just one cytokine. I presume it will drop fast *in vitro*.
Una Chen: Maybe I missed the point, but what is the effect on B cell function when you have a deficiency of BLC?
Jason Cyster: We are just getting chimeras at the moment.

A Novel CC Chemokine ABCD-1, Produced by Dendritic Cells and Activated B Cells, Exclusively Attracts Activated T Lymphocytes

C. Schaniel[1], F. Sallusto[1], P. Sideras[2], F. Melchers[1], and A. G. Rolink[1]

[1] Basel Institute for Immunology, Grenzacherstrasse 487, CH-4005 Basel, Switzerland

[2] Department of Applied Cell and Molecular Biology, Division of Tumour Biology, Umeå University, 90187 Umeå, Sweden

Cells of the immune system can migrate as single cells through blood and lymph and can organize themselves to form specific areas in primary and secondary lymphoid organs. It has become evident that chemokines and their G protein-coupled seven-transmembrane receptors play an important role in the congregation of lymphoid cells and in the reactions of T and B cells which lead to the formation of germinal centers.

Chemokines are secretory proteins of 70 to 120 amino acids that control the migration of given leukocyte populations to specific sites of immune reactions. They are divided into four families based on the presence and position of the conserved cysteines. In the CXC family, the first two cysteine residues are split by one amino acid; in the CC family they are adjacent; in the C family, only one cysteine residue is conserved; and, in the CX_3C family the two cysteines are separated by three amino acids. The chemokines can be further distinguished as either being expressed constitutively or induced by cytokines. Chemokines of the former group are of particular interest because they are likely candidates for regulating microenvironmental homing of certain leukocyte populations to and within lymphoid tissues. The repertoire of constitutively expressed chemokines has expanded rapidly and comprises thymus-expressed chemokine (TECK), secondary-lymphoid tissue chemokine (SLC), DC-CK1, EBV-induced molecule 1 ligand chemokine (ELC), thymus and activation-regulated chemokine (TARC) and B lymphocyte chemoattractant (BLC).

During a T cell-dependent immune response T and B cells get close to each other in areas of secondary lymphoid organs which are rich in interdigitating dendritic cells (DC) presenting antigen in the context of MHC. A small number of activated B cells migrate to other areas of the spleen in which follicular dendritic cells (FDC) are localized. There they proliferate, hypermutate their Ig genes, and begin Ig class switching. Extensive proliferation and maturation of B cells lead to the formation of germinal centers at the sites of the follicles.

Helper T (Th) cells are indispensable for somatic hypermutation, for class switch recombination, for the generation of memory B cells and for germinal center formation. The interaction of CD40 ligand on Th cells with CD40 on B cells is mandatory for the generation of germinal centers [1].

Follicular stroma is suspected to produce the chemokine BLC which is recognized on the B cells by the Burkitt's lymphoma receptor (BLR)-1/CXCR5 chemokine receptor [2, 3]. BLC homes B cells into the follicles, a migratory route that becomes defective in BLR-$1^{-/-}$ mice [4]. Mature, antigen-presenting DC produce DC-CK1 [5] and ELC [6] which both attract virgin T cells to be activated in the periarteriolar lymphoid sheath (PALS) of the spleen. This, in turn, allows activated T cells to be attracted from the T cell zone into the follicles for collaboration with B cells (Fig. 1).

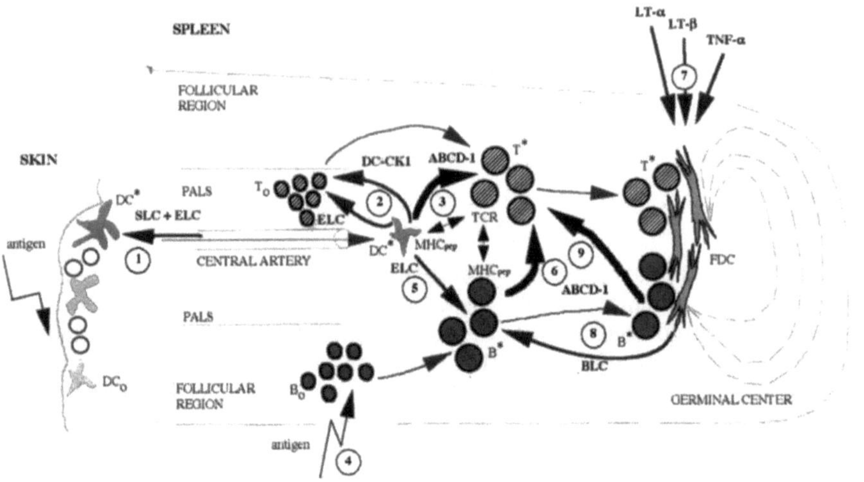

Fig. 1. Scenario for the roles of ABCD-1 in leukocyte trafficking during a T cell-dependent immune response and germinal center formation. 1) Antigen uptake in immature DC (DC_0) induces maturation of DC to become antigen-presenting cells which migrate from the site of antigen uptake, e.g. skin, to T cell-rich areas (PALS) in peripheral lymphoid organs, e.g. spleen. 2) Antigen-pulsed, mature DC in the T cell areas of secondary lymphoid organs produce DC-CK1 and ELC to attract naive, resting T cells (T_0) to be activated (T*). 3) Production of ABCD-1 by DC keeps the activated T cells attracted to the DC and, thus, continuously activated. 4) Mature resting B cells (B_0) get activated by antigen in B cell-rich follicular regions. 5) Activated B cells (B*) are now attracted by ELC to DC which are associated with activated T cells. 6) Production of ABCD-1 by activated B cells presenting MHC/peptide turns activated T cells toward the B cells. 7) Members of the TNF cytokine and receptor family activate the follicular dendritc cell network (FDC) to differentiate, 8) follicular stroma produces BLC thereby guiding the B cells into the follicles. 9) Activated T cells follow an ABCD-1 gradient to the activated B cells localized in the follicles where germinal center formation is initiated.

Here we briefly summarize the isolation and structural organization of the gene we named ABCD-1, its expression pattern, and the cell populations chemoattracted by its protein [7]. We give evidence that ABCD-1 is the mouse orthologue of the human chemokine MDC/STCP-1 [8, 9], and, thus, is a functional ligand for the chemokine receptor CCR4 [10]. Moreover, we present evidence that ABCD-1/MDC/STCP-1 can signal through a receptor(s) other than CCR4.

Identification and Characterization of a Novel CC Chemokine

We have identified a novel murine CC chemokine, named ABCD-1, by suppression subtractive hybridization. The gene was strongly upregulated and preferentially expressed in mature Sμ-Sε-switched cells generated from pro/pre-B cells stimulated with anti-CD40 and interleukin (IL) 4 [7].Three exons split by 1.2- and 2.7-kb introns encode the entire ABCD-1 gene. This gene gives rise to a ~2.2 kb transcript with a single open reading frame of 276 nucleotides. The open reading frame encodes a 92 amino acid-long unprocessed molecule consisting of a 24 amino acid-long signal peptide and a 68 amino acid-long mature protein with a predicted molecular mass of 7.8 kD [7]. The critical cysteine residues are organized as is characteristic for members of the CC family. The complete cDNA sequence of ABCD-1 can be found in EMBL/GenBank/DDBJ under the accession number AF052505.

ABCD-1 is Produced by Activated B Cells and Dendritic Cells

The expression pattern of ABCD-1 mRNA was studied by Northern blot hybridization and/or by semi-quantitative RT-PCR (Fig. 1 and [7]). All data were related to the ubiquitously expressed gene β-actin.

Relatively little message of ABCD-1 was detected in lung, spleen, thymus and lymph nodes (LN) [7]. Thus, ABCD-1 belongs to the subgroup of constitutively expressed chemokines. Expression of ABCD-1 mRNA was undetectable in brain, liver, kidney and bone marrow (BM) [7]. It was also below levels of detection in most cell lines representing distinct stages of B cell differentiation. The corresponding purified cell populations of B lineage precursors as well as immature and mature B cells from BM did not express ABCD-1 message [7]. T cell lines as well as ConA/IL-2-activated T cells, IL-3-induced macrophages and IL-2-activated natural killer (NK) cells also did not express ABCD-1 in detectable amounts [7].

High levels of ABCD-1 mRNA were seen, as expected, in pro/pre B cell lines stimulated for 3-6 days with anti-CD40 plus IL-4 (Fig. 2A). ABCD-1 mRNA was also inducible by anti-CD40/IL-4, as well as anti-CD40 alone, in mature B cells from the spleen [7]. CD40-dependent (i.e. T-cell dependent) activation induces high levels of ABCD-1 mRNA expression, while polyclonal (i.e. T cell-independent) activation induces moderate levels of ABCD-1 message in splenic (B) cells from CD3-deficient mice (Fig. 2A).

Another likely source for ABCD-1 production is DC. Freshly sorted, unstimulated, as well as anti-CD40 or GM-CSF plus TNF-α stimulated CD11c+ mesenteric LN DC expressed high amounts of ABCD-1 mRNA as did anti-CD40 activated splenic B cells (Fig. 2B and [7]). DC (> 85% CD11c+, data not shown) derived *in vitro* by culture of RAG-2 deficient bone marrow in GM-CSF-containing medium showed similarly high levels of ABCD-1 (Fig.2B).

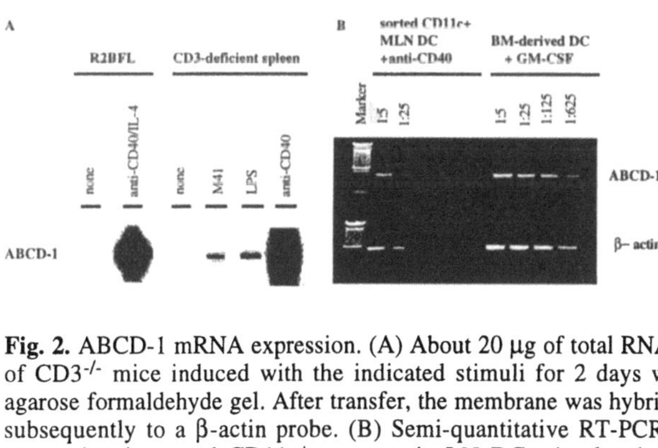

Fig. 2. ABCD-1 mRNA expression. (A) About 20 μg of total RNA from R2BFL cells and spleen of $CD3^{-/-}$ mice induced with the indicated stimuli for 2 days was electrophoresed in a 1.5% agarose formaldehyde gel. After transfer, the membrane was hybridized to an ABCD-1 probe and subsequently to a β-actin probe. (B) Semi-quantitative RT-PCR analyses of ABCD-1 mRNA expression in sorted $CD11c^{+}$ mesenteric LN DC stimulated with anti-CD40 for 24 h and DC-derived by culture of $RAG\text{-}2^{-/-}$ BM in GM-CSF-containing medium for 8 days.

ABCD-1 Exclusively Chemoattracts Activated T Cells

We used a Transwell migration assay to study the chemotactic properties of recombinant ABCD-1, produced in insect cells [7], on different cell populations. No significant migration towards ABCD-1 was seen with primary spleen cells, thymocytes, bone marrow cells, LN cells (in majority mature CD4 or CD8 single positive T cells), IL-2-activated NK cells or LPS-stimulated splenic B cells [7]. Only ConA-activated IL-2-restimulated T cell blasts were chemoattracted by ABCD-1 (Fig. 3 and [7]). Migration was concentration-dependent and showed a typical bell-shaped curve. FACS analysis of the chemoattracted T lymphoblasts revealed both CD4 and CD8 T cells (data not shown).

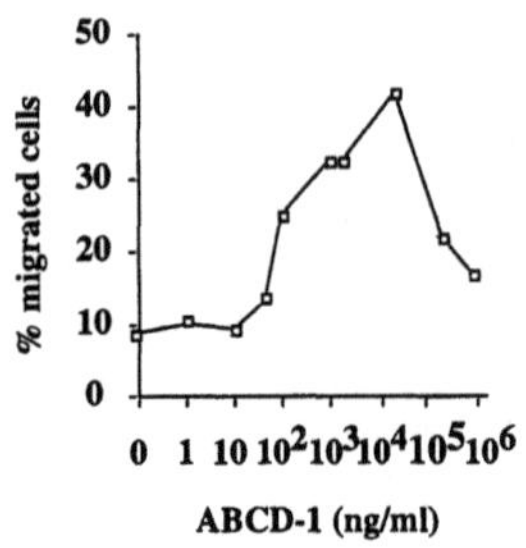

Fig. 3. ABCD-1 induced chemotaxis of ConA-activated IL-2-restimulated T lymphoblasts. One representative experiment is shown.

ABCD-1 is Most Likely the Murine Orthologue of the Human Chemokine MDC/STCP-1

The sequence of the mature ABCD-1 protein shares 64% identity and 84% similarity to the human CC chemokine MDC/STCP-1 [8,9]. We therefore suspected that ABCD-1 could be the mouse orthologue of human MDC/STCP-1. Since in both studies with the human chemokine expression of MDC/STCP-1 in activated human B cells was not investigated, we analyzed MDC/STCP-1 expression on anti-CD40 plus IL-4-stimulated human tonsillar B cells. We found them to express high levels of MDC/STCP-1 mRNA [7]. Furthermore, we synthesized cDNA from anti-CD40 plus IL-4-activated human and mouse B cells and hybridized them with an ABCD-1 or MDC/STCP-1 probe, respectively. When we used the ABCD-1-specific probe under low stringency conditions, it recognized the ~2.2 kb ABCD-1-specific sequence in the mouse cDNA and also a sequence in the human cDNA sample that comigrated with the ~2.9 kb signal detected by the MDC/STCP-1 probe [7]. These findings are consistent with the notion that ABCD-1 is most likely the murine orthologue of MDC/STCP-1.

ABCD-1 is also a potent chemoattractant for human $CD4^+$ T cells stimulated with anti-CD3/anti-CD28 and either IL-12 and anti-IL-4 to yield Th1 cells, or IL-4 and anti-IL-12 to generate Th2 cells [7]. IL-4/anti-IL-12-induced T cells migrated optimally at lower doses than did IL-12/anti-IL-4-activated T cells. ABCD-1 furthermore induced a transient increase in $[Ca^{++}]_i$ in both human Th1 and Th2 cell populations as expected from the migration assays (Fig. 4A and B). When the cells were exposed to two successive ABCD-1 challenges, the response to the second challenge was completely abrogated (Fig. 4A and B), showing homologous desensitization. The MDC/STCP-1 induced $[Ca^{++}]_i$-increase was inhibited by a prechallenge with ABCD-1, and vice versa, further supporting the idea that ABCD-1 is the murine orthologue of MDC/STCP-1 (Fig. 4C and D).

In humans, CCR4 is the only known chemokine receptor for MDC/STCP-1 [10]. On the other side, several publications have shown that expression of CCR4 is restricted to cells of Th2 type [11,12]. We, however, found that also Th1 cells, which should be devoid of CCR4, responded upon exposure to ABCD-1 (Fig. 4A). Hence, ABCD-1/MDC/STCP-1 is suspected to have a second receptor expressed on Th1 cells, and perhaps on Th2 lymphocytes. Further preliminary data strengthen this conclusion. Both human Th1 cells lacking CCR4, as revealed with an anti-human CCR4 monoclonal antibody, and Th2 cells expressing high levels of CCR4 did show a prominent $[Ca^{++}]_i$-increase upon exposure to recombinant MDC/STCP-1. Further desensitization experiments with recombinant ABCD-1/MDC/STCP-1 and other chemokines with their known cognate receptors should help us to clarify which and how many chemokine receptors function with ABCD-1/MDC/STCP-1.

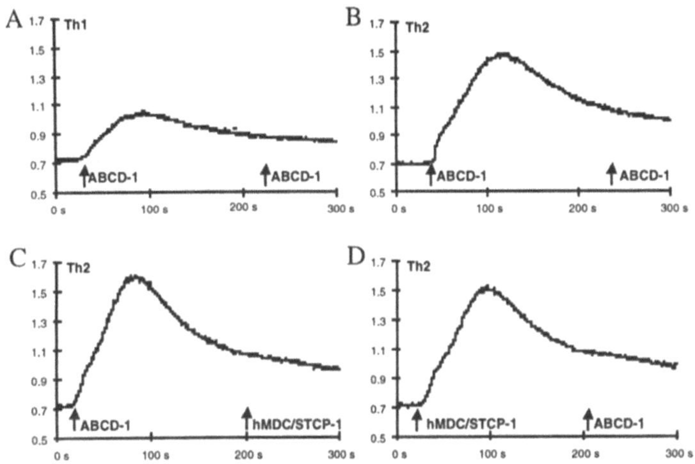

Fig. 4. Chemokine-induced $[Ca^{++}]_i$ increase in human Th1 and Th2 cells. (A) Indo-2 loaded human Th1 cells were exposed to 100 ng/ml ABCD-1 followed by a second challenge. (B) As in (A) but with human Th2 cells. (C) As in (B) but with the second exposure to 100 ng/ml recombinant human MDC/STCP-1. (D) Human Th2 cells were exposed to human MDC/STCP-1 followed by ABCD-1. Arrows show time of addition of the indicated chemokine.

A Scenario for the Roles of ABCD-1 in T Cell-dependent B Cell Responses and Germinal Center Formation

During an immune response diverse cells of the immune system follow distinct migration routes to special areas in secondary lymphoid tissues where DC-T cell and T-B cell interactions take place leading to the formation of primary and, in the end, of secondary follicles, of germinal centers (Fig. 1). The first cells involved in such a response are immature DC. When immature DC encounter antigen and are stimulated by inflammatory stimuli they get activated and mature to produce high levels of inflammatory chemokines, thereby recruiting many effector cells (immature DC, macrophages and T cells) to the site of inflammation. Maturing DC also migrate into the PALS of secondary lymphoid organs where they could present antigen in the context of MHC to naive T cells. This migration is probably organized by SLC, which attracts the DC into the tissue, and ELC, which homes them into the T cell areas. Naive T cells are likely to be attracted to the secondary lymphoid organs by SLC. Once the virgin T cells have reached the secondary tissue they have to get near antigen-presenting DC for activation. The two chemokines DC-CK1 and ELC produced by DC in the T cell zones might regulate this step. Production of ABCD-1 by DC could now keep the primed T cells attracted to the DC and, hence, continuously activated. B cells in the mantel zone also have to be activated. ELC might then attract the B cells toward the DC which are associated with activated T cells. T cell-independently activated B cells produce moderate levels of ABCD-1 which might be enough to turn the T cells away from the DC towards the B cells allowing T-B cell interactions through CD40L-CD40 . At the same time, the B cells are attracted into the follicular areas by BLC which is likely produced by follicular stroma. The activated T cells presumably follow the activated B cells through chemoattraction via ABCD-1 into the follicles, where T and B cells begin to form germinal centers.

Acknowledgements

The Basel Institute for Immunology was founded and is supported by F. Hoffmann-La Roche Ltd., Basel, Switzerland. P. Sideras was supported by the Swedish Medical Research Council (MFR), the Swedish Cancer Foundation "Cancerfonden", and the "Petrus and Augusta Heglund"-Stiftelsen. The authors thank Dr. K. Matsushima, University of Tokyo, Japan, for providing anti-human CCR4 mAb and Dr. J. Andersson for critical reading of the manuscript.

References

1. Kawabe T, Naka T, Yoshida K, Tanaka T, Fujiwara H, Suematsu S, Yoshida N, Kishimoto T, Kikutani H (1994) The immune response in CD40-deficient mice: impaired immunoglobulin class switching and germinal center formation. Immunity 1:167-178
2. Gunn MD, Ngo VN, Ansel KM, Ekland EH, Cyster JG, Williams LT (1998) A B-cell homing chemokine made in lymphoid follicles activates Burkitt's lymphoma receptor-1. Science 391: 799-803
3. Legler DF, Loetscher M, Ross RS, Clark-Lewis I, Baggiolini M, Moser B (1998) B cell-attracting chemokine 1, a human CXC chemokine expressed in lymphoid tissues, selectively attracts B lymphocytes via BLR1/CXCR5. J Exp Med 187: 655-660
4. Forster R, Mattis AE, Kremmer A, Wolf E, Brem G, Lipp M (1996) A putative chemokine receptor, BLR1, directs B cell migration to defined lymphoid organs and specific anatomic compartments of the spleen. Cell 87: 1037-1047
5. Adema GJ, Hartgers F, Verstraten R, de Vries E, Marland G, Menon S, Foster J, Xu Y, Nooyen P, McClanahan T, Bacon KB, Figdor CG (1998) A dendritic-cell-derived CC chemokine that preferentially attracts naive T cells. Nature 387: 713-717
6. Ngo VN, Tang HL, Cyster JG (1998) Epstain-Barr Virus-induced molecule 1 ligand chemokine is expressed by dendritic cells in lymphoid tissues and strongly attracts naive T cells and activated B cells. J Exp Med 188: 181-191

7. Schaniel C, Pardali E, Sallusto F, Speletas M, Ruedl C, Shimizu T, Seidl T, Andersson J, Melchers F, Rolink AG, Sideras P (1998) Activated murine B lymphocytes and dendritic cells produce a novel CC chemokine which acts selectively on activated T cells. J Exp Med 188: 451-463
8. Godiska R, Chantry D, Raport CJ, Sozzani S, Allavena P, Leviten D, Mantovani A, Gray PW (1997) Human macrophage-derived chemokine (MDC), a novel chemoattractant for monocytes, monocyte-derived dendritic cells, and natural killer cells. J Exp Med 185: 1595-1604
9. Chang M, McNinch J, Elias III C, Manthey CL, Grosshans D, Meng T, Boone T, Andrew DP (1997) Molecular cloning and functional characterization of a novel CC chemokine, stimulated T cell chemotactic protein (STCP-1), that specifically acts on activated T lymphocytes. J Biol Chem 272: 25229-25237
10. Imai T, Chantry D, Raport CJ, Wood CL, Nishimura M, Godiska R, Yoshie O, Gray PW (1998) Macrophage-derived chemokine is a functional ligand for the CC chemokine receptor 4. J Biol Chem 273: 1764-1768
11. Bonecchi R, Bianchi G, Bordignon PP, D'Ambrosio D, Lang R, Borsatti A, Sozzani S, Allavena P, Gray PA, Mantovani A, Sinigaglia F (1998) Differential expression of chemokine receptors and chemotactic responsiveness of type 1 T helper cells (Th1s) and Th2s. J Exp Med 187: 129-134
12. Sallusto F, Lenig D, Mackay CR, Lanzavecchia A (1998) Flexible programs of chemokine receptor expression on human polarized T helper 1 and 2 lymphocytes. J Exp Med 187: 875-883

Discussion

Sandy Morse: For T cell subsets within the spleen there are cells which contribute equally to some reactions, and other reactions which are dominated by one subset. Do you know if there is a difference between those subsets in terms of their nonresponsiveness to the chemokine?
Christoph Schaniel: Both CD4 and CD8 migrated with the same property: the essential difference between mouse and human studies being that others only found Th2 cells responding whereas we showed that in the human both Th1 and Th2 migrate, even though the Th2 seem to migrate better than the Th1.
Shozo Izui: You showed the migration of activated T cells in response to this new chemokine. Have you tried to see whether activated B cells also respond to it?
Christoph Schaniel: We did LPS-activated splenic B cells and they do not migrate.
Martin Lipp: Did you perform a time-course experiment to analyze the expression of the chemokine ABCD?
Christoph Schaniel: No, I did not. The analysis was done after 2 days stimulation.

Human Macrophage-Derived Chemokine (MDC) is Strongly Expressed Following Activation of both Normal and Malignant Precursor and Mature B Cells

P. Ghia[1,2], C. Schaniel[3], A.G Rolink[3], L.M. Nadler[1] and A.A. Cardoso[1].
[1]Dana-Farber Cancer Institute, Harvard Medical School, Boston, MA, [2]Istituto per la Ricerca e la Cura del Cancro, Candiolo, Italy and [3]Basel Institute for Immunology, Basel, Switzerland.

Introduction

Chemokines are a rapidly expanding group of secreted molecules that selectively control the migration and homing of leukocytes to different sites of inflammation and immune responses [1, 2]. They are believed to perform key functions in secondary lymphoid tissues, where they attract antigen-bearing dendritic cells (DC) [3, 4] and antigen-specific T and B cells, promoting interactions among them and guiding them to appropriate sites [2, 5].

Several chemokines that act on B lymphocytes have been described. They are constitutively expressed in secondary lymphoid tissues and appear to orchestrate the movement of B cells from the bloodstream, through the T zone, to the follicles [6]. The secondary lymphoid-tissue chemokine (SLC) [7-11] is a B cell chemoattractant; it is expressed by high endothelial venules (HEV) in lymph nodes (LN) and Peyer's patches, and very likely plays a prominent role in triggering lymphocyte adhesion to HEV. ELC/Mip3β [12, 13] is expressed by T zone Dcs, in particular in LN and the appendix and binds to the EBV-induced molecule 1 (EBI-1/CCR7), which was first identified as a molecule upregulated in EBV-transformed Burkitt's lymphoma cells [14]. This finding may explain the weak but significant responsiveness of resting B cells to ELC [15]. This chemokine may play an important role in attracting cells away from HEV into the T zone [15]. Two other chemokines appear to be relevant in promoting the compartmentalization of B cells into follicles. The novel BLC/BCA-1 chemokine [16, 17], the ligand for the well known Burkitt's lymphoma receptor 1 (BLR-1/CXCR5) [18], is required for the homing of B cells to follicles in the spleen and Peyer's patches. The Stroma Derived Factor-1 (SDF-1) was originally described as a growth factor and chemoattractant for B lymphocyte precursors [19, 20], but recently has been shown to attract naive and memory B cells rather than germinal center cells, suggesting another role in directing migration of B lymphocytes into follicles [21].

In contrast, expression and production of chemokines by B lymphocytes, beside the detection of low levels of Mip-1α and Mip-3α in some malignant B cell lines [12, 22], has not been previously described. Putative chemokines produced by B cells would provide a missing link to explain T cell attraction into the follicular areas and their interaction with activated B cells.

Recently, a novel murine chemokine, ABCD-1, has been isolated using a subtractive hybridization method that identifies genes preferentially expressed in activated B cells [23]. This CC chemokine, which is also expressed in activated DCs, appears to be the orthologue of the human Macrophage-Derived Chemokine (MDC) gene [24, 25]. The latter, being highly expressed in macrophages and monocyte-derived dendritic cells, appears to be synthesized specifically by cells of the macrophage lineage. In both humans and mice, these molecules are potent attractants for activated T cells, regardless of their CD8/CD4 phenotype [24, 23]. These findings have prompted us to analyze MDC expression in human bone marrow and tonsil B cell subpopulations, as well as in numerous cell lines representing different stages of B lymphocyte development.

Materials and Methods

Cells

Tonsils were obtained, as discarded tissues, from three children undergoing tonsillectomies. Human heparinized bone marrows (BM) were obtained by iliac crest aspiration from two individuals of 3 and 5 years of age, healthy or free of hematological diseases. PB monocytes from three donors were allowed to differentiate into macrophages, on plastic tissue culture dishes, *in vitro* [25]. Lymph nodes were obtained from six patients undergoing diagnostic biopsies and who were diagnosed with follicular, small cleaved cell type lymphoma (working formulation). The malignant B cells were carrying the t(14;18) translocation, as revealed by PCR [26]. Peripheral blood (PB) was drawn from seven patients diagnosed with B-cell Chronic Lymphocytic Leukemia (B-CLL) and from fourteen pediatric patients diagnosed with B-cell Acute Lymphoblastic Leukemia (B-ALL). All tissue samples from patients were obtained following appropriate informed consent and in accordance with institutional guidelines at the Dana-Farber Cancer Institute, Brigham and Women's Hospital, and the Children's Hospital, Boston, MA.

Organs were cut with a scalpel blade, incubated twice with Collagenase IV and DNAse I (Sigma, St. Louis, MO, USA), for repeated rounds of 15', at 37°C, 5% CO_2. They were then passed through a fine wire mesh to prepare a single cell suspension. Mononuclear cells from organs, PB or BM were then isolated by Ficoll-hypaque gradient (density 1.077 g/ml) (Pharmacia, Uppsala, Sweden). When not used directly for experiments at the time of preparation, samples were cryopreserved.

Cell Lines

Several cell lines reproducing different stages of B cell development have been used: pro-B ALL: Reh, 207, RS4;11; pre-B ALL: Nalm6, BLIN-1; Burkitt's lymphoma: Jijoye; bcl-2 translocated B cell lymphomas: DHL-6, DHL-16, H2, RL.

Purification of Normal and Neoplastic B Cells

Mononuclear cells were first incubated with a cocktail of anti-CD3, -CD11b, -CD14, -CD56 monoclonal antibodies, as described [27], followed by magnetic beads coated with goat anti-mouse IgG and IgM antibodies (BioMag, Perseptive Biosystems, Framingham, MA), and applied to a magnetic field. The purity of the isolated B cells was always greater than 97%. Total tonsillar B cells, CLL cells and FL cells were further FACS-sorted, as described below. BM B-cell subpopulations were directly separated by FACS sorting.

Antibodies

Surface staining of cells from normal and neoplastic tissues was performed using the following antibodies: phycoerytrin (PE) labeled anti-CD3 and fluorescein isothiocyanate (FITC) anti-CD4, biotin (BIO) labeled anti-CD8, FITC labeled anti-

CD10, PE or BIO labeled anti-CDl9, PE labeled anti-CD20 and PE labeled anti-CD5 (Coulter, Miami, FL, USA), PE labeled anti-CD38 (Becton Dickinson & Co, Mountain View, CA), polyclonal BIO-goat anti-human IgD (F(ab$_2$), streptavidin-PE (SBA, Birmingham, AL), polyclonal FITC- or PE-rabbit anti-human IgM, anti-IgG, anti-IgA and anti-IgD, anti-human kappa light chain, anti-lambda light chain (Dako, Carpenteria, CA) and streptavidin-TRICOLOR (Caltag Laboratories, San Francisco, CA).

Cell Surface Staining and Cell Sorting

Three color immunofluorescence analysis was used for the identification of neoplastic populations in the pathological samples of different B-cell populations within the tonsillar mononuclear cells and of the different B-cell precursor populations in the bone marrow. Tonsillar B cells were stained with BIO-anti-IgD (followed by streptavidin TRICOLOR), PE-anti-CD38 and FITC-anti-CD19 antibodies. Naive B-cells were identified as being CD19$^+$, IgD$^+$, CD38$^-$ cells, GC cells being CD19$^+$, IgD$^-$, CD38$^+$ and memory B-cells being CD19$^+$, IgD$^-$, CD38$^-$ [28].

BM cells were stained with BIO-anti-CD19 or anti CD10 (plus streptavidin TRICOLOR), PE-anti CD34 and FITC-anti-κL and -λL chains antibodies. Pre-B I cells were identified as being CD19$^+$, CD10$^+$, CD34$^+$, κL$^-$ or λL$^-$; pre-B II were CD19$^+$, CD10$^+$, CD34$^-$, κL$^-$ or λL$^-$. These cells were also discriminated by size on the side forward scatter profile (large and small pre-B II). Finally immature B cells could be identified as being CD19$^+$, CD10$^+$, CD34$^-$; κL$^+$ or λL$^+$ [29].

Malignant FL cells were identified as being CD19$^+$, CD38$^+$ and κL or λL chain restricted; B-CLL cells were identified as being CD19$^+$, CD5$^+$. All these different B-cell populations were isolated by FACS-sorting. Cell surface immunofluorescence, flow cytometric analysis and cell sort were performed as previously described [27] on a Coulter Elite (Coulter Co, Miami, FL), at 4°C. Only cells exhibiting low forward angle and low right angle light scattering properties (lymphoid gate) were analyzed and sorted.

Cell Culture

Purified ALL, FL and B-cell subpopulations were cultured in IMDM supplemented with 2% FBS, 0.5 mg/ml deionized BSA, 2mM L-glutamine, 50 μg/ml iron-saturated transferrin, and 5 μg/ml insulin. Cultures were performed in the presence or in the absence of soluble CD40 Ligand (sCD40L), for up to 3 days. The sCD40 ligand, a fusion protein of CD40L and CD8α chain, was kindly provided by Dr. P. Lane (Birmingham, UK) [30]. Supernatants from sCD40L stimulated B-ALL cells were collected after 3 days of culture and used for the chemotaxis assay (see below).

cDNA Preparation and PCR Analysis

To prepare cDNA, 0.5 - 1.0 x 10^6 purified or sorted cells were lysed in 1 ml of RNAzol (Biotecx Laboratories, Inc., Houston, TX), and RNA extracted according to the manufacturer's instructions. Reverse transcriptase (RT) mix (containing superscript II, GIBCO BRL, Gaithersburg, MD) was then added and incubated at 42°C for 1 h. The enzyme was inactivated for 2' at 95°C.

PCR amplification of cDNA samples was carried out, using the primers for MDC, RANTES, MIP-1 α and Actin (as control). The primers sequences are shown in Table 1. All the primer pairs are spanning intron sequences, allowing for the distinction between expressed RNA from genomic DNA. cDNAs obtained from macrophages differentiated from PB monocytes on plastic tissue culture dishes were used as positive controls [25].

Table 1. Primers sequences

GENE		PRIMERS
MDC	Fw	5' ACTGCACTCCTGGTTGTCCTCGTC 3'
	Rev	5' CACGGTCATCAGAGTAGGCTC 3'
RANTES	Fw	5' TATTCCTCGGACACCACAC 3'
	Rev	5' GCTCATCTCCAAAGAGTTGA 3'
MIP-1α	Fw	5' CTGCTGCTTCAGCTACACCTCC 3'
	Rev	5' ACCCCTCAGGCACTCAGCTCC 3'
β-ACTIN	Fw	5' GTGGGGCGCCCCAGGCACCA 3'
	Rev	5' CTCCTTAATGTCACGCACGATTTC 3'

Chemotaxis Assay

Cell migration was evaluated using 5-μm microporous Transwell inserts (Costar, Cambridge, MA). T cells were resuspended in serum-free AIM V media (GIBCO BRL, Gaithersburg, MD) and 1-2x10^5 were placed onto the inserts (upper compartment of the chemotaxis system) in a well containing 500ng/ml of recombinant MDC (R&D Systems, Minneapolis, MN) or supernatant from sCD40L stimulated B-ALL cells. After 6-hour chemotaxis at 37°C, 5% CO_2, all migrated cells were carefully resuspended, collected and counted by flow cytometry, using a Coulter XL (Coulter Co, Miami, FL). The migration percentage was calculated by dividing the number of migrated cells by the total number of input cells.

Results and Discussion

This study was conducted to test the hypothesis that activated human B cells could produce chemokines which play a role in the collaboration between B lymphocytes and T cells and in the formation of germinal centers during immune responses. It has recently been shown in mice that the chemokine ABCD-1, the orthologue of human MDC [25], is expressed in B cells activated by CD40 crosslinking [23]. MDC expression was then analyzed in B cell subpopulations obtained from human tonsils, as they represent *in vivo* activated lymphocytes.

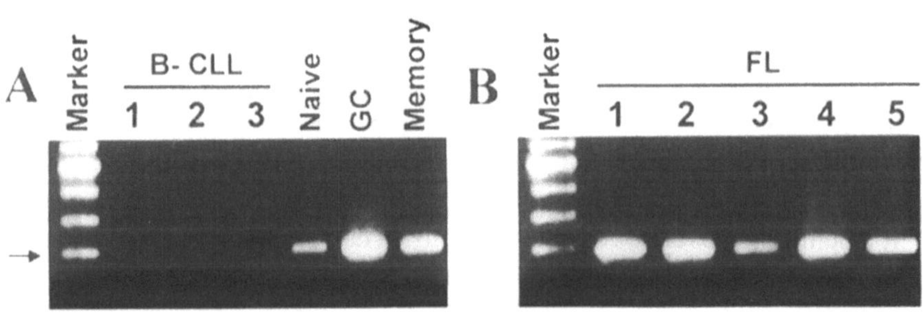

Fig. 1. Expression level of the chemokine MDC, detected by RT-PCR in A) 3 B-CLL patients and Naive, GC and Memory B cells sorted from one representative human tonsil; in B) 5 FL patients. Expected size of the amplified product (289bp) is shown by the arrow.

Naive, GC and memory B cells were FACS sorted as described in the Material and Methods section [28]. Malignant $CD38^+$ B cells, carrying the bcl-2 translocation [26], were also purified from highly invaded lymph nodes of patients diagnosed with low grade follicular lymphoma (FL). Both normal and malignant B cells showed high levels of MDC expression via RT-PCR analysis (Fig. 1A and B).
In contrast, when we analyzed five mature B cell lines, four of them derived from lymphomas carrying a bcl-2 translocation (DHL-6, DHL-16, H2, RL) did not show any presence of MDC message. Only the Burkitt lymphoma cell line Jijoye showed marked levels of expression (data not shown).
In an attempt to determine whether physiological activation signals could modify MDC expression by these cells, we cultured primary (normal and malignant) cells and cell lines in the presence of sCD40L, for 1 to 3 days. Stimulation of the cells through CD40 did not modify the level of expression of MDC, which remained stable in the primary cells and absent in the cell lines. MDC expression, then, appears to be constitutive on *in vivo* activated B cells, i.e., in secondary lymphoid tissues, regardless of their normal or malignant phenotype. This expression is not modified by further signaling through CD40.
Such a discrete pattern of expression suggests that MDC might play a relevant function in recruiting activated T cells and dendritic cells during a physiological immune response, as well as during an abnormal germinal center reaction, such as in follicular lymphoma. In such a scenario it is reasonable to speculate that MDC production could be a relevant feature of the neoplastic phenotype of lymphoma cells, as this would allow for the attraction of T cells, DCs and perhaps Follicular Dendritic Cells (FDC) which are always present in the context of the neoplastic lesions. These cell lineages have been indicated as possible contributors to the progression of the disease, contributing through different signals to the survival of the neoplastic clone [31-33]. This appears to be suggested also by our finding that none of the circulating CLL B-cells isolated from seven patients were found to express MDC (Fig. 1A).
In order to better define the relevance of MDC production during B cell ontogenesis, normal and malignant precursor B-cells were analyzed. In human BM, discrete subpopulations of B-lineage committed cells can easily be identified based on the expression of surface markers and the cell cycle status, whose changes reflect differences in the rearrangement status of the Immunoglobulin (Ig) loci [34]. According to previous reports [29, 34], we FACS sorted pre-B I cells, large and small pre-B II, and immature B cells. None of these populations showed the presence of MDC by RT-PCR analysis (data not shown).
Similar results were obtained when we purified $CD10^+$ malignant B cells from the PB of 14 children diagnosed with B-ALL at different stages of differentiation. It was not possible to detect MDC in any of these patients. Also, according to these results, several ALL cell lines resembling the pre-B I and the pre-B II stages of differentiation appeared to be negative for the expression of MDC mRNA. Among all the B-ALL cell lines analyzed (Reh, 207, RS4;11, Nalm-6, BLIN-1) only the 207 cells appeared to express high levels of mRNA.
A notable difference became evident when we cultured *in vitro* sorted $CD10^+$, $CD19^+$, κL^- or λL^- pre-B cells from normal BM, as well as malignant $CD10^+$ B-ALL cells and B-ALL cell lines. In the presence of sCD40L, MDC message was readily detected after 1 day of culture, in both normal (Fig. 2) and malignant primary B cell precursors (data not shown), and it persisted up to 3 days.
In contrast, none of the cell lines expressed MDC message after CD40 activation, with the exception of BLIN 1, which showed low levels of the message.
MDC induction by CD40 crosslinking in normal pre-B and ALL cells appears to be specific as no such effect was observed with other chemokines tested (RANTES and Mip-1α).

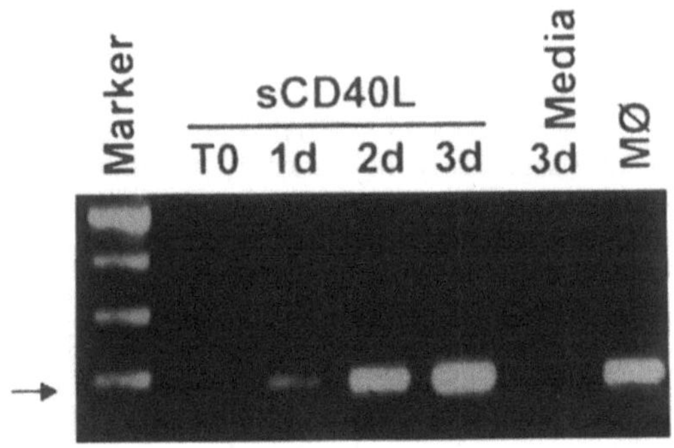

Fig. 2. Expression level of the chemokine MDC in sorted CD10⁺ pre B cells from a representative human BM (T0), upon stimulation with sCD40L (after 1, 2 and 3 days) and without any stimuli (media only after 3 days). Macrophages (Mϕ) represent the positive control.

While it is not possible to rule out the possibility that normal precursor B cells become responsive to CD40L stimulation as an effect of the inevitable maturation that happens during *in vitro* culture, this does not appear to be the case for the primary B-ALL cells, which maintained their original phenotype after the 3 days of *in vitro* culture.

Not surprisingly, supernatants from ALL cells cultured in the presence of sCD40L, but not under control conditions, induced calcium flux exclusively on T cell clones expressing the MDC receptor CCR4 (data not shown). To date, CCR4 has been shown to be the only known chemokine receptor capable of binding MDC and it has been shown to be expressed on cells responsive to MDC [35].

We have previously shown that ALL cells can be modified by CD40-crosslinking to become efficient APC and thus induce the generation and expansion of autologous anti-leukemia cytotoxic T cells (CTL) [36]. We are currently examining whether the anti-leukemia specific CTL expressed the CCR4 molecule and, more importantly, whether they could migrate in response to MDC produced by CD40-activated ALL cells. These findings would further underscore the rationale for the use of CD40-stimulated ALL cells in vaccination strategies for the treatment of ALL.

Acknowledgements

This work was supported by the NIH grants P01-CA68484-02 and P01-CA66996-01 to L.M.N. The Basel Institute for Immunology was founded and is supported by F. Hoffmann-La Roche Ltd., Basel, Switzerland. We highly acknowledge the technical assistance provided by Isabelle Grass, and Hernani M. Afonso. We are grateful to Pedro Alves for the precise help with the figures.

References

1. Rollins BJ (1997) Chemokines. Blood 90: 909-928
2. Baggiolini M (1998) Chemokines and leukocyte traffic. Nature 392: 565-568
3. Dieu MC, Vanbervliet B, Vicari A, Bridon JM, Oldham E, Ait-Yahia S, Briere F, Zlotnik A, Lebecque S, Caux C (1998) Selective recruitment of immature and mature dendritic cells by distinct chemokines expressed in different anatomic sites. J Exp Med 188: 373-386
4. Sozzani S, Allavena P, D'Amico G, Luini W, Bianchi G, Kataura M, Imai T, Yoshie O, Bonecchi R, Mantovani A (1998) Differential regulation of chemokine receptors during dendritic cell maturation: a model for their trafficking properties. J Immunol 161: 1083-1086
5. Ward SG, Bacon K, Westwick J (1998) Chemokines and T lymphocytes: more than an attraction. Immunity 9: 1-11
6. Goodnow CC, Cyster JG (1997) Lymphocyte homing: the scent of a follicle. Curr Biol 7: R219-222
7. Hedrick JA, Zlotnik A (1997) Identification and characterization of a novel beta chemokine containing six conserved cysteines. J Immunol 159: 1589-1593
8. Hromas R, Kim CH, Klemsz M, Krathwohl M, Fife K, Cooper S, Schnizlein-Bick C, Broxmeyer HE (1997) Isolation and characterization of Exodus-2, a novel C-C chemokine with a unique 37-amino acid carboxyl-terminal extension. J Immunol 159: 2554-2558
9. Nagira M, Imai T, Hieshima K, Kusuda J, Ridanpaa M, Takagi S, Nishimura M, Kakizaki M, Nomiyama H, Yoshie O (1997) Molecular cloning of a novel human CC chemokine secondary lymphoid- tissue chemokine that is a potent chemoattractant for lymphocytes and mapped to chromosome 9p13. J Biol Chem 272: 19518-19524
10. Tanabe S, Lu Z, Luo Y, Quackenbush EJ, Berman MA, Collins-Racie LA, Mi S, Reilly C, Lo D, Jacobs KA, Dorf ME (1997) Identification of a new mouse beta-chemokine, thymus-derived chemotactic agent 4, with activity on T lymphocytes and mesangial cells. J Immunol 159: 5671-5679
11. Gunn MD, Tangemann K, Tam C, Cyster JG, Rosen SD, Williams LT (1998) A chemokine expressed in lymphoid high endothelial venules promotes the adhesion and chemotaxis of naive T lymphocytes. Proc Natl Acad Sci U S A 95: 258-263
12. Rossi DL, Vicari AP, Franz-Bacon K, McClanahan TK, Zlotnik A (1997) Identification through bioinformatics of two new macrophage proinflammatory human chemokines: MIP-3alpha and MIP-3beta. J Immunol 158: 1033-1036
13. Yoshida R, Imai T, Hieshima K, Kusuda J, Baba M, Kitaura M, Nishimura M, Kakizaki M, Nomiyama H, Yoshie O (1997) Molecular cloning of a novel human CC chemokine EBI1-ligand chemokine that is a specific functional ligand for EBI1, CCR7. J Biol Chem 272: 13803-13809
14. Birkenbach M, Josefsen K, Yalamanchili R, Lenoir G, Kieff E (1993) Epstein-Barr virus-induced genes: first lymphocyte-specific G protein- coupled peptide receptors. J Virol 67: 2209-2220
15. Ngo VN, Tang HL, Cyster JG (1998) Epstein-Barr virus-induced molecule 1 ligand chemokine is expressed by dendritic cells in lymphoid tissues and strongly attracts naive T cells and activated B cells. J Exp Med 188: 181-191
16. Gunn MD, Ngo VN, Ansel KM, Ekland EH, Cyster JG, Williams LT (1998) A B-cell-homing chemokine made in lymphoid follicles activates Burkitt's lymphoma receptor-1. Nature 391: 799-803
17. Legler DF, Loetscher M, Roos RS, Clark-Lewis I, Baggiolini M, Moser B (1998) B cell-attracting chemokine 1, a human CXC chemokine expressed in lymphoid tissues, selectively attracts B lymphocytes via BLR1/CXCR5. J Exp Med 187: 655-660
18. Forster R, Mattis AE, Kremmer E, Wolf E, Brem G, Lipp M (1996) A putative chemokine receptor, BLR1, directs B cell migration to defined lymphoid organs and specific anatomic compartments of the spleen. Cell 87: 1037-1047
19. Nagasawa T, Hirota S, Tachibana K, Takakura N, Nishikawa S, Kitamura Y, Yoshida N, Kikutani H, Kishimoto T (1996) Defects of B-cell lymphopoiesis and bone-marrow myelopoiesis in mice lacking the CXC chemokine PBSF/SDF-1. Nature 382: 635-638

20. D'Apuzzo M, Rolink A, Loetscher M, Hoxie JA, Clark-Lewis I, Melchers F, Baggiolini M, Moser B (1997) The chemokine SDF-1, stromal cell-derived factor 1, attracts early stage B cell precursors via the chemokine receptor CXCR4. Eur J Immunol 27: 1788-1793
21. Bleul CC, Fuhlbrigge RC, Casasnovas JM, Aiuti A, Springer TA (1996) A highly efficacious lymphocyte chemoattractant, stromal cell-derived factor 1 (SDF-1) [see comments]. J Exp Med 184: 1101-1109
22. Sharma V, Walper D, Deckert R (1997) Modulation of macrophage inflammatory protein-1alpha and its receptors in human B-cell lines derived from patients with acquired immunodeficiency syndrome and Burkitt's lymphoma. Biochem Biophys Res Commun 235: 576-581
23. Schaniel C, Pardali E, Sallusto F, Speletas M, Ruedl C, Shimizu T, Seidl T, Andersson J, Melchers F, Rolink AG, Sideras P (1998) Activated murine B lymphocytes and dendritic cells produce a novel CC chemokine which acts selectively on activated T cells. J Exp Med 188: 451-463
24. Chang M, McNinch J, Elias Cr, Manthey CL, Grosshans D, Meng T, Boone T, Andrew DP (1997) Molecular cloning and functional characterization of a novel CC chemokine, stimulated T cell chemotactic protein (STCP-1) that specifically acts on activated T lymphocytes. J Biol Chem 272: 25229-25237
25. Godiska R, Chantry D, Raport CJ, Sozzani S, Allavena P, Leviten D, Mantovani A, Gray PW (1997) Human macrophage-derived chemokine (MDC), a novel chemoattractant for monocytes, monocyte-derived dendritic cells, and natural killer cells. J Exp Med 185: 1595-1604
26. Gribben JG, Freedman AS, Neuberg D, Roy DC, Blake KW, Woo SD, Grossbard ML, Rabinowe SN, Coral F, Freeman GJ, et al. (1991) Immunologic purging of marrow assessed by PCR before autologous bone marrow transplantation for B-cell lymphoma [see comments]. New England Journal of Medicine 325: 1525-1533
27. Ghia P, Boussiotis VA, Schultze JL, Cardoso AA, Dorfman DM, Gribben JG, Freedman AS, Nadler LM (1998) Unbalanced expression of bcl-2 family proteins in follicular lymphoma: contribution of CD40 signaling in promoting survival. Blood 91: 244-251
28. Liu YJ, Barthelemy C, de Bouteiller O, Arpin C, Durand I, Banchereau J (1995) Memory B cells from human tonsils colonize mucosal epithelium and directly present antigen to T cells by rapid up-regulation of B7-1 and B7-2. Immunity 2: 239-248
29. Ghia P, ten Boekel E, Sanz E, de la Hera A, Rolink A, Melchers F (1996) Ordering of human bone marrow B lymphocyte precursors by single-cell polymerase chain reaction analyses of the rearrangement status of the immunoglobulin H and L chain gene loci. J Exp Med 184: 2217-2229
30. Lane P, Brocker T, Hubele S, Padovan E, Lanzavecchia A, McConnell F (1993) Soluble CD40 ligand can replace the normal T cell-derived CD40 ligand signal to B cells in T cell-dependent activation. J Exp Med 177: 1209-1213
31. Petrasch S, Kosco M, Perez-Alvarez C, Schmitz J, Brittinger G (1992) Proliferation of non-Hodgkin-lymphoma lymphocytes in vitro is dependent upon follicular dendritic cell interactions. British Journal of Haematology 80: 21-26
32. Lindhout E, Mevissen ML, Kwekkeboom J, Tager JM, de Groot C (1993) Direct evidence that human follicular dendritic cells (FDC) rescue germinal centre B cells from death by apoptosis. Clinical & Experimental Immunology 91: 330-336
33. Carbone A, Gloghini A, Gruss HJ, Pinto A (1995) CD40 ligand is constitutively expressed in a subset of T cell lymphomas and on the microenvironmental reactive T cells of follicular lymphomas and Hodgkin's disease. American Journal of Pathology 147: 912-922
34. Ghia P, ten Boekel E, Rolink AG, Melchers F (1998) B-cell development: a comparison between mouse and man [In Process Citation]. Immunol Today 19: 480-485
35. Imai T, Chantry D, Raport CJ, Wood CL, Nishimura M, Godiska R, Yoshie O, Gray PW (1998) Macrophage-derived chemokine is a functional ligand for the CC chemokine receptor 4. J Biol Chem 273: 1764-1768
36. Cardoso AA, Seamon MJ, Afonso HM, Ghia P, Boussiotis VA, Freeman GJ, Gribben JG, Sallan SE, Nadler LM (1997) Ex vivo generation of human anti-pre-B leukemia-specific autologous cytolytic T cells. Blood 90: 549-561

Susceptibility Genes for AIDS and AIDS-Related Lymphoma

C.S. Rabkin[1] and S. Sei[2]
[1]Viral Epidemiology Branch, National Cancer Institute, Bethesda, MD 20892 USA
[2]HIV Clinical Interface Laboratory, Science Applications International Corporation-NCI, Frederick, MD 21702 USA

HIV-1-infected individuals are at greatly increased risk of Burkitt's and other high-grade non-Hodgkin's lymphomas, which arise as a late complication in the setting of advanced immunodeficiency [1]. Heterogeneous acquired lesions are present in varying subsets of these B-cell tumors, including activation of the c-*myc* (especially in Burkitt's lymphoma), *bcl*-6, and *ras* protooncogenes, inactivation of the p53 tumor suppressor gene, and latent infection with the Epstein-Barr virus (EBV) [2,3]. The mechanisms by which immune dysregulation leads to B-cell lymphoma are poorly understood, but may be related to disruption of cytokine control and chronic B-cell hyperactivation. Lymphomagenesis may be a multistage process progressing from polyclonal B-cell proliferation to oligoclonal expansion of antigen-selected clones to subsequent outgrowth of a monoclonal tumor [4].

Chemokines (chemotactic cytokines) are important regulators of normal B-lymphocyte maturation and proliferation [5]. In addition, chemokine receptors are coreceptors with CD4 for entry of HIV-1 into host cells, and several genetic polymorphisms in chemokine and chemokine receptor genes have been shown to modify progression of HIV-1 infection. A 32 base-pair deletion in the coding region of the CCR5 chemokine receptor gene, termed CCR5-Δ32, is protective against progression to AIDS in heterozygotes and against HIV-1 infection in homozygotes [6]. A valine to isoleucine substitution at position 64 in the transmembrane domain of the chemokine receptor gene CCR2, termed CCR2-64I, is protective against AIDS in heterozygotes but has not been shown to affect risk of infection [7]. A variant of the SDF-1 (stromal cell-derived factor 1) chemokine gene, with a G-to-A transition at position 801 of the 3' untranslated region of the SDF-1ß gene transcript (designated SDF1-3'UTR-801G-A, and abbreviated as SDF1-3'A) has been variably associated in homozygotes with slower [8] or faster [9] progression of HIV-1 infection to AIDS and death.

The variation in lymphoma occurrence in the course of HIV infection suggests host and/or environmental factors influence lymphoma risk. The chemokine and chemokine receptor genes are logical candidates, given their significance in normal B-cell development. We have therefore examined the effects of the previously reported SDF1-3'A, CCR5-Δ32, and CCR2-64I gene variants as risk factors for HIV-associated non-Hodgkin's lymphoma in three HIV-infected cohorts: 146 HIV-infected children followed at the NIH Clinical Center; 120 subjects from a cohort study of homosexual men, and 480 from a prospective cohort study of HIV-infected hemophilia patients.

Although SDF1-3'A had been initially reported to prevent progression of HIV disease [8], we found that it increased risk of HIV-associated non-Hodgkin's lymphoma (but not other AIDS-defining conditions), with homozygotes at higher risk than heterozygotes. After a median 12 years of follow-up, 19% of homozygous and 10% of heterozygous SDF1-3'A carriers developed lymphoma, compared to 5% of wild-type subjects (p<.01 for both comparisons) [10]. Overall risk of lymphoma was significantly lower in the hemophilic patients, half of whom became infected in childhood, corresponding to the slower course of HIV-1 disease in children (excluding those neonatally infected) compared to adults. Nevertheless, cumulative incidence of non-Hodgkin's lymphoma was consistently higher in SDF1-3'A carriers (heterozygous plus homozygous) compared to homozygous wildtype for all three cohorts (Fig.).

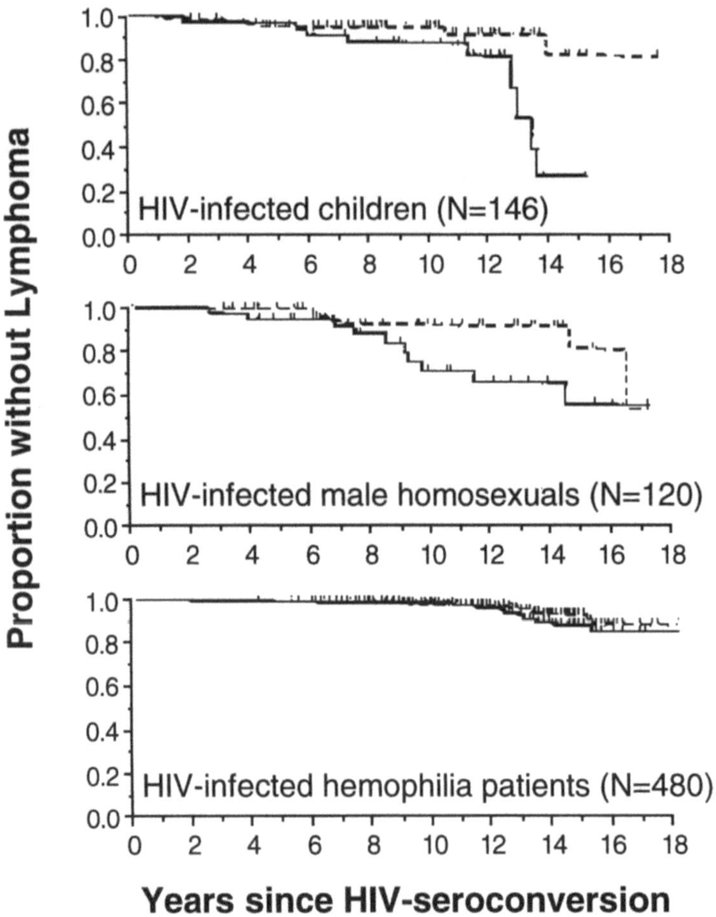

Fig. Non-Hodgkin's lymphoma risk in carriers (heterozygous plus homozygous) of SDF1-3'A (solid lines) compared to homozygous wildtype (dashed lines).

In Cox proportional hazards models (stratified by cohort to account for variation in lymphoma risk), SDF1-3'A was associated with approximate doubling of the non-Hodgkin's lymphoma hazard in heterozygotes as compared to the wildtype, and roughly a four-fold increase in homozygotes. The adjusted relative hazard of non-Hodgkin's lymphoma per copy of the SDF1-3'A allele was 2.0 (95% CI=1.3-3.1). The increased risk was particularly pronounced for Burkitt's and Burkitt-like tumors, although other high-grade systemic tumors and primary brain lymphomas were also increased.

In marked contrast, SDF1-3'A carriers were not overrepresented among 24 cases of HIV-1-negative Burkitt's and other non-Hodgkin's lymphoma that were tested for comparison [10]. This polymorphism thus appears to increase risk of non-Hodgkin's lymphoma only in the setting of HIV infection, but more cases of HIV-negative lymphoma will need to be tested to confirm this specificity.

We also found a protective association of CCR5-Δ32 against HIV-1-associated lymphoma. In the three cohorts combined, non-Hodgkin's lymphoma developed in 2% of CCR5-Δ32 carriers compared to 8% of wild-type subjects (odds ratio=0.2, p=0.03). Conversely, the protective effect of CCR2-64I against AIDS appeared to be restricted to an effect on opportunistic infection, because 6% of CCR2-64I carriers developed lymphoma compared to 5% of wild-type subjects (odds ratio=1.3, p=0.6) [10].

Burkitt's and Burkitt-like tumors uniformly have a c-myc activating chromosomal translocation [11]. We have investigated these mutations in HIV-infected individuals without lymphoma from the homosexual cohort, and previously reported that 13 (12%) of 110 subjects had detectable c-myc translocations in circulating peripheral blood mononuclear cells[12]. However, the frequency of these translocations in subjects with chemokine and chemokine receptor polymorphisms was similar to that of the overall cohort [10].

Our data seemingly explain the previous observation [13] that non-Hodgkin's lymphoma is approximately one-half as common among blacks than in whites among U.S. AIDS cases. The prevalence of SDF1-3'A varies by race, with allele frequencies of 21% in whites and 6% of blacks [8]; based on the adjusted relative hazards from the Cox model, we estimated the etiologic fraction of HIV-associated lymphoma attributable to SDF1-3'A as 36% for whites and 10% for blacks. Thus, racial differences in incidence of HIV-associated non-Hodgkin's lymphoma may in part be due to an excess of SDF1-3'A-associated cases in whites.

In summary, SDF1-3'A increases susceptibility to AIDS-related lymphoma, whereas CCR5-Δ32 is strongly protective. Lymphoma risk is greater in SDF1-3'A homozygotes than heterozygotes, indicating a co-dominant effect of this allele on AIDS-related lymphoma, in contrast to its recessive effect on overall AIDS. The adjusted hazard per copy is 2, so each copy of the variant allele doubles the risk of non-Hodgkin's lymphoma. SDF1-3'A carrier distribution may also underlie the racial difference in risk of this disorder. SDF1-3'A has a much stronger association with Burkitt's lymphoma than with other AIDS-related lymphomas. Nevertheless, SDF1-3'A does not appear to be associated with the characteristic Burkitt's lymphoma translocation in HIV-infected subjects without lymphoma, nor with Burkitt's lymphoma in the absence of HIV infection. Deciphering the genetic control of AIDS-related lymphoma may further the understanding of B-cell neoplasia and provide fundamental insights into carcinogenesis.

References

1. Biggar RJ, Rabkin CS (1996) The epidemiology of AIDS--related neoplasms. Hematol Oncol Clin North Am 10:997-1010
2. Ballerini P, Gaidano G, Gong JZ, et al (1993) Multiple genetic lesions in acquired immunodeficiency syndrome-related non-Hodgkin's lymphoma. Blood 81:166-176
3. Shibata D, Weiss LM, Hernandez AM, Nathwani BN, Bernstein L, Levine AM (1993) Epstein-Barr virus-associated non-Hodgkin's lymphoma in patients infected with the human immunodeficiency virus [see comments]. Blood 81:2102-2109
4. Przybylski GK, Goldman J, Ng VL, et al (1996) Evidence for early B-cell activation preceding the development of Epstein-Barr virus-negative acquired immunodeficiency syndrome-related lymphoma. Blood 88:4620-4629
5. Baggiolini M (1998) Chemokines and leukocyte traffic. Nature 392:565-568
6. Liu R, Paxton WA, Choe S, et al (1996) Homozygous defect in HIV-1 coreceptor accounts for resistance of some multiply-exposed individuals to HIV-1 infection. Cell 86:367-377
7. Smith MW, Dean M, Carrington M, et al (1997) Contrasting genetic influence of CCR2 and CCR5 variants on HIV-1 infection and disease progression. Hemophilia Growth and Development Study (HGDS), Multicenter AIDS Cohort Study (MACS), Multicenter Hemophilia Cohort Study (MHCS), San Francisco City Cohort (SFCC), ALIVE Study. Science 277:959-965
8. Winkler C, Modi W, Smith MW, et al (1998) Genetic restriction of AIDS pathogenesis by an SDF-1 chemokine gene variant. ALIVE Study, Hemophilia Growth and Development Study (HGDS), Multicenter AIDS Cohort Study (MACS), Multicenter Hemophilia Cohort Study (MHCS), San Francisco City Cohort (SFCC) [see comments]. Science 279:389-393
9. Mummidi S, Ahuja SS, Gonzalez E, et al (1998) Genealogy of the CCR5 locus and chemokine system gene variants associated with altered rates of HIV-1 disease progression. Nat Med 4:786-793
10. Rabkin CS, Yang Q, Goedert JJ, Nguyen G, Mitsuya H, Sei S (1999) Chemokine and chemokine receptor gene variants and risk of non-Hodgkin's lymphoma in HIV-1 infected individuals. Blood (in press)
11. Magrath IT, Bhatia K Pathogenesis of small noncleaved cell lymphomas (Burkitt's lymphoma). In: The Non-Hodgkin's Lymphomas. Magrath IT (ed)(1997) Arnold, London. 2nd ed. pp 385-409
12. Muller JR, Janz S, Goedert JJ, Potter M, Rabkin CS (1995) Persistence of immunoglobulin heavy chain/c-myc recombination-positive lymphocyte clones in the blood of human immunodeficiency virus-infected homosexual men. Proc Natl Acad Sci U S A 92:6577-6581
13. Beral V, Peterman TA, Berkelman R, Jaffe H (1991) AIDS-associated non-Hodgkin lymphoma. Lancet 337:805-809

Discussion

Martin Lipp: Does the 3' mutation in the SDF-1 gene result in any functional consequences? In the publication, it was not reported whether the mutation affects the stability of the mRNA or the level of protein expression. Do you have further information on that?
Charles Rabkin: No, it is in a non-translated region so it is unknown. Our speculation is that it would result in increased levels of the SDF1 product. We proposed a model that would be a stimulating factor that might be both protective against HIV infection but also perhaps be a driving force for lymphomagenesis, but that is pure speculation.
Richard Scheuermann: The polymorphisms in these receptors came about from resistance to HIV infection, and now you are seeing these associations in Burkitt's lymphoma, so I wonder if there is any evidence that these things might be coreceptors for EBV, or is this some type of secondary effect on activation of B cells?
Charles Rabkin: That is an excellent suggestion. I am not aware that they have been examined as a coreceptor for EBV, but they are coreceptors for HIV, and it would be a very good thing to follow up.
Katherine Siminovitch: How many of those receptor polymorphisms detected in patients with immunodeficiency diseases have been examined in the general population? Do you find those polymorphisms generally among "healthy" individuals?
Charles Rabkin: It has not been looked at.
Martin Lipp: We looked for polymorphisms within the gene of the SDF-1 receptor, CXCR4, in about 150 leukemia and lymphoma patients as well as in about 50 healthy individuals. We found only one point mutation in several members of both groups indicating a very low genetic variation within CXCR4.
Charles Rabkin: That is also the case in a large group of lymphoma patients as well as in normals.

Molecular Mechanisms of T Helper Cell Differentiation and Tissue-specific Migration

D. D'Ambrosio, P. Panina-Bordignon, L. Rogge and F. Sinigaglia
Roche Milano Ricerche, Via Olgettina 58, 20132 Milano, Italy

In different immune responses helper T lymphocytes (Th) differentiate into effectors that produce different cytokines. The two most distinct or polarized populations of Th are the Th1 and Th2 subsets. The principal effector cytokine of Th1 cells is IFN-γ. IFN-γ promotes switching of B cells to isotypes, such as IGg2a, which fix complement and promote phagocytosis by macrophages. Th1 cells have a critical role in fighting microbial and viral infections, but can also cause tissue damage if dysregulated. Th2 cells, in contrast, promote IgE production and eosinophil function, which are key players in the pathogenesis of allergic inflammation. Th2 cells may also exert an anti-inflammatory action by negatively regulating Th1 cell-mediated immune responses. Thus, understanding the molecular mechanisms controlling the differentiation of the T helper cells is crucial with regard to both the B cell regulation, particularly to heavy chain class switching, as well as to the role of Th1/Th2 cells in a variety of immunopathological conditions. In this review we outline important factors that regulate Th1/Th2 differentiation and the distinct ability of the two subsets to traffic and localize to certain tissues and sites of inflammation.

Role of cytokines in the development and regulation of T helper subsets

Th1 and Th2 cells develop from naive $CD4^+$ T cells. The differentiation process is initiated by ligation of the TCR and directed by cytokines present during the initiation of a T cell response [1]. IL-4 promotes Th2 development [2, 3], whereas IL-12 is a potent inducer of Th1 cells [4-6]. IL-4 activates Stat6 in Th2 cells [7, 8] and IL-12 induces tyrosine phosphorylation of Stat4 in developing and differentiated Th1 cells [9, 10]. The activation of these two Stat factors is essential for T cell subset development, since Stat6-deficient T lymphocytes fail to differentiate into Th2 cells in response to IL-4 [11, 12] and the analysis of $Stat4^{-/-}$-deficient mice revealed that Stat4 is essential for Th1 cell differentiation [13, 14].

Expression of the IL-12 Receptor During T Helper Cell Development
Lymphocyte response to IL-12 is dependent on the expression of high affinity IL-12R [15]. Two IL-12R subunits termed β1 and β2 have been identified [16]. The IL-12Rβ2 chain is essential for IL-12 signaling since it forms a functional, high affinity receptor in combination with IL-12Rβ1 in cotransfected Cos cells [16]. In contrast to the IL-12Rβ1, the β2 chain has a cytoplasmic domain that contains three tyrosine residues [16]. In both humans and mice, IL-12 induces tyrosine phosphorylation of Stat4 in Th1 but not Th2 cells [9, 10]. This correlates with the differential expression of the IL-12R β2 chain in these two cell types [10, 17]. The IL-12R is not present on naive T cells. Antigen stimulation induces expression of both chains of the receptor. Cells that develop along the Th1 pathway continue to

express both IL-12R subunits, but there is a selective loss of the IL-12Rβ2 transcripts during differentiation of T cells along the Th2 pathway (Fig. 1).

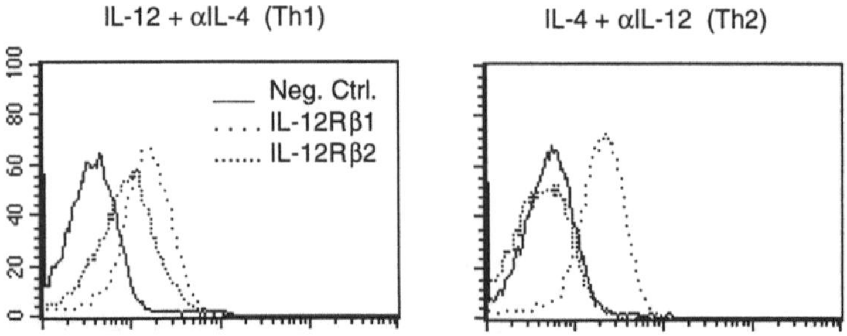

Fig. 1 IL-12R expression by in vitro polarized Th1 and Th2 cells. Cell surface expression of IL-12Rβ1 and β2 subunits was analyzed with rat-anti-huIL-12Rβ1 mAb 2B10 (dotted line), and rat-anti-huIL-12Rβ2 mAb 2B6 (dashed line). The solid line represents staining with an isotype-matched control mAb.

Regulation of IL-12R expression by IL-12 and IL-4

Since the expression of several cytokine receptors has been shown to be regulated by positive or negative feedback pathways, we asked whether IL-12 could directly influence expression of the IL-12Rβ2. IL-12 added to resting Th1 and Th2 cells resulted in a strong induction of IL-12Rβ2 transcripts in Th1 cells. We observed that naive T cells primed in the presence of IL-4 and IL-12 together, developed into cells secreting both IL-4 and IFN-γ. These cells phosphorylate Stat4 in response to IL-12 and accordingly express the IL-12Rβ2 mRNA, although to a lower level than Th1 cells [18]. In contrast, naive T cells primed in the presence of IL-4 and neutralizing anti-IL-12 mAb completely lost IL-12Rβ2 expression and, consequently, IL-12-mediated signaling. Although the mechanism by which IL-4 induces the generation of IL-12 non-responsive Th2 cells remains to be clarified, recent evidence indicates that IL-4 induces a set of transcription factors (c-Maf and GATA-3) that appear to be responsible for the development and maintenance of Th2 cells [19, 20].

Differential recruitment of T cell subsets to inflammatory sites

A critical step in the maintenance of functionally polarized immune responses is the capacity of distinct types of immune effector cells to traffic and localize to certain tissues and sites of inflammation.

Selectin ligands on helper T cells

The initial proof for the existence of mechanisms regulating the tissue-specific recruitment of Th1 and Th2 cells came from a seminal study by Austrup et al., which documented the preferential expression of P- and E-selectin ligands on Th1 cells [21]. This and a subsequent study demonstrated that expression of P- and E-selectin ligands has a critical role in recruitment of Th1 but not Th2 cells to certain inflamed tissues. Expression of P- and E-selectin ligands is controlled by the activity of α(1,3)-fucosyltransferases, a family of enzymes which modify carbohydrate moieties decorating PSGL-1 and other surface receptors [22].

Consistent with these findings, Th1 cells have been shown to express elevated levels of $\alpha(1,3)$-fucosyltransferase VII (FucTVII) resulting in high expression of P-selectin ligands in Th1 but not Th2 cells [23]. We have recently shown that IL-12 and type I IFNs, cytokines, as discussed above, with a critical role in human Th1 cell development, upregulate the expression of FucTVII on T lymphocytes (Rogge et al. manuscript in preparation).

Differential expression of chemokine receptors on Th1 and Th2 cells
The eotaxin receptor CCR3 was found to be selectively expressed on Th2 cells [24]. Eotaxin, which is found upregulated in allergic asthma [25], may act on CCR3 expressing Th2 cells and eosinophils to promote their co-localization. Several groups have subsequently reported the differential expression of several chemokine receptors on Th1 and Th2 cells. Th1 cells have been shown to preferentially express CCR5 and CXCR3 [26-28], whereas Th2 cells were reported to preferentially express CCR3, CCR4 and CCR8 [26, 28, 29]. Selective expression of chemokine receptors results in differential chemotactic responsiveness of T helper cells. MIP-1β (CCR5 ligand) and IP-10 (CXCR3 ligand) act preferentially on Th1 cells, whereas eotaxin (CCR3 ligand), I-309 (CCR8 ligand), MDC (CCR4 ligand) and TARC (CCR4 and CCR8 ligands) act predominantly on Th2 cells. These findings suggest that different chemotactic signals participate in the tissue-specific homing of Th1 and Th2 cells. Since several receptors are expressed on the same T cell subset, distinct ligand-receptor pairs may play a specific role in the localization process. Alternatively, distinct receptors (for instance CCR3, CCR4 and CCR8 on Th2 cells) may identify further specialized subsets of effector T cells or have redundant functions. We have recently found that Th2-associated CCR4 and CCR8 are strongly upregulated upon TCR and CD28-mediated activation [30], thus suggesting that upon antigen encounter Th2 cells may downregulate CCR3 and other receptors while upregulating CCR4 and CCR8. It is possible that CCR4 and CCR8 may regulate the initial extravasation of circulating Th2 cells and, upon activation, their relocalization in the tissue microenvironment. Notably, CCR4 is also expressed in TCR-activated Th1 cells, suggesting that it may also contribute to their migratory pattern. Interestingly, the chemokines TARC, MDC and I-309 (ligands of CCR4 and CCR8) are all produced by activated T cells. Taken together, these findings suggest that activated T cells may be focused and maintained at sites of antigenic challenge by the action of these ligand-receptor pairs

Integrins in Th1 and Th2 cell subsets
In addition to selectins and chemokines, adhesion molecules belonging to the integrin family are also an indispensable component in the tissue-specific recruitment of leukocytes. Recently, in a collaborative study we have found differences in the expression and function of these receptors in Th1 and Th2 cells. Among various integrin subunits, Th1 cells were found to express higher levels of $\alpha_L\beta_2$ LFA-1 (ICAM receptor) and integrin α_6 (laminin receptor) when compared to Th2 cells. Interestingly, surface expression of integrin α_6 in Th1 cells was found to be exquisitely regulated by IFN-α and IL-12, cytokines that promote human Th1 cell development (L.C. and D.D. submitted). These findings suggest that differential expression and regulation of integrins may also contribute to tissue-specific localization of T helper cells. Moreover, we found that chemokine-induced activation of integrin β_1-mediated adhesion is greatly reduced in Th2 versus Th1 cells (D. D. and R. P., manuscript in preparation). This defective integrin activation appears due to the partial uncoupling of chemokine receptor-generated signals leading to integrin β_1 activation in Th2 cells. Strong integrin β_1-mediated adhesion may promote efficient migration of Th1 cells throughout extracellular matrix (ECM) and/or may help retain extravasated Th1 cells in inflamed tissues. Thus, the differential ability of Th1 and

Th2 cells to engage integrin β_1-mediated adhesion may confer Th1 cells with a selective ability to penetrate and localize within certain tissues.

Table I. Differential Expression of Homing Receptor in Th1 and Th2 cells

Chemokine	Th1 cells		Th2 cells	
Receptors	Resting	Activated	Resting	Activated
CCR1	++	⇓	++	⇓
CCR2	++	⇓	++	⇓
CCR3	-	-	+	⇓
CCR4	-	+⇑	++	+++⇑
CCR5	++	⇓	+	⇓
CCR7	+	++⇑	+	++⇑
CCR8	-	-	+	+++⇑
CXCR3	++	⇓	-	-
CXCR4	++	⇓	++	⇓

Adhesion	Th1	Th1	Th2
Molecules		IL-12-stimulated	
P-and E-selectin ligands	++	+++⇑	+
Integrin α_6	++	+++⇑	+
LFA-1	++	++	+

The increased or decreased expression of chemokine receptors upon activation of Th1 and Th2 cells via the antigen receptor [30] is indicated by the direction of the arrow. Upregulation of adhesion molecules by stimulation with IL-12 is indicated similarly.

Extravasation thresholds and differential recruitment of helper T cells
Chronic Th1-dominated immune responses, such as in arthritic joints and DTH reaction in the skin, are often characterized by basal membrane thickening and abnormal deposition of ECM. These conditions may impose a high threshold for leukocyte extravasation. Th1 cells, by virtue of their high P- and E-selectin ligands and robust adhesion to ECM components may possess a high "extravasation potential" necessary to gain access to those inflammatory sites. In contrast, Th2 cell-driven immune responses are typified by asthma which is triggered by an acute allergic reaction characterized by vasodilatation, increased vascular permeability, edema and leukocyte extravasation. The hemodynamic changes induced by the allergic response, may significantly lower the threshold of leukocyte extravasation allowing the recruitment of cells with low "extravasation potential" such as Th2 cells.

Concluding Remarks

The diversity of T-lymphocyte function revealed by studies of T cell subsets is now a well-documented feature of the immune system. Learning how to exploit this functional dichotomy for practical applications requires greater knowledge of the molecular events that regulate the development and the effector function of these cell subsets. In this review we have discussed our own and other studies showing that the regulation of the IL-12 signaling pathway plays a crucial role for the development of Th cell subsets. Furthermore, we have discussed recent data indicating that the tissue-specific recruitment of Th1 and Th2 cells is differentially regulated by the intricate interplay of adhesion receptors and chemokines. These novel findings have extended the functional dichotomy of T cell-mediated immune responses at the level of tissue-specific homing. Given the central role of Th1 and Th2 cells in the regulation of immunity, manipulating the signals which control differentiation and/or trafficking of these cells may open new therapeutic avenues leading to the treatment of a number of immunopathological conditions.

References

1. Seder RA, Paul WE (1994) Acquisition of lymphokine-producing phenotype by $CD4^+$ T cells. Annu Rev Immunol 12:635-673
2. Seder RA, Paul WE, Davis MM, Fazekas de St. Groth B (1992) The presence of interleukin-4 during in vitro priming determines the lymphokine-producing potential of $CD4^+$ T cells from T cell receptor transgenic mice. J Exp Med 176:1091-1098
3. Hsieh CS, Heimberger AB, Gold JS, O'Garra A, Murphy KM (1992) Differential regulation of T helper phenotype development by interleukins 4 and 10 in an alpha beta T cell-receptor transgenic system. Proc Natl Acad Sci USA 89:6065-6069
4. Hsieh C-S, Macatonia SE, Tripp CS, Wolf SF, O'Garra A, Murphy KM (1993) Development of T_H1 $CD4^+$ T cells through IL-12 produced by *Listeria*-induced macrophages. Science 260:547-549
5. Seder RA, Gazzinelli R, Sher A, Paul WE (1993) Interleukin 12 acts directly on CD4+ T cells to enhance priming for interferon gamma production and diminishes interleukin 4 inhibition of such priming. Proc Natl Acad Sci USA 90:10188-10192
6. Manetti R, Gerosa F, Giudizi MG, Biagiotti R, Parronchi P, Piccinni M-P, Sampognaro S, Maggi E, Romagnani S, Trinchieri G (1994) Interleukin 12 induces stable priming for interferon γ (IFN-γ) production during differentiation of human T helper (Th) and transient IFN-γ production in established Th2 cell clones. J Exp Med 179:1273-1283
7. Schindler C, Kashleva H, Pernis A, Pine R, Rothman P (1994) STF-IL-4: a novel IL-4-induced signal transducing factor. EMBO J 13:1350-1356
8. Hou J, Schindler U, Henzel WJ, Ho TC, Brasseur M, McKnight SL (1994) An interleukin-4-induced transcription factor: IL-4 Stat. Science 265:1701-1706
9. Szabo SJ, Jacobson NG, Dighe AS, Gubler U, Murphy KM (1995) Developmental commitment to the Th2 lineage by extinction of IL-12 signaling. Immunity 2:665-675
10. Rogge L, Barberis-Maino L, Biffi M, Passini N, Presky DH, Gubler U, Sinigaglia F (1997) Selective expression of an interleukin-12 receptor component by human T helper 1 cells. J Exp Med 185:825-832
11. Takeda K, Tanaka T, Shi W, Matsumoto M, Minami M, Kashiwamura S-I, Nakanishi K, Yoshida N, Kishimoto T, Akira S (1996) Essential role of Stat6 in IL-4 signalling. Nature 380:627-630
12. Shimoda K, van Deursen J, Sangster MY, Sarawar SR, Carson RT, Tripp RA, Chu C, Quelle FW, Nosaka T, Vignalli DAA, Doherty PC, Grosveld G, Paul WE, Ihle JN (1996) Lack of IL-4-induced Th2 response and IgE class switching in mice with disrupted Stat6 gene. Nature 380:630-633
13. Thierfelder WE, van Deursen JM, Yamamoto K, Tripp RA, Sarawar SR, Carson RT, Sangster MY, Vignali DAA, Doherty PC, Grosveld GC, Ihle JN (1996) Requirement for Stat4 in interleukin-12-mediated responses of natural killer and T cells. Nature 382:171-174
14. Kaplan MH, Sun YL, Hoey T, Grusby MJ (1996) Impaired IL-12 responses and enhanced development of Th2 cells in Stat4-deficient mice. Nature 382:174-177
15. Desai BB, Quinn PM, Wolitzky AG, Mongini PKA, Chizzonite R, Gately MK (1992) IL-12 receptor. II. Distribution and regulation of receptor expression. J Immunol 148:3125-3132

16. Presky DH, Yang H, Minetti LJ, Chua AO, Nabavi N, Wu CY, Gately MK, Gubler U (1996) A functional interleukin 12 receptor complex is composed of two beta-type cytokine receptor subunits. Proc Natl Acad Sci USA 93:14002-14007
17. Szabo SJ, Dighe AS, Gubler U, Murphy KM (1997) Regulation of the interleukin (IL)-12R beta 2 subunit expression in developing T helper 1 (Th1) and Th2 cells. J Exp Med 185:817-824
18. Rogge L, D'Ambrosio D, Biffi M, Penna G, Minetti LJ, Presky DH, Adorini L, Sinigaglia F (1998) The role of Stat4 in species-specific regulation of T helper cell development by type I interferons. J Immunol in press
19. Ho I-C, Hodge MR, Rooney JW, Glimcher LH (1996) The proto-oncogene c-maf is responsible for tissue-specific expression of interleukin-4. Cell 85:973-983
20. Zheng W-P, Flavell RA (1997) The transcription factor GATA-3 is necessary and sufficient for Th2 cytokine gene expression in CD4 T cells. Cell 89:587-596
21. Austrup F, Vestweber D, Borges E, Lohning M, Brauer R, Herz U, Renz H, Hallmann R, Scheffold A, Radbruch A, Hamann A (1997) P- and E-selectin mediate recruitment of T-helper-1 but not T-helper-2 cells into inflamed tissues. Nature 385:81-83
22. Fuhlbrigge RC, Kieffer JD, Armerding D, Kupper TS (1997) Cutaneous lymphocyte antigen is a specialized form of PSGL-1 expressed on skin-homing T cells. Nature 389:978-981
23. van Wely CA, Blanchard AD, Britten CJ (1998) Differential expression of alpha3 fucosyltransferases in Th1 and Th2 cells correlates with their ability to bind P-selectin. Biochem Biophys Res Commun 247:307-311
24. Sallusto F, Mackay CR, Lanzavecchia A (1997) Selective expression of the eotaxin receptor CCR3 by human T helper 2 cells. Science 277:2005-2007
25. Lamkhioued B, renzi PM, S. A-Y, Garcia-Zepada EA, Allakhverdi Z, Ghaffar O, Rothenberg MC, Luster AD, Hamid Q (1997) Increased expression of eotaxin in brochoalveolar lavage and airways of asthmatics contributes to the chemotaxis of eosinophils to the site of inflammation. J Immunol 159:4593-4601
26. Bonecchi R, Bianchi G, Panina Bordignon P, D'Ambrosio D, Lang R, Borsatti A, Sozzani S, Allavena P, Gray PA, Mantovani A, Sinigaglia F (1998) Differential expression of chemokine receptors and chemotactic responsiveness of Th1 and Th2 cells. J Exp Med 187:129-134
27. Loetscher P, Uguccioni M, Bordoli L, Baggiolini M, Moser B (1998) CCR5 is characteristic of Th1 lymphocytes. Nature 391:344-345
28. Sallusto F, Lenig D, Mackay CR, Lanzavecchia A (1998) Flexible programs of chemokine receptor expression on human polarized T helper 1 and 2 lymphocytes. J Exp Med 187:875-883
29. Zingoni A, Soto H, Hedrick JA, Stoppacciaro A, Storlazzi CT, Sinigaglia F, DAmbrosio D, OGarra A, Robinson D, Rocchi M, Santoni A, Zlotnik A, Napolitano M (1998) The chemokine receptor CCR8 is preferentially expressed in Th2 but not Th1 cells. J Immunol 161:547-551
30. D'Ambrosio D, Iellem A, Bonecchi R, Mazzeo D, Sozzani S, Mantovani A, Sinigaglia F (1998) Selective upregulation of chemokine receptors CCR4 and CCR8 upon activation of polarized human type 2 T helper cells. J Immunol 161:5111-5115

Discussion

Federico Caligaris-Cappio: In your scenario is there a role or significance for IL-10?
Francesco Sinigaglia: Yes there is, IL-12 is clearly an anti-inflammatory cytokine in that it downregulates IL-12 production by monocytes and dendritic cells. In addition, the described ability of IL-10 to inhibit MCP-1 production in monocytes suggests that IL-10 may regulate the flux of mononuclear phagocytes to inflammatory sites. We have also looked at the ability of IL-10 to regulate a number of chemokine receptors on T helper cell subsets but we have not found any role for IL-10 there.

The Role of Chemokine Receptors in Directing Traffic of Naive, Type 1 and Type 2 T Cells

F. Sallusto, B. Palermo, A. Hoy, and A. Lanzavecchia.
Basel Institute for Immunology, Grenzacherstrasse 487, CH-4005 Basel, Switzerland

Introduction

The regulation of leukocyte migration is a complex process involving the participation of adhesion molecules, such as selectins and integrins, as well as chemokines and chemokine receptors (Baggiolini, 1998, Butcher & Picker, 1996). The combined action of adhesion molecules and chemokines is though to provide an address code for leukocyte extravasation and migration into tissues (Springer, 1994). The immune response strictly depends on the correct positioning of leukocytes at distinct anatomical sites. T cell priming occurs in the specialized confines of lymphoid tissue and requires the encounter of T cells with antigen-loaded dendritic cells (Banchereau & Steinman, 1998). Conversely, delayed type hypersensitivity or allergic reactions can occur in any tissue and result from the coordinated action of T helper (Th)1 or Th2 cells and effector leukocytes such as macrophages, basophils and eosinophils (Mosmann & Coffman, 1989, Paul & Seder, 1994, Romagnani, 1991).

As compared to naive T cells, antigen-experienced T cells are heterogeneous, reflecting their activation state and polarization. The combination of cytokines present during priming determines the pattern of cytokines produced by the effector T cells. CD4+ Th1 cells produce interferon γ (IFN-γ) and activate mononuclear phagocytes, thus protecting against intracellular microbes. In contrast, CD4+ Th2 cells produce interleukin (IL)-4 and IL-5 and are involved in responses dominated by IgE, eosinophils and basophils. It is conceivable that, as part of their different effector capabilities, Th1 and Th2 cells may also acquire the capacity to migrate to different tissues.

While selectins and integrins have long been recognized to be differentially expressed on naive and effector/memory T cells, recent data have shown that a number of chemokine receptors are also differentially expressed on T cells, depending on their antigenic experience and type of polarization (Sallusto *et al.*, 1997, 1998, Gerber *et al.*, 1997, Bonecchi *et al.*, 1998, Loetscher *et al.*, 1998). We will summarize our own work and present new data on chemokine receptor expression in vivo and its modulation upon T cell activation. Altogether, these findings indicate that T cells are flexible in regulating chemokine expression depending on the polarization program and activation state.

Th2-specific Profiles *in Vitro* and *in Vivo*

We have previously shown that CCR3, a receptor for eotaxin, eotaxin 2, RANTES, MCP-2, MCP-3 and MCP-4, originally described on eosinophils and basophils, is expressed also on human Th2 cells (Sallusto *et al.*, 1997). A specific monoclonal antibody detected CCR3 on a small percentage of CD45RO+ memory/effector T cells in adult peripheral blood (Fig. 1). These cells, when sorted and expanded *in vitro*, were enriched for Th2 cells since they produced high amounts of IL-4 and IL-5. CCR3 was also expressed on *in vitro* polarized Th2 lines, whereas it was absent in Th1 lines (Sallusto *et al.*, 1997). In general, the percentage of CCR3 positive cells was close to the percentage of IL-4 producing cells, both in the CD4 and CD8 compartment. Altogether, these results indicate that CCR3 expression identifies T cells capable of producing IL-4, the key feature of Th2.

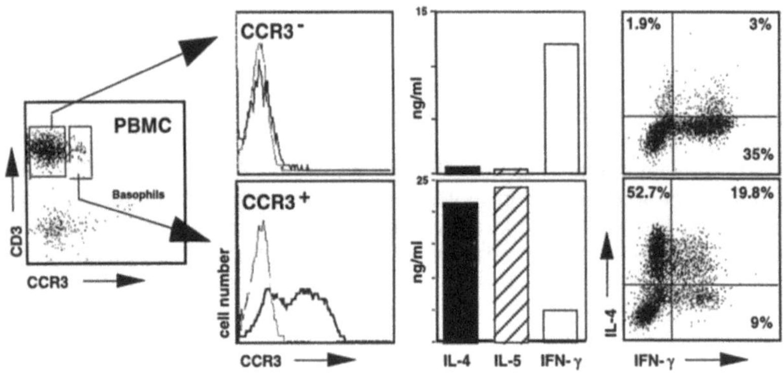

Fig. 1. CCR3 expression identifies Th2 cells in adult peripheral blood. From left to right: CCR3 expression on PBMC and polyclonal T cell lines obtained from CCR3- or CCR3+ sorted T cells. The same T cell lines were analysed for production of IL-4, IL-5 and IFN-γ by ELISA and for IL-4 and IFN-γ production at the single cell level by intracellular staining (shown are the percentages of positive cells in each quadrant).

The expression of CCR3 as a marker of Th2 cells was supported by the analysis of patients with severe allergic diseases. As shown in figure 2, a large proportion of T cells infiltrating a nasal polyp or expanded from a skin biopsy of an atopic dermatitis patient expressed high levels of CCR3 (38% and 53% respectively), while a comparable fraction produced IL-5 when stimulated with polyclonal activators (not shown).

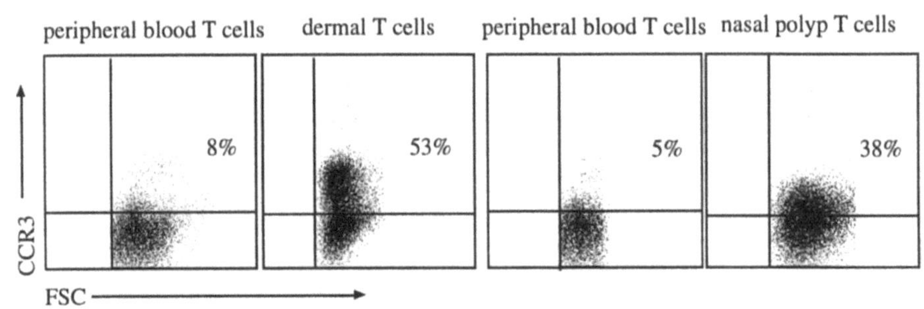

Fig. 2. CCR3 expression in peripheral blood T cells and in T cells isolated from tissue undergoing allergic reactions in patients with atopic dermatitis or nasal polyp.

CCR4, the receptor for TARC (thymus and activation-regulated chemokine) and MDC (macrophage-derived chemokine), was also found to be expressed on Th2 cells (Bonecchi *et al.*, 1998, Sallusto *et al.*, 1998). Sorting of T cells that mobilize Ca^{2+} in response to TARC allowed the isolation of IL-4-producing cells from mixed polyclonal cell lines. However, CCR4 expression can be dissociated from the IL-4-producing phenotype. Indeed, CCR4 is also expressed on T-cell lines generated in the presence of transforming growth factor-β (TGF-β) that represent nonpolarized proliferating precursors since they fail to produce IL-4 or IFN-γ (Sad & Mosmann, 1994, Sallusto *et al.*, 1998). Thus, these results indicate that CCR3 and CCR4 can be differentially regulated and that only the former correlates with the IL-4-producing Th2 phenotype.

Th1-specific Profiles

The selective expression of chemokine receptors on Th2 cells suggested that Th1 cells may also preferentially express certain chemokine receptors. CXCR3, the receptor for IP-10 (interferon-γ-inducible protein-10), Mig (monokine induced by interferon-γ) and I-TAC (interferon-inducible T cell alpha chemoattractant), all chemokines which share the property of being upregulated by IFN-γ, was found to be expressed on most peripheral blood memory T cells and at higher levels on Th1 than on Th2 cells (Bonecchi *et al.*, 1998, Sallusto *et al.*, 1998). Accordingly, Th1 cells respond to approximately one tenth the dose of IP-10 than Th2 cells do. CCR5, a receptor for RANTES, macrophage-inflammatory chemokine (MIP)-1α and MIP-1β, was found expressed on Th1 but not Th2 clones, although it was equally present on recently activated T cells, independently from their functional polarization (Bonecchi *et al.*, 1998, Loetscher *et al.*, 1998, Sallusto *et al.*, 1998). In addition, CCR5 was present only on a small fraction of peripheral blood T cells and its expression was rapidly lost from T cell lines or clones when IL-2 was withdrawn. Thus, while CXCR3 is expressed as stable markers of memory Th1 cells, CCR5 expression reflects the activation state of the T cells. This may be the reason why CCR5 is present on fewer peripheral blood memory T cells than CXCR3. One should note that some chemokine receptors such as CCR2 are equally expressed on Th1 and Th2 cells, while others, such as CCR5 and CXCR5 may reflect the T cell activation state (see below).

Flexibility in Chemokine Receptor Expression added by IFN-α or TGF-β

Polarization of T cells is regulated by the strength of antigenic stimulation, as well as by the cytokines present during priming. IFN-α and TGF-β have both been shown to affect T lymphocyte polarization. In humans IFN-α induces Th1 polarization, even in the absence of IL-12 or in the presence of IL-4 (Rogge *et al.*, 1997). In addition TGF-β prevents T cell polarization and maintains proliferating precursor cells in a semi-naive state (Sad & Mosmann, 1994). These semi-naive T cells produce only IL-2, but no other effector cytokine, and can further undergo type 1 or type 2 polarization if appropriately stimulated.

We have shown that IFN-α and TGF-β, in addition to their effects on polarization, can also affect the pattern of chemokine receptor expression (Sallusto *et al.*, 1998). When added to Th1- or Th2-polarizing conditions, IFN-α prevented the acquisition of CCR3 and CCR4, while strongly upregulating the expression of CCR1. Thus, as compared to Th1 cells polarized by IL-12, the cells polarized by IFN-α upregulate one additional chemokine receptor, CCR1, that allows them to respond to additional chemokines. In contrast, TGF-β inhibits the acquisition of CCR2, CCR3 and CCR5, while upregulating CCR4 and CCR7 expression. Thus, in line with its anti-differentiative effect, TGF-β prevents acquisition of receptors for migration to peripheral tissues, while enhancing the expression of chemokine receptors for homing to lymphoid organs. In conclusion, modulation of chemokine receptor expression by IFN-α and TGF-β provides additional flexibility for regulating leukocyte traffic, and may have profound effects on the cellular composition within a particular tissue.

Switch in Chemokine Receptors After Antigen Stimulation

Naive T cells express CXCR4, specific for SDF-1 (stromal cell-derived factor) and CCR7 specific for ELC (EBI1-ligand chemokine) and for SLC (secondary lymphoid tissue chemokine). These chemokines are produced constitutively in secondary lymphoid organs and play a role in attracting T cells to sites of antigen encounter. Once activated in the lymph nodes, T cells lose receptors for constitutive chemokines and develop into effector Th1 or Th2. These effectors, that now express distinct sets of receptors for inflammatory chemokines, circulate in the blood and extravasate at inflammatory sites, where they can recognize antigen and be activated. We have therefore investigated the effect of antigenic stimulation on chemokine receptor expression in effector Th1 and Th2 cells (Fig. 3).

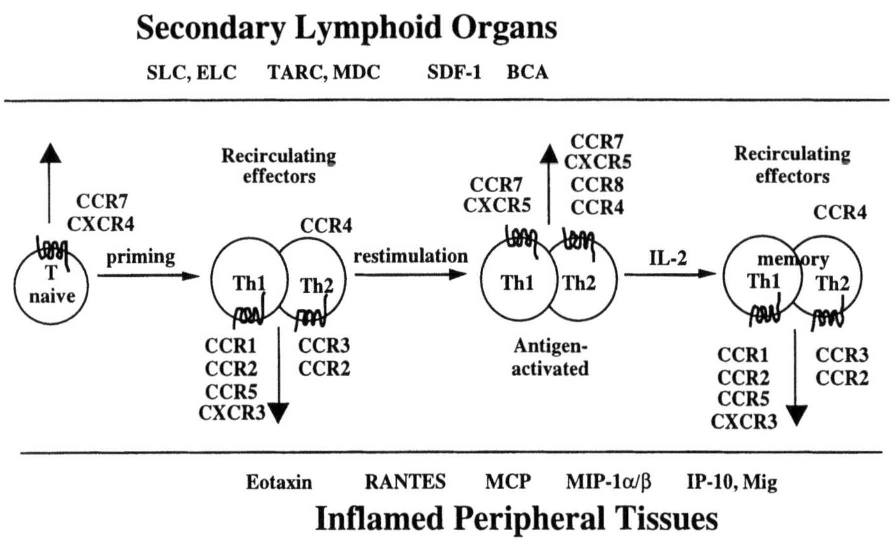

Fig. 3. Priming of naive T cells and activation of effector T cells result in a reciprocal switch in chemokine receptor expression

Within 6 hours after activation, Th2 cells downregulate CCR3 and CCR2, while upregulating CCR7, CCR4, CCR8 and CXCR5. Similarly, Th1 cells downregulate CCR1, CCR2, CCR5 and CXCR3, while upregulating CCR7 and CXCR5. Altogether these complex changes result in a global switch of receptors from those specific for inflammatory chemokines, to those specific for constitutive chemokines. These changes are compatible with the notion that, after having been attracted to inflammatory sites and activated by antigen, effector T cells might now be capable of homing back to secondary lymphoid organs or to other sites where constitutive chemokines are produced.

Concluding Remarks

A general principle that emerges from these studies is that the sharing of chemokine receptors may promote the encounter of antigen-specific T cells with the different classes of effector cells. There are two striking examples. One is the common expression of CCR3 by Th2 cells (Sallusto *et al.*, 1997), eosinophils (Ponath *et al.*, 1996) and basophils (Uguccioni *et al.*, 1997). These three cell types cooperate in the generation of allergic inflammation and, importantly, eosinophils and basophils are dependent for their activation and survival on IL-5 and IL-4 which are produced by antigen-stimulated Th2 cells (Corrigan & Kay, 1992). The second example is the common expression of CCR1 and CCR5 on Th1 cells and monocytes, which represent the precursors of dendritic cells and macrophages. This mechanism would allow the co-ordinate recruitment of antigen presenting and scavenger cells together with inflammatory T cells at sites of DTH reactions.

These scenarios are validated by immunohistochemical analysis of inflamed tissues. Thus, allergic reactions such as nasal polyps or contact dermatitis are infiltrated with T cells expressing CCR3 together with numerous eosinophils and basophils (Gerber *et al.*, 1997), while DTH reactions such as rheumatoid arthritis are infiltrated almost exclusively by CCR5 and CXCR3 expressing T cells (Loetscher *et al.*, 1998, Qin *et al.*, 1998b). One of the best examples of selective T-cell localization is the high representation of CCR5 T cells in synovial fluid (>85%) compared with the relatively low level seen in blood or lymphoid tissue (Qin *et al.*, 1998a).

The modulation of chemokine receptor expression following antigenic stimulation represents a striking example of flexibility in receptor usage and suggests the possibility that, upon activation in the tissue, T cells may be attracted to the lymphatics and secondary lymphoid organs where they may deliver help or undergo further clonal expansion. It is interesting to consider the possibility that production of constitutive chemokines such as ELC or TARC by dendritic cells in inflamed tissues may attract the recently activated T cells and in this way promote the generation and organization of chronic inflammatory reactions.

Chemokine receptors are not only useful markers of polarized T cells and tools to study T cell differentiation, but also possible targets to interfere with an immune response by inhibiting the recruitment of distinct functional subsets. Chemoattractants and their receptors are probably the most promising targets today for treating inflammatory diseases. Various types of antagonists of chemokine receptors, from monoclonal antibodies to modified chemokines or even small organic molecules have been produced to block HIV infection through chemokine receptors (Baggiolini & Moser, 1997, Wu *et al.*, 1997). There is a high probability that in coming years these compounds will emerge as effective drugs for treating autoimmune and allergic disease.

Acknowledgements

We thank Marco Colonna and Klaus Karjalainen for critical reading of the manuscript. The Basel Institute for Immunology was founded and is supported by F. Hoffmann-La Roche Ltd.

References

Baggiolini, M. (1998). Chemokines and leukocyte traffic. Nature 392, 565-568

Baggiolini, M. & Moser, B. (1997). Blocking chemokine receptors. J. Exp. Med. 186, 1189-1191

Banchereau, J. & Steinman, R. M. (1998). Dendritic cells and the control of immunity. Nature 392, 245-252

Bonecchi, R., Bianchi, G., Bordignon, P. P., D'Ambrosio, D., Lang, R., Borsatti, A., Sozzani, S., Allavena, P., Gray, P. A., Mantovani, A. & Sinigaglia, F. (1998). Differential expression of chemokine receptors and chemotactic responsiveness of type 1 T helper cells (Th1s) and Th2s. J Exp Med 187, 129-34

Butcher, E. C. & Picker, L. J. (1996). Lymphocyte homing and homeostasis. Science 272, 60-6

Corrigan, C. J. & Kay, A. B. (1992). T cells and eosinophils in the pathogenesis of asthma. Immunol Today 13, 501-507

Gerber, B., Zanni, M. P., Uguccioni, M., Loetscher, M., Mackay, C. R., Pichler, W. J., Yawalkar, N., Baggiolini, M. & Moser, B. (1997). Functional expression of the eotaxin receptor CCR3 in T lymphocytes co-localising with eosinophils. Curr. Biol. 7, 836-843

Loetscher, P., Uguccioni, M., Bordoli, L., Baggiolini, M., Moser, B., Chizzolini, C. & Dayer, J. M. (1998). CCR5 is characteristic of Th1 lymphocytes. Nature 391, 344-345

Mosmann, T. R. & Coffman, R. L. (1989). TH1 and TH2 cells: different patterns of lymphokine secretion lead to different functional properties. Annu Rev Immunol 7, 145-73

Paul, W. E. & Seder, R. A. (1994). Lymphocyte responses and cytokines. Cell 76, 241-245

Ponath, P. D., Qin, S., Post, T. W., Wang, J., Wu, L., Gerard, N. P., Newman, W., Gerard, C. & Mackay, C. R. (1996). Molecular cloning and characterization of a human eotaxin receptor expressed selectively on eosinophils. J. Exp. Med. 183, 2437-2448

Qin, S., Rottman, J. B., Myers, P., Kassam, N., Weinblatt, M., Loetscher, M., Koch, A. E., Moser, B. & Mackay, C. R. (1998a). The chemokine receptors CXCR3 and CCR5 mark subsets of T cells associated with certain inflammatory reactions. J Clin Invest 101, 746-754

Qin, S., Rottman, J. B., Myers, P., Kassam, N., Weinblatt, M., Loetscher, M., Koch, A. E., Moser, M. & MacKay, C. (1998b). The chemokine receptors CXCR3 and CCR5 mark subsets of T cells associated with certain inflammatory reactions. J. Clin. Invest. 101, 746-754

Rogge, L., Barberis-Maino, L., Biffi, M., Passini, N., Presky, D. H., Gubler, U. & Sinigaglia, F. (1997). Selective expression of an interleukin-12 receptor component by human T helper 1 cells. J Exp Med 185, 825-831

Romagnani, S. (1991). Human TH1 and TH2 subsets: doubt no more. Immunol Today 12, 256-257

Sad, S. & Mosmann, T. R. (1994). Single IL-2-secreting precursor CD4 T cell can develop into either Th1 or Th2 cytokine secretion phenotype. J Immunol 153, 3514-3522

Sallusto, F., Lenig, D., Mackay, C. R. & Lanzavecchia, A. (1998). Flexible programs of chemokine receptor expression on human polarized T helper 1 and 2 lymphocytes. J. Exp. Med. 187, 875-883

Sallusto, F., Mackay, C. R. & Lanzavecchia, A. (1997). Selective expression of the eotaxin receptor CCR3 by human T helper 2 cells. Science 277, 2005-2007

Springer, T. A. (1994). Traffic signals for lymphocyte recirculation and leukocyte emigration: the multistep paradigm. Cell 76, 301-314

Uguccioni, M., Mackay, C. R., Ochensberger, B., Loetscher, P., Rhis, S., LaRosa, G. J., Rao, P., Ponath, P. D., Baggiolini, M. & Dahinden, C. A. (1997). High expression of the chemokine receptor CCR3 in human blood basophils. Role in activation by eotaxin, MCP-4, and other chemokines. J. Clin. Invest. 100, 1137-1143

Wu, L., Paxton, W. A., Kassam, N., Ruffing, N., Rottman, J. B., Sullivan, N., Choe, H., Sodroski, J., Newman, W., Koup, R. A. & Mackay, C. R. (1997). CCR5 levels and expression pattern correlate with infectability by macrophage-tropic HIV-1, in vitro. J. Exp. Med. 185, 1681-1691.

Discussion

Fritz Melchers: What is known about maturation of macrophages? In Mike's tumors, a lot of macrophages appear to be needed to make a granuloma, sometimes T-independently.
Antonio Lanzavecchia: We do not have much experience with macrophages. In the experiments performed they did not produce ELC, even at late time points after LPS stimulation.
Gary Rathbun: In dendritic cells, inflammatory responses, IL-6 is an early cytokine and certainly is involved in inflammation. How does that fit into your scheme? Are there IL-6 receptors on non-dentritic cells?
Antonio Lanzavecchia: In dendritic cells, IL-6 has remarkably no stimulatory effect. It certainly does not induce maturation. IL-1 and TNF have much stronger effects.
Sandy Morse: For B cell interactions, are there crucial elements that you think are required for the initial activation when B cells are being exposed to antigens in the lymph nodes?
Antonio Lanzavecchia: Martin Lipp or Jason Cyster may want to answer this question, as we have not really looked at chemokine receptor expression on B cells.
Martin Lipp: We have not looked so far for the presence of all known chemokine receptors on B cells. From FACS analyses we know that on resting B cells CXCR5 is highly expressed whereas CCR7 and CXCR4 are moderately expressed. Both CXCR5 and CCR7, but not CXCR4, are transiently upregulated upon activation.
Sandy Morse: Are the complementing chemokines being made from the dendritic cells? Is this part of your spectrum? When they come, not only do they activate T cells, but participate in B cell activation?
Antonio Lanzavecchia: Mature DC produce ELC, MDC and TARC. We heard earlier that activated B cells can also make MDC. This may be a mechanism by which dendritic cells and activated B cells attract activated T cells.
Jason Cyster: We have also published that B cells respond to ELC and they respond better when they are activated.
Antonio Lanzavecchia: Along this line you may imagine that once B cells are activated, they will be attracted by dendritic cells and this way will collide with T helper cells, which having upregulated CXCR5 will move to the B cell areas. In this way T and B cells will migrate towards each other and meet at the boundary between the T and B cell areas.
Jim Kenny: I can perhaps understand how, when you put in an inflammatory reagent such as LPS or the invasion of a bacteria into the skin, you get the rapid changes in these receptors and in the chemokines. But one of the things that was very impressive at the dendritic cell meeting was that when people inject DNA, and they are vaccinating with DNA, under a situation where I do not see any real inflammatory reagents being involved, it is simply the production of a protein coming off of a DNA transcript. The most impressive thing that I took away from that meeting was that within a half hour, the dendritic cells were already off and homing to the local lymph node. How do you see that scenario in terms of chemokine receptors?
Antonio Lanzavecchia: I was not so impressed and I think there is no inconsistency since dendritic cells react and migrate quite rapidly. The downregulation of receptors for inflammatory chemokines is observed within half an hour, the upregulation of CCR7 is also rapid. So the kinetics is quite compatible with what has been observed. Concerning the requirement for inflammation, I am not sure that DNA immunization goes without inflammation. First, there is the trauma of injection. Second, the DNA that works in this system must be demethylated, and this has been shown to be sufficient to activate dendritic cells in some systems.
Manfred Kopf: TGFbeta is commonly referred to as an anti-inflammatory cytokine. Now you show data suggesting that the T cells are semi-naive when you culture them in the presence of TGFbeta. What do you mean by semi-naive?
Antonio Lanzavecchia: Semi-naive T cells are cells that cycle, can be expanded and can be kept in culture. They do not acquire the capacity to make either IL-4 or interferon gamma. Like naive T cells, they produce only IL-2.
Manfred Kopf: Do these cells express surface markers of effector/memory cells?
Antonio Lanzavecchia: I think these are the memory cells. That is our working hypotheses in the lab.
Manfred Kopf: So you say that a semi-naive cell is equivalent to a memory cell?
Antonio Lanzavecchia: Yes, that is the real memory cell. The cells that make cytokines are effector cells.

A Lymphoid Tissue-Specific Receptor, EDG6, with Potential Immune Modulatory Functions Mediated by Extracellular Lysophospholipids

Markus H. Gräler, Günter Bernhardt, and Martin Lipp
Max-Delbrück-Center for Molecular Medicine, Department of Tumor- and Immunogenetics, Robert-Rössle-Straße 10, 13092 Berlin, Germany

Introduction

Among the functionally very heterogeneous G protein-coupled receptors (GPCR) the EDG (endothelial differentiation gene) proteins define a new class of seven transmembrane proteins. The founding member, EDG1, was isolated as a PMA-inducible immediate-early transcript from human umbilical vein endothelial cells (HUVEC) [1]. Up to now six receptors belonging to the EDG family have been identified (see Table 1). As is typical for GPCRs, EDG receptors share the closest similarities in the sequences encompassing the transmembrane domain 1 (TM1) through TM7. Apart from this, EDG receptors are characterized by distinct sequence features such as a GWN/HC tetrapeptide found at the end of TM4. Furthermore all EDG proteins lack a cysteine residue in the first extracellular loop which is usually part of a disulphide bridge in GPCRs [2].

As far as it is known, these receptors utilize lipid-derived ligands in order to initiate the G protein-mediated signal cascade (see Table 1). Some of these lipid-derived ligands have recently been shown to induce migration of murine fibroblastic cells and human monocytes [3,4]. Moreover it was observed that lysophosphatidylcholine upregulates the expression of CD40 ligand on activated T cells and has mitogenic activity [5,6]. Therefore lipid-derived ligands are highly involved in immunological functions.

The divergent expression pattern of the EDG receptors (see Table 1) suggests that they serve different functions which, however, remain largely elusive. EDG1 may play an important role in the function and development of endothelial-derived tissue, whereas EDG2 was recently shown to be involved in stress fibre formation, neurite retraction, cortical neurogenesis and myelination

Table 1. Summary of some main aspects of human EDG receptors.

Receptor	Ligand	Chromosomal Localization	Main Expression	References
EDG1	S1P LPA**	1p22***	brain, spleen, heart	[1,14-17]
EDG2	LPA	?	heart, brain, placenta, small intestine, colon	[18,19]
EDG3	S1P	9q22.1-2	heart, placenta, liver, kidney, pancreas	[20,21]
EDG4	LPA	?	pancreas, testis, leukocyte, spleen, thymus, prostate	[19]
EDG5*	S1P	?	heart, lung, stomach, intestine, adrenal	[20,22]
EDG6	?	19p13.3	spleen, thymus, lymph node, peripheral leukocyte, appendix, lung	[2]

S1P, sphingosine-1-phosphate; LPA, lysophosphatidic acid.
* The symbol EDG5 is reserved by the Human Gene Nomenclature Committee for the not yet characterized human homolog of the rat H218 (AGR16) gene. Therefore the mentioned data originate from the rat H218 (AGR16) receptor.
** LPA is a low affinity agonist of EDG1.
*** *edg1* maps to this region in the constitutional translocation (1;22)(p22;q11.2) [15].

[1,7-11]. H218 (AGR16), another member of the EDG receptor subfamily isolated from rat, seems to contribute to the development of the early mammalian nervous system [12,13].

This report describes the isolation and characterization of EDG6, a novel GPCR that belongs to the EDG receptor family [2]. The cDNA coding for human EDG6 could be isolated from *in vitro* differentiated dendritic cells. EDG6-specific RNA was detected almost exclusively in cells and tissues of the lymphoid system. Moreover the expression pattern of EDG6 was found to be conserved between mouse and man. Therefore the expression of EDG6 suggests a regulatory function in immune surveillance and inflammatory responses.

Results and Discussion

With the intention of identifying novel GPCRs that are involved in the immune system, we used PCR with degenerated primers derived from the second and the seventh transmembrane domains (TMs) of five distinct chemokine receptors already known to be expressed in lymphoid tissue. Starting with an initial 648 bp fragment, the almost full length cDNA clone (1560 bp) of a novel human GPCR was isolated. This cDNA harbors an open reading frame (ORF) of 1155 bp, a 22 bp 5'-nontranslated region (NTR), and a 383 bp 3'-NTR. Based on an identity of 46% to EDG3, 44% to EDG1, 39% to EDG4 and 37% to EDG2 from the first to the seventh TM in their amino acid sequence EDG6 was assigned to the EDG receptor family. The next closest relative with 31% identity to EDG6 is the cannabinoid receptor 1 (hCB1R).

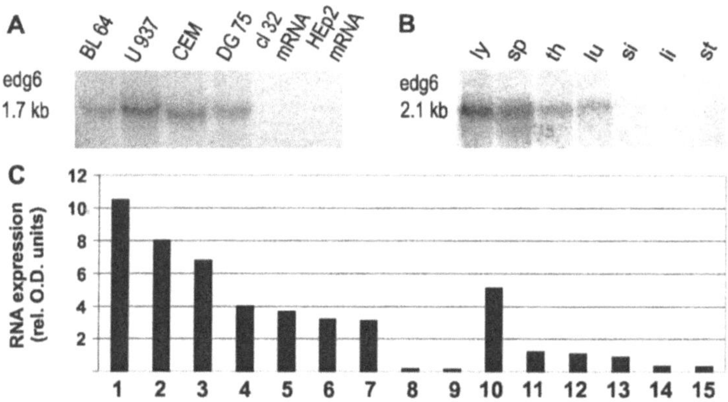

Fig. 1. *edg6* RNA expression in human cell lines and in human and murine tissues. **A.** Northern blot with total RNA of the human Burkitt lymphoma cell lines BL64 and DG 75, the promyelocytic cell line U937, and the T-cell line CEM and with mRNA of the laryngeal cell lines HEp2 and cl32. No signal was obtained with RNA of the cervical-carcinoma cell line HeLa (not shown). **B.** Northern blot with total RNA of murine tissues. ly, lymph node; sp, spleen; th, thymus; lu, lung; si, small intestine; li, large intestine; st, stomach. No signals could be detected in murine heart, liver, kidney, skeletal muscle, pancreas, cerebellum and cerebrum (not shown). **C.** Relative intensity of mRNA dot blot signals of selected human tissues (Clontech human RNA master blot). 1, spleen; 2, peripheral leukocyte; 3, lung; 4, lymph node; 5, appendix; 6, thymus; 7, bone marrow; 8, heart; 9, bladder; 10, fetal spleen; 11, fetal liver; 12, fetal thymus; 13, fetal lung; 14, fetal kidney; 15, fetal brain. No specific signals could be detected in 35 different human mRNA probes (not shown).

Interestingly the last 50 bp of the human *edg6* cDNA match with bp 13 to 62 of a short sequence encompassing the dinucleotide repeat polymorphism D19S120 (GenBank Accession No. X65642) that has been mapped to chromosome 19p13.3 [23]. Using primers derived from the 3'-end of the *edg6* cDNA and the D19S120 sequence, a DNA fragment of predicted size was obtained with human genomic DNA but not with cDNA from the *edg6* expressing Burkitt's lymphoma cell line JBL2 as a template. This sequenced fragment confirmed the close proximity between the two genomic loci. Indeed this constallation may link *edg6* to distinct disease conditions since it is known from other studies that similar repeat polymorphisms interfere with the expression of nearby located genes, thus contributing to disease [24,25].

Beside the localization of human *edg6* on chromosome 19p13.3 at the D19S120 marker, database analysis revealed that about 15.3 kb upstream of the *edg6* coding region the $G_{\alpha}16$ subunit is encoded. Whether or not this physical proximity reflects a common regulation of both genes deserves special attention since it is known that the $G_{\alpha}16$ subunit is expressed in hematopoietic cells [26-28].

To show the correct expression of EDG6 on the cell surface we tagged the receptor N-terminal with an hemaglutinin (HA) epitope tag, or C-terminal with a *myc* epitope tag, respectively [29]. FACS-analysis of transfected HEK293 cells using the corresponding antibodies against the tag confirmed the predicted orientation of EDG6 in the cell membrane with the N-terminus facing the exterior

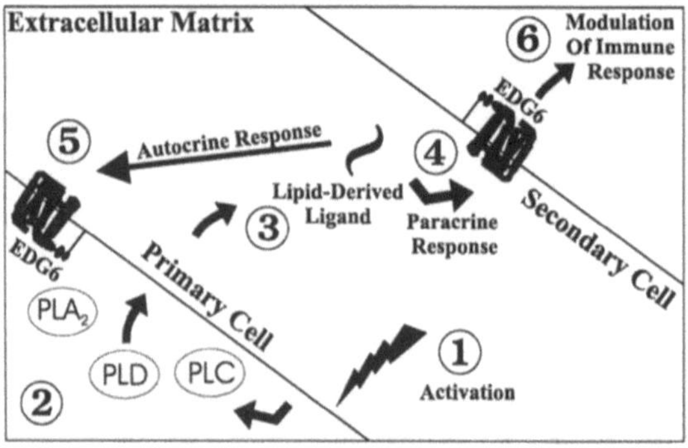

Fig. 2. Model for the putative function of EDG6 in immune surveillance. After activation (1) the involved primary cells produce diverse lipid mediators and other lipid-derived molecules via certain phospholipases (2). These messengers are released into the extracellular matrix (3). These lipid-derived molecules are able to bind specifically to EDG6 receptors expressed on the surface of secondary cells that are located close to the primary cells and induce a paracrine response (4). Another possibility is the induction of an autocrine response of the primary cells via EDG6 receptors (5). The activation of EDG6 might lead to a modulation of the immune response (6).

of the cell.

Moreover we were able to isolate the murine homolog of the human *edg6* cDNA from the fetal skin-derived dendritic cell line 18 [30]. Gene-specific primers were selected based on the murine EST sequence of the cDNA clone va16c04.r1 (GenBank Accession No. AA254425) matching the 3'-end of the coding region of the human *edg6* cDNA. The 3'-incomplete 1660 bp murine cDNA consists of a 1161 bp ORF and a 499 bp 5'-NTR with a 99 bp B1 repeat at the beginning. The murine *edg6* cDNA shares a homology of 80% to its human counterpart, the corresponding amino acid sequences are to 80% homolog and to 91% similar to each other.

Due to the lack of suitable immunological probes, the expression pattern of EDG6 was studied on the RNA level using various human as well as mouse cell lines and tissues. Northern blot analysis revealed that the human *edg6*-specific mRNA is about 1.7 kb in size (Fig. 1A), whereas its murine counterpart gives rise to a specific signal at approximately 2.1 kb (Fig. 1B). In murine tissues *edg6* RNA was present in lymph nodes, spleen, thymus and lung. There was no expression detectable in all other murine tissues examined (Fig. 1B).

A survey regarding *edg6* expression in human was done using a dot blot displaying mRNAs from 50 different tissues. The resulting expression pattern of human *edg6* matches very well with the murine RNA expression examined (Fig. 1C). A high expression level was observed in human adult and fetal spleen, in adult peripheral leukocytes, and in adult lung. Lower expression levels occurred in adult thymus, lymph node, bone marrow, and appendix as well as in fetal liver, thymus, and lung (Fig. 1C). The latter organ is the only extralymphatic tissue expressing considerable levels of *edg6* mRNA in both man and mouse. At present there is no explanation for this finding apart from the possibility that the EDG6 signal is caused by macrophages present during the preparation of lung RNA.

The observed expression pattern draws attention to a possible role of EDG6 in lymphocyte cell signalling [31]. Our working hypothesis is that EDG6 may be activated during an immunological stimulus that leads to a release of lipid-derived molecules. The activation of EDG6 could locally modulate the immune response via autocrine or paracrine mechanisms or recruit specialized cells from the pool of patroling leukocytes via secondary signalling events, e.g. induction of chemokines (Fig. 2).

Conclusion

By cloning EDG6 we identified the first receptor of this growing subfamily of GPCRs which exerts a distinct expression pattern in cells and tissues of the lymphoid system. Therefore it is conceivable to assume that EDG6 is involved in generating a suitable response to an immunological challenge. The precise role of EDG6 in this scenario is currently under investigation. Main topics include the generation of EDG6-specific monoclonal antibodies and EDG6-deficient mice.

References

1. Hla T, Maciag T (1990) An abundant transcript induced in differentiating human endothelial cells encodes a polypeptide with structural similarities to G-protein-coupled receptors. J Biol Chem 265:9308-9313
2. Gräler MH, Bernhardt G, Lipp M (1998) EDG6, a novel G-protein-coupled receptor related to receptors for bioactive lysophospholipids, is specifically expressed in lymphoid tissue. Genomics 53 (2):164-169
3. Sakai T, Peyruchaud O, Fässler R, Mosher DF (1998) Restoration of beta1A integrins is required for lysophosphatidic acid-induced migration of beta1-null mouse fibroblastic cells. J Biol Chem 273:19378-19382
4. Zhou D, Luini W, Bernasconi S, Diomede L, Salmona M, Mantovani A, Sozzani S (1995) Phosphatidic acid and lysophosphatidic acid induce haptotactic migration of human monocytes. J Biol Chem 270:25549-25556
5. Sakata Kaneko S, Wakatsuki Y, Usui T, Matsunaga Y, Itoh T, Nishi E, Kume N, Kita T (1998) Lysophosphatidylcholine upregulates CD40 ligand expression in newly activated human CD4+ T cells. FEBS Lett 433:161-165
6. Moolenaar WH (1991) Mitogenic action of lysophosphatidic acid. Adv Cancer Res 57:87-102
7. Takada Y, Kato C, Kondo S, Korenaga R, Ando J (1997) Cloning of cDNAs encoding G protein-coupled receptor expressed in human endothelial cells exposed to fluid shear stress. Biochem Biophys Res Commun 240:737-741
8. Hecht JH, Weiner JA, Post SR, Chun J (1996) Ventricular zone gene-1 (vzg-1) encodes a lysophosphatidic acid receptor expressed in neurogenic regions of the developing cerebral cortex. J Cell Biol 135:1071-1083
9. Allard J, Barron S, Diaz J, Lubetzki C, Zalc B, Schwartz JC, Sokoloff P (1998) A rat G protein-coupled receptor selectively expressed in myelin-forming cells. Eur J Neuroscience 10 (3):1045-1053
10. Fukushima N, Kimura Y, Chun J (1998) A single receptor encoded by vzg-1/lp(A1)/edg-2 couples to G proteins and mediates multiple cellular responses to lysophosphatidic acid. Proc Natl Acad Sci USA 95 (11):6151-6156

11. Weiner JA, Hecht JH, Chun J (1998) Lysophosphatidic acid receptor gene vzg-1/lp(A1)/edg-2 is expressed by mature oligodendrocytes during myelination in the postnatal murine brain. J Comp Neurol 398 (4):587-598
12. MacLennan AJ, Marks L, Gaskin AA, Lee N (1997) Embryonic expression pattern of H218, a G-protein coupled receptor homolog, suggests roles in early mammalian nervous system development. Neuroscience 79:217-224
13. Li Y, MacLennan AJ, Rogers MB (1998) A putative G-protein-coupled receptor, H218, is down-regulated during the retinoic acid-induced differentiation of F9 embryonal carcinoma cells. Exp Cell Res 239:320-325
14. Liu CH, Hla T (1997) The mouse gene for the inducible G-protein-coupled receptor edg-1. Genomics 43:15-24
15. Rhodes CH, Call KM, Budarf ML, Barnoski BL, Bell CJ, Emanuel BS, Bigner SH, Park JP, Mohandas TK (1997) Molecular studies of an ependymoma-associated constitutional t(1;22)(p22;q11.2). Cytogenet Cell Genet 78:247-252
16. Lee MJ, Thangada S, Liu CH, Thompson BD, Hla T (1998) Lysophosphatidic acid stimulates the G-protein-coupled receptor EDG-1 as a low affinity agonist. J Biol Chem 273 (34):22105-22112
17. Lee MJ, Van Brocklyn JR, Thangada S, Liu CH, Hand AR, Menzeleev R, Spiegel S, Hla T (1998) Sphingosine-1-Phosphate as a Ligand for the G Protein-Coupled Receptor EDG-1. Science 279:1552-1555
18. An S, Dickens MA, Bleu T, Hallmark OG, Goetzl EJ (1997) Molecular cloning of the human Edg2 protein and its identification as a functional cellular receptor for lysophosphatidic acid. Biochem Biophys Res Commun 231:619-622
19. An S, Bleu T, Hallmark OG, Goetzl EJ (1998) Characterization of a novel subtype of human G protein-coupled receptor for lysophosphatidic acid. J Biol Chem 273:7906-7910
20. An SZ, Bleu T, Huang W, Hallmark OG, Coughlin SR, Goetzl EJ (1997) Identification of cDNAs encoding two G protein-coupled receptors for lysosphingolipids. FEBS Lett 417:279-282
21. Yamaguchi F, Tokuda M, Hatase O, Brenner S (1996) Molecular cloning of the novel human G protein-coupled receptor (GPCR) gene mapped on chromosome 9. Biochem Biophys Res Commun 227:608-614
22. Okazaki H, Ishizaka N, Sakurai T, Kurokawa K, Goto K, Kumada M, Takuwa Y (1993) Molecular cloning of a novel putative G protein-coupled receptor expressed in the cardiovascular system. Biochem Biophys Res Commun 190:1104-1109
23. Jedlicka AE, Taylor EW, Meyers DA, Liu Z, Levitt RC (1994) Localization of the highly polymorphic locus D19S120 to 19p13.3 by linkage. Cytogenet Cell Genet 65:140
24. Risinger JI, Berchuck A, Kohler MF, Watson P, Lynch HT, Boyd J (1993) Genetic instability of microsatellites in endometrial carcinoma. Cancer Res 53:5100-5103
25. Pykett MJ, Murphy M, Harnish PR, George DL (1994) Identification of a microsatellite instability phenotype in meningiomas. Cancer Res 54:6340-6343
26. Pfeilstocker M, Karlic H, Salamon J, Kromer E, Mühlberger H, Pavlova B, Selim U, Tuchler H, Fritsch G, Kneissl S, Heinz R, Pitterman E, Paukovits MR (1996) Expression of G alpha 16, a G-protein alpha subunit specific for hematopoiesis in acute leukemia. Leukemia 10:1117-1121
27. Amatruda TT, Steele DA, Slepak VZ, Simon MI (1991) G alpha 16, a G protein alpha subunit specifically expressed in hematopoietic cells. Proc Natl Acad Sci USA 88:5587-5591
28. Mapara MY, Bommert K, Bargou RC, Leng C, Beck C, Ludwig WD, Gierschik P, Dörken B (1995) G protein subunit G alpha 16 expression is restricted to progenitor B cells during human B-cell differentiation. Blood 85:1836-1842
29. Emrich T, Förster R, Lipp M (1993) Topological characterization of the lymphoid-specific seven transmembrane receptor BLR1 by epitope-tagging and high level expression. Biochem Biophys Res Commun 197:214-220
30. Elbe A, Schleischitz S, Strunk D, Stingl G (1994) Fetal skin-derived MHC class I+, MHC class II- dendritic cells stimulate MHC class I-restricted responses of unprimed CD8+ T cells. J Immunol 153:2878-2889
31. Förster R, Mattis EA, Kremmer E, Wolf E, Brem G, Lipp M (1996) A putative chemokine receptor, BLR1, directs B cell migration to defined lymphoid organs and specific anatomic compartments of the spleen. Cell 87:1037-1047

Discussion

Jason Cyster: Would you say that one of the lipids you mentioned is the ligand for EDG6?
Martin Lipp: This is very likely but currently not known. We have tested LPA, sphingosine-1-phosphate and phosphatidic acid for binding to EDG6 expressed in HEK 293 cells. Unfortunately, the background in these cells is very high, thus we have to change the system for further binding studies.
Jason Cyster: Do all cells have at least one EDG receptor on them? Is that why the background is so high?
Martin Lipp: I do not know if all cells have at least one EDG receptor. However, the expression of these receptors in a variety of cell lineages supports our concept that the EDG family members exert an essential function in regulating the responsiveness and behavior of cells within the local microenvironment. For example, upon a primary signaling event induced by a certain cytokine, bioactive phospholipids are released into the local periphery, which then in turn may act as an "extracellular second messenger". These lipids may either amplify the signal in an autocrine fashion or may sensitize or stimulate neighboring cells. Therefore, I think that EDG6 and related receptors represent potentially very important target molecules for modulating inflammatory responses.
Dirk Eick: Do you think that LPA also regulates growth in B cells?
Martin Lipp: It is known that LPA can function as a mitogen for neutrophils, monocytes and lymphocytes. Although B cells have not been especially looked at, I think that LPA can induce proliferation in B cells during certain stages of differentiation and activation.
Michael Carroll: Is EDG6 more highly expressed on T cells than B cells? Do you think that T cells might be more crucial?
Martin Lipp: At least on the RNA level EDG6 is expressed to a similar extent in Burkitt's lymphoma cells as well as in certain T cell lines. We have not looked so far in purified primary B and T cell subsets. Thus, more functional studies are necessary to answer your question.
Michael Carroll: Have you looked in inflammatory cells?
Martin Lipp: Not yet, but we plan to do these experiments as soon as we have got monoclonal antibodies against EDG6.
Richard Scheuermann: Is it clear whether the ligand-binding domain is extracellular or intracellular?
Martin Lipp: Within the EDG receptor family the ligand binding domains have not been mapped so far. However, to me it is very likely that the hydrophobic core formed by the seven transmembrane regions, together with some extracellular parts, might be involved in this interaction.

III

Chromosomal Translocations, DNA Rearrangements and Somatic Hypermutations

Phenotypic and Molecular Characterization of Human Peripheral Blood B-cell Subsets with Special Reference to N-Region Addition and Jκ-Usage in VκJκ-Joints and κ/λ-Ratios in Naive Versus Memory B-cell Subsets to Identify Traces of Receptor Editing Processes

U. Klein, K. Rajewsky, and R. Küppers
Institute for Genetics, University of Cologne, Germany

Summary

We identified a population of IgM+IgD+ B-cells in the peripheral blood (PB) of humans that express somatically mutated V-region genes like classical class switched or IgM-only memory B-cells and comprise around 15% of PB B-cells in adults. Mutated IgM+IgD+ cells differ from unmutated naive IgM+IgD+ cells in that they express the CD27 cell surface antigen. In addition, a very small subset of IgD-only B-cells was identified in the PB that carried rearranged VH-genes with an extremely high load of somatic mutations (up to 60 mutations per gene). A common characteristic of the four somatically mutated subsets, which altogether comprise 40% of PB B-lymphocytes in adults, is the surface expression of CD27. This antigen may thus represent a general marker for memory B-cells in the human. Somatically mutated and unmutated PB B-cell subsets were analyzed for N-region addition and Jκ-usage in VκJκ-joints, and in addition for the respective κ/λ-ratios: N-nucleotides could be identified in a large fraction of Vκ-regions of all B-cell subsets, indicating that N-region insertion already occurs in the pre-germinal center (GC) phase of B-cell development. Both the Jκ-usage in expressed VκJκ-joints and the κ/λ-ratio from somatically mutated B-cells do not differ substantially from those of the unmutated cells, so that in terms of these parameters, a contribution of secondary VκJκ-rearrangements in shaping the memory B-cell repertoire is not detectable.

Introduction

Studies of the human peripheral B-cell repertoire had indicated that naive B-cells, the precursors of GC B-cells, are IgM+IgD+ and express unmutated V-regions [1-3], like CD5-positive B-cells that are not regularly driven into the GC-response [4, 5]. The post-GC, somatically mutated memory B cell repertoire consists of class switched as well as IgM-only cells [1-3, 6]. However, there is controversy as to whether a subset of IgM+IgD+ B-cells carries mutated V-regions [2, 6, 7]. So far direct evidence for the existence of such a subpopulation is missing. A recent paper describes two IgD-expressing B-cell populations in the PB which can be distinguished by the expression of the CD27 cell surface antigen, a member of the tumor necrosis factor-receptor family [8]. Since the occurrence of somatic mutations in rearranged V-genes is an indication for the developmental stage of a B-cell, i.e. pre- or post-GC, we determined the level of somatic mutation in rearranged V-genes of $CD27^+$ and $CD27^-$ IgD^+ PB B-cells by molecular single-cell analysis. Furthermore, B-cells of pre- and post-GC subsets were analyzed for the occurrence of N-region addition and Jκ-usage in expressed VκJκ-joints as well as for the respective κ/λ-ratios in order to identify traces of possible V-gene editing processes in the generation of the memory B-cell repertoire in T-dependent immune responses.

Material and Methods

The analysis of the $IgM^+IgD^+CD27^+$, $IgM^+IgD^+CD27^-$, and IgD-only PB B-cells for somatic mutation has recently been published elsewhere [9].

Analysis of N-Region Addition and Jκ-Usage in VκJκ-Joints and κ/λ-Ratios in Pre- Versus Post-GC B-cell Subsets

The VκJκ-joints analyzed were derived from references 1, 4, 6, and 9. In the case of the unmutated PB B-cell subsets, only κ-transcripts derived from IgM^+IgD^+ B-cells [1, 6] that had no or one nucleotide difference to the respective germline V-gene, and in single-cell analyses, potentially functional V-genes from $CD5^+$ B-cells [4] that showed no nucleotide differences to the corresponding germline V-genes were considered. Thus, skewing of the analysis by potentially contaminating somatically mutated B-cells in the sorted IgM^+IgD^+ and $CD5^+$ fractions was prevented. Likewise, in the case of the mutated IgM-only and class switched B-cell subsets, κ-transcripts that had two or more nucleotide differences to the respective germline V-gene [1, 6], and in single-cell analyses, potentially functional V-genes from class switched, IgM-only, and $IgM^+IgD^+CD27^+$ PB B-cells that had at least one nucleotide difference to the corresponding germline V-gene were considered [4, 6, 9].

For the analysis of the κ/λ-ratios in somatically mutated versus unmutated PB B-cell subsets, $CD19^+$ B-cells, enriched by magnetic cell separation to more than 98% from the PB of healthy volunteers, were incubated with a FITC-conjugated monoclonal antibody against CD27, and with either anti-κ-PE or anti-λ-PE (all purchased from Pharmingen) for 10 min on ice. After washing, the cell suspension was analyzed on a FACS Calibur using Cellquest software (both Becton Dickinson, Mountain View, Ca). Dead cells were excluded from the analysis by staining with propidium iodide. The percentages of λ-positive cells among the pre-GC population on the one hand and the memory cell population on the other were determined by selective gating on CD27-negative and CD27-positive cells, respectively. The percentages of κ-positive cells were determined in parallel in order to ascertain that both percentages add up to approximately 100% (not shown).

Results and Discussion

In the Human, IgD-expressing PB B-cells can be Subdivided into Somatically Mutated and Unmutated Fractions

Agematsu et al. reported that IgD-expressing PB B-cells can be separated into $CD27^+$ and $CD27^-$ subsets; IgD^- cells are $CD27^+$ [8]. Upon *in vitro* stimulation, IgD^+CD27^+ cells are rapidly activated and secrete large amounts of Ig, like IgD^-CD27^+ B-lymphocytes [8]. To investigate whether IgD^+CD27^+ cells are at a pre- or post-GC stage of development, we isolated single cells of the IgD^+CD27^+ and IgD^+CD27^- populations from the PB of three and two donors, respectively, and amplified and sequenced rearranged VH and Vκ-regions. It turned out that whereas almost all IgD^+CD27^- cells carried unmutated V-genes (31/32), most of the rearrangements derived from IgD$^+$CD27$^+$ cells showed somatic mutations (63/67) [9]. This indicates on the one hand that naive B-cells are CD27$^-$, and on the other hand that IgD$^+$CD27$^+$ cells represent a further phenotypically defined, somatically mutated B-cell subset in the human PB. IgD$^+$CD27$^+$ cells, like class switched and IgM-only cells, comprise around 15% of PB B-lymphocytes [8, 9]. One peculiarity in the sequence collection derived from the IgD$^+$CD27$^+$ cells caught our attention: some rearrangements carried an extremely high load of somatic mutations as has previously been described in normal human B-cells only for IgD-only cells of the tonsillar GC and plasma cell fractions [10, 11]. Liu and colleagues note that IgD-only cells apparently do not exist in the PB. However, we could identify a distinct albeit very small fraction (<1%) of sIg-positive IgD-only cells in the PB of most individuals analyzed. These cells are CD27$^+$ [9]. We determined the level of somatic mutation in such IgD-only cells by single-cell PCR and found that their VH-regions showed up to 60 mutations, yielding an average mutation frequency of 15% which is about three times higher than that typical for memory cells of the other subsets (Fig.1) [9]. Thus, it seems that IgD-only cells are not a peculiarity of the tonsil but that they occur also as sIg-positive cells in the PB of humans.

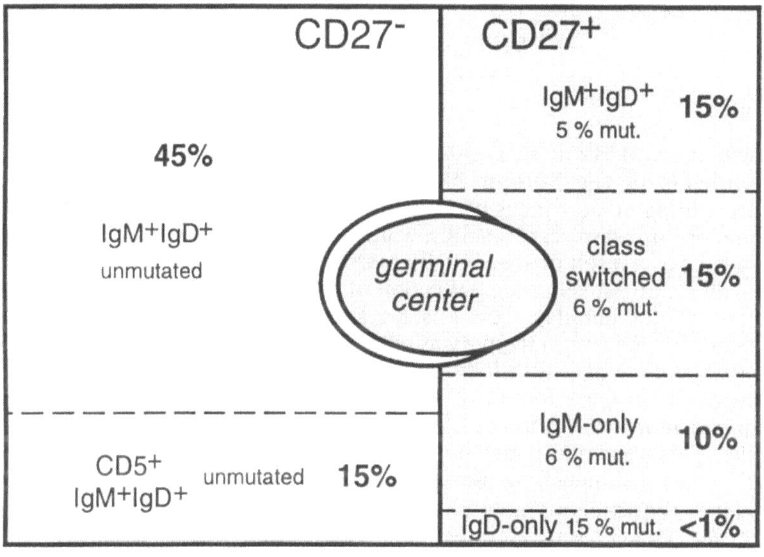

Fig. 1. Composition of the human PB B-cell repertoire. Shown are the phenotypically defined subsets, the average VH-region mutation frequencies, and the percentages of the respective subsets among all PB B-cells. See references 9 and 18 for discussion.

N-region insertion in VκJκ-joints expressed by pre- and post-GC B-cell subsets in the human PB

While in the mouse N-region addition in κ-chains has been rarely observed, a large fraction of human κ-chains contains N-nucleotides [1, 12]. It is evident from studies in the mouse that light (L) chain rearrangements occur in TdT-negative cells, which seems to be the case also in humans [13]. The recent demonstration that TdT is reexpressed in GC B-cells [14] raised the question whether N-sequences in VκJκ-joints are in fact a feature of secondary V-gene rearrangements in GC B-cells.

We had accumulated a large sequence collection of expressed Vκ-regions from pre- and post-GC B-cell subsets [1,4,6,9] which enabled us to study this question. The results are shown in Table 1 (see Material and Methods for details). In all B-cell subsets studied, a considerable fraction of Vκ-rearrangements contained N-regions. Thus, N-nucleotides are already introduced during VκJκ-rearrangements at a pre-GC stage of development, probably during B-cell differentiation in the bone marrow. Why the fraction of VκJκ-joints with N-nucleotides is so large in humans remains elusive.

Table 1. N-regions in expressed Vκ-genes derived from unmutated and mutated PB B-cell subsets

	subsets	n	Vκ-genes with N-regions
unmutated	IgM^+IgD^+	25	76%
	$CD5^+$	38	61%
mutated	IgM-only	46	54%
	IgM^+IgD^+	13	46%
	IgM^-IgD^-	20	50%

Jκ-usage in expressed VκJκ-joints and κ/λ-ratios of pre- and post-GC B-cell subsets in the human PB

If V-gene editing in the κ-locus contributes to the generation of the memory B-cell repertoire, one might observe a shift towards the use of downstream Jκ-elements in memory cells as a result of sequential κ-rearrangements. Table 2 shows the results of the analysis of our sequence collection of expressed VκJκ-joints (see Material and Methods for details). There is no substantial shift towards the use of downstream Jκ-elements in memory as opposed to unmutated B-cells.

Since rearrangements in λ-loci in general seem to occur subsequently to rearrangements in the κ-loci [15], V-gene editing processes in GC B-cells may result in an overrepresentation of λ^+ cells in the memory as opposed to the pre-GC repertoire. This was investigated by staining PB B-cells from eight normal donors for CD27, thus distinguishing pre- and post-GC B-cells, and λ or κ (see Material and Methods for details). The results of this analysis are shown in Table 3. $CD27^-$ pre-GC and $CD27^+$ post-GC cells contained comparable percentages of λ-expressing B-cells. Although these findings on the first glance seem to suggest that V-gene editing in L chain loci of GC B-cells does not play a major role in shaping the memory B-cell repertoire, it must be emphasized that B-cells have multiple possibilities for the generation of novel L chains through rearrangements at any of the four loci, making it difficult to infer from a global analysis of Jκ or λ-usage to what extent sequential L chain rearrangements occur in GC B-cells. Along this line, in a recent analysis of T-cell rich B-cell lymphoma, we encountered a case which harbored, in addition to a mutated, potentially functional Vλ-rearrangement, an in-frame, somatically mutated Vκ-region gene which was rendered non-functional by a point mutation introducing a stop codon in the Vκ-gene (manuscript submitted). This indicates that the tumor precursor had changed L chain isotype expression by V-gene editing within the GC. A similar case had been described previously for a normal PB B-cell [16].

Table 2. Jκ-usage in expressed Vκ-regions derived from unmutated and mutated PB B-cell subsets

	subsets	n	Jκ1	Jκ2	Jκ3	Jκ4	Jκ5
	IgM^+IgD^+	25	28%	28%	20%	20%	4%
unmut.	$CD5^+$	38	39.5%	18.5%	5%	24%	13%
	sum	63	35%	22%	11%	22%	9.5%
mut.	sum	74	24%	26%	15%	27%	8%

Table 3. Percentage of λ^+ B-cells among $CD27^-$ and $CD27^+$ PB B-cell subsets

		Donor							
		A	B	C	D	E	F	G	H
$\%\lambda^+$	$CD27^-$	39	38	43	36	38	40	36	43
	$CD27^+$	35	37	40	44	39	40	35	42

Concluding Remarks

Fig.1 shows the composition of the PB B-cell repertoire of humans - classified into a somatically mutated and an unmutated compartment - as it emerged from our analyses. The unmutated compartment comprises around 60% of PB B-cells and consists of $CD5^+$ and $CD5^-$ IgM^+IgD^+ B-cells [4, 17, 18]. The somatically mutated (memory) compartment, which is presumably generated in the GC-reaction, consists of four subsets, defined by their isotype [9, 18]. Strikingly, IgM-expressing memory cells outnumber classical, class switched memory cells in the PB [9, 18], and probably also in the secondary lymphoid organs [6, 19]. The somatically mutated B cells in the PB [9] and in spleen [19] (and presumably also in lymph nodes and intestine) share expression of the CD27 surface marker. The significance of CD27-expression on B-lymphocytes may be that memory B-cells, upon renewed stimulation in secondary immune responses, as the result of an additional ligation of CD27 with its ligand CD70 (found on peripheral T-cells), quickly differentiate into plasma cells [20]. Analyzing the Jκ usage in VκJκ-joints and the κ/λ-ratios in pre- versus post-GC B-cells, we do not detect a shift towards the usage of downstream Jκ-elements in expressed Vκ-regions or λ-chains in memory B-cells. Thus, in terms of these parameters, there is no evidence for a role of receptor editing in the generation of the memory B-cell receptor repertoire, leaving the case open for further investigation.

We are grateful to Michaela Fahrig and Julia Jesdinsky for excellent technical assistance. We thank Christoph Göttlinger for help with the FACS. This work was supported by the Deutsche Forschungsgemeinschaft through SFB243 and SFB502.
Address correspondence to Ulf Klein, University of Cologne, Institute for Genetics, Weyertal 121, 50931 Cologne, Germany; E-mail: Uklein@mac.genetik.uni-koeln.de

References

1. Klein U, Küppers R, Rajewsky K (1993) Human IgM+IgD+ B-cells, the major B-cell subset in the peripheral blood, express Vκ genes with no or little somatic mutation throughout life. Eur J Immunol 23:3272
2. Pascual V, Liu Y-J, Magalski A, de Bouteiller O, Banchereau J, Capra JD (1994) Analysis of somatic mutation in five B-cell subsets of human tonsil. J Exp Med 180:329
3. Klein U, Küppers R, Rajewsky K (1994) Variable region gene analysis of B-cell subsets derived from a 4-yr-old child: Somatically mutated memory B-cells accumulate in the peripheral blood already at young age. J Exp Med 180:1383
4. Fischer M, Klein U, Küppers R (1997) Molecular single-cell analysis reveals that CD5-positive peripheral blood B-cells in healthy humans are characterized by rearranged Vκ-genes lacking somatic mutation. J Clin Invest 100:1667
5. Brezinschek H-P, Foster SJ, Brezinschek RI, Dörner T, Domiati-Saad R, Lipsky PE (1997) Analysis of the human VH gene repertoire: Differential effects of selection and somatic hypermutation on human peripheral CD5+/IgM+ and CD5-/IgM+ B-cells. J Clin Invest 99:2488
6. Klein U, Küppers R, Rajewsky K (1997) Evidence for a large compartment of IgM-expressing memory B-cells in humans. Blood 89:1288
7. Paramithiotis E, Cooper MD (1997) Memory B-lymphocytes migrate to bone marrow in humans. Proc Natl Acad Sci USA 94:208
8. Agematsu K, Nagumo H, Yang FC, Nakazawa T, Fukushima K, Ito S, Sugita K, Mori T, Kobata T, Morimoto C, Komiyama A (1997) B-cell subpopulations separated by CD27 and crucial collaboration of CD27+ B-cell and helper T-cell in the immunoglobulin production. Eur J Immunol 27:2073
9. Klein U, Rajewsky K, Küppers R (1998) Human immunoglobulin (Ig)M+IgD+ peripheral blood B-cells expressing the CD27 cell surface antigen carry somatically mutated variable region genes: CD27 as a general marker for somatically mutated (memory) B-cells. J Exp Med 188:1679
10. Liu Y-J, de Bouteiller O, Arpin C, Briere F, Galibert L, Ho S, Martinez-Valdez H, Banchereau J, Lebecque S (1996) Normal human IgD+IgM- germinal center B-cells can express up to 80 mutations in the variable region of their IgD transcripts. Immunity 4:603
11. Arpin C, de Bouteiller O, Razanajaona D, Fugier-Vivier I, Briere F, Banchereau J, Liu Y-J (1998) The normal counterpart of IgD myeloma cells in germinal center displays extensively mutated IgVH gene, Cμ-Cδ switch, and λ-L chain expression. J Exp Med 187:1169
12. Klein R, Jaenichen R, Zachau HG (1993) Expressed human immunoglobulin κ genes and their hypermutation. Eur J Immunol 23:3248
13. Ghia P, ten Boekel E, Sanz E, de la Hera A, Rolink A, Melchers F (1996) Ordering of human bone marrow B lymphocyte precursors by single-cell polymerase chain reaction analyses of the rearrangement status of the immunoglobulin H and L chain gene loci. J Exp Med 184:2217
14. Meffre E, Papavasiliou F, Cohen P, de Bouteiller O, Bell D, Karasuyama H, Schiff C, Banchereau J, Liu Y-J, Nussenzweig MC (1998) Antigen receptor engagement turns off the V(D)J recombination machinery in human tonsil B-cells. J Exp Med 188:765
15. Gorman JR, Alt FW (1998) Regulation of immunoglobulin light chain isotype expression. Adv Immunol 69:113
16. Giachino C, Padovan E, Lanzavecchia A (1995) κ+λ+ dual receptor B cells are present in the human peripheral repertoire. J Exp Med 181:1245
17. Brezinschek H-P, Brezinschek RI, Lipsky PE (1995) Analysis of the heavy chain repertoire of human peripheral B-cells using single-cell polymerase chain reaction. J Immunol 155:190
18. Klein U, Goossens T, Fischer M, Kanzler H, Bräuninger A, Rajewsky K, Küppers R (1998) Somatic hypermutation in normal and transformed human B-cells. Immunol Rev 162:261
19. Tangye SG, Liu Y-J, Aversa G, Phillips JH, de Vries JE (1998) Identification of functional human splenic memory B cells by expression of CD148 and CD27. J Exp Med 188:1691
20. Agematsu K, Nagumo H, Oguchi Y, Nakazawa T, Fukushima K, Yasui K, Ito S, Kobata T, Morimoto C, Komiyama A (1998) Generation of plasma cells from peripheral blood memory B-cells: synergistic effect of interleukin-10 and CD27/CD70 interaction. Blood 91:173

Discussion

Richard Scheuermann: In the peripheral blood IgD-only cells, what is the structure of the cμ part, is it deleted at the DNA level or is it spliced out from mRNA?
Ulf Klein: We have not explicitly looked for that in the IgD-only cells of the peripheral blood described here, but Yong-Jun Liu and colleagues showed for IgD-only cells of the tonsillar germinal center and plasma cell fractions that cμ is deleted as a result of class switching events [Arpin et al., J Exp Med 187:1169, 1998].
Thomas Winkler: You just analyzed B-cells from the peripheral blood. Have you had the chance to look in spleen or lymph nodes?
Ulf Klein: The composition of the tonsillar non-germinal center B-cell fraction, consisting of naive as well as memory B cells, resembles that in the peripheral blood, although one finds fewer IgM-only memory B cells in tonsils from children [Fischer et al., J Clin Invest 100:1667, 1997]. We did not have the chance to look in spleen. (During the preparation of the present manuscript a paper was published showing that memory B cells in spleen are $CD27^+$, many of which are IgM-expressing, and otherwise phenotypically and functionally resemble memory B-cells of the tonsil and the peripheral blood [Tangye et al., J Exp Med 188:1691, 1998]).
Garnett Kelsoe: There are two famous papers from Yong-Jun Liu and colleagues, the title of the first is "Within germinal centers, isotype switching of Ig genes occurs after the onset of somatic mutation" [Immunity 4:241, 1996], that of the second "Analysis of somatic mutation in five B-cell subsets of human tonsil" [J Exp Med 180:329, 1994], describing which B-cell subsets express somatically mutated V region genes in the human tonsil. Because of the frequencies of both μδ-positive, μ-only, and class switched B-cells in the peripheral blood, I do not understand how these two analyses of the peripheral blood and the tonsil can be brought together. The original scheme proposed by Pascual et al. [J Exp Med 180:329, 1994] seems to be "broken" somewhat.
Ulf Klein: No, not at all. In contrast to our approach, they did not analyze the tonsillar germinal center and memory B-cell fractions with regard to isotype distribution. Instead, they sequenced μ, δ, and γ transcripts from the respective populations (δ, however, only from germinal center B cells). Because they observed the same mutational frequencies in μ and γ transcripts [Pascual et al., J Exp Med 180:329, 1994], which in μ-chains is about half that of γ-chains, as we found for the respective populations in the peripheral blood [Klein et al., J Exp Med 180:1383, 1994], the results of their and our analyses are largely compatible. Through our approach, that is taking into account the isotype distribution of the B-cell subsets in combination with the analysis of single cells by PCR, we could determine the sizes of the respective compartments.
Fritz Melchers: Does the ratio of $CD27^+$ versus $CD27^-$ cells ever change during life?
Ulf Klein: Yes, it does. Agematsu et al. [Eur J Immunol 27:2073, 1997] had the chance to study the frequency of $CD27^+$ B cells in cord blood, in the peripheral blood of young children, and in adults. The frequency of $CD27^+$ cells is very low at birth and increases steadily during adolescence until it seems to level at about 40% in the adult. Thus, in an 80-year-old not all B-cells are $CD27^+$.

Tuning Somatic Hypermutation by Transcription

H. Jacobs[1], A. Puglisi[1], K. Rajewsky[2] and Y. Fukita[2,3]
1 Basel Institute for Immunology, Grenzacherstr. 487, CH-4005 Basel, Switzerland
2 Institute for Genetics, University of Cologne, Weyertal 121, D-50931 Cologne, Germany
3 Present address: The First Department of Internal Medicine, Hirosaka University School of Medicine, Zaifu-cho 5, Hirosaki, Japan

Abstract

The dependence of somatic hypermutation on transcription was studied in three mutant immunoglobulin heavy chain (IgH) insertion mice in which a targeted non-functional VHB1-8 passenger transgene was either placed under the transcriptional control of a truncated DQ52 promoter (pΔ), its own RNA polymerase II dependent IgH promoter (pII) or a RNA polymerase I dependent promoter (pI). The relative mutation-frequency of the VHB1-8 passenger transgene in memory B cells of pΔ, pI and pII mice (7%, 60% and 100%) correlated with the relative levels of transgene-specific pre-mRNA expressed in germinal center B cells isolated from the mutant mice (8%, 72% and 100%, respectively). These data indicate that the mutation load of rearranged Ig genes can be tuned by transcription. The question, whether somatic hypermutation requires transcription per se or a specific component of the RNA polymerase II complex, is under investigation.

Introduction

Somatic hypermutation occurs in germinal centers (GC) and allows rearranged immunoglobulin (Ig) genes to be further diversified. Somatic hypermutation is characterized by an elevated frequency of mutations and is restricted to but not dependent on the variable regions of Ig heavy and light chain genes (see Immunol. Rev. Vol. 162, 1998). Despite the extensive knowledge of the immunobiology, experiments trying to identify critical trans-acting elements involved in the molecular mechanism(s) underlying somatic hypermutation remained speculative (Wiesendanger et al.,1998; Wood, 1998). Nevertheless, Ig-transgenic mice have provided important insights into the cis-acting DNA elements required to target somatic mutation to the V(D)J region. The V gene promoter can be exchanged by other RNA polymerase II (pol II)-dependent promoters without affecting hypermutation (Betz et al., 1994; Tumas-Brundage and Manser, 1997) . A linkage between transcription initiation and the occurrence of somatic hypermutation has been suggested by Peters and Storb who found that placing an additional Ig promoter immediately 5' to the constant portion of the Igκ chain gene leads to the occurrence of somatic hypermutation within 2 kb downstream of each promoter but not between these two areas (Peters and Storb, 1996, Rada et al 1997). Furthermore, gene targeting enabled us to demonstrate a direct correlation between the frequency of somatic hypermutation and transcription of rearranged Ig genes in GC B cells (Fukita et al., 1998). This report summarizes previously published data and includes some further characterization of the truncated DQ52 promoter, that controls transcription and somatic hypermutation of the VHB1-8 passenger transgene in B cells of pΔ mice.

Results

Somatic Hypermutation of VHB1-8 in pI, pII and pΔ mice

To study the impact of Ig transcription on somatic hypermutation we generated three IgH insertion mice that carry a rearranged VHDHJH gene segment which either lacked the IgH promoter (pΔ mice) or was placed under the control of either the Ig heavy chain gene promoter (pII mice) or a RNA polymerase I (pol I)- dependent promoter (pI mice). The pol I-dependent promoter was chosen since it might allow one to distinguish between transcription per se and the coupling of a putative mutator to a pol II specific component. Figure 1 indicates the predicted structure of the targeted IgH locus in pΔ, pI and pII mice.

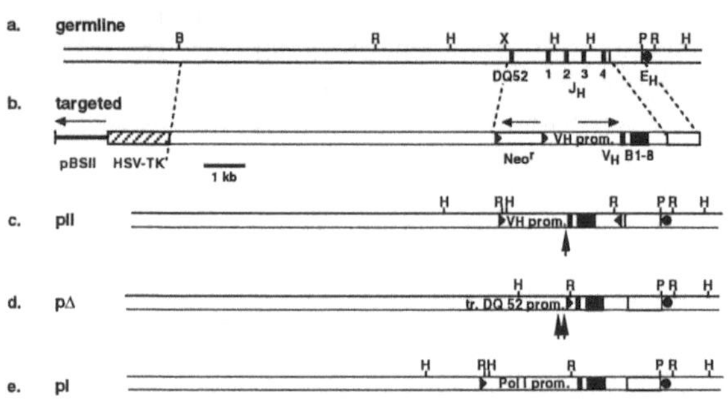

Fig. 1. Predicted structure of the targeted IgH locus (a) of the VH promoter (pII) mice before (b) and after deletion of loxP flanked neo gene (c), as well as the VH promoter deletion (pΔ) mice (d), and the pol I promoter (pI) mice (e) after deletion of the neomycin gene. Vertical arrow heads in the promoter region of pΔ and pII indicate the transcriptional start sites from the truncated DQ52 promoter and the IgH promoter, respectively.

To analyse somatic hypermutation in these mice, the VHB1-8 gene was amplified from the genomic DNA of single Vλ1+IgM-IgD- memory B cells, using primers that specifically amplify the inserted VHB1-8 gene. Coamplification and sequencing of the functionally rearranged Vλ1 gene (Jacobs et al., 1998) served as an internal control for the mutator activity.

As expected, somatic hypermutation of the VHB1-8 gene occurred normally in pII mice. About 60% of the sequenced samples contained multiple point mutations (Table 1), consistent with the finding that 64% of Vλ1 genes amplified from single cells of the same B cell fraction in wild-type mice are mutated (Jacobs et al., 1998). The mutation frequency is 0.84% (103 mutations / 12200 nt [610 nt X 20 samples]) in the VHB1-8 passenger transgene of pII mice. Taking only the mutated VHB1-8 genes into account, the mutation frequency is 1.4% (103 mutations / 7320 nt [610 nt X 12 samples]). The number of point mutations found in the amplificates of memory B cells varied from 0 to 32 (Table 1).

When analysing somatic hypermutation in memory B cells derived from pΔ mice, the percentage of mutated VHB1-8 genes was reduced to 22% compared to 60% found in pII mice (Table 1). In addition, the maximum number of point mutations detected in a mutated gene was three as compared to 32 in pII mice. To verify that we had indeed isolated memory B cells, we coamplified and sequenced the Vλ1 genes from the same single cells. Fifty-seven percent of the Vλ1 genes were found to be mutated, a value comparable to the percentage of mutated Vλ1 genes in memory B cells of wild type mice and mutated VHB1-8 genes in memory

B cells of pII mice (Table 1). Therefore, although only 22% of the analysed VHB1-8 genes were mutated, the analysis of the Vλ1 genes from the same single cells indicated that hypermutation actually occurred in 57% of the samples. Taking this finding into account, the mutation frequency of the pΔ VHB1-8 gene further decreases from 0.24% (based on 22% mutated VH genes) to 0.09% (based on 57% mutated Vλ1 genes). Thus the frequency of VHB1-8 mutations in memory B cells of pΔ mice is 15-fold lower than in memory B cells of pII mice. In contrast, the mutation frequency of 1.1% at the λ locus is consistent with a previous analysis (Jacobs et al, 1998), indicating that the hypermutator as such is unaffected in memory B cells of pΔ mice. As so far only 12 point mutations were found in the pΔ mice, the relevance of the frequent C nucleotide changes (7/12) remains unclear (Fig. 2a). These results demonstrate the importance of the VH promoter in the process of somatic hypermutation.

Table 1. Somatic Mutation Analysis and Relative Transcription Levels of VHB1-8 in pΔ, pI and pII Mice.

Mutant strain	No. of PCR products with point mutation / total no. of PCR products sequenced	Mutation frequency (1)	No. of point mutations per sequence	* Mutation frequency (2)	Normalized mutation frequency (3)	VHB1-8 pre- mRNA levels in PNA high B cells (6)	VHB1-8 mRNA levels in PNA high B cells (6)
pII mice (VHB1-8)	12 / 20 (60 %)	0.84 % (103 / 12200)	0 - 32	1.40 % (103 / 7320)	100 %	100 %	100 %
pΔ mice (VHB1-8)	8 / 35 (22 %)	0.056 % (12 / 21350)	0 - 3	0.24 % (12 / 4880) 0.092 % (12 / 12200) (4)	7 % (5)	8 %	23 %
pI mice (VHB1-8)	14 / 25 (56 %)	0.47 % (73 / 15250)	0 - 17	0.85 % (73 / 8540)	60 %	72 %	87 %
pΔ mice (Vλ1)	20 / 35 (57 %)	0.60 % (51 / 8400)	0 - 7	1.06 % (51 / 4800)			
naive B cells from p II mice	2 / 20 (10 %)	0. 030 % (3 / 12200)	0 - 2				

1) Mutation frequency = $\frac{\text{Total number of point mutations}}{\text{Total number of base pairs sequenced}}$

2) Mutation frequency * = $\frac{\text{Total number of point mutations}}{\text{Total number of base pairs of PCR products containing point mutations}}$

3) The mutation frequency * (defined in 2) of the pII mice was taken as 100%

4) This number was calculated based on the assumption that 57 % of memory B cells of the pΔ mice were under the influence of a putative somatic hypermutation machinery.

5) This number was calculated based on 4).

6) All data were first normalized on the basis of β-actin expression. For both pre-mRNA and mRNA , the amount of PCR products of the pΔ and pI mice was normalized against the PCR products of the pII mice.

To answer the question, whether the pol I dependent promoter can substitute the pol II dependent promoter, somatic hypermutation was analysed in single memory B cells isolated from pI mice. Interestingly, similar to the percentage of mutated VHB1-8 genes in pII mice and mutated Vλ1 chain genes in pΔ mice, 56% of the amplificates were mutated (Table 1). However, the range of mutations per gene (0-

17) was below that of pII mice (0-32). Similarly, the mutation frequency in memory B cells of pI mice was reduced to 0.85%, i.e., 60% of the level found in pII mice (Table 1). As indicated in Figure 2b, the pol I promoter did not have any significant impact on the distribution of point mutations compared to pol II promoter controlled hypermutation.

Identical hotspots were found in VHB1-8 genes of pII and pI mice, notably at position 31II, 65II and 105II of the VHB1-8 gene (numbering according to Kabat and Wu, (1991). These codons are typical hotspots with a RGYW consensus motif (where R is a purine base [A or G], Y a pyrimidine base [C or T], and W is A or T). This motif is a salient feature of hotspots of somatic hypermutation (Rogozin and Kolchanov, 1992, Betz et al., 1993).

As for the base exchange pattern, A and G nucleotides change to another nucleotide more frequently than C and T in both the pII mice and the pI mice (Fig. 2a). These base substitution preferences are comparable to those seen in other passenger transgenes (Betz et al., 1993).

Fig. 2. a) Base exchange pattern of hypermutation and **b)** location of somatic mutations in the modified VHB1-8 gene in pΔ, pI and pII mice. The point mutations found in the VHB1-8 gene of memory B cells are given as percentage of mutations per codons sequenced and are plotted against the position of VHB1-8 gene (numbering according to Kabat and Wu, (1991); point mutations in the leader intron and JH2 intron are also given). Percentages were calculated from 8 mutated sequences of pΔ mice, 14 of pI mice and 12 of pII mice.

a)

p II

from \ to (n=103)	A	G	C	T	%
A		7	11	14	31
G	15		10	4	28
C	3	9		14	25
T	5	6	5		16

p I

from \ to (n=72)	A	G	C	T	%
A		13	0	6	27
G	14		6	4	33
C	4	4		8	22
T	3	2	8		18

p Δ

from \ to (n=12)	A	G	C	T	%
A		1	1	1	25
G	1		0	0	8
C	1	0		6	59
T	1	0	0		8

b)

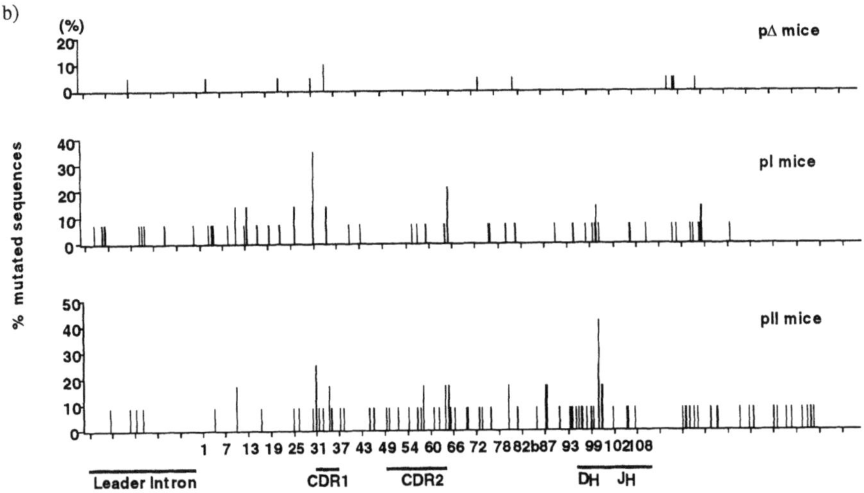

Somatic Hypermutation Correlates with the Level of Mutant VHB1-8 Specific Pre-mRNA in GC B Cells

To explore a possible relation between somatic hypermutation and transcriptional activity at the IgH locus, we determined the pre-mRNA and mRNA levels of the mutant B1-8 transgenes in GC-derived B cells by comparative RT-PCR (Klein et al., 1997). Using random hexamers, cDNA libraries were synthesised from total RNA isolated from 1 x 10^5 $CD45R^+$ PNA^{high} B cells from each of the mutant mice. Two sets of oligonucleotides were designed such that they specifically primed the mutant VHB1-8 and the β-actin cDNAs, respectively. In both cases the conditions for the amplification were chosen such that the accumulation of products was in the exponential phase. PCR products were gel-fractionated, blotted onto a nylon-membrane and hybridised with a ^{32}P-labelled VHB1-8 or β-actin probes. The 322 bp amplificates of the β-actin cDNA served as an internal standard to normalise the expression level of the VHB1-8 product. For the VHB1-8 cDNA, two PCR products of different size were observed in all three mutant strains (Fig. 3A). As confirmed by sequencing, the 265 bp fragment corresponded to the pre-mRNA of VHB1-8 and the 183 bp fragment to the mRNA, lacking the 82 bp leader intron of VHB1-8 (Fig. 3B). The ratio between the 265 bp and 183 bp fragments was similar in all samples. This argues against possible contamination of the samples by genomic DNA, as this would have favoured the amplification of the 265bp fragment only.

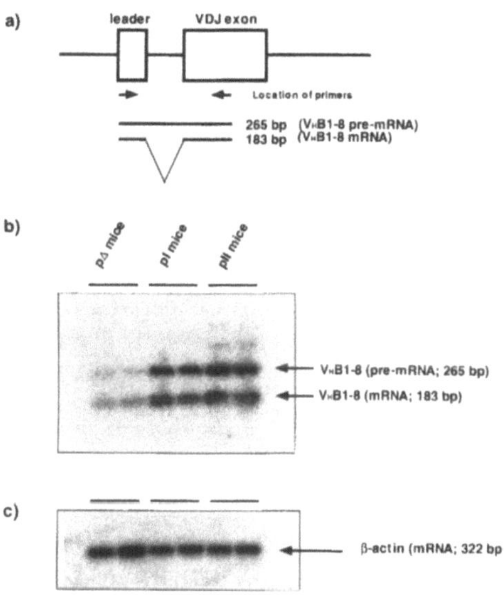

Fig. 3. Comparative PCR of cDNAs generated from splenic B220+PNAhigh B cells from pΔ, pI and pII mice. (a) Schematic figure illustrating the PCR approach to amplify the cDNA species from the mRNA and pre-mRNA of the VHB1-8 genes. Boxes indicate the leader exon and VHDHJH exon of the inserted VHB1-8 gene. Arrows indicate the location of primers used for the amplification of VHB1-8 cDNA. The thick lines labelled with 265 bp and 183 bp represent the coding sequence of the pre-mRNA and mRNA, respectively. The thin line indicates the leader intron. (b) Southern blot analysis of amplified cDNA corresponding to VHB1-8 genes from the mutant mice. Experiments were performed in duplicate. The upper band corresponds to pre-mRNA of VHB1-8 genes and the lower band to mRNA of VHB1-8 genes. The sizes of the bands are indicated. (c) Southern blot analysis of cDNA corresponding to the β-actin gene transcripts from the mutant mice. In (b) and (c), 5,000 cell equivalents of cDNA mixture were amplified in separate reaction with VHB1-8 and β-actin primers.

Normalisation of the intensity of each band of the pΔ mice and the pI mice against the corresponding bands of pII mice revealed that the level of pre-mRNA was 8% and 72% and the level of mRNA 23% and 87%, respectively (Table 1). As splicing of pre-mRNA is usually an efficient process and occurs rapidly after transcription (Zhang et al., 1994), the relatively high ratio of pre-mRNA versus mRNA levels in this study is surprising, but may be due to the premature termination codon inserted into the VHB1-8 transgene (Cheng and Maquat, 1993; Peltz et al., 1994; Maquat, 1995; Lozano et al., 1994; Aoufouchi et al., 1996).

To compare the pre-mRNA levels with the frequency of somatic hypermutation, we set the values obtained from pII mice at 100 %. The pre-mRNA- rather than the mRNA-level was chosen, since the pre-mRNA level should relate more directly to the transcription rate (Zhang et al., 1994). The resulting relative mutation frequencies of the pΔ mice and the pI mice were 7% and 60%, respectively (Table 1). These numbers correlate roughly with the relative amounts of pre-mRNA, 8% and 72%, in the pΔ mice and pI mice, respectively (Table 1).

Although the promoter of the VHB1-8 gene was completely deleted in the pΔ mice, a noticeable level of passenger transgene-specific transcripts was found in the PNAhigh B cells (Fig. 3) and LPS stimulated B cells from these mice (data not shown). In all targeting experiments the downstream portion of the DQ52 promoter (Alessandrini and Desiderio, 1991; Kottmann et al., 1992; Kottmann et al., 1994), the DQ52 element and the JH locus were replaced by the modified VHB1-8 gene. According to in vitro studies on the DQ52 promoter (Kottmann et al., 1994), the truncated form of the DQ52 promoter, as present in the targeted alleles, is transcriptionally inactive. Since somatic hypermutation occurs preferentially in a 2 kb window downstream of a defined promoter (Lebecque and Gearhart, 1990; Peters and Storb, 1996; Rogerson, 1994; Rothenfluh et al., 1993; Weber et al., 1991) we predicted that the remaining truncated DQ52 promoter fragment had preserved a low transcriptional activity (Fukita et al., 1998). To identify the transcriptional start site(s) in the pΔVHB1-8 gene, we performed 5'RACE PCR using cDNA libraries generated from LPS-stimulated B cells of pII and pΔ mice and primers that specifically hybridise to the inserted transgenes. Sequence analysis of the cloned 5'RACE PCR products revealed the presence of transgene specific restriction sites and the remaining loxP site in the case of pΔ derived as well as the presence of the introduced stop codon in the leader exon of pII and pΔ derived 5'RACE PCR products. The predominant transcription initiation sites in the pΔ locus are at position -142 and -173 bp; in the pII locus transcription initiates at position -37, -39 and -41 of the ATG start codon, see vertical arrow heads in figure 1. Therefore, in contrast to previous analysis (Kottmann et al., 1994), the upstream region of the unique XhoI restriction site in the DQ52 promoter element described by Kottmann et al. is transcriptional active in LPS blasts and GC derived B cells and likely accounts for the low level of transcription as well as somatic mutations seen in the pΔVHB1-8 transgene.

Discussion

Somatic hypermutation occurs normally in a rearranged VHDHJH gene when targeted into its physiological position in the heavy chain locus (Taki et al., 1993). Consistent with these results, somatic hypermutation of the B1-8 passenger transgene in the IgH locus occurred normally with respect to frequency and distribution of point mutations and base exchange pattern. About 60% of the IgH passenger transgenes amplified from single class switched Vλ1+ memory B cells were mutated, a value which is reproducibly found in Vλ1 genes amplified from class switched Vλ1+ B cells of wild type and other mutant mouse strains (Jacobs et al., 1998). The possibility that the unmutated amplificates are due to a contamination with naive Igμ+λ1+ B cells is unlikely, since the sorted cells expressed high levels of the Vλ1 light chain at their surface and stained negative for

IgM- and IgD- specific mAb. Therefore, ~40 % of class switched Vλ1+ B cells likely carry unmutated VλJλ or VHDHJH gene segments.

Compared to the pII mice, the mutation frequency was decreased 15 fold in the promoter-deficient passenger transgene amplified from class switched Vλ1+ B cells isolated from pΔ mice (Table 1). The 15 fold decrease in the mutation frequency of the VHB1-8 gene in pΔ mice compared to pII mice is strikingly similar to the 12.5 fold decreased frequency of somatic hypermutation in DHJH rearrangements (0.2%) in comparison to functional VHDHJH joints in hybridoma cells (2.5%) (Roes et al., 1989). This similarity can be explained by the DQ52 promoter element, which is transcriptionally active in B cells of pΔ mice and in DQ52JH rearranged Ig genes. In conclusion, the truncated DQ52 promoter element in pΔ mice is transcriptionally active and this activity likely accounts for the low level of mutations seen in the VHB1-8 gene of memory B cells isolated from pΔ mice. The finding, that transcription initiates closely to the B1-8 passenger transgene also explains the normal distribution of the point mutations in the B1-8 passenger transgene of pΔ mice.

When analysing somatic hypermutation of the pol I promoter-controlled VHB1-8 passenger gene, the mutation frequency was 60% of that found in memory B cells of pII mice. To date promoter exchange experiments have analysed somatic hypermutation of Ig genes under the control the human β globin promoter (Betz et al., 1994) and the mouse B29 promoter (Tumas-Brundage and Manser, 1997). Both promoters are pol II-dependent, the enzyme known to control the synthesis of all precursor messenger RNA (pre-mRNA) in mammalian cells (Zawel and Reinberg, 1992; Zawel et al., 1995; Orphanides et al., 1996). In contrast, the pol I promoter controls the synthesis of the ribosomal RNA precursor in the nucleolus, which subsequently is processed into the 28S, 18S and 5S ribosomal RNA (rRNA) species (Reeder, 1990).

In analogy to pol II promoters, the pol I promoter has a bipartite organisation, an upstream control element (UCE) and a start site proximal core (Grummt and Skinner, 1985; Smale and Tjian, 1985). The UCE contains 13 repeats of a 140-bp element, which enhances the activity of the pol I promoter (Kuhn et al., 1990). Exchanging UCE by pol II transactivator sequences such as GAL4 DNA binding sites, E2 protein recognition sequences or an octamer motif, did not allow transcription from the core pol I promoter (Schreck et al., 1989), suggesting that the transactivation mechanism of pol I promoter-controlled genes is different from that of pol II promoter-controlled genes. However, when placing both elements of the bipartite pol I promoter upstream of the VHB1-8 gene, a high level of polyadenylated unspliced pre-mRNA and spliced mRNA was found in GC B cells. These observations suggest, that either the pol II transcription machinery can transcribe a pol I promoter-controlled heavy chain gene in the nuclcoplasm, or the primary transcripts are indeed synthesised by thc pol I transcription machinery and the altered subnuclear localisation of the polymerase I transcripts (nucleoplasm instead of nucleolus) allows the described posttranscriptional modifications. Since we cannot exclude either possibility, the question whether thc putative mutator is physically associated with the RNA polymerase II complex or the level of transcription just reflects the accessibility of the putative mutator to the IgH locus remains to be addressed.

We compared the relative levels of RNA expressed from the mutant VHB1-8 genes in GC (CD45R+ PNAhigh) B cells, taken ex vivo, using semi-quantitative RT-PCR. In these cells somatic hypermutation is known to be ongoing (Berek et al., 1991; Jacob et al., 1991). The relative frequency of somatic hypermutation correlated well with the relative pre-mRNA level of the passenger transgenes found in CD45R+ PNAhigh B cells isolated from the mutant strains. Since nonsense codons can reduce the abundance of nuclear mRNA without affecting the abundance of pre-mRNA or the half-life of cytoplasmic mRNA (Cheng and Maquat, 1993; Maquat, 1995; Peltz et al., 1994; Lozano et al., 1994), the relatively high VHB1-8 pre-mRNA levels may be due to the presence of a termination codon in the leader exons in the various VHB1-8 transgenes, resulting in a rapid degradation of the corresponding mRNA species. Alternatively, in a cell free system, a nonsense codon was found to inhibit RNA splicing irrespective of protein synthesis (Aoufouchi et al., 1996). The mechanism for this translation independent mechanism remains unclear.

According to previous findings the 5' boundary for somatic hypermutation is located at or near the transcription start site suggesting a linkage between transcription and somatic hypermutation (Lebecque and Gearhart, 1990; Peters and Storb, 1996; Rogerson, 1994; Rothenfluh et al., 1993; Weber et al., 1991,) . Furthermore, in case of the κ light chain gene, the κ intronic and 3' enhancers are critical cis-elements for hypermutation (Betz et al., 1994; Yelamos et al., 1995). The results presented in this report indicate that somatic hypermutation correlates with the transcriptional activity in the IgH locus. This result is expected, if the transcription machinery is physically associated with (part of) the hypermutator (Peters and Storb, 1996; Goyenechea et al., 1997). We had hoped to support this model by the demonstration that hypermutation is only seen in the case of pol II- and not pol I-dependent transcription. Its occurrence in both cases and the ambiguity of that result makes us unable to exclude the possibility that the apparent correlation of somatic hypermutation with the pre-mRNA levels might simply reflect the accessibility of the putative mutator to the IgH locus.

Acknowledgement

The authors like to thank Cell Press for permission to reproduce data described by Fukita et al., 1998. The authors are grateful to Dr I. Grummt for providing the mouse rDNA promoter/enhancer fragment. This work was supported by the Deutsche Forschungsgemeinschaft through SFB 243, the Land Nordrhein-Westfalen and the European Community (B104-CT96-0077). Y.F. and H.J. were supported by postdoctoral fellowships of the Alexander von Humboldt Foundation and the European Molecular Biology Organization, respectively. At present H.J. is working as a member at the Basel Institute for Immunology, which was founded and is supported by F. Hoffmann-La Roche Ltd, Basel, Switzerland.

Experimental Procedures

Identification of transcription initiation sites by 5'RACE PCR

Total RNA was isolated from LPS stimulated spleen cells derived from pI, pII and pΔ mice using anion exchange columns (Qiagen, Hilden, Germany). The transcription initiation sites were identified by 5'RACE PCR using the MarathonTM cDNA Amplification System (Clontech, Palo Alto, CA) in combination with the transgene specific primer (GSP) TGCTACCAAGAAGAGGATGAGT. PCR products were cloned into the pCR 2.1-TOPO Vector (Invitrogen, Leek, The Netherlands) and sequenced by dye terminator cycle sequencing (Perkin Elmer, Foster City, CA) and analysed using the Lasegene Navigator software (DNAstar).

Other methods
The generation of pI, pII and pΔ mice, cell separation, fluorescence activated cell sorting, single-cell PCR, and comparative RT-PCR analysis are described in detail (Fukita et al., 1998; Jacobs et al., 1998).

References

Alessandrini A, Desiderio SV (1991) Coordination of immunoglobulin DJH transcription and D-to-JH rearrangement by promoter-enhancer approximation. Mol Cell Biol 11: 2096-2107

Aoufouchi S, Yelamos J, Milstein C (1996) Nonsense mutations inhibit RNA splicing in a cell-free system: recognition of mutant codon is independent of protein synthesis. Cell 85:415-422

Betz AG, Milstein C, Gonzalez-Fernandez A, Pannell R, Larson T, Neuberger M S (1994) Elements regulating somatic hypermutation of an immunoglobulin kappa gene: critical role for the intron enhancer/matrix attachment region. Cell 77:239-248

Betz AG, Neuberger MS, Milstein C (1993) Discriminating intrinsic and antigen-selected mutational hotspots in immunoglobulin V genes. Immunol Today 14: 405-411

Cheng J, Maquat L E (1993) Nonsense codons can reduce the abundance of nuclear mRNA without affecting the abundance of pre-mRNA or the half-life of cytoplasmic mRNA. Mol Cell Biol 13:1892-1902

Fukita Y, Jacobs H, Rajewsky K (1998) Somatic Hypermutation in the Heavy Chain Locus Correlates with Transcription. Immunity 9: 105-114

Gonzalez-Fernandez A, Gupta SK, Pannell R, Neuberger MS, Milstein C (1994) Somatic mutation of immunoglobulin lambda chains: a segment of the major intron hypermutates as much as the complementarity-determining regions. Proc Natl Acad Sci U S A 91:12614-12618

Goyenechea B, Klix N, Yelamos J, Williams GT, Riddell A, Neuberger MS, Milstein C (1997) Cells strongly expressing Ig(kappa) transgenes show clonal recruitment of hypermutation: a role for both MAR and the enhancers. Embo J 16:3987-3994

Grummt I, Skinner JA. (1985) Efficient transcription of a protein-coding gene from the RNA polymerase I promoter in transfected cells. Proc Natl Acad Sci U S A 82:722-726

Jacobs H, Fukita Y, van der Horst GTJ, de Boer J, Weeda G, Essers J, de Wind N, Engelward BP, Samson L, Verbeek S, Ménissier de Murcia J, de Murcia G, te Riele H, Rajewsky K (1998) Hypermutation of Immunoglobulin Genes in Memory B cells of DNA repair-deficient Mice. J Exp Med 187:1735-1743

Kabat EA, Wu TT (1991) Identical V region amino acid sequences and segments of sequences in antibodies of different specificities. Relative contributions of VH and VL genes, minigenes, and complementarity-determining regions to binding of antibody-combining sites. J Immunol 147: 1709-1719

Klein U, Küppers R, Rajewsky, K (1997) Evidence for a large compartment of IgM-expressing memory B cells in humans. Blood 89:1288-1298

Kottmann AH, Brack C, Eibel H, Köhler, G (1992) A survey of protein-DNA interaction sites within the murine immunoglobulin heavy chain locus reveals a particularly complex pattern around the DQ52 element. Eur J Immunol 22:2113-2120

Kottmann AH, Zevnik B, Welte M, Nielsen PJ, Köhler G (1994) A second promoter and enhancer element within the immunoglobulin heavy chain locus. Eur J Immunol 24:817-821

Kuhn A, Deppert U, Grummt I (1990) A 140-base-pair repetitive sequence element in the mouse rRNA gene spacer enhances transcription by RNA polymerase I in a cell-free system. Proc Natl Acad Sci U S A 87:7527-7531

Lozano F, Maertzdorf B, Pannell R, Milstein C (1994). Low cytoplasmic mRNA levels of immunoglobulin kappa light chain genes containing nonsense codons correlate with inefficient splicing. Embo J 13:4617-4622

Maquat LE (1995) When cells stop making sense: effects of nonsense codons on RNA metabolism in vertebrate cells. Rna 1:453-465

Orphanides G, Lagrange T, Reinberg D (1996) The general transcription factors of RNA polymerase II. Genes Dev 10:2657-2683.

Peltz SW, He F, Welch E, Jacobson A (1994) Nonsense-mediated mRNA decay in yeast. Prog Nucleic Acid Res Mol Biol 47:271-298

Peters A, Storb U (1996) Somatic hypermutation of immunoglobulin genes is linked to transcription initiation. Immunity 4:57-65

Rada C, Yélamos J, Dean W, Milstein C (1997) The 5' hypermutation boundary of k chains is independent of local and neighbouring sequences and related to to the distance from the initiation of transcription. Eur J Immunol 27:3115-3120

Reeder RH (1990) rRNA synthesis in the nucleolus. Trends Genet 6:390-395

Roes J, Huppi K, Rajewsky K, Sablitzky F (1989) V gene rearrangement is required to fully activate the hypermutation mechanism in B cells. J Immunol 142:1022-1026

Rogerson BJ (1994) Mapping the upstream boundary of somatic mutations in rearranged immunoglobulin transgenes and endogenous genes. Mol Immunol 31:83-98

Rogozin IB, Kolchanov NA (1992) Somatic hypermutagenesis in immunoglobulin genes. II. Influence of neighbouring base sequences on mutagenesis. Biochim Biophys Acta 1171, 11-18

Rothenfluh HS, Taylor L, Bothwell AL, Both GW, Steele E.J (1993) Somatic hypermutation in 5' flanking regions of heavy chain antibody variable regions. Eur J Immunol 23, 2152-2159

Schreck R, Carey MF, Grummt I (1989) Transcriptional enhancement by upstream activators is brought about by different molecular mechanisms for class I and II RNA polymerase genes. Embo J 8:3011-3017

Smale ST, Tjian R (1985) Transcription of herpes simplex virus tk sequences under the control of wild-type and mutant human RNA polymerase I promoters. Mol Cell Biol 5:352-362

Taki S, Meiering M, Rajewsky K (1993) Targeted insertion of a variable region gene into the immunoglobulin heavy chain locus [see comments]. Science 262:1268-1271

Tumas-Brundage K, Manser, T (1997) The transcriptional promoter regulates hypermutation of the antibody heavy chain locus. J Exp Med 185:239-250

Wiesendanger M, Scharff MD, Edelman W (1998) Somatic Hypermutation, Transcription, and DNA Mismatch repair. Cell 94:415-418

Wood RD (1998) DNA repair: Knockouts still mutating after the first round. Curr Biology 8: 757-760

Yelamos J, Klix N, Goyenechea B, Lozano F, Chui YL, Gonzalez-Fernandez A, Pannell R, Neuberger MS, Milstein C (1995) Targeting of non-Ig sequences in place of the V segment by somatic hypermutation. Nature 376:225-229

Zawel L, Kumar, KP, and Reinberg, D (1995) Recycling of the general transcription factors during RNA polymerase II transcription. Genes Dev 9:1479-1490

Zawel L, Reinberg D (1992) Advances in RNA polymerase II transcription. Curr Opin Cell Biol 4:488-495

Zhang G, Taneja KL, Singer RH, Green MR (1994) Localization of pre-mRNA splicing in mammalian nuclei [see comments] Nature 372:809-812

Discussion

Una Chen: Regarding the vector design for targeting on the hypermutation, does that have a distance or orientation effect?
Heinz Jacobs: So far, in our targeting experiments we did not change the distance or the orientation of the promoter. But based on data published by A. Peters and U. Storb, it seems that the distance between promoter and enhancer is not so critical. The orientation of the promoter seems to be more critical, it has to point towards the enhancers.
Andreas Radbruch: If you interfere with the processing of the transcript, do you modulate the frequency of hypermutation? For example by splicing, what happens if you delete the splice acceptor site?
Heinz Jacobs: Yosho Fukita made one VHB1-8 knock-in mouse carrying an Ig gene with a mutated splice donor and acceptor and there was no effect on somatic hypermutation. This result fits with the finding that you can basically insert any DNA into this region – for instance a neo-gene which is not spliced but will undergo somatic hypermutation. So it is not at all dependent on splicing.
Riccardo Dalla-Favera: In your Pol-1 system, are you sure that transcription actually occurs where Pol-1 transcription occurs? Maybe the presence of the enhancer and the matrix attachment sites, and the distance enhancer, has made Pol-1 look like a Pol-2 terminal site?
Heinz Jacobs: That is exactly what I think. I don't expect that the Pol I heavy chain gene locates in the nucleolus. Most likely it is outside of the nucleolus and possibly transcribed by RNA polymerase I. We still have to address this issue. If the Pol I system is sensitive to alpha amanitin, this would argue for RNA polymerase II transcription. If, however, it is insensitive, we could argue that somatic hypermutation depends on transcription but not on the RNA polymerase II. This will exclude many factors, such as components of the TFIIH complex which have been implicated in somatic hypermutation.
Dirk Eick: Is something known about the transcription rate of Pol I and Pol II?
Heinz Jacobs: We haven't analyzed this yet in our system, but based on the literature the average Pol I activity is about two fold higher than Pol II (which is one reason why I chose it and not a Pol-III promoter). The fact that the pre-mRNA level in Pol II is somewhat higher than Pol I could be due to the relative high transcription rate of the heavy chain locus or due to an altered subnuclear localization of the Pol I promoter controlled heavy chain gene.
Jacques van Dongen: Can you say something about somatic hypermutation on the second allele, the non-functional allele, whether it occurs, whether the size of this mutational window is also 1.5kb? For instance, what happens in a D-J rearrangement, or a V-D rearrangement?
Heinz Jacobs: The targeted alleles are nonfunctional so-called 'passenger transgenes' and therefore the second allele must be functional and will mutate as well. In principle any transcribed and rearranged gene-segment should mutate in this 1.5 window if it is in a certain proximity to the enhancers.
Jacques van Dongen: If somatic hypermutation starts from the promoter site, would this mean that the D-J rearrangement can never be affected by somatic hypermutation?
Heinz Jacobs: It will be affected if the D segment has a promoter, as for example DQ52 in the mouse, which has a promoter.

Immunoglobulin Gene Associated Chromosomal Translocations in B-Cell Derived Tumors

G. Klein
Microbiology and Tumor Biology Center (MTC), Karolinska Institute, Stockholm, Sweden

My talk will be quite similar to the talk of Riccardo Dalla Favera, but while he emphasized diversity, I shall focus on common, unifying features.

It is quite extraordinary that certain B-cell derived tumors in three different species, Burkitt lymphoma (BL) in humans, plasmacytomas in mice (MPC) and the spontaneous immunocytomas (RIC) of the Louvain rat, although different with regard to cell type and developmental history, carry highly homologous Ig/myc translocations. Another rare feature is the virtually 100% association between each of the three tumor types and its translocations. The few exceptional MPCs that were translocation free on cytogenetic examination turned out to carry cryptic and often complex translocations that have led to the same result: juxtaposition of c-myc and Ig sequences.

Are there any common denominators in the pathogenetic history of the three tumors?

Chronic stimulation of cell division in the preneoplastic target cell appears as the only common feature. In BL, the combined action of EBV, known to immortalize activated immunoblasts and to persist, with a different expression pattern, in long lived resting B-cells, may act in concert with chronic hyper- or holoendemic malaria that can stimulate B and suppress T cells. In MPC, intraperitoneal, mineral oil induced or other foreign body granuloma is an essential prerequisite for tumor development. Only genetically susceptible BALB/c mice respond. RIC originates from the ileocoecal lymph nodes that drain the intestines of helminth infested rats. It produces mainly IgE, indicating that hypersensitization to parasite antigens may have triggered the proliferation of the small IgE+ B cell subfraction.

There is an interesting difference between B and T-cell lymphoma/leukemia associated translocations. Only some genes, mainly myc, bcl-1 and bcl-2, (and, more occasionally, bcl-3 or bcl-9) are involved in the human B cell translocations. Ig/myc is found in BL, Ig/bcl-1 in mantle cell lymphoma, Ig/bcl-2 in follicular lymphoma. A larger number and variety of genes can be juxtaposed to TCR sequences in acute T-cell leukemia. Myc is one of them but is only infrequently involved. Other partners include transcription factors, homeobox and other developmental genes.

Comparisons between lymphoma associated human and murine translocations reveal interesting similarities and contrasts. The myc gene is juxtaposed to a switch region in sporadic BL, MPC and RIC. In endemic BL, a D or J (and sometimes a V) region is preferentially affected. This has no known counterpart in the mouse. Another difference is provided by the fact that the extensively studied murine T-cell lymphomas have no known chromosome translocations. Numerical chromosome changes are frequent.

There is a curious geometrical difference between the typical and the variant Ig/myc translocations. The same difference is found in mice and in humans. In the typical (IgH/myc) translocations, the myc-carrying telomeric chromosome fragment moves to the broken end of the IgH chromosome. Since c-myc is oriented "head up", with its 5' end towards the centromere whereas IgH is "hanging down", with the 5' end towards the telomere, the two juxtaposed genes face each other head to head. Both are constitutively active in the translocation carrying cell. In variant translocations, c-myc stays in its original location. The chromosome break occurs 3' of the gene, often in the pvt-1 region, and the kappa or lambda carrying chromosome fragment joins the intact myc gene in a head to tail orientation. The reasons for this topographical difference may be sought in the fact that both kappa and lambda are oriented "head up" on the chromosome, like c-myc. Reciprocal exchanges of terminal chromosome fragments generate the configurations that are actually found.

The typical or IgH/myc translocations are in majority (about 80%) in both BL and MPC. In BL, the kappa and the lambda/myc translocations occur in about 10% each. Most of the variant translocations are kappa/myc in the mouse. The murine lambda/myc translocations were only discovered when MPCs were induced by a combination of pristane oil treatment and Abelson virus infection. Also, v-abl has increased the ratio of variant/to typical MPC associated translocations from about 10 to 40%. An exceptional N-myc/kappa translocation, the only known case where N-myc but not c-myc was activated, was also found in a pristane oil + Abelson virus treated mouse. The role of v-abl is not understood. It may be related to its strong immortalizing effect on pre-B cells. In that capacity, it might increase the number and life span of translocation-prone precursor cells. Neither v-abl, nor the Ig/myc translocations appear to interfere with plasma cell differentiation. Alternatively, or in addition, v-abl may rescue translocation carrying myc-driven cells from apoptotic death. It is known that v-abl has a bcl-2 independent antiapoptotic effect.

Fine Structure of the IgH/myc Translocations

There is a systematic difference in the IgH breakpoint distribution between the African, largely EBV carrying, and the sporadic, predominantly EBV negative BLs (see 1 for review). In endemic BL, the break usually affects a site in the VDJ region, whereas in sporadic BL, a switch region is most commonly involved. HIV-associated BL resembles sporadic BL. This difference may point to the stage in the B-cell life cycle when the translocations occur. The VDJ region may become translocation prone at the time of somatic V gene hypermutations, whereas an S region may be affected at the time of, or in preparation for class switching. In the mouse and rat plasmacytomas, a switch region is affected as a rule. Involvement of VDJ is extremely rare, if it occurs at all.

There is a certain statistical correlation between the preferably affected switch site and the most frequently produced immunoglobulin heavy chain class in the tumor. Smu is the preferred myc translocation site in sporadic BLs and IgM is the most frequent product. Most MPCs make IgA and Salpha is the most common breaksite. The majority of the RICs make IgE, with Sepsilon as the most frequent breaksite. This is in line with the established fact that the switch recombinases affect both IgH alleles in parallel and with the idea that translocations are generated by faulty class switching.

New Hypotheses on Translocation Mechanisms

Two new mechanisms have been proposed to explain two kinds of translocations that involve the VDJ region. The first hypothesis is based on the findings of Gellert's group [2] and the parallel, independent findings of Schatz' group [3]. They have shown that the VDJ recombinase can function as a transposase, by catalyzing the intermolecular transposition of DNA segments *in vitro*. Pieces of DNA can be inserted into other DNA molecules in a RAG-dependent fashion. Gellert and his colleagues have suggested that the RAG enzymes may be responsible for some types of chromosomal translocations. Previously, it has been assumed that translocations may occur when a DNA double strand break occurs within an IgH locus during VDJ recombination (as also in class switching), concomitantly with a DNA double strand break on another chromosome, e.g. in the major breakpoint regions of the bcl-1 or the bcl-2 gene. The new findings offer another explanation. It was suggested [2] that intermediate products of the RAG-mediated VDJ recombination with DNA double strand breaks can attack other, **intact** DNA molecules. The RAG enzymes can catalyze their insertion into other DNA sites. This may result in a chromosomal translocation. The DNA break would occur within a few bp of a recombination signal sequence (RSS). The lymphoid specific RAG-1 and 2 factors initiate VDJ recombination by introducing a double strand DNA break adjacent to the RSS at the border with the coding DNA, producing a blunt cut signal end and a hairpin coding end. The later processing and joining of cleaved signal ends and coding ends is carried out largely by cellular factors involved in the repair of double strand DNA breaks. Coding ends are processed and joined rapidly, forming imprecise coding joints. In contrast, signal ends can persist for many hours before they are ligated to form precise signal joints, possibly because they remain bound by the RAG proteins.

The 11;14 (bcl-1/IgH) translocations in mantle cell lymphoma and the 14;18 (bcl-2/IgH) translocations in follicular cell lymphoma join the partner gene directly to an RSS equipped JH segment. This is consistent with the postulated mechanism. A similar mechanism may occur in T cell lymphomas where a TCR alpha, beta or delta locus is affected. Both types of translocations are conceivably generated by a transposition of an RSS of an Ig or TCR locus to a random site on another chromosome. Tumor development then becomes a matter of secondary changes and selection.

The IgH/myc translocations in endemic BL are different. The translocation breakpoints are widely scattered . They affect V genes and adjacent regions that serve as the site of somatic hypermutation. They are usually **not** near to any RSS or RSS-like elements or any other characteristic motifs but are located in J intron sequences or within rearranged VJ genes. Küppers and his colleagues have suggested that translocations targeted into fully rearranged and somatically mutated V region genes occur as the consequences of aberrant somatic hypermutation [4]. The frequent occurrence of deletions and duplications in mutated V region genes, generated by DNA strand breaks, may involve the danger of chromosomal translocations, probably occurring in the germinal center. A similar mechanism may be responsible for bcl-8 translocations.

Interestingly, VDJ-involving myc translocations of the type seen in endemic BL have not been encountered in the mouse. This may relate to the fact that the somatic hypermutations of the mouse V genes are largely due to point mutations.

Translocations in Non-neoplastic Tissues

If potentially tumorigenic translocations are continuously generated by the accidents of normal immunoglobulin rearrangement, they should be detectable in non-neoplastic tissues. PCR technology has permitted the full verification of this postulate. Limpens et al [5] have detected 14;18 IgH(bcl2) translocations in the majority of healthy blood donors. Some individuals have carried 2 to 5 different 14;18 translocation carrying B-cell clones. Ig/myc translocations have also been detected in HIV-infected and, to a lesser extent, in normal persons [6] but the most extensive information is available in the mouse [7,8,9]. IgH/myc (12;15) translocations have been found not only in normal, plasmacytoma susceptible BALB/c mice, but also in MPC-resistant strains. In BALB/c they were detected in a higher frequency, but it could not be decided whether this is due to a difference in translocation incidence, and/or the expansion of translocation carrying clones.

If it is assumed that the Ig/myc translocations occur in both MPC induction susceptible and resistant strains, the extraordinary susceptibility of BALB/c must have posttranslocational reasons. The first question is whether the major BALB/c susceptibility factor acts at the level of the tumor precursor cell or at some modifying, extracellular level (e.g. at the cytokine secretion pattern from the oil granuloma). This was answered by an experiment of Silva et al several years ago [10]. Reciprocal chimeras between BALB/c and the MPC resistant DBA/2 strain were treated with pristane. They were susceptible to MPC induction, but the plasmacytomas originated exclusively from the BALB/c cells. The susceptibility of the BALB/c mice must be therefore determined at the cellular level.

Three or four genes influencing MPC susceptibility are segregating in crosses between BALB/c and resistant strains [10] but the p16 variant carried by BALB/c and deficient in its ability to bind to CDK4 is currently the most important candidate at the cellular level [12] , and Beverly Mock, this volume). The findings suggest an impaired tumor suppressor function of the BALB/c variant. p16 is known to act through the pRB system. Its dysfunction may increase the resistance of the myc-driven cells to growth-arresting signals. This may not be the only relevant difference, however. It is also noteworthy that the IgH/myc translocations detected by PCR in normal or precancerous BALB/c tissues show little or any sequence losses around the breakpoint. In contrast, the developing MPCs show extensive remodellings and losses. This may relate to the DNA repair defects found in BALB/c [14].

It thus appears that myc activation by chromosomal translocation and at least one additional, apoptosis antagonizing event are the **minimum requirements** for MPC development. They are not sufficient, however. As shown by Silva (this volume), pristane treated MPC resistant bcl-2 transgenic C57Bl mice carry detectable 12;15 translocation carrying plasma cells in their peritoneal fluid but fail to develop MPC, in spite of the fact that the bcl-2 transgene is known to raise the apoptotic threshold and to favor MPC development in pathogen free BALB/c mice. Additional, BALB/c associated genetic factors may be required as also indicated by the analysis of segregating crosses [11], as already mentioned. The telomeric portion of chromosome 4 that contains p16 has two additional, linked but distinct susceptibility genes (Beverly Mock, this volume).

Susceptibility to Burkitt lymphoma is not known to be influenced by genetic factors. The Ig/myc translocation is associated with the tumor in virtually 100% and must be therefore seen as a bottleneck, **sine qua non** event. There are several, potentially relevant additional changes in most BL tumors. They include p53 mutations [15], p16 silencing by methylation [16], and bax mutations [17]. They may counteract apoptosis and/or remove cell cycle regulatory controls. This is probably mandatory for BL development. The cell of origin, a GC centroblast or centrocyte, is programmed for apoptotic death, unless it receives an antiapoptotic signal. In contrast to EBV-transformed B blasts of normal origin where apoptosis is counteracted by the activation of the CD40 pathway by LMP2 and the elevation of the bcl-2 level, the myc driven BL cell is highly apoptosis prone. This cell phenotype dependent contrast is also reflected by the fact that even long propagated LCLs lack p53 mutations and p16 silencing.

Conclusions

1. Human and rodent B-cell tumor associated translocations appear to be generated continuously, as accidents of normal immunoglobulin rearrangement. The following three mechanisms have been identified so far:

   i. Recombination signal sequence (RSS)-led, transposon like invasion of other chromomes by VDJ sequences. Examples: IgH/bcl-1 and IgH/bcl-2 only found in humans.

   ii. V-gene hypermutation associated rearrangements in memory B-cells, postulated to generate IgH/myc translocations in endemic BL. Not found in mice where point mutations, not associated with rearrangements, are responsible for somatic hypermutation.

   iii. IgH/myc translocations involving an S region, attributed to faulty class switching. Examples: sporadic BL, AIDS-associated BL, mouse plasmacytoma, rat immunocytoma.

2. If translocations are continuously generated, tumor development must depend on posttranslocational changes. The exceptional susceptibility of the BALB/c mouse strain to MPC may be due, at least in part, to a functionally defective p16 isoform. In BL, p53 mutations, p16 silencing and bax deletions may contribute to apoptosis resistance and/or the escape from cell cycle regulatory controls.

References

1. Magrath, I. (1990) The pathogenesis of Burkitt's lymphoma. Advances in Cancer Research, 55:133-270.
2. Hiom K. Melek M, Gellert M (1998) DNA transposition by the RAG1 and RAG2 proteins: a possible source of oncogenic translocations. Cell 94:463-470.
3. Agrawall A. Eastman Q. Schatz D. (1998) Transposition mediated by RAG1 and RAG2 and its implications for the evolution of the immune system. Nature 394:744-751.
4. Goossens T. Klein U. Küppers R. (1998) Frequent occurrence of deletions and duplications during somatic hypermutation:Implications for oncogene translocations and heavy chain disease. Proc. Natl. Acad. Sci.USA 95:2463-2468.
5. Limpens J. Stad R. Vos C. de Vlaam C. de Jong D. van Ommen GJ. Schuuring E. Kluin PM. (1995) Lymphoma-associated translocation t(14;18) in blood B cells of normal individuals. Blood 85;2528-36.
6. Müller J. Janz S. Goedert J. Potter M. Rabkin C. (1995) Persistence of immunoglobulin heavy chain/c-*myc* recombination-positive lymphocyte clones in the blood of human immunodeficiency virus-infected homosexual men. Proc. Natl. Acad. Sci. USA 92:6577-6581.
7. Janz S. Muller J. Shaughnessy J. Potter M. (1993) Detection of recombinations between c-myc and immunoglobulin switch alpha in murine plasma cell tumors and preneoplastic lesions by polymerase chain reaction. Proc. Natl. Acad. Sci. USA 90:7361-5.
8. Müller J. Mushinski E. Williams J, Hausner P. (1997) Immunoglobulin/myc recombinations in murine Peyer's patch follicles. Genes, Chromosomes & Cancer 20:1-8.
9. Roschke V. Kopantzev E. Dertzbaugh M. Rudikoff S. (1997) Chromosomal translocations deregulating c-myc are associated with normal immune responses. Oncogene 14:3011-3016.
10. Silva, S. Sugiyama H. Babonits M. Wiener F. Klein G. (1991) Differential susceptibility of BALB/c and DBA/2 cells to plasmacytoma induction in reciprocal chimeras. International Journal of Cancer 49:224-228.
11. Mock BA. Krall MM. Dosik JK. (1993) Genetic mapping of tumor susceptibility genes involved in mouse plasmacytomagenesis. Proc. Natl. Acad. Sci. USA 90:9499-94503.
12. Zhang S. Ramsay E. Mock B. (1998) Cdkn2a, the cyclin-dependent kinase inhibitor encoding $p16^{INK4a}$ and $p19^{ARF}$, is a candidate for the plasmacytoma susceptibility locus, Pctr1. Proc. Natl. Acad. Sci. USA 95: 2429-2434.
13. Müller J. Janz S. Potter M. (1995) Differences between Burkitt's lymphomas and mouse plasmacytomas in the immunoglobulin heavy chain/c-myc recombinations that occur in their chromosomal translocations. Cancer Research 55:5012-5018.
14. Beecham EJ. Mushinski JF. Shacter E. Potter M. Bohr VA. (1991) DNA repair in c-myc proto-oncogene locus: possible involvement in susceptibility or resistance to plasmacytoma induction in BALB/c mice. Molecular & Cellular Biology 11:3095-104.
15. Wiman KG. Magnusson KP. Ramqvist T. Klein G. (1991) Mutant p53 detected in a majority of Burkitt lymphoma cell lines by monoclonal antibody Pab240. Oncogene 6:1633.
16. Klangby U. Okan I. Magnusson KP. Wendland M. Lind P. Wiman KG. (1998) p16/INK4a and p15/INK4b gene methylation and absence of p16/INK4a mRNA and protein expression in Burkitt's lymphoma. Blood 91:1680-1687.
17. Brimmell M. Mendiola R. Mangion J. Packham G. (1998) BAX frameshift mutations in cell lines derived from human haemopoietic malignancies are associate with resistance to apoptosis and microsatellite instability. Oncogene 16:1803-1812.

Analysis of B-cell Neoplasias by Spectral Karyotyping (SKY)

E. Hilgenfeld[1,2], H. Padilla-Nash[1], E. Schröck[1] and T. Ried[1]
[1]Genetics Department, Division of Clinical Sciences, National Cancer Institute (NCI), National Institutes of Health (NIH), Bethesda, MD, USA
[2]Innere Medizin A, Westfälische Wilhelms-Universität Münster, Germany

Abstract

B-cell neoplasias represent a heterogeneous group of diseases, including acute lymphocytic leukemia (ALL) and the broad spectrum of non-Hodgkin's lymphomas (NHL). Conventional cytogenetic analysis has revealed specific chromosomal aberrations in ALL as well as in NHL. Spectral karyotyping (SKY) is a novel molecular cytogenetic technique which allows the visualization of all human chromosomes in different colors, therefore greatly facilitating the recognition of chromosomal aberrations. The potential of SKY is exemplified by the fact that in our experience, 70% of the cases analyzed resulted in karyotypes where the majority of aberrations were either refined or new aberrations were detected when compared to their G-banding karyotypes. This also applies to the analysis of B-cell neoplasias. In hematologic malignancies, especially acute leukemias, specific chromosomal aberrations are of etiologic as well as diagnostic and prognostic importance. The identification of new recurrent chromosomal aberrations could therefore lead to a better characterization of disease entities or subgroups in ALL and NHL and further improve diagnosis, treatment stratification and ultimately prognosis. Interestingly, the comparison of the pattern of chromosomal aberrations in hematological neoplasias and carcinomas revealed striking differences. While about 50% of the aberrations in hematological malignancies are balanced translocations, such aberrations are exceedingly rare in epithelial cancers in which unbalanced structural and numerical aberrations prevail.

Introduction

In contrast to epithelial neoplasias, balanced translocations are frequently detected in hematological malignancies. Two main mechanisms have been observed by which these balanced translocations detected in leukemias and lymphomas result in an altered gene function. The first mechanism leads to a fusion of coding sequences of, in most instances, a transcription factor or receptor tyrosine kinase gene to an unrelated gene resulting in a chimeric protein with oncogenic properties. This mechanism is most common in myeloid leukemias. The second mechanism, characteristic of lymphoid neoplasias, repositions transcriptional control genes to the vicinity of promoter/enhancer elements of the immunoglobulin genes, thereby leading to deregulated gene expression (Ong and Le Beau, 1998, Look, 1998).

The importance of this latter mechanism has become clear by the detection of the activation of the *MYC* proto-oncogene through its juxtaposition to the immunoglobulin heavy chain locus (IgH) in the translocation t(8;14)(q24;q32) first detected in Burkitt's lymphoma (Taub et al., 1982).
In acute lymphocytic leukemia (ALL) as well as non-Hodgkin's lymphoma (NHL) recurrent specific somatically acquired genetic alterations have been detected. In ALL these specific chromosomal aberrations correlate with immunophenotypical features, response to therapy as well as clinical course and are therefore of diagnostic, prognostic and therapeutic importance. The detection of these chromosomal aberrations at diagnosis has become crucial for risk-adapted therapy in childhood as well as adult ALL (review in Faderl et al., 1998).
The most common genetic abnormality occurring in pediatric lymphoid leukemias of B-lineage (approx. 25%) is the recently detected translocation t(12;21)(p13;q22), which gives rise to the TEL-AML1 fusion gene (Golub et al., 1995). This translocation is rarely detected by routine karyotyping because the telomeric segments of 12p and 21q are indistinguishable in G-banded metaphases. This aberration is associated with a good prognosis and is a prognostic factor independent of other features associated with a favorable course in ALL (Look, 1998).
In B-NHL, approximately 90% of the cases exhibit chromosomal aberrations and in 70 % of the translocations described in B-cell neoplasias, the IgH-locus (14q32) is involved. A number of non-random abnormalities correlate with clinical, morphologic and immunophenotypic features, but this relationship is further advanced in leukemias than in any other malignancy. In NHL specific genetic correlates have not been identified in every currently recognized clinical entity (Ong and Le Beau, 1998).
Historically, cytogenetic analysis has relied solely on chromosome banding techniques. SKY is a new molecular cytogenetic method which greatly assists in the identification of marker chromosomes, subtle translocations and complex chromosomal rearrangements (Schröck et al., 1996). The value of SKY for improved karyotyping of malignant cells has been amply demonstrated (Veldman et al., 1997, Ning et al., 1998, Rao et al., 1998, Sawyer et al., 1998, Macville et al., 1999, Padilla-Nash et al., submitted). SKY has proven invaluable for the reconstruction of highly rearranged karyotypes in epithelial cancers as well as leukemias and lymphomas.

Material and Methods

Metaphase preparation was performed according to standard cytogenetic protocols. The multiple myeloma cell lines and fixed cell suspensions of the clinical cases were kindly provided by Drs. Michael Kuehl and Oskar Haas.
SKY painting probes were prepared from flow-sorted chromosomes kindly supplied by Dr. Johannes Wienberg and Prof. Malcolm Ferguson-Smith. The labeling, hybridization and detection protocols used were described in Macville et al. (1997). SKY image acquisition was performed as previously described in Schröck et al. (1996). Aberrations were designated according to the guidelines in ISCN 1995 (Mitelman et al. 1995).

Results and Discussion

There are technological limitations in evaluating malignant cells when relying exclusively on conventional cytogenetic banding techniques. For example, the discovery of the translocation t(12;21), the most common translocation in pediatric ALL, became only possible by chromosome painting (FISH) (Romana et al., 1994) and, by G-banding analysis, 44% of ALL cases appear to be karyotypically normal or display no recurrent translocations (Look, 1998). As SKY continues to uncover new translocations, balanced as well as unbalanced, with unprecedented accuracy, the identification of new aberrations and new recurring breakpoints becomes feasible. Thus far, 35 % of all aberrations detected in 30 cases of hematological malignancies and 45 % of the aberrations described in 115 solid tumors and the respective cell lines were newly identified when comparing the SKY data with the results of the G-banding analysis (Fig.1).

Fig. 1:

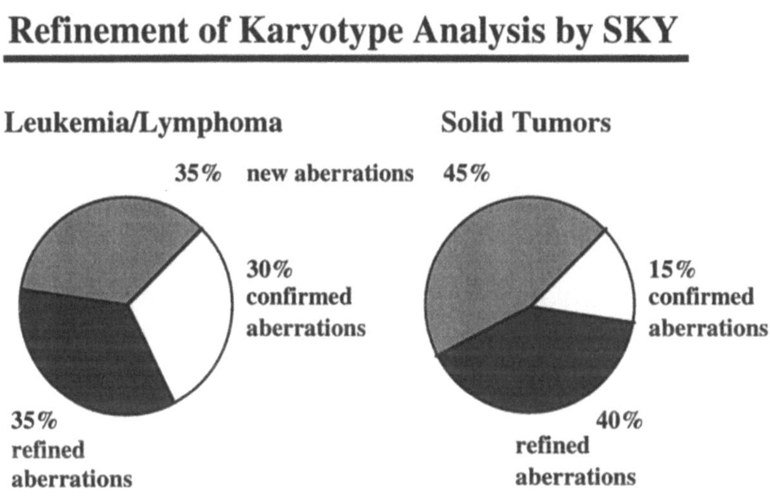

Within our series of hematological malignancies studied by SKY, we analyzed six cases of B-ALL and NHL. Five of them were previously studied by G-banding elsewhere and revealed a complex karyotype. Furthermore, two multiple myeloma cell lines, H929 and OPM2, have been characterized. The G-banding analysis of these cell lines has previously been described (Katagiri et al., 1985, Gazdar et al., 1986).

In the ALL/NHL cases, 64 structural and 13 numerical aberrations were detected by SKY in comparison to 58 structural and 19 numerical aberrations identified by G-banding. In total, 41 new aberrations (53 %) were identified, 24 were refined (31 %) and 12 aberrations (16 %) were confirmed. 36 structural aberrations (56 % of the structural aberrations, 47 % of all aberrations) were newly detected by SKY and 22 structural aberrations were redefined (34 % of the structural aberrations, 29 % overall). Only 4 structural aberrations described by G-banding were confirmed (6 %, overall 5 %).

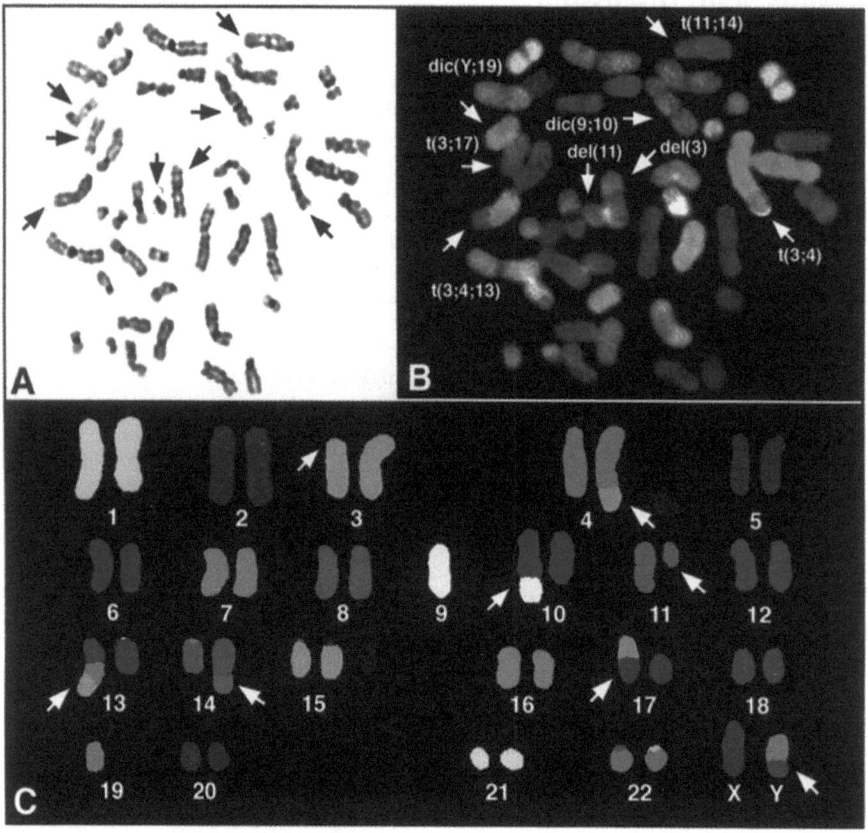

Fig. 2. SKY karyotype of a patient with Non-Hodgkin's Lymphoma (NHL). In (A) a G banded metaphase spread is shown. Arrows point to the abnormal chromosomes. (B) is the same metaphase spread following hybridization with 24 color, combinatorially labeled chromosome paints prepared from flow-sorted human chromosomes. In C the metaphase spread has been karyotyped and is displayed in classification colors. Arrows identify the numerous translocations and deletions.

In our cases SKY detected 17 balanced and 28 unbalanced translocations in comparison to only 5 balanced and 1 unbalanced translocation identified by G-banding. These results again confirm the power of this technique to detect novel structural aberrations, especially chromosomal translocations, and resolve complex karyotypes. Figure 2 presents the SKY-Analysis of a NHL-case whose complex karyotype was fully clarified by SKY. Of note, the add(14q) seen by G-banding analysis was identified as a t(11;14)(q13;q32).
Conversely, our SKY analysis of 9 cell lines from pancreatic carcinomas revealed 144 aberrations, only 6 of which were balanced translocations, none of them recurring (Ghadimi et al., in press). In our hands, the application of SKY to metaphase chromosomes prepared from breast, cervical, pancreatic and colorectal carcinomas (Schröck et al., 1996, Macville et al., 1999, Ghadimi et al., in press) and the comparison of the SKY results with data obtained by comparative genomic hybridization (CGH) has identified a pattern of chromosomal aberrations that is clearly distinct from the one observed in acute leukemias. It has become obvious that balanced chromosomal translocations are rare in carcinomas. This could indicate that the translocation induced activation of oncogenes or generation of a chimeric protein with oncogenic properties is less important for carcinogenesis, and that gains or losses of function of oncogenes or tumor suppressor genes, respectively, via unbalanced structural or numerical chromosomal aberrations, define the disturbance of the genetic equilibrium that triggers malignant transformation in epithelial cancers.
However, in hematological malignancies recurring numerical and unbalanced structural aberrations, especially deletions, have also been detected. Therefore, especially in NHL, the relevance of tumor suppressor genes and a resulting multistep process has been proposed for lymphomagenesis (Ong and Le Beau, 1998).
As SKY allows a comprehensive cytogenetic analysis of unprecedented accuracy, the identification of new recurrent chromosomal aberrations in B-cell neoplasias could lead to a better characterization of disease entities or subgroups and further improve diagnosis, treatment stratification and ultimately prognosis. Furthermore, SKY contributes to the clarification of specific patterns of chromosomal aberrations and therefore to our understanding of malignant transformation and biological course of the disease.

Acknowledgements

The authors wish to thank Dr. O. Haas and Dr. T. Gribbon for providing the clinical cases as well as Dr. W.M. Kuehl for kindly providing material of the multiple myeloma cell lines.

References

Faderl S, Kantarjian HM, Talpaz M, Estrov Z (1998) Clinical significance of cytogenetic abnormalities in adult acute lymphoblastic leukemia. Blood 91: 3995-4019

Gazdar AF, Oie HK, Kirsch IR, Hollis GF (1986) Establishment and characterization of human plasma cell myeloma culture having rearranged cellular *myc* proto-oncogene. Blood 67: 1542-1549

Ghadimi BM, Schröck E, Walker RL, Wangsa D, Jauho A, Meltzer PS, Ried T Specific chromosomal aberrations and amplification of the AIB1 nuclear receptor coactivator gene in pancreatic carcinomas Am J Path (in press)

Golub TR, Barker GF, Bohlander SK, Hiebert SW, Ward DC, Bray-Ward P, Morgan E, Raimondi SC, Rowley JD, Gilliland DG (1995) Fusion of the TEL gene on 12p13 to the AML 1 gene on 21q22 in acute lymphoblastic leukemia. Proc Natl Acad Sci USA 92: 4917-4921

Katagiri S, Yonezawa T, Kuyama J, Kanayama Y, Nishida K, Abe T, Tamaki T Ohnishi M, Tarui S (1985) Two distinct human myeloma cell lines originating from one patient with myeloma. Int J Cancer 36: 241-246

Look AT (1998) Genes altered by chromosomal translocations in leukemias and lymphomas. in: Vogelstein B, Kinzler KW (eds.) The genetic basis of human cancer. McGraw-Hill, New York

Macville M, Veldman T, Padilla-Nash H, Wangsa D, O'Brien P, Schröck E, Ried T (1997) Spectral karyotyping, a 24-colour FISH technique for the identification of chromosomal rearrangements. Histochem Cell Biol 108: 299-305

Macville M, Schröck E, Padilla-Nash H, Keck C, Ghadimi B, Zimonjic D, Popescu N, Ried T (1999): Comprehensive and definitive molecular cytogenetic characterization of HeLa Cells by spectral karyotyping. Cancer Res 59: 141-150

Mitelman F (ed) (1995): ISCN 1995: An international system for human cytogenetic nomenclature. Karger AG, Basel

Ning Y, Liang JC, Nagarajan L, Schröck E, Ried T (1998) Characterization of 5q deletions by subtelomeric probes and spectral karyotyping. Cancer genet Cytogenet 103: 170-172

Ong ST, Le Beau MM (1998) Chromosomal abnormalities and molecular genetics of non-Hodgkin's lymphoma. Semin Oncol 25: 447-460

Padilla-Nash H, Pirc-Danoewinata H, Hilgenfeld E, Ried T, Haas O, Schröck E Spectral Karyotyping resolves complex karyotypes in acute leukemias (submitted)

Rao PH, Cigudosa JC, Ning Y, Calasanz MJ, Iida S, Tagawa S, Michaeli J, Klein B, Dalla-Favera R, Jhanwar SC, Ried T, Chaganti RSK (1998) Multicolor Spectral Karyotyping identifies new recurring breakpoints and translocations in multiple myeloma. Blood 92: 1743-1748

Romana SP, Le Coniat M, Berger R (1994) t(12;21): A new recurrent translocation in acute lymphoblastic leukemia. Genes Chrom Cancer 9: 186-191

Sawyer JR, Lukacs JL, Munshi N, Desikan KR, Singhal S, Mehta J, Siegel D, Shaughnessy J, Barlogie B (1998) Identification of new nonrandom translocations in multiple myeloma with multicolor spectral karyotyping. Blood 92, 4269-4278

Schröck E, du Manoir S, Veldman T, Schoell B, Wienberg J, Ferguson-Smith MA, Ning Y, Ledbetter DH, Bar-Am I, Soenksen D, Garini Y, Ried T (1996) Multicolor Spectral Karyotyping of human chromosomes. Science 273: 494-497

Taub R, Kirsch I, Morton C, Lenoir G, Swan D, Tronick S, Aaronson S, Leder P (1982) Translocation of the c-myc gene into the immunoglobulin heavy chain locus in human Burkitt lymphoma and murine plasmocytoma cells. Proc Natl Acad Sci USA 79: 7837-7841

Veldman T, Vignon C, Schröck E, Rowley JD, Ried T (1997) Hidden chromosome abnormalities in haematological malignancies detected by multicolour spectral karyotyping. Nature Genetics 15: 406-410

Recurrent Non-reciprocal Translocations of Chromosome 5 in Primary T(12;15)-positive BALB/c Plasmacytomas

A. E. Coleman, T. Ried and S. Janz

Laboratory of Genetics, Division of Basic Sciences, NCI, NIH, Bethesda, MD, USA

Genome Technology Branch, NCHGR, NIH, Bethesda, MD, USA

Abstract

The majority of inflammation-induced peritoneal BALB/c plasmacytomas (≈ 90 %) harbor a balanced T(12;15) chromosomal translocation that deregulates the expression of the proto-oncogene c-*myc*. Recent evidence suggests that the T(12;15) is an initiating tumorigenic mutation that occurs in early plasmacytoma precursor cells. However, plasmacytomas take a long time to develop (average tumor latency ≈ 220 days), which suggests that additional tumor progression events may be required to complete oncogenesis. We hypothesized that such tumor progression events may take the form of secondary chromosomal aberrations that can be detected by spectral karyotyping (SKY). We screened the entire chromosome complement of 18 primary BALB/c plasmacytomas carrying the T(12;15) and found in nine tumors (50 % recurrence) secondary cytogenetic aberrations that involved bands D, E and F of chromosome (Chr) 5. The Chr 5D-F rearrangements were manifested predominantly as unbalanced translocations with various partner chromosomes. This finding led us to propose the existence of an important plasmacytoma progression locus in the central region of Chr 5, which presumably becomes involved in peritoneal plasmacytoma development by promiscuous chromosomal translocations.

Introduction

Secondary genetic changes have been postulated to occur in the course of inflammation-induced plasmacytoma development that takes place in the peritoneal cavity of genetically susceptible inbred BALB/c mice or hypersusceptible congenic C.D2-Idh1-Pep3 mice after treatment with the C19-isoalkane pristane [1] or certain tumorigenic silicone gels [7]. It seemed reasonable to hypothesize that secondary genetic alterations may include chromosomal aberrations that occur subsequently to the widely known c-*myc*-activating chromosomal translocation, T(12;15). The T(12;15) translocation has been shown to comprise a very early, if not initiating, oncogenic event during plasmacytoma development [3,5]. However, the postulated chromosomal abnormalities could not be detected thus far by conventional karyotype analysis. In fact, the only recurrent secondary cytogenetic change that has been found by G-banding is the trisomy 11 in a subset of virally induced plasmacytomas [6,11]. The main reason for the failure to detect additional chromosomal aberrations in inflammation-induced plasmacytomas might have been a technical one, namely the inherent difficulty and insensitivity of G-banding in the mouse. Mouse cells contain 20 acrocentric chromosomes that are similar in shape and size, and it is generally accepted that they are much harder to identify unambiguously than their human counterparts. To overcome the limitations of conventional cytogenetic analysis in the mouse, we applied a recently developed molecular cytogenetic method; i. e., spectral karyotyping (SKY). SKY is a genome-wide screening method that permits the visualization of each mouse chromosome in a different color [4,8]. All mouse chromosomes, including large chromosomal or extrachromosomal fragments, can be objectively identified by SKY, thus eliminating many of the uncertainties and ambiguities of conventional karyotyping of mouse tumors. In the study presented here, we utilized SKY to assess the entire chromosome complement of 18 primary inflammation-induced plasmacytomas harboring the balanced chromosomal translocation, T(12;15). The analysis revealed a diverse picture with respect to secondary cytogenetic changes: some tumors contained none but others contained one or several additional aberrations. The most interesting finding was that 9 out of 18 primary plasmacytomas contained alterations of Chr 5, which took predominantly the form of non-reciprocal translocations that joined Chr 5D-F with variable partner chromosomes in unbalanced promiscuous translocations.

Methods

Inflammation-induced Peritoneal Plasmacytomas

Plasmacytomas were induced by i.p. applications of pristane (2,6,10,14-tetramethylpentadecane) or small fragments of silicone gels. The tumors originated in genetically susceptible BALB/c or hypersusceptible C.D2-Idh1-Pep3 mice that were included in various plasmacytoma induction protocols. All plasmacytomas were subjected to cytogenetic analysis in consecutive order and no attempt was made to select for or exclude tumors, with the exception of those plasmacytomas for which a sufficient number of metaphase plates could not be obtained. SKY was performed to detect the presence of one of the c-*myc*-activating chromosomal translocations, the hallmark mutations of BALB/c plasmacytomas. A total of 18 tumors were found to contain the T(12;15) translocation and 9 tumors were shown to harbor the T(6;15) translocation. The T(12;15)$^+$ tumors were scrutinized for secondary cytogenetic aberrations, which were scored on the basis of 10 to 20 matching metaphase plates per tumor. We are still collecting the $T(6;15)^+$ plasmacytomas, which were less numerous during the sample acquisition period, to generate a group of tumors for cytogenetic analysis that is similar in size to the T(12;15)-harboring plasmacytomas.

Spectral Karyotyping (SKY)

SKY was performed as described elsewhere [4,8]. Briefly, mouse metaphase chromosomes were prepared from plasmacytoma cells obtained from the peritoneal exudate cell pellet of mice harboring primary tumors. Chromosome-specific painting probes were generated from flow-sorted chromosomes. DNA prepared from sorted chromosomes was amplified by DOP-PCR (degenerate oligonucleotide-primed PCR) incorporating haptenized or fluorochrome-conjugated nucleotides [9]. Labeled probes were hybridized *in situ* for three nights in the presence of a large excess of unlabelled Cot-1 fraction of mouse genomic DNA (BRL). Biotin- and digoxigenin-haptenized nucleotides of chromosome-specific probes were detected with avidin-conjugated Cy5 and antibody-conjugated Cy5.5 (using mouse anti-digoxigenin antibody sandwiched by goat anti-mouse antiserum), respectively. Chromosomes were counterstained with DAPI. Spectral analysis of chromosomes was carried out on an epifluorescence microscope (Leica DMRBE) that was equipped with a SD200 spectral cube (Applied Spectral Imaging) and a custom-designed filter cube (SKY1, Chroma Technology, Brattleboro, VT). This set-up permits the simultaneous excitation of all dyes and the measurement of their emission spectra. The spectral measurement of the hybridization was visualized by assigning a red, green and blue (RGB) look-up table to specific sections of the emission spectrum. The RGB display allows the assessment of important parameters of the hybridization, e.g., intensity and homogeneity. Based on the measurement of discrete emission spectra at all pixels of the image, the hybridization colors are then converted by applying a spectral classification algorithm that results in the assignment of a discrete color to all pixels with identical spectra. The spectral classification is the basis for chromosome identification and spectral karyotyping [2].

Results and Discussion

The entire chromosome complement of 18 peritoneal mouse plasmacytomas harboring the c-*myc*-deregulating chromosomal translocation, T(12;15), was analyzed by spectral karyotyping (SKY). Most tumors were analyzed at the G0 stage, except the plasmacytoma, TEPC 3610, which was examined in three consecutive *in vivo* passages in pristane-primed BALB/c mice in order to collect a sufficient number of metaphase plates for a reliable karyotype analysis. Both products of the reciprocal chromosomal translocation, T(12;15), were visualized readily by SKY in all 18 tumors; i. e., the large Chr T(12;15) containing the deregulated c-*myc* gene and the small Chr (15;12) thought to be irrelevant for plasmacytomagenesis. Most plasmacytomas contained two copies of Chr T(12;15) and/or Chr T(15;12), which can be explained most plausibly by a tetraploidization event subsequent to the translocation, as suggested earlier [10]. This explanation was strengthened by conventional karyotype analysis using DAPI- and G-banded metaphase spreads, which were prepared to complement SKY and determine the modal chromosome number. The plasmacytomas were found to be in the hyperdiploid to subtetraploid range. In 9 out of 18 tumors, recurrent aberrations were found in the central region of Chr 5 (Fig. 1). Four of the tumors were induced by silicone gels (SIPCs) and the remaining five were induced by tetramethylpentadecane (TEPCs). The Chr 5 aberrations occurred with a prevalence of 50 %. They appeared to cluster in the central region of the chromosome spanning bands D through F. The mapping of the aberrations to this region was based on the comparison of SKY-painted chromosomes with the inverted DAPI counterstains. This permitted in most situations the confident assignment of the affected chromosomal band. In some instances, however, the precision of that determination was not fully satisfactory and should be augmented in future studies with high-resolution G-banding, FISH and fiber FISH. The following commonalities among the Chr 5 alterations were noted. First, the great majority of aberrations involving Chr 5D-F took the form of non-reciprocal translocations; i. e., only one product of translocation was retained in the cell in which the illegitimate genetic exchange occurred. The exception to this observation was the balanced translocation, T(5;5), found in TEPC 3610. Second, most plasmacytomas were monoclonal with respect to aberrations involving Chr 5. The unusual tumor in that regard was plasmacytoma, TEPC 836, that contained two distinct clones of tumor cells with different types of Chr 5 rearrangements; i. e., a $T(5;6)^+$ clone and a $T(2;5)^+$ clone were co-detected. Third, all but one plasmacytomas harbored a single copy of the translocated Chr 5. The only exception to this rule was tumor, TEPC 420, which contained two copies of Chr T(5;X). Taken together, our findings suggest that Chr 5 harbors in its central portion a tumor progressor gene that appears to get involved in peritoneal plasmacytoma development by non-reciprocal translocation events. The identification of the putative plasmacytoma progressor locus on Chr 5 will be the subject of future studies in our laboratory.

References

1. Anderson PN, Potter M (1969) Induction of plasma cell tumors in BALB/c mice with 2,6,10,14-tetramethylpentadecane (pristane). Nature 222:994-995
2. Garini Y, Macville M, du Manoir S, Buckwald RA, Lavi M, Katzir N, Wine D, Bar-Am I, Schröck E, Cabib D, Ried T (1997) Spectral karyotyping. Bioimaging 5:1-8
3. Janz S, Müller J, Shaughnessy J, Potter M (1993) Detection of recombinations between c-*myc* and immunoglobulin switch α in murine plasma cell tumors and preneoplastic lesions by polymerase chain reaction. Proc Natl Acad Sci USA 90:7361-7365

4. Liyanage M, Coleman A, du Manoir S, Veldman T, McCormack S, Dickson RB, Barlow C, Wynshaw-Boris A, Janz S, Wienberg J, Ferguson-Smith MA, Schröck E, Ried T (1996) Multicolour spectral karyotyping of mouse chromosomes. Nat Genet 14:312-315
5. Müller JR, Potter M, Janz S (1994) Differences in the molecular structure of c-*myc*-activating recombinations in murine plasmacytomas and precursor cells. Proc Natl Acad Sci USA 91:12066-12070
6. Ohno S, Migita S, Wiener F, Babonits M, Klein G, Mushinski JF, Potter M (1984) Chromosomal translocations activating *myc* sequences and transduction of v-*abl* are critical events in the rapid induction of plasmacytomas by pristane and abelson virus. J Exp Med 159:1762-1777
7. Potter M, Morrison S, Wiener F, Zhang XK, Miller F W (1994) Induction of plasmacytomas with silicone gel in genetically susceptible strains of mice. J Natl Cancer Inst 86:1058-1065
8. Schröck E, du Manoir S, Veldman T, Schoell B, Wienberg J, Ferguson-Smith MA, Ning Y, Ledbetter DH, Bar-Am I, Soenksen D, Garini Y, Ried T (1996) Multicolor spectral karyotyping of human chromosomes. Science 273:494-497
9. Telenius H, Pelmear AH, Tunnacliffe A, Carter NP, Behmel A, Ferguson-Smith MA, Nordenskjold M, Pfragner R, Ponder BA (1992) Cytogenetic analysis by chromosome painting using DOP-PCR amplified flow-sorted chromosomes. Genes Chromosomes Cancer 4:257-263
10. Wiener F (1984) Chromosomal aberrations in murine plasmacytomas. Curr Top Microbiol Immunol 113:178-182
11. Wiener F, Coleman A, Mock BA, Potter M (1995) Nonrandom chromosomal change (trisomy 11) in murine plasmacytomas induced by an ABL-MYC retrovirus. Cancer Res 55:1181-1188

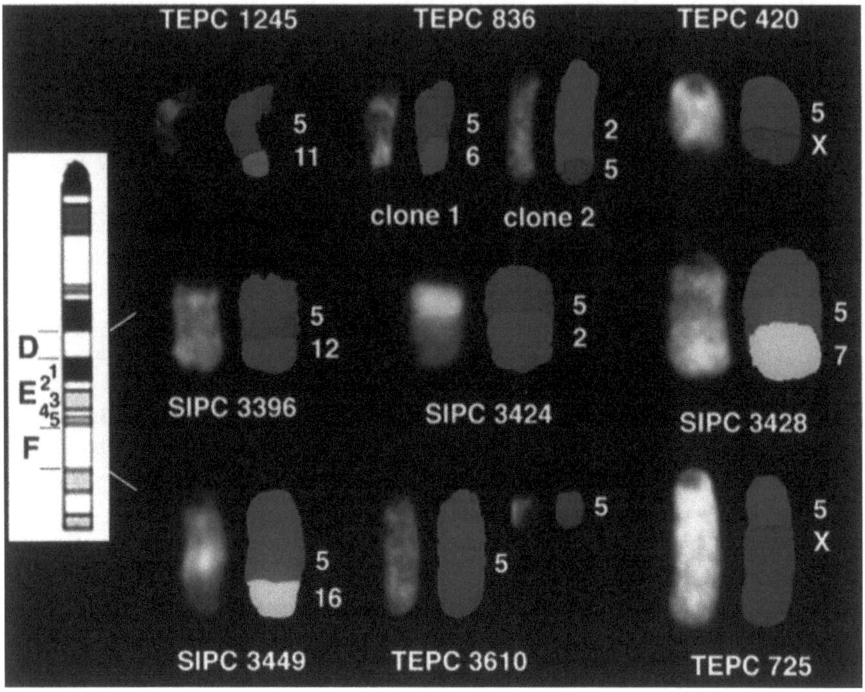
TEPC 1245
5
11
TEPC 836
5
6
2
5
clone 1
clone 2
TEPC 420
5
X
D
E
F
5
12
SIPC 3396
5
2
SIPC 3424
5
7
SIPC 3428
5
16
SIPC 3449
5
5
TEPC 3610
5
X
TEPC 725

Figure 1.

Discussion

Sandy Morse: You have defined in the precursor lesions the foci of expanded cells by PCR the presence of the T(12;15). Are there enough mitotic figures, etc. there, and can you get hold of those cells so that you can begin to develop a sense of ordering for the abnormalities that you see?
Siegfried Janz: It would be great to identify the cytogenetic aberrations in foci of atypical plasma cells because these foci comprise the precursor lesions of mouse plasmacytomas, as you indicated correctly in your question. However, very little is known in that regard. Mitotic figures are rarely seen in plasmacytic foci; thus, SKY cannot be performed. Based on our PCR studies, it is reasonable to suspect that the focal plasma cells contain the T(12;15) translocation, but this has not been demonstrated yet. I believe it will be difficult to discern all cytogenetic changes in foci; in fact, we may have a long way to go before the sequence of cytogenetic aberrations in the course of mouse plasmacytomagenesis can be established. An additional but altogether different problem is that it is currently unclear whether malignant plasma cell tumor development utilizes a unified tumor progression pathway, or not. It is possible that several, distinct progression pathways exist in BALB/c plasmacytomagenesis; one subgroup of tumors may utilize the putative progressor gene on Chr 5 and another subgroup of tumors may employ other, yet unknown genetic changes.
Thomas Ried: I have technical comment: once you know these translocations, because you have successfully applied screening tests for aberrations like chromosome banding, SKY or CGH, you can then develop specific DNA probes that you can use in non-dividing interface cells, and actually correlate chromosome abnormalities to genetic abnormalities with immunophenotype or tissue morphology, or whatever you want.
Fritz Melchers: I understand that there is this dominant 12;15 translocation, but who says that this would not be the bottleneck-selecting mutation that you need in order to get a plasmacytoma? What tells you that that was first?
Siegfried Janz: The T(12;15) was found to be present in all tumors included in this study. In most plasmacytomas, two copies of both products of translocation were detected; i. e., two copies of Chr T(12;15) and two copies of Chr T(15;12). The most likely explanation for this finding is that the T(12;15) translocation preceded the tetraploidization of tumor cells, a characteristic feature of most mouse plasmacytomas. In contrast to the T(12;15) translocation, the products of the non-reciprocal translocations involving Chr 5 were found to exist as single copies in the majority of tumors. Thus, it is likely that the Chr 5 aberrations occurred after the T(12;15) translocation and the tetraploidization event.
George Klein: A single visible change?
Siegfried Janz: Yes, in all but one tumor only a single copy of the rearranged Chr 5 was detected. In the exceptional tumor, two such copies were found. Furthermore, in all but one tumor, the reciprocal product of the translocation of recombining Chr 5 was lost. Again, there was one exceptional tumor in which the reciprocal product was retained.

MYC-Induced *Cyclin D2* Genomic Instability in Murine B Cell Neoplasms

J.F. Mushinski[1], J. Hanley-Hyde[1], G.J. Rainey[1,2], T.I. Kuschak[3], C. Taylor[3], M. Fluri[5], L.M. Stevens[1,4], D.W. Henderson[1] and S. Mai[3,5]

[1] Molecular Genetics Section, Laboratory of Genetics, National Cancer Institute, Bethesda MD 20892-4255; [2] Present address: Department of Biochemistry, Tufts University Medical Center, Boston, MA 02111; [3] Manitoba Institute of Cell Biology, University of Manitoba, Winnipeg, MB, Canada R3E OV9; [4] Degree candidate in the Molecular & Cell Biology Program, University of Maryland, College Park, MD; [5] The Basel Institute for Immunology, Grenzacherstrasse 487, CH-4005 Basel, Switzerland

Introduction

I would like to begin by reiterating two important truisms of neoplasia. First, carcinogenesis, including B-cell neoplasia, is a multi-step phenomenon. That is, it involves a series of mutations. Second, these mutations must accumulate in a single cell, so it is critical that the susceptible cell be a stem cell or a cell with stem cell-like potential to self-replicate with the mutations as they accumulate. I will be considering the actions of the proto-oncogene, c-*Myc*, which may contribute to both these steps.

I will focus on the role the *Myc* gene plays in genomic instability in B-cell neoplasia. Genomic instability is another way of saying accumulation of mutations. We are all aware that in many B lymphocytic neoplasms, c-*Myc* expression is constitutively upregulated as a result of any of three processes associated with genomic instability: 1) gene amplification (Citri et al. 1987; Feo et al. 1994); 2) insertion of retrovirus (Hayward et al. 1981) or transposon (Morse et al. 1988); or 3) chromosomal translocation of c-*Myc* to one of the immunoglobulin loci (Shen-Ong et al. 1982). What has not yet been clarified is what role c-*Myc* expression, whether over-expression or constitutive expression, plays in the multi-step process of carcinogenesis. Previous studies have suggested that MYC protein contributes to neoplasia by affecting the cell cycle (Steiner et al. 1995). Cells with c-*Myc* overexpression may show shortened G1-phases (Karn et al. 1989), while cells with one disrupted c-*Myc* allele have a prolonged G1-phase (Hanson et al. 1994). Disruption of both c-*Myc* alleles also prolonged the G2-phase in a cell line (Mateyak et al. 1997), suggesting that c-*Myc* expression and cell cycle progression are linked through the activation of G1 cyclins and cyclin-dependent kinases (cdks) (Steiner et al. 1995). The cdk-activating phosphatase gene, cdc 25a, is thought to be a target of MYC transactivation (Galaktionov et al. 1996), which offers a plausible mechanism for this linkage, but not necessarily the only one. In the present study, we show evidence of MYC-dependent genomic instability of the *cyclin D2* gene, with an increase in intrachromosomal copy numbers or extrachromosomal elements bearing *cyclin D2* sequences and attendant increased *cyclin D2* gene products. These findings link c-*Myc* overexpression and cell cycle regulation for the first time at the level of genomic instability of this G1 cyclin.

Results

Cyclin D2 Expression in Murine B-lymphocytic Lines

We wished to examine the relationship between c-*Myc* expression and expression of regulatory molecules that control the passage of cells through the G1 phase of the cell cycle. To this end my lab cloned cDNAs for the mouse D-family cyclins and used them to study the expression of the G1 cyclins in mouse B-cell lines. Figure 1 shows a blot of poly $(A)^+$ RNA from a series of mouse B-cell lymphoma cell lines arrayed from left to right in increasing maturation (Mushinski et al. 1988).

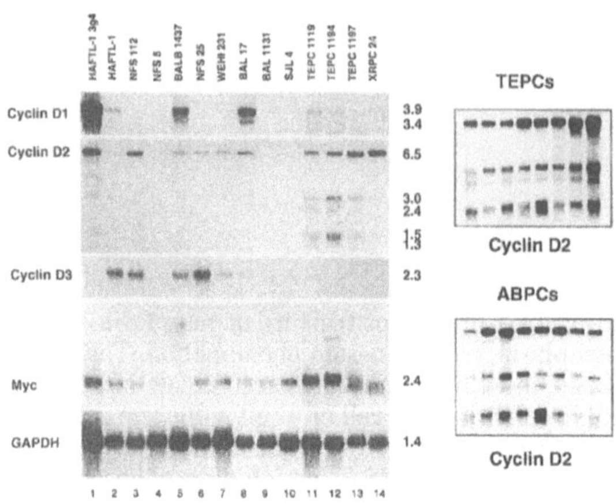

Fig. 1 Cyclin expression in mouse B-lymphocytic tumors.
Left panel. Poly $(A)^+$ RNAs (5 μg) from HAFTL-1 3g4 and HAFTL-1, related clones of pro-B lymphocytes, the former more myeloid than the second; NFS 112, NFS 5, BALB 1437, pre-B cell lines; NFS 25, WEHI 231, BAL 17, BAL 1131. mature B-cell lines, SJL 4, plasmablast; and TEPC 1119, TEPC 1194, TEPC 1197, XRPC 24, plasmacytoma lines. The blot was hybridized first with *cyclin D2* cDNA and then sequentially with other probes, as indicated. Sizes of major hybridizing bands are indicated on the right. **Right panels.** mRNAs from additional plasmacytomas hybridized with *cyclin D2* cDNA.

This blot was sequentially hybridized with the four murine G1 cyclin probes (Hamel and Hanley-Hyde, 1997). *Cyclin E* transcripts were virtually undetectable, so they are not shown. When normalized to the *GAPDH* control hybridization signals (Fort et al. 1985), the highest level of expression of the predominant *cyclin D2* mRNA (6.5-kb) was seen in the four plasmacytomas (lanes 11 - 14). In addition, a characteristic quartet of smaller *cyclin D2* mRNAs is prominent in these four lanes. These plasmacytomas bear *Myc*-activating chromosome translocations and are the B cells with the highest *Myc* mRNA content, although there is not a direct correlation between the steady-state level of *Myc* and that of *cyclin D2* mRNAs. This pattern of high c-*Myc* and *cyclin D2* mRNAs was also seen in northern blots of RNA from dozens of additional plasmacytomas, 16 of which are shown in the inset panels on the right.

The *Cyclin D2* Gene in B-cell Neoplasia

These results inspired us to study the structure and expression of the *cyclin D2* gene in B-cell neoplasms. We cloned the 5.4-kb upstream region of mouse *cyclin D2* and determined its sequence. We noted a high degree of conservation between the mouse sequence and that published for the 1.5 kb upstream of the human *cyclin D2* gene (Brooks et al. 1996). We observed that there were four canonical MYC/MAX binding "E box" motifs (CACGTG) upstream of exon one, suggesting that MYC/MAX might play a role in the function of this gene. Data from a direct test of MYC on *cyclln D2* promoters are not yet complete, but we do not believe that MYC upregulates *cyclin D2* expression, for reasons that will become clear later.

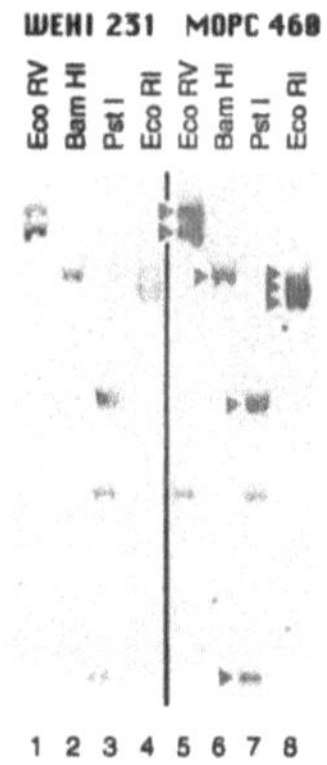

Fig. 2. Cyclin D2-hybridized Southern blot of 10μg of DNA from WEHI 231 and MOPC 460 digested with the indicated restriction endonucleases.

Instead, we found very intriguing results when we used our *cyclin D2* genomic probe to examine the gene dose in certain human and mouse malignancies. Here we will present the data only for mouse plasmacytoma MOPC 460D (Jaffe et al. 1967), in which the c-*Myc* gene has been deregulated by a t(12;15) chromosome translocation. The Southern blot of DNA from this tumor, digested with four different restriction endonucleases, is shown in Figure 2. Here we see stronger *cyclin D2*-hybridizing bands (indicated by arrowheads) in most of the lanes of DNA from MOPC 460D, compared with similar digests of DNA from WEHI 231, in which the c-*Myc* gene is single-copy. The same membrane was also hybridized with a probe for mouse *ribonucleotide reductase*, subunit 1, a gene that is neither amplified nor translocated in these tumors (not shown). These results indicate that the lanes were loaded equally and that the *cyclin D2* gene is amplified in MOPC 460D, in which expression of the c-*Myc* gene has been deregulated. Similar evidence of *cyclin D2* amplification can be found in human tumors, e.g., COLO320HSR, in which *Myc* is amplified (Mai et al. submitted).

We looked at the state of the *cyclin D2* gene in MOPC 460D with a finer degree of resolution using fluorescent *in situ* hybridization (FISH) analysis of metaphase chromosomes (Mai et al. 1996). Figure 3 shows FISH analysis of a typical MOPC 460D metaphase in which the background DNA in the chromosomes is stained red with propidium iodide, while *cyclin D2* hybridization is indicated by green spots on extra-chromosomal elements (EEs), shown with large white arrowheads, or by brown dots when superimposed on the red-stained chromosomes, indicated by white arrows. Thus, amplification of the *cyclin D2* gene in this tumor takes both an intra- and extra-chromosomal form.

MYC-induced *Cyclin D2* Instability Demonstrated *in vitro*

We felt that it was important to test whether the genomic instability of *cyclin D2* was a direct result of c-*Myc* upregulation, rather than one of many genetic epiphenomena that may have occurred during the long-term passage of these established tumors. So we established an *in vitro* system in which c-*Myc* could be upregulated under our control. This involved the immortalization of BALB/c bone marrow-derived pre-B lymphocytes by infection with Abelson virus (Rosenberg and Baltimore 1976) and the subsequent addition of overexpressed mouse *bcl-2* (Gurfinckel et al. 1987). The *Myc* expression vector was pBabePuroMycER^{TM}, expressing a chimeric protein in which human c-MYC is coupled to a mutated estrogen receptor (Littlewood et al. 1995). Although this protein is constitutively expressed, the MYC portion of the chimeric protein is only active in the presence of 4-hydroxytamoxifen (4HT). Figure 4 shows an RNA blot of a time course of pre-B cells in which the exogenous MYC-ER^{TM} protein has been activated by 4HT. *Cyclin D2* mRNA, but not *cyclin D3*, is upregulated after 3-4 days of exposure to 100 nM 4HT. This upregulation does not occur in pre-B cells that do not bear the pBabe-PuroMycER^{TM} (not shown). Since this increase in *cyclin D2* expression took 3-4 days of increased MYC activity, the equivalent of about 4 or 5 cell doublings, we feel that MYC does not upregulate *cyclin D2* expression as a transactivation factor. Instead, we postulate that *cyclin D2* amplification, in the form of extra- and intra-chromosomal elements, was responsible for the increased expression. Steady-state levels of cyclin D2 protein, as determined by western blotting of cell lysates collected after 3-4 days of exposure to 4HT (not shown) was also upregulated.

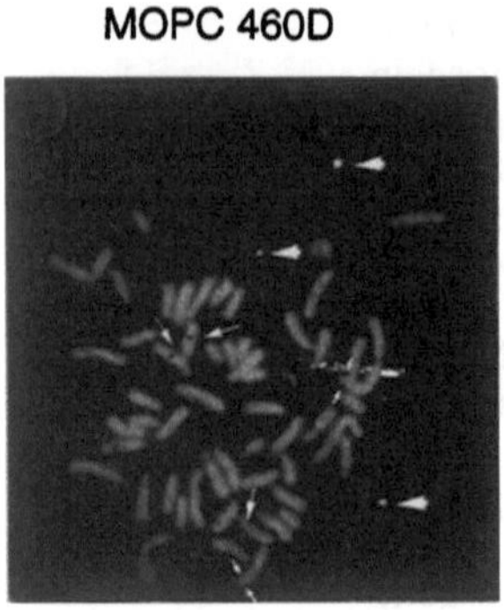

Fig. 3. Fluorescent *in situ* hybridization (FISH) of a MOPC 460D metaphase spread. Chromosomes are stained red with propidium. Hybridization by the mouse *cyclin D2* genomic probe is shown by green dots with large white arrowheads (extrachromosomal) and brown spots with white arrows (intrachromosomal).

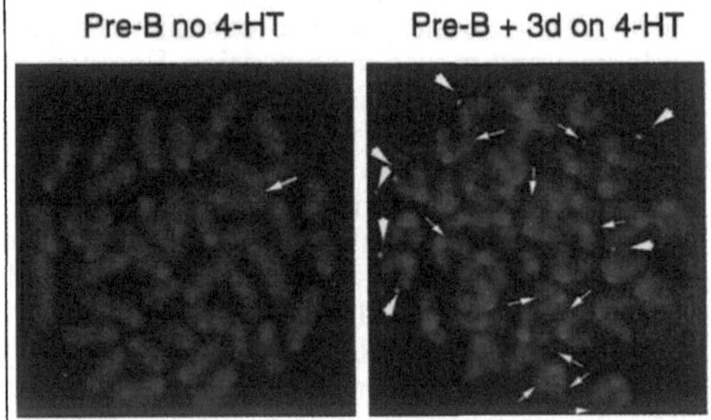

Fig. 5. Fluorescent *in situ* hybridization (FISH) study of pre-B lymphoma cells containing stably integrated pBabePuroMycER™. DAPI-stained DNA chromosomes are blue. Sites of *cyclin D2* hybridization are green. Large white arrowheads and small white arrows show large and small green-fluorescing spots.

Left panel: before 4-hydroxytamoxifen treatment;

Right panel: after 3 days of growth on 4-hydroxytamoxifen.

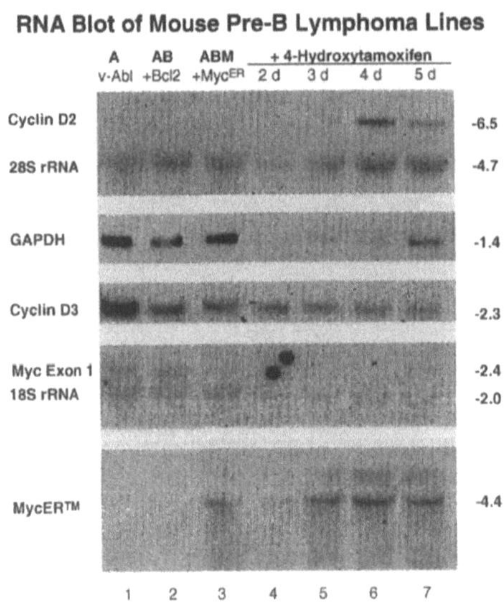

Fig. 4. Northern blot of 20 μg of total RNA from BALB/c pre-B lymphoma cells with or without stably integrated pBabePuroMycER™. Each lane contains RNA from cells that had been treated with 4-hydroxytamoxifen for the indicated number of days. Hybridizing bands are identified on the left, and their sizes (in Kb) are indicated on the right.

To see whether this upregulation of *cyclin D2* expression was connected with changes at the genomic level, we studied the nuclei of these cells with FISH, using *cyclin D2* as a probe. As shown in Figure 5, after 3 days of 4HT activation of MycER™ there were distinct EEs that hybridized with the genomic *cyclin D2* probe. This time the chromosomal counterstain was DAPI, which appears blue, and the *cyclin D2* genes are identified by green spots. Before 4HT treatment, no more than four hybridizing spots could be seen on the chromosomes, indicating the endogenous, normal *cyclin D2* loci. After Myc activation by 4HT, a dozen or more spots of hybridization could be seen, either extrachromsomally or intrachromosomally. An analogous experiment was performed with the same *Myc* expression vector in the ψ2 line of mouse fibroblasts (Mann et al. 1983). Both upregulation at the mRNA level and EEs as evidence of genomic instability were detected after 3 days of *Myc* activation by 4HT (data not shown). Thus this phenomenon of MYC-induced *cyclin D2* instability may be a general one.

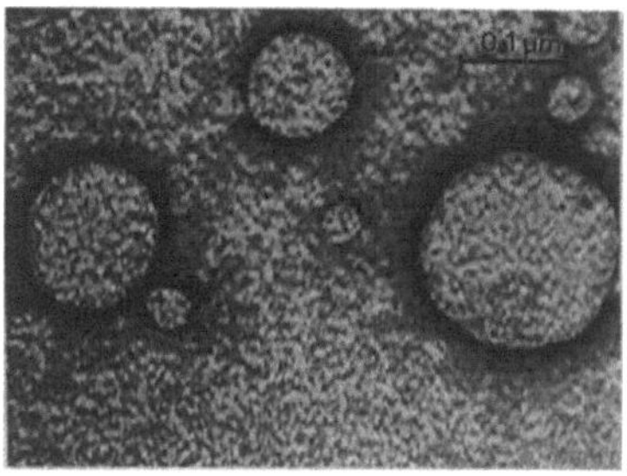

Fig. 6. Electron micrograph of Hirt supe from Pre-B lymphoma cells containing stably integrated pBabePuroMycER^{TM} after 3 days of activation by 4-hydroxytamoxifen. The grid was stained with uranyl acetate and shadowed with tungsten.

Extrachromosomal elements are DNA-containing circles

We wanted to learn more about these extrachromosomal elements and sought ways to isolate them. The best way we found was using the method or Hirt (1967) in which chromosomal material is coagulated by lysis of cells with 0.6% sodium dodecyl sulfate (SDS) in 0.01 M EDTA, pH 7.5, followed by precipitation of the SDS in 1 M NaCl. The supernatant ("Hirt supe") is enriched for EEs, which can be visualized under the electron microscope. Figure 6 shows an electron micrograph of a typical Hirt supe preparation of pre-B cells after 3 days of 4HT treatment. This material was placed on a grid, stained with uranyl acetate and shadowed with tungsten. Circles of this size, sometimes including "buds" that could be replication bubbles, are not seen in pre-B cells before 4HT treatment. Normal cells do contain much smaller circles (usually <0.05 µm in diameter) that contain repetitive DNA motifs only (Gaubatz, 1990). They are too small to be seen by FISH (light microscopy). We, of course, are interested in knowing 1) how many of these larger circles hybridize to *cyclin D2*? 2) are these *cyclin D2* genes complete enough to yield translatable mRNA? 3) how many other genes are similarly represented in EEs after MYC activation? So, we plan to study them further in the coming months.

Discussion

The *cyclin D2* amplification that was detected in mouse plasmacytomas *in vivo* and 4HT-activated Myc ER^{TM} *in vitro* was accompanied by enhanced mRNA and protein levels on RNA and protein blots. The data obtained to date do not require upregulation of either RNA transcription or changes in RNA stability. In fact, our data suggest that, despite the presence of at least three canonical E box motifs upstream of the promoter of *cyclin D2*, MYC does not directly transactivate *cyclin D2* transcription. The delay of 3-4 days before steady-state levels increase is also not consistent with MYC's action as transcription-activating factor in this case. It is possible that simple *status-quo* rates of expression would yield increased steady-state levels of mRNA and protein if the template were increased, such as by the amplification that we have demonstrated. Our electron microscopy studies have demonstrated that 4HT-activated MYC induces the generation of circular extra-chromosomal elements that contain *cyclin D2* sequences. We do not know at this juncture whether the *cyclin D2* mRNAs are synthesized directly on these EEs, but we hope to find out in the coming months. Such a mechanism could also be responsible for the high levels of *cyclin D2* mRNA in plasmacytomas, secondary to their constitutive expression of high levels of c-*Myc* mRNA and protein.

This MYC-associated genomic instability may have another possible consequence: the frequent aneuploidy seen in plasmacytomas (and other cancer cells) that express high MYC levels and have been passaged for extended periods of time *in vivo* or *in vitro*. However, it is important to emphasize that this MYC-associated tendency to amplification appears to be locus-specific. Gene amplification has been shown previously for *Dhfr* (Mai 1994) and in this paper for *cyclin D2*, but we have determined that high c-*Myc* expression produces no such amplification in the genes encoding *ornithine decarboxylase*, *syndecan-2*, *glyceraldehyde-3-phosphate-dehydrogenase* or *cyclin C* (Mai et al. 1996).

Acknowledgements

This work was supported by grants to S M from the National Science and Engineering Research Council (NSERC), the Manitoba Health and Research Council (MHRC), and the Thorlakson Foundation Fund. The Basel Institute for Immunology was founded and is supported by F. Hoffmann-La Roche, Basel, Switzerland.

References

Brooks AR, Shiffman D, Brooks EE and Milner PG (1996) Functional analysis of the human cyclin D2 and cyclin D3 promoters. J Biol Chem 271: 9090-9099

Citri Y, Braun J and Baltimore D (1987) Elevated myc expression and c-*myc* amplification in spontaneously occurring B lymphoid cell lines. J Exp Med 165: 1188-1194

Feo S, Liegro CD, Jones T, Read M and Fried M (1994) The DNA region around the c-*myc* gene and its amplification in human tumour cell lines. Oncogene 9: 955-961

Fort P, Marty L, Piechaczyk M, El Sabrouty S, Dani C, Jeanteur P and Blanchard JM (1985) Various rat adult tissues express only one major mRNA species from the glyceraldehyde-3-phosphate-dehydrogenase multigenic family. Nucl Acids Res 13: 1431-1437

Galaktionov K, Chen X and Beach D (1996) Cdc25 cell-cycle phosphatase as a target of c-*myc*. Nature 382: 511-517

Gaubatz, JW Mutation Res (1990) Extrachromosomal circular DNAs and genomic sequence plasticity in eukaryotic cells. 237: 271-292

Gurfinkel N, Unger T, Givol D and Mushinski JF (1987) Expression of the *bcl-2* gene in mouse B lymphocytic cell lines is differentiation stage specific. Eur J Immunol 17: 567-570

Hamel PA and Hanley-Hyde J (1997) G1 cyclins and control of the cell division cycle in normal and transformed cells. Cancer Investigation 15: 143-152

Hanson KD, Shichiri M, Follansbee MR and Sedivy JM (1994) Effects of *c-myc* expression on cell cycle progression. Mol Cell Biol 14: 5748-5755

Hayward WS, Neel BG and Astrin SM (1981) Activation of a cellular onc gene by promoter insertion in ALV-induced lymphoid leukosis. Nature 290: 475-480

Hirt, B (1967) Selective extraction of polyoma DNA from infected mouse cell cultures. J Mol Biol 26: 365-369

Jaffe BM, Eisen HN, Simms ES and Potter M (1969) Myeloma proteins with anti-hapten antibody activity: epsilon-2,4- dinitrophenyl lysine binding by the protein produced by mouse plasmacytoma MOPC-460. J Immunol 103: 872-874

Jansen-Duerr P, Meichle A, Steiner P, Pagano M, Finke K, Botz J, Wessbecher J, Draetta G and Eilers M (1993) Differential modulation of cyclin gene expression by MYC. Proc Natl Acad Sci USA 90: 3685-3689

Karn J, Watson JV, Lowe AD, Green SM and Vedeckis W (1989) Regulation of cell cycle duration by c-*myc* levels. Oncogene 4: 773-787

Littlewood TD, Hancock DC, Danielian PS, and Evan GI (1995) A modified oestrogen receptor ligand-binding domain as an improved switch for the regulation of heterologous proteins. Nucl Acids Res 23: 1686-1690

Mai S (1994) Overexpression of c-*myc* precedes amplification of the gene encoding dihydrofolate reductase. Gene 148: 253-260

Mai S, Hanley-Hyde J and Fluri M (1996) c-*Myc* overexpression associated DHFR gene amplification in hamster, rat, mouse and human cell lines. Oncogene 12: 277-288

Mann R, Mulligan RC and Baltimore D (1983) Construction of a retrovirus packaging mutant and its use to produce helper-free defective retrovirus. Cell 33: 153-159

Mateyak MK, Obaya AJ, Adachi S and Sedivy JM (1997) Phenotypes of c-*Myc*-deficient rat fibroblasts isolated by targeted homologous recombination. Cell Growth Differ 8: 1039-1048

Morse B, Rotherg PG, South VJ, Spandorfer JM and Astrin SM (1988) Insertional mutagenesis of the *myc* locus by a LINE-1 sequence in a human breast carcinoma. Nature 333: 87-90

Mushinski JF, Davidson WD and Morse HC (1987) Activation of cellular oncogenes in human and mouse leukemia-lymphomas: spontaneous and induced oncogene expression in murine B lymphocytic neoplasms. Cancer Invest 5: 345-368

Rosenberg N and Baltimore D (1976) A quantitative assay for transformation of bone marrow cells by Abelson murine leukemia virus. J Exp Med 143: 1453-1463

Shen-Ong GLC, Keath EJ, Piccoli SP and Cole MD (1982) Novel *myc* oncogene RNA from abortive immunoglobulin-gene recombination in mouse plasmacytomas. Cell 31: 443-480

Steiner P, Philipp A, Lukas J, Godden-Kent D, Pagano M, Mittnacht S, Bartek J and Eilers M (1995) Identification of a *Myc*-dependent step during the formation of active G1 cyclin-cdk complexes. EMBO J 14: 4814-4826

Discussion

Sandy Morse: In terms of this very interesting phenomenon, do you find it in naturally occurring Burkitt's, in primary plasmacytomas, and in Abelson virus-induced plasmacytomas, or how generalizable is it?
Fred Mushinski: Well, one out of three is not bad. We have not done the Burkitt's, we want to do them; we have not done the primary plasmacytomas, we want to do them; but we have looked at Abelson-induced plasmacytomas, and, yes, the D2 effects are seen in the ABPCs as well as non-abl PCTs.
George Klein: In the early work on gene amplification in mouse leukemic cells, it was found that the amplified DHFR genes, responsible for methotrexate resistance, were only maintained as long as selection was maintained. When selection was relaxed they waned. This led Michael Bishop to suggest that oncogene amplification in tumors must reflect selective advantage. Your amplification and maintained extrachromosomal elements in mouse plasmacytomas must therefore give the cell a selective advantage. What could this be in a cell that is already myc-driven? My second point is that it would be interesting to look at EBV-negative Burkitt's because they express cyclin D3 instead of D2. Would you get D3 amplification? Is the cyclin D2 amplification induced by your construct maintained when you relax the tamoxifen stimulation and passage the cells *in vitro* and *in vivo*, or does it wane?
Fred Mushinski: Working backwards, if we stop stimulation of the cells with 4-hydroxy-tamoxifen the expression and the extrachromosomal elements wane over the course of another 4 or 5 days. They have not gone away completely but they have diminished substantially. What is the selective advantage? I am not quite sure. There is a similar question about myc. We know myc is dysregulated in the plasmacytomas by chromosome translocation, and these do not go away during transplantation or culturing. This implies that constitutive myc expression needs to be maintained. We surmise that because it is maintained, we continue to see the substantially larger cyclin D2-containing extrachromosomal and inter chromosomal elements in long-established tumors, and these do not seem to go away. I think that what myc, and perhaps cyclin D2, may mediate is keeping cells in cycle so that they do not die. It must be a careful balance because if you over-express myc you might end up killing the cells. If you underexpress myc they might stop growing, but I think that perhaps through the cyclin D2 (although we don't know for sure) the cells will be kept in cycle, allowing them to accumulate mutations. We believe that myc probably stimulates this form of instability, and perhaps other kinds of instability, which we hope to check in the future. Regarding cyclin D3 amplification in Burkitt lymphomas, we are eager to test this possibility.
Richard Scheuermann: Have you looked at some of the putative myc targets, like ornithine decarboxylatase or CDC25a?
Fred Mushinski: Yes we have looked at both, but are you asking if they are also involved in amplification?
Richard Scheuermann: Are you are getting gene amplification rather than direct effects on transcription?
Fred Mushinski: No, we don't. But I am not really sure whether the CDC25a is actually a good target of myc in these cells, because we hybridized that same northern blot and did not see excess CDC25a, b, or c transcripts. The ODC is a well established myc target, but does not seem to be involved in the amplification. This makes the important point that the genes targeted for myc-induced genomic instability do not have to be the same genes targeted for myc-induced trans-activation of expression.
Michael Reth: If one expresses myc in an inducible fashion in the B lymphoma cells WEHI 231, the cells go rapidly into apoptosis. Formerly it was thought that myc prevents apoptosis in WEHI 231, as cells stably transfected with myc are resistant to apoptosis. However, due to the inducible system, it is now clear that myc did the opposite (including apoptosis) and resulted in a strong selection for variant WEHI 231 cells which survived the transfection and are subsequently resistant to apoptosis. Did you ever check for apoptosis in your cells when you induced myc?
Fred Mushinski: Yes, I think these cells are teetering on a delicate balance, because when Sabine Mai was making all the preparations for a study of the nuclei for hybridization, she thought the cells looked as if they were going to die. That is they appeared to be apoptosing. In fact they do not die, but they look as if they are trying to die. So I suspect that it is going to be very diffi-

cult to sort out why the cells appear to be teetering on death but instead grow and proliferate. I do think that would be an important area for further study.

Riccardo Dalla-Favera: Did you look at enough cells under basal conditions to exclude selection as opposed to induction?

Fred Mushinski: Of the preB cells?

Riccardo Dalla-Favera: Or any system. I am asking if it is a minority of cells carrying amplified targets there and you are simply selecting those cells when you overexpress myc as opposed to inducing amplification?

Fred Mushinski: Well, since they are in culture they select themselves to some extent. However, it seems hard to invoke this sort of explanation for the extrachromosomal elements that were seen in so many cells. After all, they appeared after only 3 or 4 days in culture in the presence of 4-OH tamoxifen during which time they could have multiplied only a few times. Nonetheless, I don't think I can exclude your postulate

Riccardo Dalla-Favera: More specifically, how many cells did you count under known tamoxifen conditions?

Fred Mushinski: Hundreds, with and without tamoxifen treatment.

Riccardo Dalla-Favera: And they don't have extrachromosomal copies in the absence of tamoxifen?

Fred Mushinski: Yes, that is certain. However, I might point out that there is a certain plasticity to the genome, and that repetitive sequences exist outside the chromosomes in every cell, even normal ones. Large extrachromosomal elements bearing unique sequences are only seen in tumor cells.

Riccardo Dalla-Favera: Secondly, can you exclude an induction of myc expression of cyclin? Those Northern and Western blots could also reflect their being myc-responsive genes, so how much is induction of transcription versus amplification?

Fred Mushinski: I don't really know why the transcription is upregulated. I think, as you pointed out with your identification of e-box motifs yesterday, that there are e-boxes in lots of places, and probably all are not really myc-max targets. Typically, if you have a myc-max-responding e-box-containing gene, it is upregulated within a few minutes or a few hours of myc expression. We do not really see our D2 upregulation before a matter of days. So it very much parallels the appearance of the extrachromosomal elements, and we think they are connected. Unfortunately, to be able to prove that RNA transcripts actually come off those circles is a really big challenge.

Dirk Eick: I have a question on the origin of the circles. High c-myc expression can induce apoptosis. Is it possible that these circles originate from apoptotic events?

Fred Mushinski: I would think that an apoptotic event that would generate those things would be catastrophic for that nucleus, and it seems as though the rest of the chromosomes are pretty well intact. We see quite a few extrachromosomal elements, but I do not believe that they could have come from neighboring cells that had completely shattered. I think there are too many there to think of that, and the morphology of apoptotic bodies is clearly different from that of extrachromosomal elements. Fragments of genomic DNA typically appear as linear fragments of DNA or chromatin, rather than the circular forms that we routinely see. It's a thoughtful question, however.

Dirk Eick: Fragmented DNA may be re-ligated to circles and phagozytized by neighboring cells.

Fred Mushinski: To be sure, phagocytosis is a key aspect of apoptosis, but that is usually a feature of macrophages and not by the B cells.

Dirk Eick: I do not know about B cells, but normal fibroblasts can take up apoptotic bodies.

Sandy Morse: An extension of the question is, do you see the presence of double minute-like structures that do not have the cyclin or DHFR, which you said is also amplified, and they are multiple, and you are just seeing a subset of those?

Fred Mushinski: We need to do the study on a more global basis to find this out rather than just picking DHFR, which Sabine Mai started with, or cyclin D2, which we are now working with. There is another enzyme called ribonucleotide reductase which we are also studying, of which one subunit is upregulated and amplified, and the other is not. We need to figure out a way to use some of the more high-tech screening processes to find out whether expression and amplification happens on a large number of genes or a small number of genes.

Heinz Jacobs: Can you exclude the pre-existence of these amplification products in a certain frequency of these cells before the induction of myc?

Fred Mushinski: I don't think they preexist.

Gary Rathbun: Have you cloned some of these circles and sequenced them, and is there anything about the joins that is unique?
Fred Mushinski: We are working on that, but the circles are hard to deal with and we have not learned how to make them routinely. Our intent is to clone them and sequence them, and to find out something about their nature. They don't digest nicely with restriction endonucleases, so we have a lot to learn about them.
Una Chen: I understood that with the pre-B cells, stimulation of the estrogen receptor-myc chimera leads to amplification. Is that amplification effect reversible?
Fred Mushinski: Yes, you take away the 4-hydroxytamoxifen and they tend to go away in the course of 4 - 6 days, not completely gone. but they go down a lot. Both the amplification as extrachromosomal elements, and messenger RNA.
Una Chen: After you have seen the amplifications, can you withdraw 4HT and the cells will return to the original state, i.e. not amplified?
Fred Mushinski: Yes.
Martin Lipp: Did you analyze the amplified extrachromosomal material by multicolor karyotyping (SKY)? Possibly, the circles do not only contain the cyclic D2 region but also sequences from other chromosomes indicating a selection for additional functional genes on the extrachromosomal material.
Fred Mushinski: I think that is very likely. To the first part of your question, no, but we are eager to do SKY analysis or to ask a similar question with CGH, as we heard from Thomas Ried. I think that is a very important question, and we are eager to do both those projects.
Fritz Melchers: From the FISH pictures that you showed, is the cyclin D2 gene also on a chromosomal element?
Fred Mushinski: Yes.
Fritz Melchers: Is the cyclin D gene simply cut out and then replicated extrachromosomably, or is the amplification assumed to be from the chromosomal element and thereby creating all the circles?
Fred Mushinski: The latter is my assumption. Would you propose an alternative?
George Klein: It seems that part of your audience is somewhat puzzled by your findings and is seeking non-specific explanations. A specific explanation appears more attractive to us. Do you find the extrachromosomal bodies in most cells? Is that right?
Fred Mushinski: Yes.
George Klein: That speaks for a specific phenomenon. Cyclin D2 amplification could provide the cells with an advantage. The amplicons could be of different sizes because they would incorporate various sequences around the selectively favored gene. The real question is at the biological level. Is the amplification restricted to B cell-derived lines? Have you tried others?
Fred Mushinski: Yes, we have put the same construct in fibroblasts and did the same induction with 4-hydroxytamoxifen, and found exactly the same thing. After 3-4 days, we got upregulation. Since there is some baseline expression in these fibroblasts the level of cyclin D2 mRNA started a little higher than in the pre-B cells, but it went up after 3-4 days, and the FISH analysis showed similar kinds of extrachromosomal elements.
Riccardo Dalla-Favera: Your interpretation is unique: myc induces some kind of instability in the locus, brings cyclin D2 out of the chromosome and makes it replicate. I am trying to see whether you can exclude that there are some low copy number circles already out, and myc simply increases their replication. I mention that because there is the story of myc favoring DNA replication, particularly as the chromosomal site is not a new one. I think George Klein published a paper 10 years ago on the effect of myc on replication of SV40. I am trying to address whether myc is inducing instability and then this amplicon replicates, or they are preexisting and this is another example in which myc can increase the copy number.
Sandy Morse: He should be able to find out from analysis of Hirt DNA from the starting population.
Bart Barlogie: Can you check this with BrdU in some ways?
Fred Mushinski: I don't know how we can better look at it than the way we have done it. It could be that they are too small to be seen by FISH.
Riccardo Dalla-Favera: I think mechanistically it makes a whole lot of difference.
Fred Mushinski: I think the mechanism is really important to get at and I value your thoughts, but we don't see those round circles before the amplification, in fact there aren't any really beautiful circles at all, just these sort of cruddy-looking things. So I don't think that is the case.

The Role of Somatic Hypermutation in the Generation of Deletions and Duplications in Human Ig V Region Genes and Chromosomal Translocations

R. Küppers, T. Goossens, and U. Klein
Institute for Genetics, University of Cologne, Germany

Introduction

In the course of T-cell dependent immune responses, antigen-activated B-lymphocytes migrate into B-cell follicles of secondary lymphoid organs and establish germinal centers (GC). In these structures, the proliferating GC B-cells activate the mechanism of somatic hypermutation, which introduces somatic mutations into rearranged immunoglobulin (Ig) V region genes [1, 2]. These mutations are (with rare exceptions) specific for Ig V genes and occur with a high rate of about 1 in 10^3-10^4 bp/cell cycle [1, 2]. In a selection process taking place within the GC, only GC B-cells which acquired favourable mutations, i.e. mutations that result in an increased affinity to the immunizing antigen, are allowed to survive and finally differentiate into either plasma cells or memory B-cells.

Deletions and Duplications in Rearranged V Region Genes of Human GC and post-GC B Cells

It was generally believed that the process of somatic hypermutation is largely restricted to the generation of somatic point mutations [1, 3]. However, in our studies on V region genes carried by human B-cell lymphomas, we repeatedly encountered V gene sequences harbouring deletions and/or insertions (mostly duplications) of variable length (summarized in [4]). To address the question whether these events are a peculiarity of transformed B-cells, we amplified rearranged V region genes from various subsets of normal human B-cells by single cell PCR. This experimental strategy has the advantage that the PCR products can be directly sequenced, avoiding potential PCR or cloning artifacts which might pose problems in the interpretation of the results. Moreover, by amplifying V gene rearrangements from genomic DNA, both in- and out-of-frame rearrangements are amplified. The latter are particularly informative for studying the occurrence of deletions/duplications (del/dup) in rearranged V genes: since these rearrangements are not expressed, del/dup accumulate in these genes without being subject to counterselection.

The analysis of human tonsillar GC B-cells revealed the occurrence of del/dup in 4% of the in-frame and 43% of the out-of-frame VH rearrangements (Table 1; [4]). Similar values were obtained for human intestinal IgM- or IgA-secreting plasma cells (9% of in-frame and 38% of out-of-frame VH gene rearrangements show del/dup) and a collection of human peripheral blood memory B-cells (4% of in-frame and 60% of non-functional rearrangements show del/dup)

[5,6]. Comparing these frequencies to those previously observed in V region genes of human B-cell lymphomas, it becomes evident that del/dup are not overrepresented in malignant B-cells (Table 1).

Table 1. Frequency of deletions/duplications in human V region genes

Population	Mutated V Genes	Genes Sequenced	Mutation Frequency#	V Genes with Del./Dup. Pot. Functional	Non-functional
HD and NHL	yes	V_H	10.0%	7/54 (13%)	5/8 (63%)
HD and NHL	yes	V_L	5.6%	2/39 (5%)	2/6 (33%)
GC B-cells	yes	V_H	6.3%	3/70 (4%)	12/28 (43%)
plasma cells	yes	V_H	8.7%	5/58 (9%)	3/8 (38%)
memory B-cells*	yes	V_H	5.2%	5/117 (4%)	9/15 (60%)
naive B-cells	no	V_H		0/73	0/14
unmutated V_κ genes from mutated NHL and HD	no	V_κ			0/18

Sequences were taken from ref. [4-6] and references therein.
*collection of VH sequences from IgD^+CD27^+ B-cells (84 pot. functional, 12 non-functional), IgG B-cells (16 pot. functional, 2 non-functional) and IgM-only B-cells (17 pot. functional, 1 non-functional) [6]. #average value

At which developmental stage and by which process are such del/dup generated? The finding that these events were completely absent from V region genes amplified from naive B-cells with unmutated V genes (Table1), and that all sequences with del/dup in addition harboured somatic point mutations, strongly suggests that del/dup occur in the course of the GC reaction, likely as a byproduct of somatic hypermutation. This is further supported by the observation that there is a correlation between the average frequency of somatic point mutations and del/dup in our sequence collection (Table 1), and by the lack of recombination signal sequences (RSS) at the borders of deletions or duplications (which might have argued for an involvement of the V gene recombination "machinery" in the generation of del/dup). Moreover, del/dup were found throughout the region that is target for somatic hypermutation, and duplicated segments of DNA harboured shared as well as unique point mutations [4]. This latter observation strongly argues that the duplications were generated in the GC-reaction while the cell was acquiring somatic point mutations. Taken together, there is strong evidence that del/dup are generated in GC B-cells as a byproduct of somatic hypermutation. Overall, 6% of somatic mutations in out-of-frame rearrangements represent del/dup [4].

Since B-cells undergoing somatic hypermutation are selected for expression of a functional antigen receptor, it is not surprising that del/dup were found less frequently in productive than in out-of-frame rearrangements, because many of the del/dup will "cripple" an originally functional V region gene (e.g. when a deletion removes large parts of a V gene or leads to loss of the correct reading frame). Almost all del/dup in the productive rearrangements are either three, six or nine basepairs long and are found in the complementarity determining regions (CDRs) which are involved in antigen binding. Perhaps the generation of antibody variants with aminoacid-del/dup in the antigen-binding sites represents an additional mechanism (besides nucleotide exchanges) to generate antibody variants in the GC-reaction [4, 7, 8].

The occurrence of del/dup in rearranged human Ig genes was also studied by other groups. Wilson and colleagues analyzed heavy chain transcripts from human tonsillar B-cell subsets and identified del/dup in about 2% of V region genes amplified from GC and memory B-cells [7]. In agreement with our findings, the del/dup events in the in-frame rearrangements were largely restricted to the CDRs and either three or six basepairs long. Ohlin & Borrebaeck presented four examples of antibodies with known specificity that harboured del/dup in the expressed heavy chain genes, further supporting that such events can be tolerated in or near the CDRs and may even contribute to high affinity antigen binding [8]. In a recent V gene mutation study by Levy et al. [9], VH gene transcripts as well as a genomic fragment of the JH intron were amplified from memory B-cells. Del/dup were identified in about 5% of the transcripts and the frequency of del/dup in the JH intron was calculated to represent around 3% of all somatic mutations [9].

Why have Deletions and Duplications Previously been Observed only Rarely?

In the light of the studies discussed above, it may appear surprising why del/dup events have previously been observed only rarely in rearranged V genes. Several reasons are likely to contribute to this. First, most studies focused on the analysis of productive rearrangements, in which del/dup are found much less frequently than in non-productive rearrangements (see above). Second, if V gene rearrangements are amplified from populations of cells, cloning steps are involved prior to sequencing. Since cloned PCR products may contain cloning or PCR artifacts, unusual rearrangements obtained from such experiments are usually disregarded in a mutation analysis. Third, if PCR products obtained from cell populations are isolated from agarose gels before sequencing, V gene rearrangements of unusual length will be lost if only the band of expected length is cut out from the gel. Fourth, many of the one, two or three aminoacid deletions or duplications in the CDRs of productive rearrangements are at or near positions where other germline genes of the same V gene family show length variation. Since some of the computer programs used for sequence evaluation are designed such that mismatches in a homology search reduce the homology "score value" less than del/dup, a mutated V gene with a small del/dup in a CDR may be mistakenly assigned to a different member of the respective V gene family, thus showing no del/dup but several additional point mutations in the homology comparison.

Del/ins have also been described only rarely in human Vκ light chain genes. This is likely due to the following reasons. First, human Vκ genes show on average a two to threefold lower frequency of somatic point mutations than heavy chain genes [6]. Consequently, the frequency of del/dup is expected to be proportionally lower in Vκ as opposed to VH genes (as is evident from our comparative analysis of rearranged VH and VL genes derived from HD and NHL cases; Table 1). Second, most non-functional Vκ gene rearrangements are inactivated by rearrangement of the κ deleting element. This rearrangement not only deletes the Cκ gene, but also the κ enhancers which are known to be indispensable for somatic hypermutation (discussed in [10]). Thus, non-functional Vκ genes almost always lack somatic mutations [6]. It should be noted that the lack of del/dup and somatic point mutations in non-productive Vκ gene rearrangements derived from somatically mutated B-cells (Table 1) further supports the association of somatic point mutations and del/dup.

Implications of the Presence of Deletions/Duplications in Mutated V Genes for the Mechanism of Somatic Hypermutation

Since the generation of del/dup is intimately associated with DNA strand breaks, the frequent occurrence of these events has implications for the (so far unknown) mechanism of somatic hypermutation. In the collection of VH transcripts analyzed by Wilson et al. [7], del/dup were restricted to CDR I and II, and often associated with hotspots of somatic hypermutation. Interestingly, these in-frame del/dup were found at tracks of either direct repeats or palindromes [7]. Based on this feature of the del/dup, the authors propose a model for the generation of del/dup that is based on slippage of DNA polymerase at repetitive tracks of DNA [7]. Clearly, this model is very attractive for explaining the generation of codon del/dup in CDRs. The problem with this model is, however, that codon del/dup in CDRs account for only a small fraction of all del/dup events. As outlined above, most del/dup that are introduced into the DNA of mutating GC B-cells do not fit into this picture, as turned out from the analysis of not-selected out-of-frame V gene rearrangements which harbour five to ten times more del/dup (Table 1). In those rearrangements, no particular DNA-pattern, like direct or inverted repeats, was found at the borders of the del/dup, and the length of the del/dup was highly variable, with some deletions being more than 200 bp long [4]. Thus, the occurrence of the vast majority of del/dup events cannot easily be explained by DNA polymerase slippage at positions with direct or inverted repeats. However, the generation of del/dup as they are found in non-productive rearrangements is compatible with previously proposed models of somatic hypermutation. For example, if somatic hypermutation is initiated by DNA single or double strand breaks, additional strand breaks or the removal of nucleotides at the breakpoints could result in deletions. On the other hand, duplications might be generated if two staggered single strand breaks occur at opposite DNA strands, followed by separation of the strands, fill-in of the single strands, and finally religation of the DNA ends.

Implications for an Involvement of Somatic Hypermutation in B-cell Lymphomagenesis

Studies on V region genes expressed by human B-cell malignancies revealed that most types of lymphomas carry somatically mutated V region genes and are thus likely to be derived from GC or post GC B-cells (reviewed in [10]). In many B-cell lymphomas, characteristic chromosomal translocations involving Ig loci were identified, which have been assumed to result from erroneous class switch or V gene recombination. Many chromosome translocations involving the Ig-loci most likely result from erroneous class switching events; one well-described example is the frequent translocation of c-myc into the IgH-switch regions in sporadic Burkitt's lymphoma. Recently, Knight and colleagues demonstrated that isotype switching in B-cells of rabbits occasionally occurs by interchromosomal recombination [11], making it conceivable how oncogene translocations into the IgH-locus may occur as an accident of class switching. That chromosome translocations may take place during V gene rearrangement in the bone marrow, and perhaps also during the GC-reaction, is exemplified by the bcl-2 translocation in follicular lymphoma which is dependent on the recombination signal sequence (RSS). Gellert and colleagues suggest how such a chromosome translocation involving the Ig-locus may come about in mechanistic terms, as the RAG enzymes can mediate transposition events between the Ig-locus and non-Ig DNA [12].

Our observation of a high frequency of deletions and duplications throughout V regions of GC and GC-derived B-cells, implying that potentially recombinogenic strand breaks occur during somatic hypermutation, led us to conclude that probably also somatic hypermutation plays a so far unrecognized role in B-cell lymphomagenesis [4]. An example for the generation of chromosomal translocations involving Ig-loci that most likely happened as a byproduct of somatic hypermutation (and not V(D)J-recombination or class switching) represents the c-myc translocation in endemic Burkitt's lymphoma. In this B-cell malignancy, c-myc is often translocated into the V region or the J intronic region which are both targets for the hypermutation "machinery". There is no association with RSS-sites at the breakpoints of recombination, therefore distinguishing it from the bcl-1 and bcl-2 translocations that (almost) always occur at the 5' ends of the DH or JH gene segments. Exemplified in Fig.1 is a case in which the V region has been translocated into the c-myc region on chromosome 8. The V region shows somatic mutations, and the fact that it was separated by the translocation from the Ig enhancers, which are indispensable for somatic hypermutation, strongly indicates that the translocation took place after the B-cell had already acquired somatic mutations within the GC, and that many chromosomal translocations in endemic Burkitt's lymphoma probably represent byproducts of somatic hypermutation. Thus, it seems that besides misdirected V gene and class switch recombination, somatic hypermutation represents a third mechanism that is involved in the generation of transforming events contributing to B-cell lymphomagenesis. It will be interesting to see whether this is not only by causing translocations, but also through the erroneous introduction of somatic point mutations into non-Ig genes [14, 15].

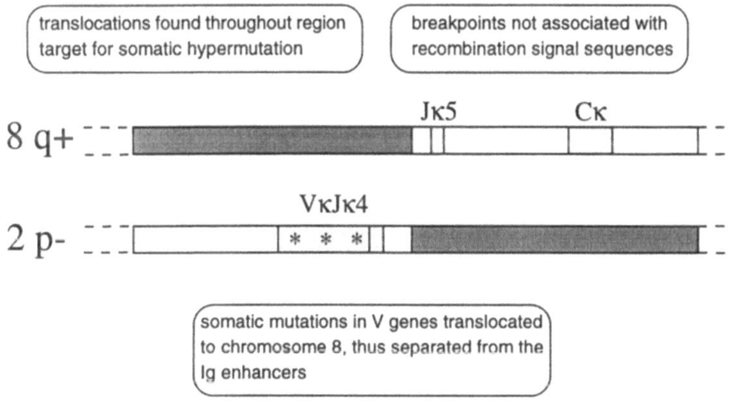

Fig. 1. Translocation of a VκJκ-joint into the c-myc region on chromosome 8 in a case of endemic Burkitt's lymphoma [13].

We are grateful to Michaela Fahrig and Julia Jesdinsky for excellent technical assistance. We thank Klaus Rajewsky for many stimulating and helpful discussions. This work was supported by the Deutsche Forschungsgemeinschaft through SFB502.
Address correspondence to Ralf Küppers, University of Cologne, Institute for Genetics, Weyertal 121, 50931 Cologne, Germany; E-mail: rkuppers@mac.genetik.uni-koeln.de

References

1. Kocks C, Rajewsky K (1989) Stable expression and somatic hypermutation of antibody V regions in B-cell developmental pathways. Annu Rev Immunol 7:537-559
2. Rajewsky K (1996) Clonal selection and learning in the antibody system. Nature 381:751-758
3. Neuberger MS, Milstein C (1995) Somatic hypermutation. Curr Opin Immunol 7:248-254
4. Goossens T, Klein U, Küppers R (1998) Frequent occurrence of deletions and duplications during somatic hypermutation: Implications for oncogene translocations and heavy chain disease. Proc Natl Acad Sci USA 95:2463-2468
5. Fischer M, Küppers R (1998) Human IgA- and IgM-secreting intestinal plasma cells carry heavily mutated VH region genes. Eur J Immunol 28:2971-2977
6. Klein U, Rajewsky K, Küppers R (1998) Human immunoglobulin (Ig)$M^{+}IgD^{+}$ peripheral blood B-cells expressing the CD27 cell surface antigen carry somatically mutated variable region genes: CD27 as a general marker for somatically mutated (memory) B-cells. J Exp Med 188:1679-1689
7. Wilson PC, de Bouteiller O, Liu Y-J, Potter K, Banchereau J, Capra J D, Pascual V (1998) Somatic hypermutation introduces insertions and deletions into immunoglobulin V genes. J Exp Med 187:59-70
8. Ohlin M, Borrebaeck CAK (1998) Insertions and deletions in hypervariable loops of antibody heavy chains contribute to molecular diversity. Mol Immunol 35:233-238
9. Levy Y, Gupta N, Le Deist F, Garcia C, Fischer A, Weill J-C, Reynaud C-A (1998) Defect in IgV gene somatic hypermutation in common variable immuno-deficiency syndrome. Prot Natl Acad Sci USA 95:13135-13140
10. Klein U, Goossens T, Fischer M, Kanzler H, Braeuninger A, Rajewsky K, Küppers R (1998) Somatic hypermutation in normal and transformed human B-cells. Immunol Rev 162:261-280
11. Kingzette M, Spieker-Polet H, Yam P-C, Zhai S-K, Knight KL (1998) Trans-chromosomal recombination within the Ig heavy chain switch region in B-lymphocytes. Prot Natl Acad Sci USA 95:11840-11845
12. Hiom K, Melek M, Gellert M (1998) DNA transposition by RAG1 and RAG2 proteins: a possible source of oncogenic translocations. Cell 94:463-470
13. Kato S, Tachibana K, Takayama N, Kataoka H, Yoshida MC, Takano T (1991) Genetic recombination in a chromosomal translocation t(2;8) (p11;p24) of a Burkitt's lymphoma cell line, KOBK101. Gene 97:239-244
14. Shen HM, Peters A, Baron B, Zhu X, Storb U (1998) Mutation of BCL-6 gene in normal B-cells by the process of somatic hypermutation of Ig genes. Science 280:1750-1752
15. Pasqualucci L, Migliazza A, Fracchiolla N, William C, Neri A, Baldini L, Changanti RSK, Klein U, Küppers R, Rajewsky K, Dalla-Favera R (1998) BCL-6 mutations in normal germinal center B-cells: Evidence of somatic hypermutation acting outside Ig loci. Prot Natl Acad Sci USA 95:11816-11821

Chromosome 13 Deletion in Myeloma

J. Shaughnessy and B. Barlogie
Myeloma and Transplantation Research Center, University of Arkansas for Medical Sciences and Arkansas Cancer Research Center, Little Rock, Arkansas 72205 USA
(Supported in part by CA55819 from the National Cancer Institute, Bethesda, Maryland.)

Introduction

Multiple myeloma (MM) is characterized by a tremendous "genomic chaos" unique to this hematopoietic neoplasm. The lack of readily identifiable dominant cytogenetic abnormalities has presented an obstacle to molecular genetic research attempting to define lesions critical for myelomagenesis (Sawyer, et al., 1995). In addition, due to the hypoproliferative nature of this malignancy presenting with a terminally differentiated phenotype, informative karyotypes are available in only one-third of patients studied. Yet, DNA cytometric and, more recently, fluorescence in situ hybridization (FISH) studies of interphase cells have revealed genetic alterations in virtually all myeloma cases examined (Latreille et al., 1980; San Miguel et al., 1995; Flactif et al., 1995; Drach et al., 1995). The frequent involvement of chromosome 14q32, the site of the Ig heavy chain genes, in chromosome translocations of myeloma has led several groups to identify the partner chromosomes involved. Unlike most B-cell leukemias and lymphomas in which 14q32 translocations have recurrent partner chromosomes, molecular investigations of these translocations in myeloma have revealed considerable heterogeneity of partner loci (Bergsagel et al., 1996; Chesi et al., 1997; Iida et al., 1997; Chesi et al., 1998; Stec et al., 1998). None of these 14q32 translocations has yet been associated with a distinct clinical disease course in myeloma. Thus, it is unclear whether these translocations play a critical role in myelomagenesis.

Results

Our long term commitment to performing karyotype analyses in each and every patient enrolled in high dose therapy trials with autologous hematopoietic stem cell support has finally paid off in that a grave prognosis could be traced to the presence of partial or complete deletions of chromosome 13 (c13) (Tricot et al., 1997). A more recent analysis of 231 newly diagnosed patients receiving Total Therapy (multi-regimen induction and myeloablative therapy in the tandem transplant setting), the presence of G-band metaphase evidence of complete or partial deletion of c13, present in 18% prior to first transplant, was associated with markedly inferior event-free and overall survival (Fig. 1). The 18% patients exhibiting c13 deletions had significantly shorter median duration of event-free survival (EFS) and overall survival (OS) of 22 and 32 months compared to 49 and 84+ months, respectively, among the remaining 82% patients. The adverse consequences of c13 deletion are also apparent in previously treated patients. Similar observations have since been reported with standard therapy using both metaphase and FISH techniques (Perez-Simon et al., 1998; Seong et al., 1998).

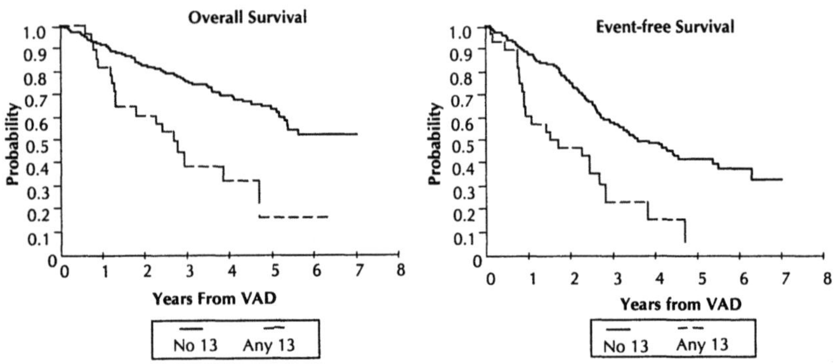

Fig. 1. Survival curves for event-free and overall survival for 231 myeloma patients receiving total therapy, with the variable being the presence or absence of chromosome 13 abnormalities as determined by conventional G-banding metaphase cytogenetic analyses. Broken line represents patients with abnormalities of chromosome 13. Solid line represents patients with normal chromosome 13.

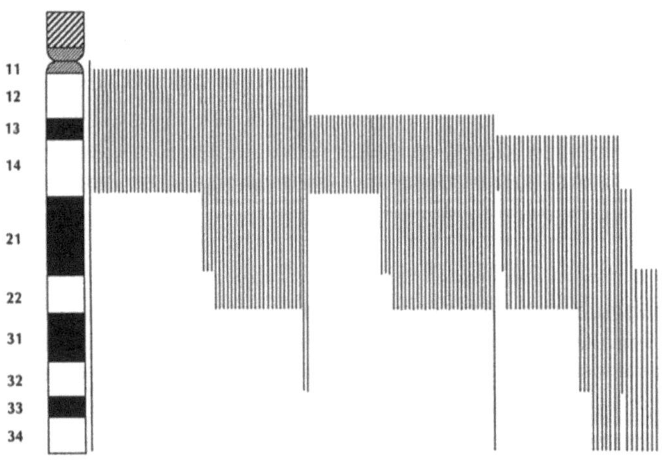

Fig. 2. Schematic view of cytogenetic deletions of the q arm of chromosome 13 in 145 myeloma patients. Each black line to the right of the chromosome indicates the part of chromosome 13 that has been deleted in one patient. Note that virtually every patient has deletion of 13q14.

Scrutiny of 145 karyotypes with c13q deletions showed 137 (94%) involved 13q14 and 100 (68%) had deletions of the 13q21-q22 region (Fig. 2). 13q14 was the minimally deleted region in the analysis. These observations are consistent with recent data obtained by comparative genomic hybridization experiments which also showed 13q14 to 13q21 deletions (Cigudosa et al., 1998).

Interphase FISH analysis was performed to fine-map c13q deletions in more detail. Using a panel of P1 artificial chromosomes (PACs) spanning the entire q arm, triple-color interphase FISH (TRI-FISH) (Ahmann et al., 1998), was applied to mononuclear cells from bone marrow aspirates of myeloma patients. In these experiments, we simultaneously hybridized cells with one of 11 probes located along the q arm of c13 and a chromosome 10 probe to control for ploidy (rarely deleted or amplified in myeloma). Cells were also hybridized with a fluorophore-labeled antibody against immunoglobulin light chains to identify clonal plasma cells. Of 39 patients analyzed to date, whole arm or interstitial deletions have been observed in 76%. All but 2 had deletion of the marker D13S272 which was sole deletion in 3 patients (flanking markers showed presence of 2 signals). Nullisomy for markers D13S272 and D13S21 was relatively high at 18% and 15%, respectively. Nullisomy for BRCA2 was seen in 10% of the cases. Nullisomy for all other markers was found to be 2.5% or less. (Table 1).

Table 1. Comparison of Chromosome 13 Deletion Using G-banding, TRI-FISH, and Deletion Frequencies of Selected Loci

G-banding		% Monoallelic Deletion (% Biallelic Deletion)			
Del 13	**N**	**BRCA2**	**RB1**	**D13S272**	**D13S31**
No	23	39 (9)	48 (4)	83 (22)	61 (22)
Yes	15	67 (13)	67 (0)	67 (13)	60 (7)
Total	38	50 (10)	55 (2)	76 (18)	61 (15)

Discussion

Preliminary data presented here indicate that molecular deletions of c13 are almost universal in myeloma and that TRI-FISH represents a powerful new method for identifying numeric chromosome abnormalities in this hypoproliferative malignancy. We have been able to demonstrate that the incidence of c13 abnormalities rises from 18% by conventional G-banding to 76% by TRI-FISH. The TRI-FISH method is also able to identify microscopically unrecognizable c13 abnormalities in samples with clear myeloma karyotypes and, more importantly, identify deletions in cells not analyzable by metaphase cytogenetics. TRI-FISH has also demonstrated that several deletion hotspots exist and likely harbor one or more genes important to controlling myeloma growth and or apoptosis.

Detailed molecular studies of c13 deletions are in progress to determine the clinically critical regimen(s) of deletion with both standard and high dose therapy regimens. Evolution of c13 deletion is envisioned that may involve several critical suppressor genes and may lead to a more aggressive clinical course. The adverse prognostic implications of c13 deletion in myeloma contrast with findings in chronic lymphocytic leukemia, where c13 deletions also occur commonly without, however, conferring a deleterious prognosis (Juliusson et al., 1990; Dohner et al., 1997). Furthermore, there is considerably less genetic heterogeneity in CLL, although Ig hypermutations, albeit of a lesser degree than in myeloma, have been reported in this B cell malignancy as well (Fais et al., 1998). Interestingly, somatic mutation of other loci i.e. BCL6, thought to result from Ig hypermutation mechanisms, has been shown to occur in the B-cell lineage (Shen et al., 1998). With this important observation in mind it is possible to envision that critical tumor suppressor genes on c13 could also be affected by somatic hypermutation. This phenomenon, in combination with the high incidence of c13 deletion as demonstrated by TRI-FISH, could have dramatic consequences in myeloma.

References

Ahmann GJ, Jalal SM, Juneau AL, Christensen ER, Hanson CA, Dewald GW, Greipp PR. (1998) A novel three-color, clone-specific fluorescence in situ hybridization procedure for monoclonal gammopathies. Cancer Genet. Cytogenet. 101:7-11

Bergsagel PL, Chesi M, Nardini E, Brents LA, Kirby SL, Kuehl WM. (1996) Promiscuous translocations into immunoglobulin heavy chain switch regions in multiple myeloma. Proc. Natl. Acad. Sci. USA. 93:13931-13936

Chesi M, Bergsagel PL, Shonukan OO, Martelli ML, Brents LA, Chen T, Schrock E, Ried T, Kuehl WM. (1998) Frequent dysregulation of the c-maf proto-oncogene at 16q23 by translocation to an Ig locus in multiple myeloma. Blood 91:4457-4463.

Chesi M, Nardini E, Brents LA, Schrock E, Ried T, Kuehl WM, Bergsagel PL. (1997) Frequent translocation t(4;14)(p16.3;q32.3) in multiple myeloma is associated with increased expression and activating mutations of fibroblast growth factor receptor 3. Nat. Genet. 3:260-264.

Cigudosa JC, Rao PH, Calasanz MJ, Odero MD, Michaeli J, Jhanwar SC, Chaganti RS. (1998) Characterization of nonrandom chromosomal gains and losses in multiple myeloma by comparative genomic hybridization. Blood 91:3007-3010.

Dohner H, Stilgenbauer S, Fischer K, Bentz M, Lichter P. (1997) Cytogenetic and molecular cytogenetic analysis of B cell chronic lymphocytic leukemia: specific chromosome aberrations identify prognostic subgroups of patients and point to loci of candidate genes. Leukemia Suppl. 2:S19-S24.

Drach J, Schuster J, Nowotny H, Angerler J, Rosenthal F, Fiegl M, Rothermundt C, Gsur A, Jager U, Heinz R, et al. (1995). Multiple myeloma: high incidence of chromosomal aneuploidy as detected by interphase fluorescence in situ hybridization. Cancer Res. 55:3854-3859.

Fais F, Ghiotto F, Hashimoto S, Sellars B, Valetto A, Allen SL, Schulman P, Vinciguerra VP, Rai K, Rassenti LZ, Kipps TJ, Dighiero G, Schroeder HW, Ferrarini M, Chiorazzi N. (1998) Chronic lymphocytic leukemia B cells express restricted sets of mutated and unmutated antigen receptors. J. Clin. Invest. 102:1515-25.

Flactif M, Zandecki M, Lai JL, Bernardi F, Obein V, Bauters F, Facon T. (1995) Interphase fluorescence in situ hybridization (FISH) as a powerful tool for the detection of aneuploidy in multiple myeloma. Leukemia 912:2109-2114.

Iida S, Rao PH, Butler M, Corradini P, Boccadoro M, Klein B, Chaganti RS, Dalla-Favera R. (1997) Deregulation of MUM1/IRF4 by chromosomal translocation in multiple myeloma. Nat. Genet. 2:226-230.

Juliusson G, Oscier DG, Fitchett M, Ross FM, Stockdill G, Mackie MJ, Parker AC, Castoldi GL, Guneo A, Knuutila S, et al. (1990) Prognostic subgroups in B-cell chronic lymphocytic leukemia defined by specific chromosomal abnormalities. N. Engl. J. Med. 323:720-724.

Kalachikov S, Migliazza A, Cayanis E, Fracchiolla NS, Bonaldo MF, Lawton L, Jelenc P, Ye X, Qu X, Chien M, Hauptschein R, Gaidano G, Vitolo U, Saglio G, Resegotti L, Brodjansky V, Yankovsky N, Zhang P, Soares MB, Russo J, Edelman IS, Efstratiadis A, Dalla-Favera R, Fischer SG. (1997) Cloning and gene mapping of the chromosome 13q14 region deleted in chronic lymphocytic leukemia. Genomics 42:369-377.

Latreille J, Barlogie B, Dosik G, Johnston DA, Drewinko B, Alexanian R. (1980) Cellular DNA content as a marker of human multiple myeloma. Blood 55:403-8.

Perez-Simon JA, Garcia-Sanz R, Tabernero MD, Almeida J, Gonzalez M, Fernandez-Calvo J, Moro MJ, Hernandez JM, San Miguel JF, Orfao A. (1998) Prognostic value of numerical chromosome aberrations in multiple myeloma: A FISH analysis of 15 different chromosomes. Blood 91: 3366-3371.

San Miguel, JF., Garcia-Sanz, R., Gonzalez, M., Orfao, A. (1995) Immunophenotype and DNA cell content in myeloma. Baillieres Clin. Haematol. 8:735-59.

Sawyer JR, Waldron JA, Jagannath S, Barlogie B. (1995) Cytogenetic findings in 200 patients with Multiple Myeloma. Cancer Genet. Cytogenet. 82:41-9.

Seong C, Delasalle K, Hayes K, Weber D, Dimopoulos M, Swantkowski J, Huh Y, Glassman A, Champlin R, Alexanian R. (1998) Prognostic value of cytogenetics in multiple myeloma. Br. J. Haematol. 101:189-194.

Shen HM, Peters A, Baron B, Zhu X, Storb U. (1998) Mutation of BCL-6 gene in normal B cells by the process of somatic hypermutation of Ig genes. Science. 280:1750-2

Stec I, Wright TJ, van Ommen GJB, de Boer PAJ, van Haeringen A, Moorman AFM, Altherr MR, den Dunnen JT. (1998) WHSC1, a 90 kb SET domain-containing gene, expressed in early development and homologous to a drosophila dysmorphy gene maps in the wolf-hirschhorn syndrome critical region and is fused to IgH in t(4;14) multiple myeloma. Hum. Mol. Genet. 7:1071-1082.

Tricot, G., Barlogie, B., Jagannath, S., Bracy, D., Mattox, S., Vesole, D., Naucke, S., Sawyer, J. (1995) Poor prognosis in multiple myeloma is associated only with partial or complete deletions of chromosome 13 or abnormalities involving 11q and not with other karyotypes abnormalities. Blood 86:4250-4256.

Unusual Immunoglobulin and T-cell Receptor Gene Rearrangement Patterns in Acute Lymphoblastic Leukemias

T. Szczepański[1,2], M. J. Pongers-Willemse[1], A. W. Langerak[1], and J. J. M. van Dongen[1]

[1] Dept. of Immunology, University Hospital Rotterdam/Erasmus University Rotterdam, Rotterdam; The Netherlands, and [2] Dept. of Pediatrics and Hematology, Silesian Medical Academy, Zabrze, Poland.

Abstract

Immunoglobulin (Ig) and T-cell receptor (TCR) genes are rearranged in virtually all acute lymphoblastic leukemia (ALL) cases. However, the recombination patterns display several unusual features as compared to normal lymphoid counterparts. Cross-lineage gene rearrangements occur in more than 90% of precursor-B-ALL and in ~20% of T-ALL, whereas they are rare in normal lymphocytes. Approximately 25-30% of the Ig and TCR gene rearrangements at diagnosis are oligoclonal, and can undergo continuing or secondary recombination events during the disease course. Based on our extensive molecular studies we hypothesize that the unusual Ig and TCR gene rearrangements in ALL occur as an early postoncogenic event resulting from the continuing V(D)J recombinase activity on accessible gene loci. This hypothesis is on the one hand supported by the virtual absence of cross-lineage gene rearrangements in normal lymphocytes and mature lymphoid malignancies and on the other hand by the presence of oligoclonality and secondary Ig and TCR gene rearrangements in ALL.

Introduction

Acute lymphoblastic leukemia (ALL) is a malignancy of immature lymphoid cells. Leukemic lymphoblasts are considered as the malignant counterparts of normal bone marrow B-cell precursors and thymic T-cell precursors that have undergone malignant transformation resulting in precursor-B-ALL and T-ALL, respectively. The oncogenic events block further differentiation, freezing the cell in a particular stage of the development, and subsequently enable uncontrolled proliferation. In virtually all ALL cases leukemic cells contain rearranged immunoglobulin (Ig) and/or T-cell receptor (TCR) genes [1,2]. This is probably related to the fact that Ig and TCR gene rearrangements take place very early during lymphoid differentiation i.e. before surface expression of the pan-B-cell marker CD19 in B-cell progenitors and in $CD34^+/CD1a^-$ thymocytes, respectively [3,4]. In exceptional ALL cases, most probably derived from very immature progenitor cells, the Ig and TCR gene loci are preserved in germline configuration.

In contrast to normal lymphoid development, Ig and TCR gene rearrangements in ALL have several unusual characteristics. Owing to the observation of cross-lineage TCR gene rearrangements in precursor-B-ALL and in some mature B-cell malignancies together with the finding of rearranged Ig heavy chain (*IGH*) genes in some T-ALL, Ig and TCR gene rearrangements cannot be regarded as specific markers for B-lineage and T-lineage, respectively [5]. In contrast, cross-lineage gene rearrangements are not observed in normal human thymocytes, whereas their frequency in normal B-cells is very low (below 0.5%) [3,6]. Other unusual characteristics of Ig and TCR gene rearrangements in ALL as compared to their normal counterparts are the overrepresentation of particular rearrangement types, e.g. the restriction to certain gene segments, the usage of pseudogenes, the presence of "end-stage" rearrangements, and the occurrence of asynchronous combinations of gene rearrangements [1,2,7].

Since a leukemic clone originates from a single malignantly transformed lymphoid cell, all lymphoblasts in principle have identically rearranged Ig and TCR genes i.e. monoclonal gene rearrangements. However, in a substantial proportion of ALL there is evidence of oligoclonality. Subclones frequently show junctional region sequences related to the major clone, reflecting a continuing rearrangement process. Ongoing recombinations may also result in changes of leukemia-specific rearrangements at relapse of the disease [8-11].

The occurrence of unusual gene rearrangements in ALL can be explained in several ways. It could be that cross-lineage gene rearrangements occur in early lymphoid progenitors leading to a stop in further differentiation and maturation. As a consequence, a large fraction of such proliferating, immature lymphoid precursor cells without functional lineage-specific rearrangements and/or with cross-lineage gene rearrangements would normally undergo apoptosis unless they become neoplastic. An alternative explanation could be that unusual and cross-lineage gene rearrangements in ALL represent postoncogenic events resulting from the ongoing activity of the common B and T-cell V(D)J recombinase system on gene loci, which are accessible at the stage of maturational arrest and initial proliferation. Secondary and ongoing rearrangements would then take place during the proliferative phase as well. Here we present the results of our extensive studies on Ig and TCR gene rearrangements patterns in ALL, which in our opinion favour the hypothesis of unusual gene recombination in ALL as a predominantly postoncogenic event.

Results & Discussion

Lineage-specific Gene Rearrangements in ALL

During the last years we performed detailed analysis of Ig and TCR gene rearrangements in 340 ALL patients at diagnosis (Table 1) [1,12-16]. In virtually all precursor-B-ALL cases (>95%) Southern blot analysis revealed clonal *IGH* gene rearrangements. In a significant proportion of these patients (~40%) obvious differences in density of two or more rearranged bands were found, reflecting oligoclonality at the *IGH* locus [12]. Since PCR analysis is more sensitive than Southern blotting, one can expect that *IGH* oligoclonality might in fact even concern a larger fraction of precursor-B-ALL cases. Fig. 1 illustrates a case with multiple clonal *IGH* gene rearrangements at diagnosis as detected by heteroduplex PCR analysis [17]. Furthermore, PCR studies have already shown that the vast majority of *IGH* gene rearrangements were not functional, and that DH-DH-JH fusions could be identified in ~20% of patients [18,19].

Ig light chain gene rearrangements were found in 60% of cases (Table 1). Rearrangements of the Ig kappa light chain (*IGK*) gene occur more frequently than in the Ig lambda light chain (*IGL*) gene locus and often concern deletional rearrangements to the kappa deleting element (Kde) [20]. In contrast to normal B cells we observed an unusually high frequency of *IGK* deletional rearrangements compared to *IGK* and *IGL* gene rearrangement frequencies. Oligoclonality of *IGK* gene rearrangements was observed in <10% of precursor-B-ALL patients [12].

Table 1. Relative frequencies of Ig and TCR gene rearrangements in ALL [a]

	IGH		*IGK*		*IGL*	*TCRB*	*TCRG*	*TCRD*	
	R	D	R	D				R	D
Precursor-B-ALL (children)	95%	3%	30%	30%	20%	30%	60%	55%	35%
T-ALL	20%	0%	0%	0%	0%	90%	95%	70%	25%
Total ALL	85%	2%	25%	25%	15%	45%	65%	60%	35%

[a] Gene configurations as determined by interpretation of Southern blot results: R, rearrangement of at least one allele; D, deletion on both alleles or one allele deleted and the other in germline configuration.

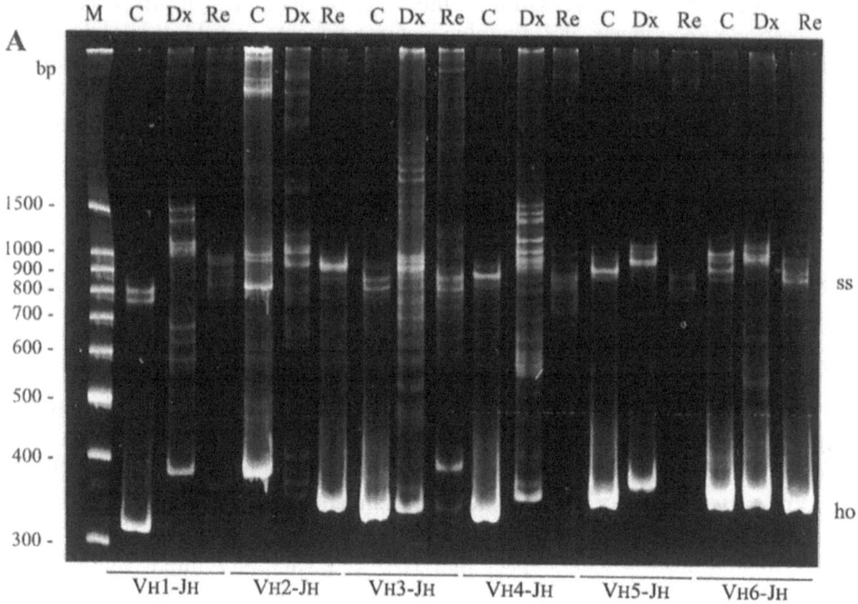

B

	VH	N-REGION	VH/DH	N-REGION	DH	N-REGION	JH
(Dx)	VH6-1(-6)	GAGGGAGGG	(-14) DH2-2 (-1)	AAG	(-7) DH6-13 (0)	CGGGGATG	(-6) JH6b
(Re)			VH2-70 (-2)	CCGCCG	(-10) DH6-13 (0)	CGGGGATG	(-6) JH6b

Fig. 1. (A) Heteroduplex PCR analysis of bone marrow DNA from a precursor-B-ALL patient at diagnosis (Dx) and at relapse (Re) using six VH family-specific primers together with a JH consensus primer. The results illustrate oligoclonality both at diagnosis (five *IGH* gene rearrangements) and at relapse (three *IGH* gene rearrangements). None of the rearrangements was identical between diagnosis and relapse. ss, Single-strand fragments; ho, homoduplexes; C, positive control; M, 100 bp molecular weight marker **(B)** Fluorescent sequencing of clonal PCR products at diagnosis and relapse showed that two different rearrangements shared an identical DH6-13-JH6b junctional region, thereby proving the clonal relationship between the diagnosis and relapse cell samples.

Interestingly, a significant proportion (~20%) of *IGL* gene rearrangements in precursor-B-ALL involves the non-functional J-Cλ6 gene region (Tümkaya et al., submitted for publication).

Analysis of a small group of adult precursor-B-ALL patients revealed several intriguing differences as compared to childhood patients [21]. Firstly, we observed a lower level of *IGH* oligoclonality (~20% versus ~40% in children) despite a comparable incidence of *IGH* gene rearrangements. Secondly, all detected *IGK* gene deletions concerned rearrangements of the Kde to Vκ gene segments, which represent two thirds of the Kde rearrangements in pediatric precursor-B-ALL and only half of the Kde rearrangements in mature B-cell leukemias [20,21].

TCR gene rearrangements occur in more than 95% of T-ALL cases (Table 1). The TCR delta (*TCRD*) locus first undergoes rearrangement in normal thymocyte development and likewise is the most frequently rearranged gene in T-ALL (~95%). In contrast to frequent subclone formation in Ig genes in precursor-B-ALL, this phenomenon is rarely observed for TCR gene rearrangements in T-ALL (Langerak et al., unpublished data).

Interestingly, in several T-ALL patients an atypical TCR gamma (*TCRG*) gene rearrangement was demonstrated showing an interstitial deletion of ~170 bp of the downstream part of the Vγ2 gene segment [22].

Cross-lineage TCR Gene Rearrangements in Precursor-B-ALL

Our analysis of a large group of 202 pediatric precursor-B-ALL patients revealed TCR beta (*TCRB*), *TCRG*, and *TCRD* gene rearrangements in 35%, 59%, and 89% of cases, respectively (Table 1) [15]. In total, in 93% of the precursor-B-ALL cases one or more TCR genes were rearranged and/or deleted, indicating that cross-lineage TCR gene rearrangements are ubiquitously present in malignant B-lineage lymphoblasts. However, the spectrum of cross-lineage TCR gene rearrangements in precursor-B-ALL is very limited (Table 2). *TCRB* gene rearrangements are restricted to the Jβ2 region. This is in contrast to normal T-cells and T-ALL, which employ both Jβ1 and Jβ2 gene regions. *TCRG* gene rearrangements in precursor-B-ALL most frequently (~70%) concern rearrangements to Jγ1 region gene segments. Curiously, 80% of *TCRD* gene rearrangements represent incomplete Vδ2-Dδ3 or Dδ2-Dδ3 joinings, whereas complete rearrangements to the Jδ1 gene segment, characteristic for normal T-cells and T-ALL blasts (particularly TCRγδ$^+$ [23]) have never been reported in precursor-B-ALL. Apparently, only certain parts of the *TCRB* and *TCRD* genes are accessible for continuing activity of the V(D)J recombinase in precursor-B-ALL. Using a transgenic mouse model, Lauzurica et al. [24] showed that V-D to J recombination in human *TCRD* genes is controlled by the *TCRD* enhancer, whereas rearrangements to the Dδ3 gene segment are controlled by a separate mechanism. It seems highly probable that in precursor-B-ALL *TCRD* gene

Table 2. Unusual TCR gene rearrangements in precursor-B-ALL as compared to normal T-cells and T-ALL

	Precursor-B-ALL	Normal T-lymphocytes/T-ALL
TCRB genes	exclusively to Jβ2: Vβ-Jβ2: 53% Dβ-Jβ2: 35%	both to Jβ1 and Jβ2
TCRG genes	Vγ-Jγ1.3: 40% Vγ-Jγ2.3: 28% Vγ-Jγ1.1: 27%	TCRαβ$^+$ T cells: mainly to Jγ1.3/2.3 TCRγδ$^+$ T cells: mainly VγII-Jγ1.2 T-ALL blasts: mainly to Jγ1.3/2.3
TCRD genes	Vδ2-Dδ3: 40-70% Dδ2-Dδ3: 10-40%	TCRαβ$^+$ T cells/T-ALL: mainly biallelic deletion TCRγδ$^+$ T cells: mainly Vδ2-Jδ1 TCRγδ$^+$ T-ALL: mainly Vδ1-Jδ1

rearrangements are restricted to those that are independent of the *TCRD* enhancer. Furthermore, Vδ2 and Dδ2 gene segments in precursor-B-ALL can further undergo rearrangements to Jα gene segments and the majority of *TCRD* gene deletions reflect secondary Vα-Jα rearrangements [6,15].

The analysis of combinations of cross-lineage TCR gene rearrangements in precursor-B-ALL patients showed that *TCRD* gene rearrangements and/or deletions occurred in the majority of cases (~90%) and that 27% of childhood precursor-B-ALL had *TCRD* gene rearrangements and/or deletions with germline *TCRG* and *TCRB* genes [15]. This implies that the hierarchy of cross-lineage TCR gene events is similar to early T-cell development, where rearrangements in the *TCRD* locus occur first, followed by *TCRG*, and subsequently by *TCRB* gene rearrangements. Nevertheless, in a few cases we found rearranged *TCRB* genes with *TCRD* and *TCRG* loci in germline configuration. Furthermore, the frequencies of cross-lineage TCR gene rearrangements seem to be related to the maturation stages of malignant B cells. The frequency of TCR gene rearrangements is lower in immature precursor-B-ALL (pro-B-ALL) as compared to $CD10^+$ precursor-B-ALL (common ALL and pre-B-ALL). When comparing common ALL and pre-B-ALL subgroups, it is striking that in the "mature" ($CyIg\mu^+$) pre-B-ALL group a higher frequency of patients have their TCR genes in germline configuration (15% versus 2% in common ALL). TCR gene rearrangements are still present in the most mature precursor-B-ALL subgroup with simultaneous cytoplasmic and membrane Igμ expression (transitional-pre-B-ALL). However, in mature B-cell malignancies cross-lineage TCR gene rearrangements are rare (<5%) [1,25].

Based on combined Southern blotting and heteroduplex PCR analysis we showed oligoclonality in 38% and 30% of precursor-B-ALL patients with *TCRG* and *TCRD* gene rearrangements, respectively, which is comparable to the frequency of oligoclonality found in the *IGH* locus [15].

In adult precursor-B-ALL a striking predominance of immature Dδ2-Dδ3 cross-lineage recombinations was observed (44%), whereas the more mature Vδ2-Dδ3 gene rearrangements occurred less frequently (38%). This is in contrast to the high frequency (>70%) of the more mature Vδ2-Dδ3 gene rearrangements in childhood precursor-B-ALL. Together with the characteristic *IGH* and *IGK* gene rearrangement patterns this suggests that the Ig and TCR genotype of precursor-B-ALL in adults is less mature than in children [21].

Cross-Lineage *IGH* Gene Rearrangements in T-ALL

In contrast to the frequent cross-lineage TCR gene rearrangements in precursor-B-ALL, *IGH* gene rearrangements in T-ALL occur in ~20% of patients (19% of $CD3^-$ T-ALL, 50% of $TCR\gamma\delta^+$ T-ALL, and only 4% of $TCR\alpha\beta^+$). Using heteroduplex PCR analysis we found a high frequency (~80%) of incomplete DH-JH rearrangements as well as preferential usage of DH6-19 and the most downstream DH7-27 gene segment together with the most upstream JH1 and JH2 gene segments. We have not found VH gene restriction in the complete VH-JH recombinations, which comprised 18% of cross-lineage *IGH* gene rearrangements in T-ALL patients. Furthermore, oligoclonality in the *IGH* locus was found in

27% of T-ALL patients with rearranged *IGH* genes (Szczepański et al., submitted for publication). Cross-lineage *IGH* gene rearrangements are rare in mature T-cell malignancies and Ig light chain gene rearrangements have only been reported anecdotally in malignant T lymphoblasts [1].

Secondary and Ongoing Gene Rearrangements in ALL
Another striking feature of Ig and TCR gene rearrangements in ALL is the occurrence of secondary recombination events. Secondary rearrangements via continuing VH to DH-JH joining, VH gene replacements, and "de novo" *IGH* gene rearrangements have frequently been reported for precursor-B-ALL (Fig. 1) [26,27]. Southern blot comparison between *IGH* configuration at diagnosis and at relapse provided evidence for clonal changes in 40% of precursor-B-ALL cases [8]. A few limited PCR studies estimated the frequency of *IGH* clonal evolution at ~30% of cases [9,28].

Recently, we found evidence for continuing VH to DH-JH recombination in T-ALL, while VH replacement has been described previously during disease progression of a T-lymphoblastic lymphoma [29].

Based on Southern blot analysis, differences in *TCRB*, *TCRG*, and *TCRD* gene rearrangements between diagnosis and relapse were found in 30%, 20%, and 10% of T-ALL, respectively [8]. Limited PCR studies estimated the frequency of *TCRG* and *TCRD* clonal evolution at 10-40% of T-ALL cases [10,11]. Interestingly, we demonstrated in several T-ALL cases ongoing, polyclonal δREC-ψJα gene rearrangements within otherwise monoclonal leukemic populations[30].

Cross-lineage *TCRG* and *TCRD* gene rearrangement patterns in precursor-B-ALL were found discordant between diagnosis and relapse in 30-50% of cases by Southern blotting. However, in a few cases seemingly clonal Vδ2-Dδ3 rearrangements appeared to be oligoclonal upon PCR analysis [15,21]. Moreover, ongoing Vδ2-Dδ3 to Jα recombination was demonstrated in the vast majority of Vδ2-Dδ3-positive precursor-B-ALL [6]. Finally, in a few precursor-B-ALL cases with clonal *TCRG* rearrangements at diagnosis the disease recurred with *TCRG* genes in germline configuration (clonal regression) [8,10].

Conclusions

ALL blasts display a variety of characteristic gene rearrangements. The majority of lineage-specific rearrangements probably reflect the gene configuration status of the lymphoid precursor cell that was transformed at a particular stage of differentiation. Cross-lineage gene rearrangements that are found in ALL could potentially be acquired before malignant transformation as well. However, then one would expect them to occur in normal lymphocytes at much higher frequencies. Since the majority of cross-lineage gene rearrangements are monoclonal and not oligoclonal, they should have occurred early after malignant transformation. The rare occurrence of cross-lineage gene rearrangements in TCRαβ$^+$ lineage T-ALL as well as in mature B-cell and T-cell malignancies can be explained by the absence of recombinase activity in these more mature types of lymphoid malignancies. Oligoclonality at diagnosis, clonal regression, ongoing and secondary recombination are unequivocally later postoncogenic events. Taken together, we hypothesize that the unusual gene rearrangements in ALL are caused by post-transformation continuing activity of the V(D)J recombinase enzyme system on accessible gene loci.

References

1. Van Dongen JJM, Wolvers-Tettero ILM (1991) Analysis of immunoglobulin and T cell receptor genes. Part II: Possibilities and limitations in the diagnosis and management of lymphoproliferative diseases and related disorders. Clin Chim Acta 198:93-174.
2. Felix CA, Poplack DG (1991) Characterization of acute lymphoblastic leukemia of childhood by immunoglobulin and T-cell receptor gene patterns. Leukemia 5:1015-1025.
3. Bertrand FE, III, Billips LG, Burrows PD, Gartland GL, Kubagawa H, Schroeder HW, Jr. (1997) Ig D(H) gene segment transcription and rearrangement before surface expression of the pan-B-cell marker CD19 in normal human bone marrow. Blood 90:736-744.
4. Ktorza S, Sarun S, Rieux-Laucat F, de Villartay JP, Debre P, Schmitt C (1995) CD34-positive early human thymocytes: T cell receptor and cytokine receptor gene expression. Eur J Immunol 25:2471-2478.
5. Greaves MF, Chan LC, Furley AJ, Watt SM, Molgaard HV (1986) Lineage promiscuity in hemopoietic differentiation and leukemia. Blood 67:1-11.
6. Steenbergen EJ, Verhagen OJ, van Leeuwen EF, van den Berg H, von dem Borne AE, van der Schoot CE (1995) Frequent ongoing T-cell receptor rearrangements in childhood B-precursor acute lymphoblastic leukemia: implications for monitoring minimal residual disease. Blood 86:692-702.
7. Biondi A, Francia di Celle P, Rossi V, Casorati G, Matullo G, Giudici G, Foa R, Migone N (1990) High prevalence of T-cell receptor V delta 2-(D)-D delta 3 or D delta 1/2-D delta 3 rearrangements in B-precursor acute lymphoblastic leukemias. Blood 75:1834-1840.
8. Beishuizen A, Verhoeven MA, van Wering ER, Hählen K, Hooijkaas H, van Dongen JJM (1994) Analysis of Ig and T-cell receptor genes in 40 childhood acute lymphoblastic leukemias at diagnosis and subsequent relapse: implications for the detection of minimal residual disease by polymerase chain reaction analysis. Blood 83:2238-2247.
9. Marshall GM, Kwan E, Haber M, Brisco MJ, Sykes PJ, Morley AA, Toogood I, Waters K, Tauro G, Ekert H, Norris MD (1995) Characterization of clonal immunoglobulin heavy chain and T cell receptor gamma gene rearrangements during progression of childhood acute lymphoblastic leukemia. Leukemia 9:1847-1850.
10. Taylor JJ, Rowe D, Kylefjord H, Chessells J, Katz F, Proctor SJ, Middleton PG (1994) Characterisation of non-concordance in the T-cell receptor gamma chain genes at presentation and clinical relapse in acute lymphoblastic leukemia. Leukemia 8:60-66.
11. Baruchel A, Cayuela JM, MacIntyre E, Berger R, Sigaux F (1995) Assessment of clonal evolution at Ig/TCR loci in acute lymphoblastic leukaemia by single-strand conformation polymorphism studies and highly resolutive PCR derived methods: implication for a general strategy of minimal residual disease detection. Br J Haematol 90:85-93.
12. Beishuizen A, Hählen K, Hagemeijer A, Verhoeven MA, Hooijkaas H, Adriaansen HJ, Wolvers-Tettero ILM, van Wering ER, van Dongen JJM (1991) Multiple rearranged immunoglobulin genes in childhood acute lymphoblastic leukemia of precursor B-cell origin. Leukemia 5:657-667.
13. Beishuizen A, Verhoeven MA, Mol EJ, Breit TM, Wolvers-Tettero ILM, van Dongen JJM (1993) Detection of immunoglobulin heavy-chain gene rearrangements by Southern blot analysis: recommendations for optimal results. Leukemia 7:2045-2053.

14. Breit TM, Wolvers-Tettero ILM, Beishuizen A, Verhoeven M-AJ, van Wering ER, van Dongen JJM (1993) Southern blot patterns, frequencies and junctional diversity of T-cell receptor δ gene rearrangements in acute lymphoblastic leukemia. Blood 82:3063-3074.
15. Szczepański T, Beishuizen A, Pongers-Willemse MJ, Hählen K, van Wering ER, Wijkhuijs JM, Tibbe GJM, De Bruijn MAC, van Dongen JJM (1999) Cross-lineage T-cell receptor gene rearrangements occur in more than ninety percent of childhood precursor-B-acute lymphoblastic leukemias: alternative PCR targets for detection of minimal residual disease. Leukemia 13 (in press).
16. Pongers-Willemse MJ, Seriu T, Stolz F, d'Aniello E, Gameiro P, Pisa P, Gonzalez M, Bartram CR, Panzer-Grumayer ER, Biondi A, San Miguel JF, van Dongen JJM (1999) Primers and protocols for standardized MRD detection in ALL using immunoglobulin and T cell receptor gene rearrangements and *TAL1* deletions as PCR targets. Report of the BIOMED-1 Concerted Action: Investigation of minimal residual disease in acute leukemia. Leukemia 13 (in press).
17. Langerak AW, Szczepański T, van der Burg M, Wolvers-Tettero ILM, van Dongen JJM (1997) Heteroduplex PCR analysis of rearranged T cell receptor genes for clonality assessment in suspect T cell proliferations. Leukemia 11:2192-2199.
18. Height SE, Swansbury GJ, Matutes E, Treleaven JG, Catovsky D, Dyer MJ (1996) Analysis of clonal rearrangements of the Ig heavy chain locus in acute leukemia. Blood 87:5242-5250.
19. Steenbergen EJ, Verhagen OJ, van Leeuwen EF, Behrendt H, Merle PA, Wester MR, von dem Borne AE, van der Schoot CE (1994) B precursor acute lymphoblastic leukemia third complementarity-determining regions predominantly represent an unbiased recombination repertoire: leukemic transformation frequently occurs in fetal life. Eur J Immunol 24:900-908.
20. Beishuizen A, Verhoeven MA, Mol EJ, van Dongen JJM (1994) Detection of immunoglobulin kappa light-chain gene rearrangement patterns by Southern blot analysis. Leukemia 8:2228-2236.
21. Szczepański T, Langerak AW, Wolvers-Tettero ILM, Ossenkoppele GJ, Verhoef G, Stul M, Petersen EJ, de Bruijn MAC, van't Veer MB, van Dongen JJM (1998) Immunoglobulin and T cell receptor gene rearrangement patterns in acute lymphoblastic leukemia are less mature in adults than in children: implications for selection of PCR targets for detection of minimal residual disease. Leukemia 12:1081-1088.
22. Castellanos A, Martin-Seisdedos C, Toribio ML, San Miguel JF, Gonzalez Sarmiento R (1998) TCR-gamma gene rearrangement with interstitial deletion within the TRGV2 gene segment is not detected in normal T-lymphocytes. Leukemia 12:251-253.
23. Langerak AW, Wolvers-Tettero ILM, van den Beemd MWM, van Wering ER, Ludwig W-D, Hählen K, Necker A, van Dongen JJM (1999) Immunophenotypic and immunogenotypic characteristics of TCRγδ$^+$ T cell acute lymphoblastic leukemia. Leukemia 13 (in press).
24. Lauzurica P, Krangel MS (1994) Enhancer-dependent and -independent steps in the rearrangement of a human T cell receptor delta transgene. J Exp Med 179:43-55.
25. Szczepański T, Langerak AW, van Dongen JJM, van Krieken JHJM (1998) Lymphoma with multi-gene rearrangement on the level of immunoglobulin heavy chain, light chain, and T-cell receptor beta chain. Am J Hematol 59:99-100.
26. Kitchingman GR (1993) Immunoglobulin heavy chain gene VH-D junctional diversity at diagnosis in patients with acute lymphoblastic leukemia. Blood 81:775-782.
27. Steenbergen EJ, Verhagen OJ, van Leeuwen EF, von dem Borne AE, van der Schoot CE (1993) Distinct ongoing Ig heavy chain rearrangement processes in childhood B-precursor acute lymphoblastic leukemia. Blood 82:581-589.
28. Steward CG, Goulden NJ, Katz F, Baines D, Martin PG, Langlands K, Potter MN, Chessells JM, Oakhill A (1994) A polymerase chain reaction study of the stability of Ig heavy-chain and T-cell receptor delta gene rearrangements between presentation and relapse of childhood B-lineage acute lymphoblastic leukemia. Blood 83:1355-1362.
29. Rosenquist R, Lindh J, Roos G, Holmberg D (1997) Immunoglobulin VH gene replacements in a T-cell lymphoblastic lymphoma. Mol Immunol 34:305-313.
30. Breit TM, Verschuren MCM, Wolvers-Tettero ILM, van Gastel-Mol EJ, Hählen K, van Dongen JJM (1997) Human T cell leukemias with continuous V(D)J recombinase activity for TCR-delta gene deletion. J Immunol 159:4341-4349.

Discussion

Kenneth Nilsson: Are these patients all children or do the adults also have the same type of unusual rearrangements?
Jacques van Dongen: Yes, adult ALL also have comparable unusual rearrangements. Only a few studies have been performed in adults. We have found exactly the same phenomena in adult ALL at a slightly lower frequency than in childhood ALL. For instance, 30% instead of 40% *TCRB* gene rearrangements in precursor-B-ALL, etc. The rearrangements in adult ALL also tend to be more immature, e.g. more incomplete Dδ2-Dδ3 rearrangements in adults versus children. So there are some differences (see: Szczepanski et al. Leukemia 1998;12:1081-1088).
Kenneth Nilsson: Is anything known about the cytogenetics?
Jacques van Dongen: We did not correlate our data with cytogenetics. However, the frequencies of the Ig and TCR gene rearrangements are very high whereas the characteristic cytogenetic aberrancies occur at lower frequencies, together 30-40% with a predominance of the t(12;21) in children and in adults at frequencies of 35-40% with a predominance of t(9;22).
Kenneth Nilsson: So could it be that you have randomly selected only the normal diploid ones?
Jacques van Dongen: No, these were mainly consecutive patients, there was no selection.
Federico Caligaris-Cappio: What about the possible diagnostic or prognostic significance of the unusual Ig and TCR gene rearrangements? Did you correlate them within a large series?
Jacques van Dongen: Not in this large series yet, but in the first series of precursor-B-ALL that we analyzed for *IGH* gene oligoclonality, we found that oligoclonal precursor-B-ALL had a poorer prognosis than the ALL with two clones, versus the ones that consisted of only one clone, as detected by Southern blotting (see: Beishuizen et al., Leukemia 1991;5:657-667). So there seems indeed to be a difference in prognosis, but this was not statistically significant.
George Klein: Since you are asking for similar models, isn't the pre-B Abelson leukemia, which is monoclonal by retroviral insertion but then keeps rearranging its Ig genes, a model for this?
Jacques van Dongen: That may well be, yes. These murine leukemias indeed also represent early differentiation stages. Do they also develop *TCR* gene rearrangements?
George Klein: No, only Ig gene rearrangements.
Jacques van Dongen: So they apparently are at a stage of transformation where the *TCR* genes are not accessible for the recombinase enzyme system.
Michael Reth: Where did you get the material from? Was it the whole tumor?
Jacques van Dongen: These are typical blood and bone marrow samples that arrive in our laboratory from newly diagnosed patients. The immunophenotyping and the Ig and TCR gene analyses are performed in our laboratory on freshly obtained patient material. The patients arrive consecutively from the hospital, and the tumor loads, especially in children, are high (generally >80%).
Michael Reth: Were the rearrangements, analysed in DNA, derived from a cell population or did you use single cell PCR?
Jacques van Dongen: The Southern blotting is performed on DNA from all blood or bone marrow cells together, but the background of normal cells is low. If you perform PCR, you may nevertheless amplify the gene rearrangements from normal cells. However, even then you can distinguish between monoclonal and polyclonal (normal) rearrangements by use of heteroduplex analysis of the obtained PCR products (see Langerak et al. Leukemia 1997; 11:2192-2199). Even in case of the ongoing "polyclonal" δREC-ψJα rearrangements in otherwise monoclonal T-ALL, we could prove that these polyclonal rearrangements were derived from the monoclonal leukemic T-cells and not from normal T-cells (Breit et al. J Immunol 1997; 159:4341-4349). This was based on our finding that all δREC-ψJα rearrangements were exclusively occurring on one *TCRD* allele (with a Vδ2-Jδ1 rearrangement), which was identified via a C/T polymorphism at 87 bp upstream of the recombination signal sequence of the δREC gene segment. So this polymorphism could be used as an allele-specific marker.

Heinz Jacobs: The V gene segments which are used in the V to DJ rearrangements, are these the proximal ones?

Jacques van Dongen: I presume that you are referring to the cross-lineage *IGH* gene rearrangements in T-ALL. We looked carefully at the various gene segments and found that D gene segments are used preferentially with a relatively high frequency of the most proximal DQ52 (D7-27 in the new nomenclature) and it was also curious to see the high frequency of D6-19 usage: together they constituted over 60% of all the D_H gene segments used in T-ALL. So there is a real preference for particular gene segments. This also concerns the most upstream J_H gene segments. However, V gene segments were used randomly.

Analysis of Variable Heavy and Light Chain Genes in Follicular Lymphomas of Different Heavy Chain Isotype

W.M. Aarts, R.J. Bende, S.T. Pals and C.J.M. van Noesel
Department of Pathology, Academic Medical Center, Meibergdreef 9, 1105 AZ, Amsterdam, the Netherlands

Introduction

Follicular lymphomas (FLs) are considered prototypes of germinal center derived B-cell malignancies. This contention is based on histomorphological characteristics [1] as well as on the presence of somatic mutations in the variable heavy and light chain genes (VH and VL genes) [2,3]. FLs are believed to have retained two important features of germinal center B cells, *i.e.* their capability of ongoing somatic hypermutation [4-6] and heavy chain isotype switching [7-9]. To investigate somatic mutation in relation to heavy chain isotype expression, we analyzed the immunoglobulin variable genes (IgV genes) of a panel of IgM-expressing and isotype-switched FLs. We find elevated frequencies of somatic mutation compared to normal B cells, but FLs resemble normal B cells in VH family gene usage, patterns of somatic mutation and differences in mutation frequency found between IgM-expressing and isotype-switched FLs. Our study questions the capacity of at least some FLs to undergo somatic hypermutation.

Results and Discussion

We screened 51 FLs by RT-PCR. Clonality had already been determined immunohistochemically in these FLs. To assess clonality and isotype expression at molecular level, the complementarity determining region 3 (CDR3) was amplified, with a primer that anneals to the framework 3 region (FR3) combined with primers specific for either the JH genes or for the constant regions of different heavy chain isotypes [10]. Because of the highly variable length of CDR3 regions [11], the CDR3-specific PCR applied on a polyclonal B-cell population yields products of variable size, visible as a smear pattern after electrophoresis. In contrast, a single band is obtained in case of a monoclonal B-cell population. In 23 FLs (45%) we observed a sharp band on a high resolution agarose gel with a JH primer and one of the primers specific for the constant heavy chain (CH) regions as downstream primers. In another 13 cases we could establish clonality only with use of a Cμ, Cγ or Cα downstream primer, and not with the JH primer, most likely due to the presence of somatic mutations at the annealing site of the JH primer. In summary, in 36 of 51 FLs (71%) we could confirm clonality with a CDR3-specific PCR, which is in accordance with literature. Using DNA extracted from frozen tissue material, Lozano *et al.* could establish clonality in 9 of 13 cases of FL (69%) [12]. Diss *et al.* detected clonal CDR3-PCR products in 8 out of 10 FLs (80%) when DNA from frozen tissue was used [13]. Segal *et al.* could assess clonality in 31 out of 60 FLs (52%) by amplifying the CDR3 region from DNA [14]. The cases in which clonality could not be established may either contain too many non-neoplastic normal B cells, or somatic mutations in their VH genes at the primer annealing sites. As our results show, the usage of downstream primers specific for the CH genes, which is only possible if cDNA is used, can significantly improve clonality analyses. In only one of these 36 cases, expression of more than one isotype could be demonstrated: lymphoma no. 8 was shown to contain both a clonal IgM, IgD and IgG population, as determined by CDR3-specific PCR.

Nineteen FLs were selected from the FLs with a clonal CDR3-PCR pattern. In this selection, isotype-switched FLs were relatively overrepresented. Of these 19 FLs the complete VH genes were amplified using RT-PCR with family-specific VH leader primers. PCR products were sequenced directly, or independent molecular clones were sequenced after introduction of the PCR fragments into a TA cloning vector [10]. Of 9 of these 19 FLs, the Vκ genes were also analyzed [15]. The sequences found were compared to the most homologous germline VH sequences [16] and Vκ sequences [17].

The usage of VH genes of FLs was similar to the VH gene usage of normal B cells [18,19]. We found that 63% used VH3 genes, 21% used VH4 genes, 11% used VH1 genes and 5% (1 FL) used the VH5 gene (Table 1), which is in accordance with frequencies found by Bahler *et al.*, who analyzed a selection of 36 FLs [2]. Of 9 of the FLs the Vκ genes were also sequenced: 56% used the Vκ3 gene, 33% used the Vκ1 gene and 11% used the Vκ4 gene. This differs from a selection of 10 FLs described in literature, of which 90% used Vκ1 genes, and 10% used the Vκ4 gene [3]. Normal B-cells are reported to use Vκ1 genes in 50% of cases, followed by Vκ3 (25%) and Vκ4 (19%). Vκ2 genes are only used in 6% of cases [20]. The differences we find in Vκ gene usage may be related to the low number of FLs analyzed.

In accordance with literature, high numbers of somatic mutations were found in the IgV genes of the FLs [2,3]; on average 28 (9.5%) and 17 (5.9%) mutations were found in the VH genes and Vκ genes, respectively. It has been reported for FLs as well as for normal antigen-experienced B cells, that Vκ genes are less mutated than VH genes [3,21]. The Vκ genes contained less somatic mutations than their partner VH genes, with exception of case no. 25 (Fig. 1). In this FL the amount of somatic mutation was found to be lower in the VH gene than in the Vκ gene, which indicates that this relation between the amount of somatic mutation in VH and Vκ genes is not absolute. Also the amount of intraclonal variation was found to be lower in the VH-gene than in the Vκ-gene of FL no. 25 (0.4 versus 4.9 mutations per clone, respectively; Table 1).

The mutation patterns in the VH genes of the FLs were suggestive of selection for preservation of the structure of the immunoglobulin molecule, since low ratios of replacement versus silent mutations (R/S ratios) were found in the frame-

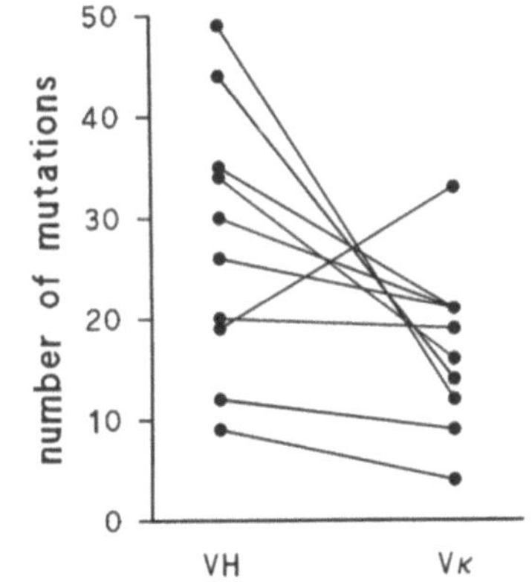

Fig. 1. Correlation between amount of somatic mutation in VH and Vκ sequences of the same FLs.

work regions (FRs; Table 1). Low R/S ratios in the FRs were independent of the total amount of somatic mutation or the presence of intraclonal variation. In normal antigen-selected B cells, the R/S ratio in the FRs is about 1.5 [22]. In one case, no. 59, the R/S ratio of the FRs was found to be significantly higher (Table 1).

The FLs were shown to have a variable degree of intraclonal variation when amplified VH molecules were sequenced individually. Of 16 FLs analyzed at the clonal level, 11 showed intraclonal variation above the Taq error frequency [10], ranging from 0.7 to 14.8 mutations per clone, compared to the consensus sequence. Five FLs did not show significant intraclonal variation in their VH genes ($\leq$0.4 mutations per clone). The shared mutations found in 9 of these 11 FLs are indicative of true intraclonal variation rather than Taq error (data not shown). The occurrence of intraclonal variation is generally thought to be a reflection of ongoing somatic hypermutation [4-6,9].

Heavy chain isotype expression of the FLs was determined both immunohistochemically and by PCR. Eight FLs expressed IgM, nine expressed IgG, one FL expressed IgA and in one FL both IgM- and IgG-positive cells were found (case 8). It was remarkable that in 7 out of 8 IgM-positive FLs, coexpression of IgD was found. The VH genes of IgG- and IgA-expressing FLs were found to contain 32.5 somatic mutations (11%) on average, whereas 22.4 somatic mutations (7.6%) were found in IgM-sequences. A relation between the amount of somatic mutations and isotype expression is also found in normal antigen-experienced B cells: IgM-derived VH sequences carry on average 3.7-5.7 somatic mutations (1-2%) and IgG-derived VH sequences contain approximately 10 somatic mutations (3%) [21,23]. The observation that a difference between IgM- and IgG-derived V genes still seems present, in spite of substantially elevated mutation frequencies and in spite of supposed ongoing somatic hypermutation in most FLs, is noteworthy. As yet however, this difference does not reach statistical significance (p=0.068; Mann-Whitney U test). More cases are currently being analyzed to settle this issue. For the Vκ sequences a similar picture was found: Vκ sequences derived from IgG-expressing FLs contained on average 20.6 somatic mutations (7.1%), whereas Vκ sequences derived from IgM-expressing FLs contained 13.4 somatic mutations (4.7%).

As mentioned, in only one FL isotype switch variants were found (case 8).

Table 1.: VH and Vκ gene analysis of FLs

FL	HC isotype	VH gene	no. of mutations	R/S_{FR}	intraclonal variation (clones)*	Vκ gene	no. of mutations	R/S_{FR}	intraclonal variation (clones)*
1†	μ	V3-23	12	1.0	nd	L8	9	2.0	nd
3	μ, δ	V3-7	26	1.1	0.4 (5)	L6	21	2.0	nd
13	μ, δ	V4-34	9	1.5	3.2 (5)	nd			
15	μ	V4-34	9	0.5	0.3 (4)	A27	4	0	nd
16	μ, δ	V3-11	49	1.1	nd	A30	12	1.0	nd
17	μ, δ	V3-23	16	0	0.3 (3)	nd			
57	μ, δ	V3-7	25	0.5	0.2 (9)	nd			
58	μ, δ	V4-34	26	0.8	2.0 (5)	nd			
8‡	μ, δ	V3-23	30	1.0	5.0 (7)	L16	21	0.7	2.3 (4)
8‡	γ	V3-23	35	0.9	4.0 (5)	L16	21	0.7	2.3 (4)
2	γ	V3-30	37	1.2	0.7 (3)	nd			
4	γ	V3-23	49	1.1	14.8 (5)	nd			
5	γ	V3-30.3	20	1.8	nd	B3	19	1.3	nd
6	γ	V3-23	44	0.5	3.0 (4)	L6	14	1.3	5.6 (5)
25	γ	V3-30	19	0.6	0.4 (5)	L12a	33	1.1	4.9 (7)
35	γ	V1-69	34	1.1	1.8 (8)	L2	16	1.0	nd
52	γ	V3-7	41	0.9	3.2 (6)	nd			
59	γ	V5-51	11	9.0	3.8 (4)	nd			
66	γ	V4-39	39	1.7	3.0 (6)	nd			
49	α	V1-18	29	0.9	6.3 (6)	nd			

nd: not determined

R/S_{FR}: the ratio of replacement versus silent mutations was determined for the framework regions

* the intraclonal variation is indicated as the number of mutations observed per clone, compared to the consensus sequence; in brackets is the number of clones analyzed

† IgD expression was not assessed

‡ The isotype switch variants of lymphoma no. 8 were counted in our analyses as separate lymphomas; the Vκ genes of the IgM- and IgG-expressing cells were not sequenced independently.

The IgM- and IgG-derived VH genes contained the same VDJ rearrangement, indicating that they originated from the same tumor clone. Compared to the germline gene, V3-23, the IgM-derived sequence was already extensively mutated: 30 somatic mutations were found compared to V3-23. The IgG-derived sequence contained 35 somatic mutations, of which 30 were shared with the IgM-sequence. The finding that the IgM-derived sequence of this FL was already extensively mutated, indicates that somatic mutation started before the isotype switch, like in normal B cells [24]. Recently, we analyzed a relapse of this lymphoma, which developed nine years later. The relapse sample contained IgG-expressing tumor cells only. The IgG-derived sequence of this second timepoint also contained 35 somatic mutations compared to V3-23. Of these mutations, 30 were shared with the IgM- and the IgG-derived sequences of the first timepoint. The 5 additional mutations were different from those of the IgG-derived sequence of the first timepoint (data not shown). Interestingly, at both timepoints substantial intraclonal variation was found, ranging from 5 mutations per clone at the first timepoint (Table 1) to 1.3 mutations per clone at the second timepoint (data not shown). It is noteworthy that, despite this intraclonal variation, which is generally thought to be a reflection of ongoing somatic hypermutation, there is no significant increase in the number of somatic mutations over time. Instead, it seems that other subclones became predominant. For the Vκ sequences from the first and second timepoints a similar picture emerges: Compared to the germline gene, L16, 21 somatic mutations were present at the first timepoint, whereas at the second timepoint only one additional mutation was found. These findings are in accordance with published data, in which patients are described who suffered from a relapse of a FL. Also in these cases no clear accumulation of somatic mutations was found over time despite presumed ongoing somatic hypermutation [6,9,25]. These observations question the current lymphomagenesis model, which describes transformation of a single cell that retains the capacity to acquire somatic mutations and undergo isotype switch. Alternatively, it can be hypothesized that final transformation occurs in more than one member of the offspring of a genetically instable, but not yet fully transformed, clone. In this model, tumor cells may have lost the capacity to acquire somatic mutations and intraclonal variation is ascribed to heterogeneity already present in a proliferating clone before the final transformation. The question whether FLs are capable of ongoing somatic hypermutation is significant, as it has direct implications for the concept of antigen-driven tumorigenesis.

Acknowledgment

This study was supported by a grant from the Dutch Cancer Society (AMC 95-957).

References

1. Harris, N.L., Jaffe, E.S., Stein, H., Banks, P.M., Chan, J.K.C., Cleary, M.L., Delsol, G., de Wolf-Peeters, C., Falini, B., Gatter, K.C., Grogan, T.M., Isaacson, P.G., Knowles, D.M., Mason, D.Y., Muller-Hermelink, H.-K., Pileri, S.A., Piris, M.A., Ralfkiaer, E. and Warnke, R.A. (1994) A revised European-American classification of lymphoid neoplasms: A proposal from the international lymphoma study group. Blood 84, 1361-1392.
2. Bahler, D.W., Campbell, M.J., Hart, S., Miller, R.A., Levy, S. and Levy, R. (1991) Ig VH gene expression among human follicular lymphomas. Blood 78, 1561-1568.
3. Stamatopoulos, K., Kosmas, C., Papadaki, T., Pouliou, E., Belessi, C., Afendaki, S., Anagnostou, D. and Loukopoulos, D. (1997) Follicular lymphoma immunoglobulin κ light chains are affected by the antigen selection process, but to a lesser degree than their partner heavy chains. Brit. J. Haematol. 96, 132-146.
4. Levy, S., Mendel, E., Kon, S., Avnur, Z. and Levy, R. (1988) Mutational hot spots in Ig V region genes of human follicular lymphomas. J. Exp. Med. 168, 475-489.

5. Zelenetz, A.D., Chen, T.T. and Levy, R. (1992) Clonal expansion in follicular lymphoma occurs subsequent to antigen selection. J. Exp. Med. 176, 1137-1148.
6. Zhu, D., Hawkins, R.E., Hamblin, T.J. and Stevenson, F.K. (1994) Clonal history of a human follicular lymphoma as revealed in the immunoglobulin variable region genes. Brit. J. Haematol. 86, 505-512.
7. Raghoebier, S., Broos, L., Kramer, M.H.H., van Krieken, J.H.J.M., Kluin-Nelemans, J.C., van Ommen, G.J.B. and Kluin, P.M. (1995) Histological conversion of follicular lymphoma with structural alterations of t(14;18) and immunoglobulin genes. Leukemia 9, 1748-1755.
8. Zelenetz, A.D., Chen, T.T. and Levy, R. (1991) Histologic transformation of follicular lymphoma to diffuse lymphoma represents tumor progression by a single malignant B cell. J. Exp. Med. 173, 197-207.
9. Ottensmeier, C.H., Thompsett, A.R., Zhu, D., Wilkins, B.S., Sweetenham, J.W. and Stevenson, F.K. (1998) Analysis of VH genes in follicular and diffuse lymphoma shows ongoing somatic mutation and multiple isotype transcripts in early disease with changes during disease progression. Blood 91, 4292-4299.
10. Aarts, W.M., Willemze, R., Bende, R.J., Meijer, C.J.L.M., Pals, S.T. and van Noesel, C.J.M. (1998) VH gene analysis of primary cutaneous B-cell lymphomas: Evidence for ongoing somatic hypermutation and isotype switching. Blood 92, 3857-3864.
11. Sanz, I. (1991) Multiple mechanisms participate in the generation of diversity of human H chain CDR3 regions. J. Immunol. 147, 1720-1729.
12. Lozano, M.D., Tierens, A., Greiner, D.C., Wickert, R.S., Weisenburger, D.D. and Chan, W.C. (1996) Clonality analysis of B-lymphoid proliferations using the polymerase chain reaction. Cancer 77, 1349-1355.
13. Diss, T.C., Pan, L., Peng, H., Wotherspoon, A.C. and Isaacson, P.G. (1994) Sources of DNA for detecting B cell monoclonality using PCR. J. Clin. Pathol. 47, 493-496.
14. Segal, G.H., Jorgensen, T., Scott, M. and Braylan, R.C. (1994) Optimal primer selection for clonality assessment by polymerase chain reaction analysis: II. Follicular lymphomas. Hum. Pathol. 25, 1276-1282.
15. For the Vκ-family specific PCR the following upstream primers were used: Vκ1: 5'-AAATCG ATACCACCATGGACATGAGGGTCCCC-3', Vκ1b: 5'-AAATCGATACCACCATGGACAT GAG(A/G)GTCC(C/T)(C/T)G-3', Vκ2: 5'-AAATCGATACCACCATGAGGCTCCCTGCTC AG-3', Vκ3: 5'-AAATCGATACCACCATGGAAACCCCAGCGCA, Vκ3b: 5'-AAATCGATA CCACCATGGAA(G/A)CCCCAGC(G/T/A)CAG, Vκ4: 5'-AAATCGATACCACCATGGTGT TGCAGACCCAG-3'. As downstream primers a consensus Jκ primer was used:5'-GCGGCCG CCACTTACGTTTGATCTCCACCTTG-3', or a Cκ primer: 5'-GGGAATTCAACAGAGGCA GTTCCAGACTT-3'. PCR conditions were the same as for the VH family-specific PCR.
16. Tomlinson, I.M., Walter, G., Marks, J.D., Llewelyn, M.B. and Winter, G. (1992) The repertoire of human germline V_H sequences reveals about fifty groups of V_H segments with different hypervariable loops. J. Mol. Biol. 227, 776-798.
17. Schäble, K.F. and Zachau, H.G. (1993) The variable genes of the human immunoglobulin κ locus. Biol. Chem. Hoppe-Seyler 374, 1001-1022.
18. Brezinschek, H.P., Brezinschek, R.I. and Lipsky, P.E. (1995) Analysis of the heavy chain repertoire of human peripheral B cells using single-cell polymerase chain reaction. J. Immunol. 155, 190-202.
19. Logtenberg, T., Schutte, M.E.M., Inghirami, G., Berman, J.E., Gmelig-Meyling, F.H.J., Insel, R.A., Knowles, D.M. and Alt, F.W. (1989) Immunoglobulin VH gene expression in human B cell lines and tumors: biased VH gene expression in chronic lymphocytic leukemia. Int. Immunol. 1, 362-366.
20. Cuisinier, A.M., Fumoux, F., Moinier, D., Boubli, L., Guigou, V., Milili, M., Schiff, C., Fougereau, M. and Tonelle, C. (1990) Rapid expansion of human immunoglobulin repertoire (VH, V kappa, V lambda) expressed in early fetal bone marrow. The New Biologist 2, 689-699.
21. Tomlinson, I.M., Walter, G., Jones, P.T., Dear, P.H., Sonnhammer, E.L.L. and Winter, G. (1996) The imprint of somatic hypermutation on the repertoire of human germline V genes. J. Mol. Biol. 256, 813-817.
22. Shlomchik, M.J., Marshak-Rothstein, A., Wolfowicz, C.B., Rothstein, T.L. and Weigert, M.G. (1987) The role of clonal selection and somatic mutation in autoimmunity. Nature 328, 805-811.
23. Pascual, V., Liu, Y.-J., Magalski, A., de Bouteiller, O., Banchereau, J. and Capra, J.D. (1994) Analysis of somatic mutation in five B cell subsets of human tonsil. J. Exp. Med. 180, 329-339
24. Liu, Y.J., Malisan, F., de Bouteiller, O., Guret, C., Lebecque, S., Banchereau, J., Mills, F.C., Max, E.E. and Martinez-Valdez, H. (1996) Within germinal centers, isotype switching of immunoglobulin genes occurs after the onset of somatic mutation. Immunity 4, 241-250.
25. Bahler, D.W. and Levy, R. (1992) Clonal evolution of a follicular lymphoma: Evidence for antigen selection. Proc. Natl. Acad. Sci. USA 89, 6770-6774.

Discussion

Isaac Witz: In the lymphoma which you analyzed following an interval of nine years, was the grade of malignancy higher than nine years previously?
Mijntje Aarts: No, it was the same.
Isaac Witz: So whatever you could measure was more or less the same?
Mijntje Aarts: Yes, it was still the same kind of follicular lymphoma, not a diffuse lymphoma.
Richard Scheuermann: What percent of your patients showed this intraclonal variation?
Mijntje Aarts: We tested 16 patients, 11 of them had intraclonal variations, and five did not have significant intraclonal variation.
Richard Scheuermann: So 11 had intraclonal variations and you only sequenced four clones from each?
Mijntje Aarts: For some we sequenced three, the minimum, and for some we sequenced nine.
Richard Scheuermann: But what that is implying is that you have these two clones, or multiple clones, that had to get their second hits about the same time, and then grow at the same rate in order to give that kind of effect, according to your second model.
Mijntje Aarts: Yes, about two at the same time, you are right.
Heinz Jacobs: Since B cells usually die if they lose their Ig receptor, would you expect, if you mutate further on, that these cells would need an additional oncogene just to compensate for the loss of surface Ig?
Mijntje Aarts: Yes.
Heinz Jacobs: Since there is no argument that the primary tumor cells are not allowed to differentiate, one could also explain your data as follows: some of the primary tumor cells differentiate further, switch, and become memory B cell-like. So what you end up with after nine years is basically a selective outgrowth of those cells which stopped hypermutation and became memory-like B cells.
Mijntje Aarts: Yes, but even in the last time-point, after nine years we found intraclonal variation and although it was lower than at the first time-point, it was still 1.3 mutations per clone. So above Taq error. If this intraclonal variation is really due to ongoing somatic hypermutation, we would have expected more mutations to accumulate in these years.
Heinz Jacobs: But at a certain moment you can always say it stops, because they just leave the hypermutation process and you end up with a few clones which still show intraclonal variation.
Richard Scheuermann: I think that is a more likely explanation. After it gets the final oncogenic hit, it has a certain window of time where it can still somatically hypermutate, but then that gets shut off and you see this kind of effect.
Mijntje Aarts: Yes, you would say that then maybe more than one clone would survive the chemotherapy and that is why we still have intraclonal variation. That is also a good hypothesis.
Carel van Noesel: This is a significant point then, because people consider this important as it is an argument for antigen-driven lymphomagenesis: that in spite of ongoing somatic hypermutation the antigen receptor keeps in shape. If this process had already stopped long before nine years, that would make this argument less valuable.
Richard Scheuermann: But if in the intraclonal variation, you still get targeted mutations to CDRs and you get this replacement to silent skewing, that also argues that there has to be some selection, even during this process, right?
Mijntje Aarts: Yes, if you look at the so-called new mutations, the mutations that we find in the different clones, we still find a low R/S ratio in the framework region. So if this is really ongoing somatic hypermutation, then selection still takes place.
Carel van Noesel: The idea you get is that you look at a prolonged germinal center reaction and that that is the final situation. That is the feeling that we get from our study, but also from what is published. So we very much doubt whether the majority of new clones are still capable of somatic hypermutation.

Jacques van Dongen: It is curious that follicular lymphomas in particular apparently escape the anti-idiotype therapy in the long-term. You could say that already at initial diagnosis very tiny clones exist that have another idiotype and that over the years they can escape from the anti-idiotype therapy. Do you think that they do not develop during treatment, but that they are already there at the start of treatment?
Carel van Noesel: I think so.
Jacques van Dongen: And that is the selection of the minor clone.
Carel van Noesel: There is a paper in which it is suggested that a minor clone is predominant after this kind of therapy. [Caspar et al. (1997) Idiotype vaccines for non-Hodgkin's lymphoma induce polyclonal immune responses that cover mutated tumor idiotypes: comparison of different vaccine formulations. Blood 90(9):3699-3706]
Jacques van Dongen: Could it be proven that the selected minor clone was already there at diagnosis?
Carel van Noesel: If you are lucky.
Mijntje Aarts: It could be found as a minor clone.

Regulation of c-*myc* and Immunoglobulin κ Gene Transcription by Promoter-proximal Pausing of RNA Polymerase II

E.-E. Schneider, T. Albert[1], D.A. Wolf[2], and D. Eick

Institute for Clinical Molecular Biology and Tumor Genetics, GSF-Research Center for Environment and Health, Marchioninistrasse 25, D-81377 Munich, Germany; present addresses: [1]Laboratory for Physiological Chemistry, Utrecht University, The Netherlands; [2]Department of Cancer Cell Biology, Harvard School of Public Health, Boston, MA 02115, USA

In normal cells, the proto-oncogene c-*myc* is regulated by promoter-proximal pausing of RNA polymerase II (pol II). In Burkitt lymphoma cells, c-*myc* is chromosomally translocated to one of the three immunoglobulin (Ig) gene loci and its transcription is driven constitutively by Ig enhancers. Promoter-proximal pausing of pol II is abolished on the translocated c-*myc* allele. This raised the question whether induction of Ig gene transcription also involves activation of promoter-proximal paused pol II. Here we have studied the transcriptional activation of a functionally rearranged Igκ gene in the mouse pre B cell line 70Z/3. We show that pol II pauses approximately 50 bp downstream of the transcriptional start site of the uninduced Igκ gene.

Introduction

Promoter-proximal pausing of pol II at c-*myc* gene promoters in man and mouse has been described (Krumm et al., 1992; Strobl and Eick, 1992, Kohlhuber et al., 1993). Transcription complexes pause at variable positions approximately 1-50 bp downstream of the RNA cap site. (Krumm et al., 1992, 1995; Strobl and Eick, 1992; Kohlhuber et al., 1993; Wolf et al., 1995; Albert et al., 1997).

In Burkitt lymphoma (BL) and mouse plasmacytoma, the c-*myc* gene is chromosomally translocated to either the Ig heavy chain gene locus, or one of the two Ig light chain gene loci. The translocated c-*myc* allele is highly expressed, while the normal allele is usually transcriptionally silent (Spencer and Groudine, 1991). Several studies indicated that the Ig enhancers are responsible for activation of the translocated c-*myc* (Polack et al., 1991, 1993; Hörtnagel et al., 1995; Madisen et al., 1994). A detailed analysis of two c-*myc*/Igλ light chain translocations with chromosomal breakpoints downstream of the c-*myc* transcription unit showed that promoter-proximal pausing of pol II is abolished at the c-*myc* promoter of the translocation chromosome suggesting that Ig enhancers are able to induce processivity of promoter-proximal paused pol II (Strobl et al., 1993). This was further supported by the observation that Igκ gene enhancers can activate c-*myc* and abolish promoter-proximal pausing of pol II on episomal constructs (Hörtnagel et al., 1995).

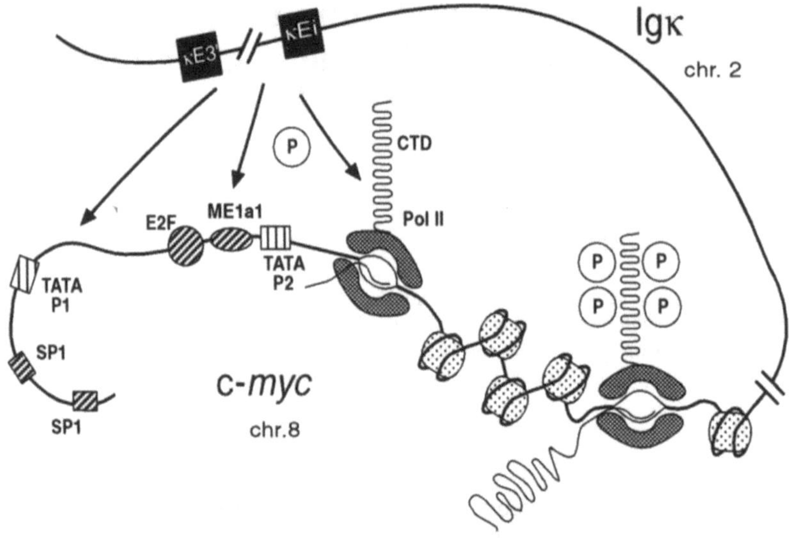

Fig. 1. Model of c-*myc* activation by the Igκ gene enhancers *in vivo* and on episomal constructs. The BL specific t(2;8) translocation with the c-*myc* promoter and the Igκ gene enhancers is depicted. The TATA-boxes of the c-*myc* P1 and P2 promoters, SP1, E2F and ME1a1 binding sites as well as the positions of mapped nucleosomes are indicated (Pullner et al., 1996; Albert et al., 1997). Episomal constructs containing only the 3' enhancer (κE3') establish a paused pol II downstream of the P2 promoter without expressing the gene in the BL cell line Raji (Strobl et al., 1993). A construct containing additionally the intron enhancer (κEi) and the matrix attachment region (MAR, not shown) expresses high levels of c-*myc* RNA and promoter proximal pausing of pol II is abolished (Hörtnagel et al., 1995). This construct expresses also high levels of P1-specific RNA. The CTD of pol II at the pause site is assumed to be hypophosphorylated, while the CTD of a transcribing pol II is assumed to be hyperphosphorylated. For further details see in the text.

The signals leading to activation of paused pol II at the c-*myc* promoter are not well defined but probably involve phosphorylation and acetylation signals (Wolf et al., 1995, Madisen et al., 1998). A likely target for phosphorylation is the carboxy-terminal domain (CTD) of the large subunit of pol II containing the consensus hepta-peptide Ser-Pro-Thr-Ser-Pro-Ser-Tyr. In cells, two forms of pol II are detectable containing a hypophosphorylated CTD (pol IIa) and hyperphosphorylated CTD (pol IIo). Studies with different promoters suggested that the hypophosphorylated form of pol II is involved in the initiation process and in the establishment of a promoter-proximal paused complex (for review see Greenblatt, 1997). Hyperphosphorylation of CTD occurs at later time points, e.g. when pol II undergoes the transition into a processive transcription mode that is thought to be mediated by transcriptional transactivators (Yankulov et al., 1994). Thus, the Ig enhancers and factors binding to sites within these enhancers might be involved in regulation of CTD-phosphorylation thereby conferring processivity to the paused pol II downstream of the c-*myc* promoter (see Fig. 1. for the current model). This raised the question whether Ig enhancers regulate Ig transcription from Ig promoters by activation of a promoter-proximal paused pol II.

The Igκ gene in pre-B cells can be activated and transcribed in response to bacterial lipopolysaccharide (LPS), interleukin-1 (IL-1), gamma interferon (IFN-γ), and various physiological inducers which mimic different intracellular second messengers. The induction of the Igκ gene by IFN-γ occurs independently

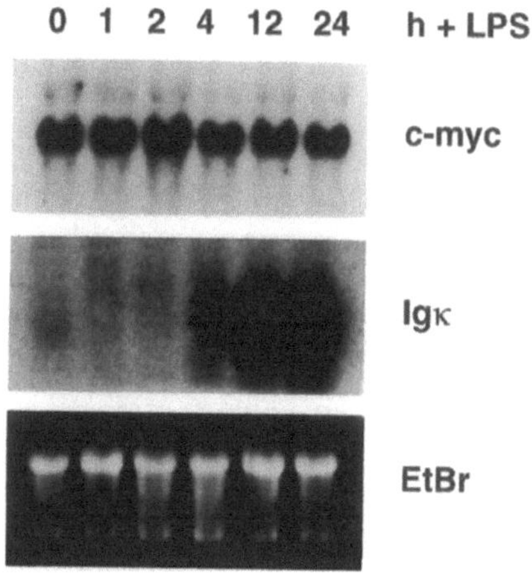

Fig. 2. Levels of c-*myc* and Igκ RNA in 70Z/3 cells after NF-κB activation by LPS. Northern blot analyses were performed with c-*myc* and Igκ constant region specific probes. The ethidium bromide-stained gel before RNA transfer is shown at the bottom. Methods: 70Z/3 cells were induced with 10 μg/ml of bacterial LPS (Salmonella typhosa, Sigma) and total cellular RNA was isolated at the indicated time points. Ten μg RNA were separated on a 1% formaldehyde-agarose gel, transferred onto a nylon membrane (Hybond N+, Amersham), and hybridized with ^{32}P-labeled DNA probes as described in Sambrook et al. (1989).

of NF-κB, whereas the induction of Igκ gene transcription by LPS, IL-1 and other inducers requires NF-κB activation and binding of NF-κB to the Igκ gene intron enhancer (κEi) (Sen and Baltimore, 1986a, b; Briskin et al., 1988; Baeuerle and Henkel, 1994). Upon activation by a wide range of signals NF-κB is translocated from the cytoplasm into the nucleus and functions as a potent transcriptional activator of various genes (Baeuerle and Henkel, 1994; Baldwin, 1996). Here, we have studied the molecular level at which NF-κB activates Igκ gene transcription.

Results and Discussion

In the mouse pre-B cell line 70Z/3 with a functionally rearranged Igκ gene addition of LPS led to an accumulation of mature Igκ transcripts between 4 and 12 hours (Fig. 2) (Parslow et al., 1984). The previously suggested transcriptional start site ~30 bp upstream of the ATG start codon (Parslow et al., 1984) was confirmed by primer extension experiments (data not shown).

To examine whether the functionally rearranged Igκ gene harbors a paused pol II proximal to its promoter, we performed high resolution nuclear run-on experiments, which allow the detection of pol II distribution along the gene (Wolf et al., 1995). A set of ten antisense oligonucleotides, each 50 bases long, spanning the Igκ gene promoter-proximal region was immobilized on membranes and used for hybridization to ^{32}P-CTP labeled nuclear run-on RNA (Figure 3). After hybridization, filters were washed with RNAse A to digest non-hybridized RNA and exposed to X-ray films. A strong hybridization signal corresponding to

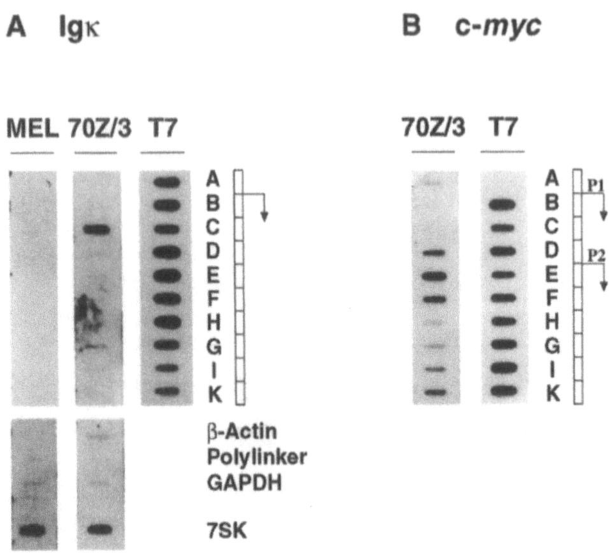

Fig. 3. Nuclear run-on analysis of the promoter region of the functionally rearranged Igκ gene and of the c-*myc* gene in 70Z/3 cells. (**A**) Labeled RNAs of nuclear run-on reactions were hybridized to a set of antisense oligonucleotides (A-K) comprising the Igκ promoter and its downstream region. MEL cells served as non-B cell control, homogeneously labeled T7 RNA of the Igκ gene as hybridization standard. Oligonucleotides complementary to the β-actin and GAPDH gene served as pol II control, an oligonucleotide complementary to the 7SK RNA as pol III control; a polylinker was used as negative control. (**B**) Labeled nuclear run-on RNAs were also hybridized to a set of antisense oligonucleotides (A-K) comprising the c-myc P2 promoter and its downstream region. The transcriptional start sites of the Igκ and c-*myc* promoters are indicated by arrows. Methods: Isolation of nuclei, run-on reaction, purification of labeled RNA, hybridization of RNA to membrane bound oligonucleotides, washing of the membranes including digestion of single stranded RNA with RNAse A, and mouse c-*myc* and control oligonucleotides have been described (Kohlhuber et al., 1993; Wolf et al., 1995). Oligonucleotides were synthesized complementary to the Igκ gene promoter, 50 nucleotides long, starting with oligonucleotide A 50 bp upstream of the RNA cap site. All transcription signals detected in the run-on assay, except the signal for the pol III specific 7SK probe, were sensitive to 250 nM α-amanitin.

oligonucleotide C downstream of the Igκ gene promoter was obtained in 70Z/3 cells while signals on oligonucleotide D and oligonucleotides further downstream were not detectable in the run-on experiment (Fig. 3A, lane 2). The strong run-on signal on oligonucleotide C was not observed for mouse erythroleukemia (MEL) cells that do not contain a rearranged Igκ gene (lane 1). The signals obtained for the pol II transcribed β-actin and GAPDH genes as well as for the pol III transcribed 7SK gene showed the same intensities in 70Z/3 and MEL cells. This indicates that the Igκ gene in 70Z/3 cells harbors a paused pol II in the region 50 to 100 bp downstream of the transcriptional start site. This pol II has not received all factors or signals for its release and for productive transcription of the Igκ gene. However, in the nuclear run-on reaction the paused pol II becomes artificially activated probably by the addition of detergents and transcribes a short piece of RNA. The signal pattern obtained with run-on RNAs derived from LPS-induced 70Z/3 cells was almost identical to the pattern of uninduced cells, except that the signals

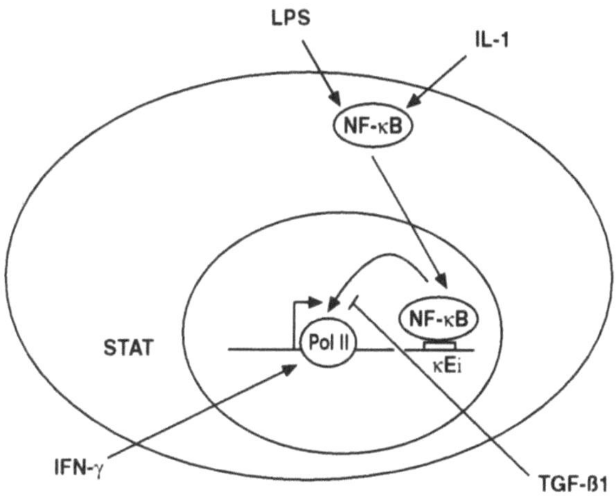

Fig. 4. Model of Igκ gene activation by NF–κB.

for oligos D to K were slightly increased (data not shown). This is comparable with observations for other genes with a promoter-proximal paused pol II, as e.g. for the c-*myc* P2 promoter where the pause site remains occupied even if the gene is expressed. Downstream of the c-myc P2 promoter, a paused pol II has been described in MEL cells (Kohlhuber et al., 1993). The pause site was determined to the sequence corresponding to oligonucleotide E, which was confirmed for 70Z/3 cells (Fig.3B, lane 1). Pausing of pol II proximal to the Igκ promoter was also shown in *in vivo* footprint experiments by demonstration of a transcription bubble at the pause site. Unpaired T-residues in the transcription bubble were hypersensitive to oxidation by potassium permanganate (data not shown).

The finding of a paused pol II proximal to the Igκ gene promoter has major implications for our understanding of the Ig enhancer functions and the role of binding of the transcription factor NF-κB to κEi. Activation of the E-selectin (Lewis et al., 1994), β-interferon (Thanos and Maniatis, 1995), and VCAM-1 genes (Neish et al., 1995) by NF-κB requires promoter-proximal binding sites of NF-κB and co-operative binding of NF-κB to other transcription factors which results in the formation of higher order complexes. If and how these complexes contribute to recruitment of pol II to the promoter and later to processive transcription of pol II is not yet understood. Here we have shown that NF-κB activates Igκ gene transcription in 70Z/3 cells at the level of RNA elongation. NF-κB acts from a distant enhancer in response to LPS and activates a paused pol II after having transcribed already a short piece of RNA. Interestingly, TGF-β1 can inhibit activation of the Igκ gene by LPS without affecting binding of NF-κB to DNA, indicating that TGF-β1 may specifically interfere with a signal pathway/interaction of κEi and the paused pol II. Since Igκ gene transcription induced by IFN-γ is not sensitive to TGF-β1 (Briskin et al., 1988), different signal cascades with different sensitivity to TGF-β1 appear to converge at paused pol II complexes. Whether these pathways converge in CTD-signalling remains to be demonstrated. Other signals such as histone acetylation can be considered as well (Madisen et al., 1998).

The finding of a promoter-proximal paused pol II at an Igκ gene supports predicted models linking transcription to the process of somatic hypermutation at the Ig genes (Neuberger and Milstein, 1995; Peters and Storb, 1996; Jacobs et al., 1998; Fukita et al., 1998). Whereas the 3´ boundary of hypermutations is not well defined and lies about 1.5 kb downstream of the transcriptional start site, the 5´ boundary of mutations is located between 100 and 150 bp downstream of the transcriptional start site within the leader intron (Rada et al., 1994; Rogerson, 1994). Pausing of pol II might have a functional relevance for somatic hypermuation of the Ig variable region, thus providing an explanation for the defined start site of mutator activity downstream of the pause site.

Acknowledgements
We are grateful to R. Mocikat for providing 70Z/3 cells. This work was supported by the Deutsche Forschungsgemeinschaft (SFB190), Deutsche Krebshilfe, EU-Biomed II, and Fonds der Chemischen Industrie.

References

Albert T, Mautner J, Funk JO, Hortnagel K, Pullner A, Eick D (1997) Nucleosomal structures of c-myc promoters with transcriptionally engaged RNA polymerase II. Mol Cell Biol 17:4363-4371

Baeuerle PA, Henkel T (1994) Function and activation of NF-kappa B in the immune system. Annu Rev Immunol 12:141-179

Baldwin AS (1996) The NF-kappa B and I kappa B proteins: new discoveries and insights. Annu Rev Immunol 14:649-683

Briskin M, Kuwabara MD, Sigman DS, Wall R (1988) Induction of kappa transcription by interferon-gamma without activation of NF-kappa B. Science 242:1036-1037

Fukita Y, Jacobs H, Rajewsky K (1998) Somatic hypermutation in the heavy chain locus correlates with transcription. Immunity 9:105-114

Greenblatt J (1997) RNA polymerase II holoenzyme and transcriptional regulation. Curr Opin Cell Biol 9:310-319

Hörtnagel K, Mautner J, Strobl L J, Wolf DA, Christoph B, Geltinger C, Polack A (1995) The role of immunoglobulin kappa elements in c-myc activation. Oncogene 10:1393-1401

Jacobs H, Fukita Y, van der Horst GT, de Boer J, Weeda G, Essers J, de Wind N, Engelward BP, Samson L, Verbeek S, de Murcia JM, de Murcia G, te Riele H, Rajewsky K (1998) Hypermutation of immunoglobulin genes in memory B cells of DNA repair-deficient mice. J Exp Med 187:1735-1743

Kohlhuber F, Strobl LJ, Eick D (1993) Early down-regulation of c-myc in dimethylsulfoxide-induced mouse erythroleukemia (MEL) cells is mediated at the P1/P2 promoters. Oncogene 8:1099-1102

Krumm A, Hickey LB, Groudine M (1995) Promoter-proximal pausing of RNA polymerase II defines a general rate-limiting step after transcription initiation. Genes Dev 9:559-572

Krumm A, Meulia T, Brunvand M, Groudine M (1992) The block to transcriptional elongation within the human c-myc gene is determined in the promoter-proximal region. Genes Dev 6: 2201-2213

Lewis H, Kaszubska W, DeLamarter JF, Whelan J (1994) Cooperativity between two NF-kappa B complexes, mediated by high-mobility-group protein I(Y), is essential for cytokine-induced expression of the E-selectin promoter. Mol Cell Biol 14:5701-5709

Madisen L, Groudine M (1994) Identification of a locus control region in the immunoglobulin heavy-chain locus that deregulates c-myc expression in plasmacytoma and Burkitt's lymphoma cells. Genes-Dev 15:2212-2226

Madisen L, Krumm A, Hebbes TR, Groudine M (1998) The immunoglobulin heavy gene locus control region increases histone acetylation along linked c-myc genes. Mol Cell Biol 18:6281-6292

Neish AS, Read MA, Thanos D, Pine R, Maniatis T, Collins T (1995) Endothelial interferon regulatory factor 1 cooperates with NF-kappa B as a transcriptional activator of vascular cell adhesion molecule 1. Mol Cell Biol 15:2558-2569

Neuberger MS and Milstein C (1995) Somatic hypermutation. Curr Opin Immunol 7:248-254

Parslow TG, Blair DL, Murphy WJ, Granner DK (1984) Structure of the 5' ends of immunoglobulin genes: a novel conserved sequence. Proc Natl Acad Sci U S A 81:2650-2654

Peters A, Storb U (1996) Somatic hypermutation of immunoglobulin genes is linked to transcription initiation. Immunity 4:57-65

Polack A, Feederle R, Klobeck G, Hortnagel K (1993) Regulatory elements in the immunoglobulin kappa locus induce c-myc activation and the promoter shift in Burkitt's lymphoma cells. Embo J 12:3913-3920

Polack A, Strobl L, Feederle R, Schweizer M, Koch E, Eick D, Wiegand H, Bornkamm GW (1991) The intron enhancer of the immunoglobulin kappa gene activates c-myc but does not induce the Burkitt-specific promoter shift. Oncogene 6:2033-2040

Pullner A, Mautner J, Albert T, Eick D (1996) Nucleosomal structure of active and inactive c-myc genes. J Biol Chem 271:31452-31457

Rada C, Gonzalez Fernandez A, Jarvis JM, Milstein C (1994) The 5' boundary of somatic hypermutation in a V kappa gene is in the leader intron. Eur-J-Immunol. 24:1453-457

Rogerson BJ (1994) Mapping the upstream boundary of somatic mutations in rearranged immunoglobulin transgenes and endogenous genes. Mol-Immunol 31:83-98

Sambrook J, Fritsch EF, Maniatis, T (1989) *Molecular Cloning: A Laboratory Manual* . Cold Spring Harbor Laboratory Press, Cold Spring Harbor, NY, ed. 2

Sen R, Baltimore D (1986a) Inducibility of kappa immunoglobulin enhancer-binding protein Nf-kappa B by a posttranslational mechanism. Cell 47:921-928

Sen R, Baltimore D (1986b) Multiple nuclear factors interact with the immunoglobulin enhancer sequences. Cell 46:705-716

Spencer CA, Groudine M (1991) Control of c-myc regulation in normal and neoplastic cells. Adv Cancer Res 56:1-48

Strobl LJ, Eick D (1992) Hold back of RNA polymerase II at the transcription start site mediates down-regulation of c-myc in vivo. Embo J 11:3307-3314

Strobl LJ, Kohlhuber F, Mautner J, Polack A, Eick D (1993) Absence of a paused transcription complex from the c-myc P2 promoter of the translocation chromosome in Burkitt's lymphoma cells: implication for the c-myc P1/P2 promoter shift. Oncogene 8:1437-1447

Thanos D, Maniatis T (1995) NF-kappa B: a lesson in family values. Cell 80:529-532

Wolf DA, Strobl LJ, Pullner A, Eick D (1995) Variable pause positions of RNA polymerase II lie proximal to the c-myc promoter irrespective of transcriptional activity. Nucleic Acids Res 23:3373-3379

Yankulov K, Blau J, Purton T, Roberts S, Bentley DL (1994) Transcriptional elongation by RNA polymerase II is stimulated by transactivators. Cell 77:749-759

Discussion

Gary Rathbun: In the sequence that is between the rearranged J region, the kappa and the enhancer where the mutations fall off, are there any sequences that look like a secondary structure or something else that would prevent somatic mutations from operating?

Dirk Eick: I have not looked at the sequence, maybe the people working with immunoglobulin genes can answer this question.

Heinz Jacobs: It has always been suggested that there are some secondary structures. There are a lot of programs, and depending on which model the program is based, you always find a secondary structure. But it has not been figured out experimentally whether one of these models is correct.

Siegfried Janz: Does the well-established promoter shift in the transcription of the c-myc gene in Burkitt's lymphomas contribute in any way to the targeting of the hypermutation machinery to the first exon of the c-myc gene?

Dirk Eick: It is not known whether the different promoter usage in Burkitt lymphomas does contribute to a lower or higher mutation rate in the first exon of c-myc.

IV

Biology of Lymphomagenesis, B-CLL, Autoimmunity

Epidemiology of B-Cell Lymphomas

C. S. Rabkin
Viral Epidemiology Branch, National Cancer Institute, Bethesda, MD 20892 USA

The B-lineage lymphomas are a diverse set of neoplasms that vary in their clinical and histologic appearance. Epidemiologic data on the non-Hodgkin's lymphomas generally obscure distinctions among these tumors, presenting an additional challenge to interpretation. Nevertheless, observations about their similarities and differences may provide important clues to the etiology of these disorders.

The incidence of non-Hodgkin's lymphoma epidemiology increases dramatically with age. Incidence rates rise exponentially, going from about 1 per 100,000 per year, up to 100 per 100,000 in the oldest age groups. In most countries, males tend to have higher rates than females; in the United States, for example, female rates are about 70-80% of male rates (Fig. 1).

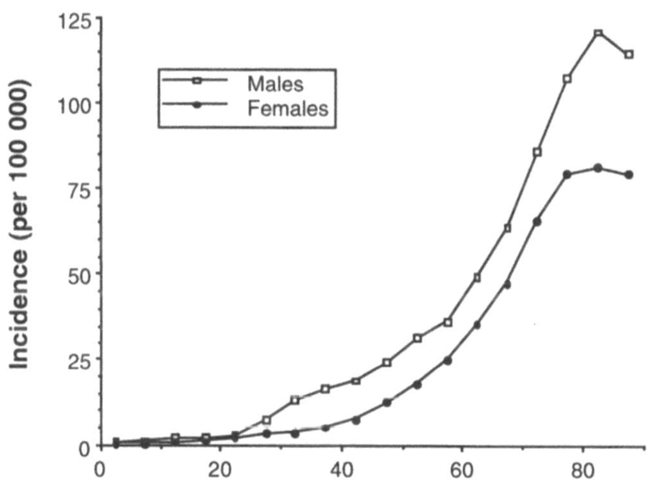

Fig. 1. Annual incidence of non-Hodgkin's lymphoma by age and sex, U.S. Surveillance, Epidemiology, and End Results (SEER) Program, 1991-1995.

Non-Hodgkin's lymphoma incidence varies only moderately between countries, in contrast to the 30-fold variation in B-cell leukemia incidence. Lymphoma incidence tends to be higher in developed countries, as in Western Europe, North America and Australia, and lower in South America, Africa, and parts of Asia [1]. In the United States, non-Hodgkin's lymphoma rates vary by race, with African-Americans and Asian-Americans having about 70% of the rates of whites [2].

A striking feature in lymphoma epidemiology worldwide has been an inexorable increase in incidence. In the United States, non-Hodgkin's lymphoma incidence has increased approximately 3% each year from 1935 to the present [1,3] (Fig. 2). It is the third fastest increasing tumor in both sexes [4]. Mortality rates have increased somewhat more slowly, about 2% annually [4]. The reasons for this long-standing temporal increase are generally not known [5]. However, in certain population subgroups, HIV-associated cases explain some of the increase since 1980. For example, San Francisco (USA) has had a major epidemic of HIV infection among males since the late 1970s, and as a consequence has a non-Hodgkin's lymphoma incidence rate more than twice the national average (Fig. 3).

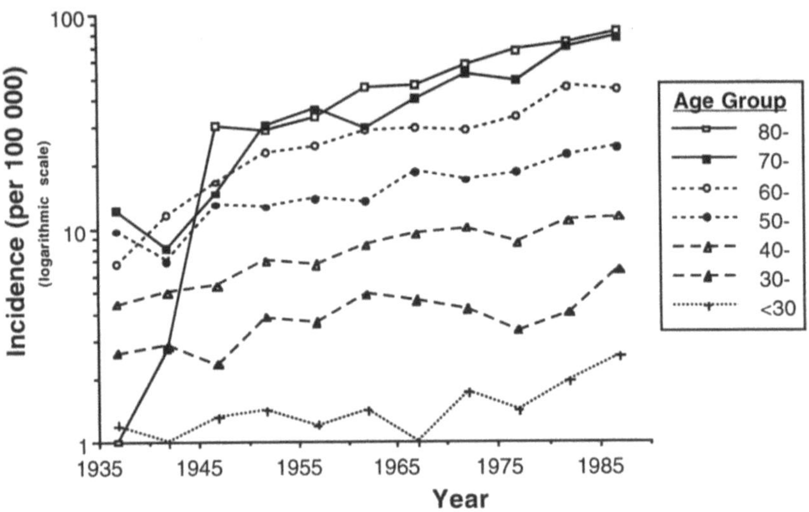

Fig. 2. Age-specific incidence of non-Hodgkin's lymphoma in males, Connecticut (USA) Tumor Registry, 1935-88. Data from Zheng et al. (1992).

These trends in non-Hodgkin's lymphoma incidence are nearly universal. Increases are present in both men and women, in all races, and are seen in virtually every country that has reliable cancer registration data. Incidence rates have been increasing in every age group, with the greatest increases found in the oldest age groups (Fig. 2).

Interpretation of trends in individual subtypes of lymphoma is complicated by shifts in classification, but it appears that increases have been more pronounced in higher

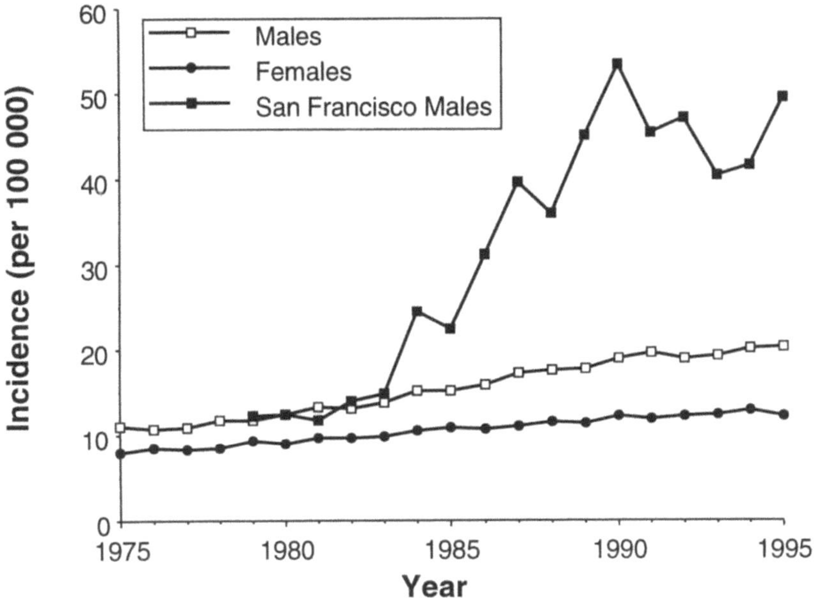

Fig. 3. Age-adjusted incidence of non-Hodgkin's lymphoma by sex, San Francisco and U.S. Surveillance, Epidemiology, and End Results (SEER) Program, 1975-1995.

histologic grades [6]. In United States incidence data for the past 20 years, high-grade and unclassified tumors have increased by 9% and 7% per year, respectively, whereas low-grade and intermediate-grade tumors have each increased by 1.5% per year (Fig. 4). Among recent influences on lymphoma incidence, HIV-associated tumors are primarily of high histologic grade [7], which may in part explain this difference.

What does the epidemiology of non-Hodgkin's lymphoma indicate about the etiology of these tumors? HIV has had a substantial impact on lymphoma incidence and is an informative model for lymphoma development. Other risk factors have been noted in case-control studies, including certain foods, nitrate in drinking water, and hair dye use, as well as a number of occupational exposures, including benzene, vinyl chloride, and herbicides [8]. There are also some occupational groups at elevated risk for which the exposures are undefined, including farmers, grain handlers, refinery workers, chemists, and pathologists [9]. Several rare genetic syndromes of altered immunity, particularly ataxia-telangiectasia, Wiskott-Aldrich syndrome, and common variable immunodeficiency, have a very high incidence of non-Hodgkin's lymphomas as an important aspect of these disorders [10]. Family history of lymphoma is associated with a slight increase in risk, suggesting a component of inheritable predisposition accounting for a minor proportion of disease [9]. With the exception of the various causes of immunodeficiency, the relative risks associated with other lymphoma risk factors are relatively modest.

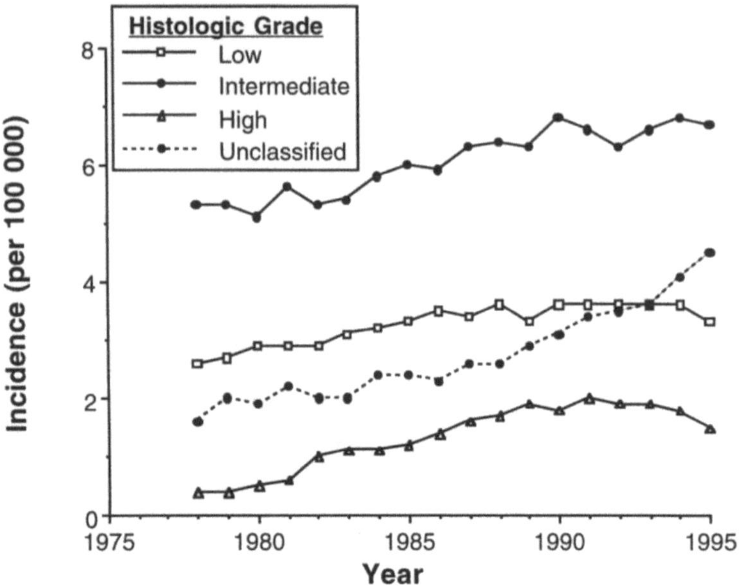

Fig. 4. Age-adjusted incidence of non-Hodgkin's lymphoma by histologic grade, U.S. Surveillance, Epidemiology, and End Results (SEER) Program, 1978-1995.

It is important to note that the increasing trend in non-Hodgkin's lymphoma predates the AIDS epidemic, so it is not just due to HIV. Furthermore, the increases do not appear to be artifactual. Although there has been some re-classification of diseases that were not previously considered non-Hodgkin's lymphoma, such as some types of Hodgkin's disease, such changes can explain only a small part of the increase [6]. Improved diagnosis is also only responsible for a small amount [5]. The changes in lymphoma incidence appear to be real, and identifying the explanation for them remains a challenge for better understanding of these diseases.

References

1. Devesa SS, Fears T (1992) Non-Hodgkin's lymphoma time trends: United States and international data. Cancer Res 52:5432s-5440s
2. Non-Hodgkin's lymphoma. In: Cancer Statistics Review: 1973-1995, National Cancer Institute. Ries LAG, Kosary CL, Miller BA, Hankey BF, Edwards BK (ed) (1998) U.S. Department of Health and Human Services, Bethesda.
3. Zheng T, Mayne ST, Boyle P, Holford TR, Liu WL, Flannery J (1992) Epidemiology of non-Hodgkin lymphoma in Connecticut. 1935-1988. Cancer 70:840-849
4. Overview. In: Cancer Statistics Review: 1973-1995, National Cancer Institute. Ries LAG, Kosary CL, Miller BA, Hankey BF, Edwards BK (ed) (1998) U.S. Department of Health and

Human Services, Bethesda.
5. Hartge P, Devesa S (1992) Quantitation of the impact of known risk factors on time trends in non-Hodgkin's lymphoma incidence. Cancer Res 52:5566s-5569s
6. Rabkin CS, Devesa SS, Zahm SH, Gail MH (1993) Increasing incidence of non-Hodgkin's lymphoma. Semin Hematol 30:286-296
7. Rabkin CS, Yellin F (1994) Cancer incidence in a population with a high prevalence of infection with human immunodeficiency virus type 1. J Natl Cancer Inst 86:1711-1716
8. Rabkin CS, Ward MH, Manns A, Blattner WA (1995) Epidemiology of non-Hodgkin's lymphoma. In: The non-Hodgkin's lymphomas. Magrath IT (ed) Edward Arnold, London. 2nd ed. pp 171-186
9. Scherr PA, Meuller NE (1996) Non-Hodgkin's lymphomas. In: Cancer epidemiology and prevention. Schottenfeld D, Fraumeni JF,Jr. (ed) Oxford University Press, New York. 2nd ed. pp 920-945
10. Filipovich AH, Mathur A, Kamat D, Shapiro RS (1992) Primary immunodeficiencies: genetic risk factors for lymphoma. Cancer Res 52:5465s-5467s

Discussion

Sandy Morse: It is well established in mice that pristane exposure results in developing plasmacytomas, is there any evidence in humans for a similar effect, for example do pathologists get exposure to pristane from analyzing samples, etc.
Charles Rabkin: Not that I've heard of. But no one has tried injecting pathologists intraperitoneally.
Riccardo Dalla-Favera: So AIDS is responsible or is associated with an increase in Burkitt's and diffuse immunoblastic lymphomas?
Charles Rabkin: That is right.
Riccardo Dalla-Favera: So any increase in follicular lymphoma would be AIDS-independent. But is there an increase in follicular lymphoma?
Charles Rabkin: There is a small increase in follicular lymphoma; some of it is due to spill-over because the reported cases are not perfectly classified, but most of the increase is not due to HIV.
Riccardo Dalla-Favera: So there is an increase in follicular and also in the high-grade independent of AIDS?
Charles Rabkin: Yes.
Federico Caligaris-Cappio: So if you take away AIDS the increase is in both categories, low grade and high grade?
Bart Barlogie: I thought it was a plateau for follicular lymphoma, with age.
Charles Rabkin: Yes, a plateau with age, but no, the absolute incidence has been increasing. High grade lymphoma is so rare outside of HIV it is hard to say whether there has been an increase or not, and that again the diagnostics show that the big change is from HIV.
Richard Scheuermann: The problem that I have is that if you see this increase in the different lymphomas, besides from AIDS, and it is present in all countries around the world, you cannot really explain that by changes in exposure, or changes in genetic makeup, or things like that. So what seems more likely to me would be that it is improvement in diagnostics or being able to recognize the disease worldwide.
Charles Rabkin: You can hypothesize some exposures and there is one study by Nat Rothman about a very ubiquitous exposure to PCBs which really can be detected in all parts of the world. He showed that that was a risk factor in one study. That study needs to be replicated and it is not clear that that really explains the increase, but it certainly is a provocative finding. In terms of whether it is just diagnostic, there is some evidence in age-specific rates and socio-economic differentiation of rates that some of that contributes, but it by no means explains everything. Even in areas where there is very rudimentary autopsy data, it appears that there is an increase independent of the changes in diagnostic practices.
Gary Rathbun: It also seems that some of the insights you might be able to gain from the analysis of these various subtypes of non-Hodgkin's are hampered a little, as you pointed out, by the systematics, i.e. what is being used to define a specific subtype. It may be that you are missing a trend simply because the systematics break down or are insufficient.
Charles Rabkin: Certainly. I don't think the Revised European-American Lymphoma (Real) classification is going to end that either. It is a constant problem that hampers us. It is not just within non-Hodgkin's lymphoma but, as was pointed out, undiagnosed cases are now being called non-Hodgkin's lymphoma, so it is a very difficult set of statistics to work out.
Paolo Ghia: To be provocative, a big change in exposure all over the world happened with the change in using unleaded fuel and you said that benzene is one of the factors that can induce lymphoma worldwide. Now that we use unleaded fuel with benzene we have all been exposed for 15 years.
Charles Rabkin: Again, these trends go back much farther than that, but it certainly will be an important thing to follow now.

Alternative Splicing of CD79a (Igα) and CD79b (Igβ) Transcripts in Human B-CLL Cells

A. Alfarano, P. Circosta, A. Vallario, C. Camaschella*, S. Indraccolo^, A. Amadori^ and F. Caligaris-Cappio.
Dipartimento di Scienze Biomediche e Oncologia Umana, Università di Torino; Laboratorio di Immunologia Oncologica, IRCC, Candiolo, Italy; * Dipartimento di Scienze Cliniche e Biologiche, Università di Torino; ^ Dipartimento di Scienze Oncologiche e Chirurgiche, Sezione di Oncologia, Università di Padova , Italy

B-chronic lymphocytic leukemia (B-CLL) is an accumulative disease of resting CD5+ B lymphocytes that present a number of distinctive features including the expression of faint to virtually undetectable amounts of monoclonal surface immunoglobulins (sIg), an unusual kinetic hyporesponsiveness, an extended cell survival due to defective apoptosis and a failure to present soluble and allo antigens (1). It is conceivable that abnormalities of the B cell receptor (BCR) may play a prominent role in causing these functional anomalies. The BCR of mature B cells is a multimeric complex formed by the sIg homodimer and the noncovalently bound heterodimer Igα/Igβ (CD79a/CD79b) encoded by the mb-1 and the B29 genes (2,3). CD79a and CD79b have an extracellular part that forms an Ig-like domain and binds to sIg, a transmembrane and a cytoplasmic domain (4). The heterodimer, which is both essential and sufficient for Ig to reach the membrane (2-5), is the signal transducing unit of the BCR (6-8). CD79a and CD79b function synergistically to induce the apoptosis mediated via the BCR (9), influence Ag internalization and increase the efficiency of Ag presentation (10). RNA truncated forms (ΔCD79a and ΔCD79b) which arise by alternative splicing have been described in a variety of human B cells and B cell lines (11,12). ΔCD79a lacks a portion of the extracellular domain encoded by exon 2 (13) and ΔCD79b lacks the entire extracellular Ig-like domain encoded by exon 3 (11).

B-CLL cells have a defective signal transduction via the BCR (14). The monoclonal antibody (MAb) SN8, which identifies an epitope on the extracellular domain of CD79b, fails to react with malignant B cells in most B-CLL patients (15). The diminished display of BCR on the membrane of B-CLL cells has been ascribed to the occurrence of somatic mutations predicted to affect CD79b expression (16). This finding has not been confirmed by subsequent studies (17, 18). Rather, an alternative explanation has been offered by the detection of the ΔCD79b truncated form in B-CLL cells as well as in SN8 negative activated normal B cells (18).

In the present work we have investigated the RNA transcripts of CD79a and CD79b in CLL and show that all cases analysed are characterized by the presence of the ΔCD79a that lacks a major portion of the CD79a extracellular domain and the

ΔCD79b mRNA that results in the deletion of the entire CD79b extracellular domain. We propose a role for the alternative splicing of CD79a and CD79b genes in causing a disturbed BCR assembly process that may be responsible for its reduced expression on the surface of B-CLL cells.

Material and Methods

Cells and Cell Lines

Peripheral blood lymphocytes (PBL) from 35 patients with B-CLL were studied. According to the Rai staging system (19) 5 patients were stage 0, 5 stage I, 10 stage II, 5 stage III and 10 stage IV. Two B-CLL cell lines, MEC1 and MEC2 (20) were analysed. The controls were: a) Daudi, Raji, Jurkatt and U266 cell lines; b) four EBV-induced cell lines (lymphoblastoid cell lines: LCL) obtained from 4 different normal donors; c) fresh unstimulated PBL from 18 normal donors; d) B lymphocytes purified from the PB of 3 normal donors and stimulated *in vitro* with murine fibroblastic L cells stably expressing both human CD40 ligand (L) and CD32/FcgRII (CD40L/CD32-L cells, gift of Dr. J. Banchereau, Dardilly, France).

Cell Separation and Phenotyping

PBL were obtained by separation on Ficoll-Hypaque (FH; Pharmacia-LKB, Uppsala, Sweden) gradient and washed twice in phosphate buffered saline (PBS).

Different combinations of Abs were used in direct or indirect immunofluorescence. Goat antisera to human (h) μ, δ, κ and λ chains were directly conjugated with fluorescein-isothiocyanate (FITC, Tago, Burlingame, CA). The mouse MAbs used were CD5-FITC (Leu1, Becton-Dickinson, Mountain View, CA), CD19-phycoerythrin (PE) (Leu12, Becton Dickinson,), CD23-PE (Leu20, Becton Dickinson), CD3-FITC (Leu 4, Beckton Dickinson), HLA-DR-PE (Becton Dickinson), CD79a-PE (clone HM57, Dako), CD79b-FITC (clone SN8; Dako, Glostrup, Denmark) and CB3-1 (ref 21; kind gift of MD Cooper, Howard Hughes Medical Inst., Birmingham, AL).

An aliquot of cells was stained with an appropriate amount of fluorochrome-labelled antibody (Ab) and resuspended for flow cytometric analysis. Cell populations were considered CD79b positive if > 30% of the cells stained with the MAb (15). To evaluate the expression of CD79a in the cytoplasm, cells were washed with staining medium, fixed and permeabilized with the Caltag Fix and Perm Cell Permeabilization kit (Caltag Laboratories, San Francisco, Ca). Permeabilized cells were incubated with 10 μl CD79a-PE for 30 min at 4 °C, washed and resuspended for flow cytometric analysis. Negative controls were performed by incubating cells with isotype irrelevant Abs. All samples were analysed using a FACScan Research cytometer (Becton-Dickinson) equipped with a 488 nm argon ion laser (BDIS). Data acquisition was performed using the FACScan Research Software (BDIS). Analysis of the fluorescence histograms was performed by the Kolmogorov-Smirnov test (22).

RT-PCR and cDNA Analysis.

Two μg of total cellular RNA were reverse-transcribed using 12.5 U of AMV-RT (Promega, Madison, WI) and 0.5 μg of (oligo)dT as primer for 45 min at 42°C.

PCR was performed in a 50 μL volume with 25 pmol of primers, 1U of *Thermus Aquaticus* (Taq) polymerase (AmpliTaq, Perkin Elmer, Branchburg, NJ) and 200 mM of dNTPs (Pharmacia Biotech, Uppsala, Sweden) and GENE Amp 10xPCR Buffer II (Perkin-Elmer). The conditions of PCR were as previously described (18). Primers used to amplify CD79b cDNA (Fig. 1) were synthesized with sequences corresponding to nucleotides 11-35 (A: forward) and nucleotides 696-719 (B: reverse) (23). Primers used to amplify CD79a cDNA (Fig. 1) were synthesized with sequences corresponding to nucleotides 25-44 (C: forward) and nucleotides 576-595 (D: reverse) (13).

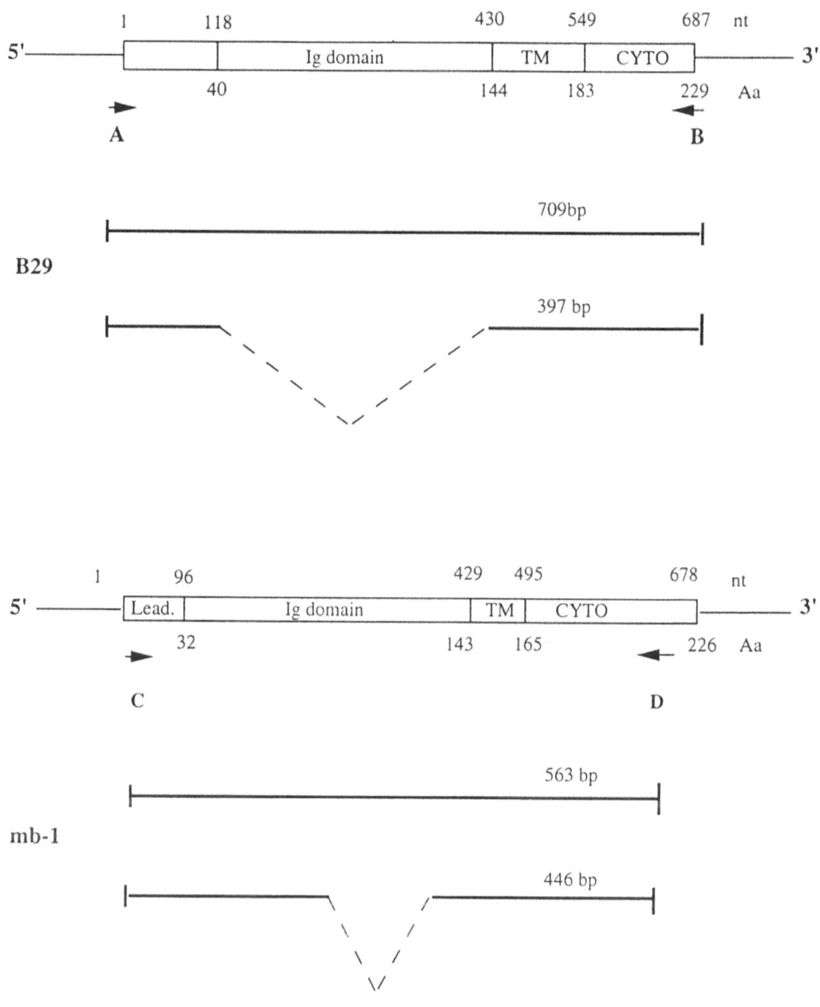

Fig. 1. Schematic representation of the alternative splicing of CD79b (B29) and CD79a (mb-1) cDNA. Primer's positions are indicated by arrows.

Results

CD79a and CD79b Protein Expression

We used SN8 and HM57MAb in double staining with CD19 to evaluate samples of MEC1, MEC2 cell lines and of 35 CLL fresh samples. MEC1, MEC2 and their parental cells were HM57 positive, SN8 negative. All fresh samples were HM57 positive while, consistent with the observation of a larger study (15), 30/35 CLL cases (85%) were SN8 and CB3-1 negative.

Unstimulated CD19+ cells from 18 normal donors were > 85% HM57, SN8 and CB3-1 positive; the expression of HM57 and SN8 was equally distributed in CD5+ and CD5- PBL B cells. In normal CD19 positive B cell samples stimulated by the CD40L/CD32-L cell system the percentage of CD19 positive, SN8 positive cells was < 20%, while the expression of HM57 remained > 80%. The proportion of SN8 positive cells of the four LCL cell lines from normal individuals was < 5%, while, again, the proportion of HM57 positive cells was >80%.

Daudi and Raji cells reacted very strongly with SN8, while Jurkatt cells were completely negative. U266 was the negative control for HM57.

CD79a and CD79b Transcript Analysis

Total RNA from 35 fresh B-CLL samples was retrotranscribed to cDNA and amplified by PCR using primers able to detect the alternatively spliced versions of CD79a and CD79b (Fig. 1).

The transcript analysis of CD79a revealed two fragments of different size (563bp and 446bp) in all samples. The 563bp band corresponds to the entire transcript analysed; the 446bp band corresponds to the alternative spliced form lacking Aa 266-328 (Fig. 1) in the membrane anchoring region (17, 19). Both fragments were absent in the U266 cell line. A comparison of normal and B-CLL samples revealed that the 563bp fragment was more evident in all B-CLL samples examined.

As for CD79b, two fragments of different size (709bp and 397bp) were found. The 709bp band corresponds to the expected CD79b entire transcript and the 397bp band corresponds to the alternative spliced form lacking exon 3, which codes for Aa 40 - 143 of the extracellular domain (Fig. 1) (24). In all samples examined, as well as in MEC1 and MEC2 cell lines, the 397bp band was always detectable. The 397bp fragment was virtually undetectable in the Raji cell line that shows very high levels of SN8 reactivity. A comparison of normal and B-CLL samples revealed that the 397bp fragment was generally more evident in B-CLL. In normal B cells stimulated *in vitro* by the CD40L/CD32-L cell system as well as in the 4 LCL examined the level of expression of the 397bp fragment was increased (not shown).

Discussion

The majority of CLL cells express low to undetectable amounts of the extracellular epitope of CD79b. As the integrity of the CD79a/CD79b heterodimer is essential for the transport of Ig to the membrane, the signal transduction and the process of apoptosis (2-10), it is reasonable to predict that abnormalities of the BCR have a central role in the pathophysiology of the disease. In this work we demonstrate that B-CLL cells consistently have two mRNA forms, which are the product of an alternative splicing, for both CD79a and CD79b. The ΔCD79a lacks a portion of the extracellular domain encoded by exon 2 and the ΔCD79b lacks the extracellular Ig-like domain. Both ΔCD79a and ΔCD79b have been demonstrated in a variety of human B cells and B cell lines using an RNAse protection assay (11, 12). Experiments of BCR reconstitution in murine fibroblast L cells have established an unequivocal relationship between the presence of internally deleted mRNA and the absence of detectable CD79b on the membrane (12). On these bases it becomes tempting to speculate that the formation of CD79b mRNA lacking the extracellular domain plays a role in the BCR phenotypic abnormalities in B-CLL.

The possibility that alternative splicing may have a role in the mechanisms that lead to the abnormalities of BCR expression in B-CLL is supported by the observations on normal B lymphocytes. Resting normal B cells, that express the CD79b extracellular epitope in more than 80% of the elements, present low amounts of ΔCD79b (12), irrespective of the expression of CD5 indicating that SN8 and ΔCD79b are not restricted to a phenotypically distinct B cell subset (18). Activated B cells have higher levels of internally deleted mRNA (12): in these cells the proportion of elements that fail to express the extracellular epitope of CD79b is also increased (18). High levels of ΔCD79b are observed in activated B cells irrespective of the activation stimuli delivered, suggesting that the process of B cell activation *per se* favours the posttranscriptional negative regulation of CD79b. Several observations (23-27) lead to suggest that the mechanism of alternative splicing which produces a CD79b form lacking the Ig-like extracellular domain is a physiological mechanism during B cell activation. Thus, it is reasonable to conclude that the abnormalities of BCR in B-CLL likely reflect the state of activation of the B cell where the malignant transformation has occurred. The biochemical properties of the protein encoded by the ΔCD79 transcripts are unknown as are the dynamics and the features of the assembly of the BCR components in human fresh malignant B cells. The assembly of the different BCR components has been explored in detail in Ramos cell line, where it has been shown that the association of Ig heavy and light chains together with CD79a and CD79b is required and sufficient to permit the exit of BCR complex out of the endoplasmic reticulum (28). It is plausible that, because of the presence of alternatively spliced versions, the process of assembly of the BCR components is disturbed in CLL cells, thereby leading to the abnormalities of BCR organization that influence the behaviour of malignant B-CLL cells.

Acknowledgements

This work was supported by A.I.R.C. and by MURST. P.C. and A.V. are recipients of a G. Ghirotti fellowship. The helpful secretarial assistance of Mrs. Giuliana Tessa, Fondazione R. Favretto, is greatly acknowledged.

References

1. Caligaris-Cappio F (1996) B-chronic lymphocytic leukemia: a malignancy of anti-self B cells. Blood 87:2615-2620
2. Reth M (1992) Antigen receptors on B lymphocytes. Annu Rev Immunol 10:97-121
3. van Noesel CJM, van Lier RAW (1993) Architecture of the human B-cell antigen receptors. Blood 82:363-373
4. Pleiman CM, D'Ambrosio D, Cambier JC (1994) The B-cell antigen receptor complex: structure and signal transduction. Immunol Today 15:393-399
5. Venkitaraman AR, Williams GT, Dariavach P, Neuberger MS (1991) The B-cell antigen receptor of the five immunoglobulin classes. Nature 352:777-781
6. Clark MR, Campbell KS, Kazlauskas A, Johnson SA, Hertz M, Potter TA, Pleiman C, Cambier JC (1992) The B cell antigen receptor complex. Association of Iga and Igb with distinct cytoplasmic effectors. Science 258:123-126
7. Lin J, Justement LB (1992) The MB-I/B29 heterodimer couples the B cell antigen receptor to multiple src family protein tyrosine kinases. J Immunol 149:1548-1555
8. Sanchez M, Misulovin Z, Burkhardt AL, Mahajan S, Costa T, Franke R, Bolen IB, Nussenzweig M (1993) Signal transduction by immunoglobulin is mediated through Iga and Igb. J Exp Med 178: 1049-1057
9. Tseng J, Eisfelder BJ, Clark MR (1997) B-cell antigen receptor-induced apoptosis requires both Iga and Igb. Blood 89:1513-1520
10. Bonnerot C, Lankar D, Hanau D, Spehner D, Davoust J, Salamero J, Fridman WH (1995)

Role of B cell receptor Igα and Igβ subunits in MHC class II-restricted antigen presentation. Immunity 3:335-360
11. Hashimoto S, Chiorazzi N, Gregersen PK (1995) Alternative splicing of CD79a (Ig-alpha/mb-1) and CD79b (Ig-beta/B29) RNA transcripts in human B cells. Mol Immunol 32:651-659
12. Koyama M, Nakamura T, Higashihara M, Herren B, Kuwata S, Shibata Y, Okumura K, Kurokawa K (1995) The novel variants of mb-1 and B29 transcripts generated by alternative mRNA splicing. Immunol Lett 47:151-156
13. Leduc I, Preud'homme JL, Cogné M (1990) Structure and expression of the mb-1 transcript in human lymphoid cells. Clin exp Immunol 90,141-146
14. Lankester AC, van Schijndel GMW, van der Schoot CE, van Oers MHJ, van Noesel CJM, van Lier RAW (1995) Antigen receptor nonresponsiveness in chronic lymphocytic leukemia B cells. Blood 86:1090-1097
15. Zomas AP, Matutes E, Morilla R, Owusu-Ankomah K, Seon BK, Catovsky D (1996)Expression of the immunoglobulin-associated protein B29 in B cell disorders with the monoclonal antibody SN8 (CD79b). Leukemia 10:1966- 1970
16. Thompson AA, Talley JA, Do HN, Kagan HL, Kunbel L, Berenson J, Cooper MD, Saxon A, Wall R (1997) Aberrations of the B-Cell receptor B29 (CD79b) gene in chronic lymphocytic leukemia. Blood 90:1387-1394
17. Rassenti LZ, Padmanabha S, Kipps TJ (1997) Expression of the B cell receptor Ig beta (CD79b) in chronic lymphocytic leukemia. Blood (Suppl.) 90:2016
18. Alfarano A, Indraccolo S, Circosta P, Minuzzo S, Vallario A, Zamarchi R, Fregonese A, Calderazzo F, Faldella A, Aragno M, Camaschella C, Amadori A, Caligaris-Cappio F (1999) An alternatively spliced form of CD79b gene may account for altered B cell receptor expression in B-chronic lymphocytic leukemia. Blood, in press.
19. Rai KR, Sawirsky A, Cronkite EP, Chanana AD, Levy RN, Pasternack BS (1975) Clinical staging of chronic lymphocytic leukaemia. Blood 46:219-234
20. Stacchini A, Aragno M, Vallario A, Alfarano A, Circosta P, Gottardi D, Faldella F, Rege-Cambrin G, Thunberg U, Nilsson K, Caligaris-Cappio F (1998) MEC1 and MEC2: two new cell lines derived from B-chronic lymphocytic leukaemia in prolymphocytoid transformation. Leuk Res, in press.
21. Nakamura T, Kubagawa H, Cooper MD (1992) Heterogeneity of immunoglobulin-associated molecules on human B cells identified by monoclonal antibodies. Proc Natl Acad Sci USA 89:8522-8526
22. Young IT (1977) Proof without prejudice: use of the Kalmogorov-Smirnov test for the analysis of the histograms from flow systems and other sources. J Histochem Cytochem 25:935-941
23. Muller B, Cooper L, Terhorst C (1992) Cloning and sequencing of the cDNA encoding the human homologue of the murine immunoglobulin-associated protein B29. Eur J Immunol 22:1621-1625
24. Hashimoto S, Chiorazzi N, Gregersen PK (1994) The complete sequence of the human CD79b (Igb/B29) gene: identification of a conserved exon/intron organization, immunoglobulin-like regulatory regions, and allelic polymorphism. Immunogenetics 40: 145-151
25. Verschuren MCM, Comans-Bitter WM, Kapteijn CAC, Mason DY, Brouns GS, Borst J, Drexler HG, van Dongen JJM (1993) Transcription and protein expression of mb-1 and B29 genes in human hematopoietic malignancies and cell lines. Leukemia 7: 1939-1947
26. Mason DY, van Noesel CJ, Cordell JL, Comans-Bitter WM, Micklem K, tse Ag, van Lier RA, van Dongen JJ (1992) The B29 and mb-1 polypeptides are differentially expressed during human B cell differentiation. Eur J Immunol 22:2753-2756
27. Mori S, Takanashi M, Shiota M, Choi SH, Yamanashi Y, Watanabe T, Koike M (1994) Down-regulation of membrane immunoglobulin-associated proteins, mb-1, B29 and3 Lyn, in AIDS-lymphomas and related conditions. Virchows Arch 424: 553-561
28. Brouns GS, de Vries E, Borst J (1995) Assembly and intracellular transport of the human B cell antigen receptor complex. Int Immunol 7:359-368

Discussion

George Klein: Did I understand you to say that the CLL cells are largely resting and not activated B cells because of the defectiveness of BCR?
Federico Caligaris-Cappio: Yes.
George Klein: My wife Eva has been studying the EBV activability of CLL cells. This is independent of the BCR since activation is triggered by the EBV-specific CD21 receptor. This activation is also blocked, at least partially. Would you comment on that?
Federico Caligaris-Cappio: I must admit that we have spent too many years and too much money trying to obtain EBV cell lines in CLL and we always failed, apart from a couple of exceptions. In other words, it is extremely difficult to obtain CLL cell lines, even if the CD21 is there, even if there are no apparent defects in the receptor. I can't explain it. I can only say that in general terms CLL cells appear to be phenotypically activated, but they lack all the functional features of activated B cells, including the ability to be transformed by EBV.
Sandy Morse: I have a question relating to the CD5 nature of it, in the current debate that, in the mouse anyhow, ranges around whether or not this is a lineage-identifying protein or one which simply reflects activation. Do you see the presence of CD5 on these cells as being another evidence of activation or perhaps reflecting their origin from mantle cells?
Federico Caligaris-Cappio: In humans, certainly, $CD5^+$ B cells can be found in the mantle zone of lymph nodes. The properties of malignant $CD5^+$ B cells are somehow similar to those of the purified $CD5^+$ B cells, with a number of differences. They also produce polyreactive autoantibodies, but for instance normal $CD5^+$ B cells from the mantle zone can be transformed by EBV, while a malignant B-CLL cell cannot. Taking all the data together, I think that it is reasonable to state that in humans the $CD5^+$ B cell population – in functional terms – is rather independent and I do not think that you can consider it simply as the result of the activation of normal B cells.
Sandy Morse: So you favor an origin from mantle zone cells?
Federico Caligaris-Cappio: Yes.
Katherine Siminovitch: In your PCR analysis it looked as if you had amplified not only the splice variant but also the normal form of the CD79. Therefore, should you not expect to see a mixed population of receptors?
Federico Caligaris-Cappio: I think that we still do not know that. We are trying to analyze that at the single-cell level in order to answer that question.
Kasuo Ohnishi: Is it possible to immunoprecipitate a spliced variant of CD79?
Federico Caligaris-Cappio: We are trying to and it is not an easy task.
Kasuo Ohnishi: Are there any differences in associated molecules for spliced variants of CD79b?
Federico Caligaris-Cappio: The data are too preliminary so I cannot say anything about that.
Bart Barlogie: What happened to the experimental approach to push CLL cells towards hairy cells and plasma cells? I think hairy cells to plasma cells is possible. What happens to the BCR?
Federico Caligaris-Cappio: I can say that the hairy cells have normal expression of surface CD79b, as do most non-Hodgkin's lymphomas. The reason why we concentrated on CLL is that this lack of expression of the extracellular portion of CD79b, at least on phenotypic grounds, appeared to be a window strictly limited to CLL. That is why we investigated the molecular basis of this defect. I don't know what would happen to BCR if we try to push CLL *in vitro* toward hairy cells because we have not done these experiments.
Bart Barlogie: Can you restore it?
Federico Caligaris-Cappio: I do not know because the experiments that we have done are too limited in this direction.
Georg Bornkamm: My question also concerns stimulation by CD40, since EBV reflects, in a way, physiological activation of B cells. Do the cells respond to CD40 ligand by upregulation of costimulatory molecules and activation markers?
Federico Caligaris-Cappio: Yes, absolutely. If you analyze freshly drawn CLL cells they are CD80 and CD86 negative, but if you stimulate them with CD40 ligand, they upregulate CD80

and CD86, and also even if in normal conditions they are lousy antigen-presenting cells, they become good APCs after CD40 ligand stimulation.

Georg Bornkamm: So it is not a general block?

Federico Caligaris-Cappio: No, it is a reversible block and it can be reversed in those experimental conditions.

Fritz Melchers: Regarding this restoration, can you take a wild-type Igα (CD79) and transfect it into the tumor cell and see whether it now gains normal function?

Federico Caligaris-Cappio: You can, but we have not done it.

Fritz Melchers: Do you know the autoantigen in some of these cases?

Federico Caligaris-Cappio: In some instances the surface Ig on CLL cells has rheumatoid factor activity.

Fritz Melchers: So you would even have an antigen?

Federico Caligaris-Cappio: Yes.

Fritz Melchers: Then you can test whether it goes back to normal?

Federico Caligaris-Cappio: Yes, it may be experimentally tested.

Heinz Jacobs: So would transgenic mice expressing the truncated version develop tumors?

Federico Caligaris-Cappio: No, I am not saying that this is the oncogenic event.

Heinz Jacobs: Then you are saying it is a lack of activation.

Carel van Noesel: Perhaps it is good to mention a study by a Japanese group [Koyama et al. (1995) The novel variants of mb-1 and B29 transcripts generated by alternative mRNA splicing. Immunol Lett 47:151-156] who did reconstitution studies. They failed to get a B cell receptor complex on the surface with these truncated CD79 molecules.

Federico Caligaris-Cappio: That was done in the Raji cell line.

Fritz Melchers: May be dominant negative?

Federico Caligaris-Cappio: Yes.

Novel Aspects of Murine B Cell Lymphomas

H. C. Morse III,[1] C.-F. Qi,[1] L. Tadesse-Heath,[1] S. K. Chattopadhyay,[1] J. M. Ward,[2] A. Coleman,[3] J. W. Hartley,[1] and T. N. Fredrickson[4]
[1]Laboratory or Immunopathology, National Institute of Allergy and Infectious Diseases; and [2]Veterinary Pathology, [3]Laboratory of Genetics, and [4]Registry of Experimental Cancers, National Cancer Institute, National Institutes of Health, Bethesda, Maryland

Marginal Zone Lymphoma (MZL)

Introduction of ecotropic murine leukemia virus (MuLV) induction loci onto the low-lymphoma, ecotropic MuLV-negative strain, NFS, yielded strains of mice (NFS.V$^+$) that develop a high incidence of hematopoietic neoplasms (1, 2) comprising primarily lymphomas of B cell origin. Histopathologic studies of 645 lymphomas yielded morphologic diagnoses compatible with synonyms provided by the Kiel (3) and REAL (4) classifications of human B lymphomas but applied to the mouse (Table 1). The "Bethesda/Kiel" terminology will be used here. The speculative "LIP/REAL" classification is based on studies suggesting uniting parallels with human neoplasms of these types (e.g., Siminovitch, this volume, for mouse MCL equivalent). MZL, diagnosed only once previously, in NZB (5), were unexpectedly most common in our series, at 36% (Hartley et al., manuscript in preparation).

The average age at diagnosis for MZL was 400 days. Although spread beyond the spleen was rare, MZL demonstrated progression from a benign-appearing expansion of the marginal zone (EMZ) to low-grade lymphoma (MZL → MZL+)

Table 1. Morphologic diagnoses of B cell lymphomas in NFS.V$^+$ mice

Diagnosis: Bethesda/Kiel	LIP/REAL—speculative	Percent of tumors
Marginal zone (MZL)	MZL	36
Centroblastic-centrocytic (CBCCL)	Follicular center (FCL), follicular	5
Centroblastic, follicular (CBL)	FCL	4
Immunoblastic (IBL)	Diffuse large cell (DLCL)	6
Diffuse CBL (CBLdiff)	DLCL	9
Lymphoblastic (B-LL)	?Burkitt's type (BTL)	20
Small lymphoblastic (SLL)	SLL/[?Mantle cell (MCL)]/CLL	8
Centrocytic (CCL)	MCL	< 1

and then high-grade (MZL++ → CBLdiff) (Fig. 1). The strongest evidence for this progression came from biopsy-necropsy studies in which the splenic lesions of single mice could be examined at one time point and compared with material obtained weeks to months later (Fig. 1; Table 2; Fredrickson et al., submitted for publication).

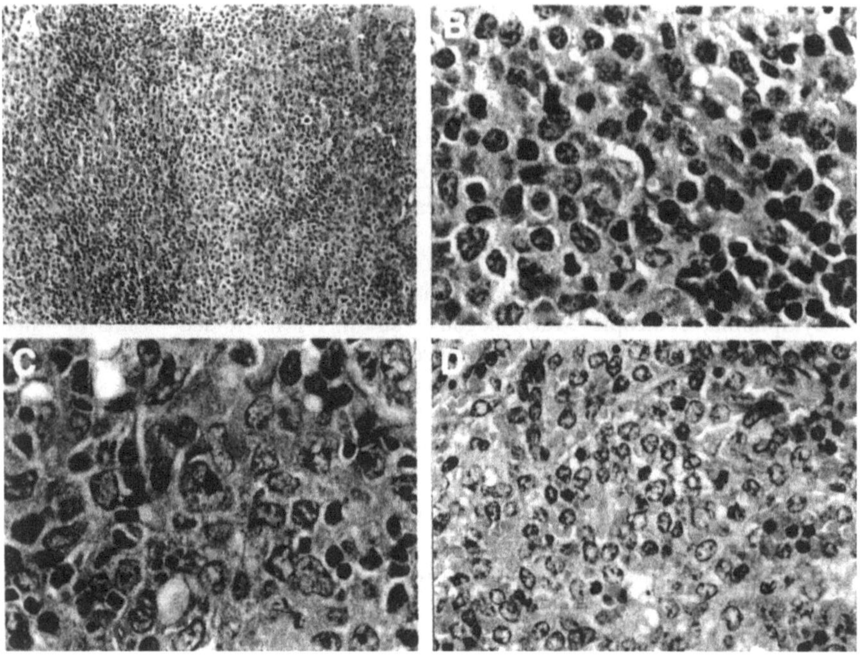

Figure 1. Progression of MZL in NFS.V^{+} mice. **A.** Earliest discernable proliferation of the marginal zone (EMZ) between the splenic follicle (left) and the red pulp (right) (H+E: ×50). **B.** Cytologic detail of marginal zone cells shown in **A**. Nuclei contain stippled chromatin and variable numbers of small nucleoli (H+E: ×250). **C.** Necrosy sample of spleen showing advanced MZL++—mainly composed of centroblasts but also immunoblasts (center)—that had progressed in 47 days from typical MZL+ (H+E: ×250). **D.** CBLdiff, typical of entire spleen, that had progressed from MZL in 148 days after biopsy (H+E: ×150).

These studies showed that most cases diagnosed at biopsy as EMZ, MZL, or MZL+ progressed to higher grade. A relation between MZL and CBLdiff was also revealed in transplants of primary CBLdiff to immunodeficient mice that grew out as MZL. When CBLdiff is diagnosed only at autopsy, however, we do not feel it is possible to determine whether it derived from a MZL or a follicular lymphoma of centroblastic type.

Southern blot analyses of DNAs from cases ranging from EMZ to CBLdiff revealed a progression from poly- or oligoclonal to monoclonal as judged by the organization of IgJ_H genes (Table 2). In the biopsy-necropsy series, one or more

Table 2. Biopsy-necropsy studies of marginal zone lymphoma progression

Biopsy diagnosis	Autopsy diagnosis (%) EMZ	MZL	MZL+	MZL++	Percent progression
EMZ →	25	25	16	33	75
MZL →		50	30	50	80
MZL+ →			66	33	33
MZL++ →				100	0

Diagnosis	Percent of cases EMZ	MZL	MZL+	MZL++	CBL diffuse
Spleen weight > 800 mg	0	5	30	56	88
Oligo/polyclonal	43	26	5	6	0
Mono/oligoclonal	57	74	95	94	100

clones detected in the biopsy sample was usually found in the DNA obtained at autopsy, demonstrating that the lesions differing in stage derived form the same clone. More than 90% of MZL were also judged to be clonal based on the presence of clonal, somatically acquired ecotropic proviral insertions. The role of ecotropic MuLV in lymphomagenesis is usually thought of in terms of insertional mutagenesis of proto-oncogenes or tumor suppressor genes. A series of these insertions has been molecularly cloned, and cellular sequences adjacent to the viral integrations are being used to determine whether the altered sites are seen frequently in our series and if the insertions affect gene expression (Chattopadhyay et al., unpublished observations). Transplantation studies (Table 3) demonstrated

Table 3. Transplantation of marginal zone-related lymphomas in immunodeficient and immunocompetent mice

Primary Lymphoma				Characteristics of Outgrowths* G1 scid		G1 NFS.V+	
NFS.V+	SW (g)	Diagnosis	J_H	Diagnosis	J_H	Diagnosis	J_H
1	2.6	CBLdif	2	CBLdif	2	MZL++	2
2	1.2	MZL/CBCC/My	2	CBLdif/My	2	MZL+/CBCC/My	2
3	0.2	MZL	2			MZL	2
4	0.4	MZL	2			MZL+	2
5	1.0	SLL/MZL	4	CBLdif	2		
6	0.9	CBCC/MZL	1	CBLdif	2		

* Diagnosis and number of non-germline hybridization bands (J_H) revealed in Southern blots of *Eco*RI-digested DNA and J_H probe.

that the tumors were malignant in both immunologically competent and incompetent hosts. The appearance of a MZL++ in a recipient of a CBLdiff primary tumor reinforces the relationship between these two pathologic entities. In addition, all clonal J_H bands seen in primary lymphomas were observed, with one exception, in the first generation (G1) transplants. Finally, the homing characteristics of MZL were demonstrated by their growth in the splenic marginal zones of transplant recipients.

The opportunity to understand the contribution of altered gene expression to development of MZL came from the recognition of EMZ and MZL in spleens of B6 $p53^{-/-}$ mice (Table 4; Ward et al., submitted for publication). Previous studies showed these mice to be at high risk for early-onset thymic lymphoma (T-LL), also observed in our series (6, 7).

Table 4. Development of marginal zone abnormalities in $p53^{-/-}$ mice

	Percent of mice	
Spleen diagnosis	12 weeks	5 to 8 months
Normal	57	4
EMZ	43	38
MZL	0	34
MZL + T-LL	0	12

MZL in $p53^{-/-}$ mice likely follow the pattern seen in NFS.V$^+$ of histologic progression from EMZ → MZL and molecular progression from oligoclonal to clonal. By 5 to 8 months, over 40% of mice exhibited MZL either alone or in concert with splenic T-LL (Table 4). Of note, ecotropic proviral insertional mutagenesis could not be implicated in the genesis of these tumors, as DNAs contained only the single endogenous virus of B6 mice. MZL develop at a much later age in non-mutant B6 mice (J. M. Ward, unpublished observations), indicating that p53 mutations act to accelerate this disease. This observation also shows that MZL occur in unmanipulated, aging mice other than NFS.V$^+$ and NZB.

Based on studies of solid tumors, Kinzler and Vogelstein suggested that oncogenes involved in their development could be subdivided into the categories of caretakers and gatekeepers (8). Caretakers are responsible for maintaining genomic integrity and include genes such as *Ptprc* (scid), *Ku70*, and *Atm*. In contrast, gatekeepers are responsible for inducing growth arrest or apoptotic death of tumor cells; *p16* and *p53* are representative of genes in this category. Extending these concepts to the pathogenesis of MZL, we suggest first that EMZ results from chronic antigenic stimulation resulting in poly/oligoclonal proliferation of normal MZ cells. Mutation of both copies of yet-unidentified caretakers results in widespread, unrepaired DNA breaks or mutations in genes yielding oligoclonal outgrowth of MZL → MZL+. Eventually, these mutations involve caretakers, leading to irreversible progression to MZL++ and CBLdiff. The plentiful MZL of NFS.V$^+$ mice provide a rich resource for examining this model.

The Role of *Bcl6* in Large Cell B Lymphomas

Expression of BCL6, a transcriptional repressor required for germinal center formation (9, 10), is frequently altered in human DLCL and follicular lymphomas due to chromosomal translocations that result in promoter substitution (11, 12). Immunohistochemical and western blot analyses of BCL6 expression in NFS.V$^+$ B-lineage lymphomas demonstrated that only high-grade lymphomas had a high proportion of cells that expressed BCL6 at elevated levels (Table 5; Qi et al., submitted for publication).

Southern blot analyses of *Bcl6* structure in the same lymphomas revealed changes in DNAs from one immunoblastic lymphoma and three B-LL. Studies of cultured lymphoma cell lines representing B cells at differentiation also showed an alteration of *Bcl6* structure in WEHI 231. Further studies of this line demonstrated that BCL6 transcripts and protein were of normal size (Qi et al.).

Table 5. Expression and genomic organization of BCL6 in mouse lymphomas

		Immunocytochemistry		Immunoblotting		
Grade	Classification	% positive	% high expression	% positive	% high expression	Altered *Bcl6* DNA
Low	MZL	0	0	0	0	0 / 10
	SLL	30	0	40	0	0 / 10
	CBCCL	45	0	33	17	0 / 10
High	CBL	80	80	90	90	0 / 10
	IBL	90	90	90	90	1 / 10
	B-LL	95	95	100	100	3 / 20

The observation that WEHI 231 had no somatically acquired clonal ecotropic MuLV integrations suggested that insertional mutagenesis was not responsible for the change in *Bcl6* structure and that chromosomal translocation could be involved. This possibility was initially assessed by chromosome painting (13), which revealed a balanced T(5;16) translocation affecting the region of chromosome 16 known to carry *Bcl6* (Qi et al., submitted for publication). We extended these studies using FISH combined by painting of chromosomes 5 and 16. *Bcl6* was localized to the translocation breakpoint and found to reside only on chromosome 16. These findings provide striking parallels to the human translocations that affect BCL6 expression in human DLCL and follicular lymphomas. Molecular identification of the abnormalities in WEHI 231 will allow us to determine whether the other tumors with alterations in *Bcl6* structure have also undergone translocations. If translocations are a regular feature of mouse high-grade diffuse lymphomas, this will follow plasmacytomas with T(12;14) as the second lymphoma type with a characteristic translocation.

Discussion

Analyses of lymphomas occurring in NFS.V^+ and $p53^{-/-}$ mice have demonstrated that there are likely mouse counterparts for the majority if not all B cell-lineage lymphoma types described in humans. The homologies include histopathologic, cytologic, and molecular features of these neoplasms (Fredrickson et al., manuscript in preparation). It has been shown that human MZL bearing p53 mutations have a worse prognosis than those without, and we report here that MZL of the mouse are accelerated in $p53^{-/-}$ mice. In addition, we have shown that mouse high-grade lymphomas carry mutations of BCL6, a recurring translocation in human DLCL and follicular lymphomas. As reported elsewhere in this volume, abnormalities in SHP-1 may contribute to both mouse and human MCL. The mouse thus provides a powerful model system for dissecting the pathogenesis of various B-lineage tumors as well as opportunities to evaluate prevention and treatment strategies.

References

1. Fredrickson TN, Morse HC III, Rowe WP (1984) Spontaneous tumors of NFS mice congenic for ecotropic murine leukemia virus induction loci. JNCI 73:521–524
2. Fredrickson TN, Hartley JW, Morse HC III, Chattopadhyay SK, Lennert K (1995) Classification of mouse lymphomas. Curr Top Microbiol Immunol 194:109–116
3. Lennert K, Feller A (1992) Histopathology of non-Hodgkin's lymphomas, 2d ed. Springer-Verlag, New York
4. Harris NL, Jaffe ES, Stein H, Banks PM, Chan JKC, Cleary ML, Delsol G, deWolf-Peeters C, Falini B, Gatter KC, Grogan TM, Isaacson PG, Knowles DM, Mason DY, Muller-Hermelink H-K, Pileri SA, Piris MA, Ralfkiaer E, Warnke RA (1994) A revised European-American classification of lymphoid neoplasms: a proposal from the International Lymphoma Study Group. Blood 5:1361–1392
5. Yumoto T, Yoshida Y, Yoshida H, Ando K, Matsui K (1980) Prelymphomatous and lymphomatous changes in splenomegaly of New Zealand black mice. Acta Pathol Jpn 30:171–186
6. Donehower LA, Harvey M, Slagle BL, McArthur MJ, Montgomery CA Jr, Butel JS, Bradley A (1992) Mice deficient for p53 are developmentally normal but susceptible to spontaneous tumours. Nature 356:215–221

7. Purdie CA, Harrison DJ, Peter A, Dobbit L, White S, Howie SEM, Salter DM, Bird CC, Wyllie AH, Hooper ML, Clarke AR (1994) Tumour incidence, spectrum and ploidy in mice with a large deletion in the p53 gene. Oncogene 9:603–609
8. Kinzler KW, Vogelstein B (1997) Gatekeepers and caretakers. Nature 386:761–762
9. Ye BH, Cattoretti G, Shen Q, Zhang J, Hawe N, deWaard R, Leung C, Mouri-Shirazi M, Orazi A, Chaganti RSK, Rothman P, Stall AM, Pandolfi P-P, Dalla-Favera R (1997) The *BCL-6* proto-oncogene controls germinal-centre formation and Th2-type inflammation. Nat Genet 16:161–170
10. Dent AL, Shaffer AL, Yu X, Allman D, Staudt LM (1997) Control of inflammation, cytokine expression, and germinal center formation by BCL-6. Science 276:589–592
11. Ye BH, Chaganti S, Chang C-C, Niu H, Corradini P, Chaganti RSK, Dalla-Favera R (1995) Chromosomal translocations cause deregulated *BCL6* expression by promoter substitution in B cell lymphoma. EMBO J 14:6209–6217
12. Onizuka T, Moriyama M, Tamochi T, Kuroda T, Kazama A, Kanazawa N, Sato K, Kato T, Ota H, Mori S. BCL-6 gene product, a 92- to 98 kD nuclear phosphoprotein, is highly expressed in germinal center B cells and their neoplastic counterparts. Blood 86:28–37
13. Rabbitts P, Impey H, Heppell-Parton A, Langford C, Tease C, Lowe N, Bailey D, Ferguson-Smith M, Carter N (1995) Chromosome specific paints from a high resolution flow karyotype of the mouse. Nat Genet 9:369–375

Molecular Pathogenesis of B Cell Malignancy: the Role of BCL-6

R. Dalla-Favera, A. Migliazza, C.-C. Chang, H. Niu, L. Pasqualucci, M. Butler, Q. Shen, and G. Cattoretti
Departments of Pathology and Genetics & Development, College of Physicians and Surgeons, Columbia University, New York, NY 10032, USA

Human malignancies displaying a mature B cell phenotype include non-Hodgkin lymphoma, (NHL), chronic lymphocytic leukemia (CLL), and multiple myeloma (MM). Analogous to most cancer types, the pathogenesis of these malignancies represents a multistep process involving the progressive and clonal accumulation of multiple genetic lesions affecting proto-oncogenes and tumor suppressor genes. However, several important features distinguish the mechanism and type of genetic alterations associated with NHL, CLL, and MM (Table 1).

Table 1. Genomic instability and type of cytogenetic lesions in mature B cell malignancies

Tumor	Non-Clonal Lesions		Clonal Lesions		
	General Instability	Microsatellite Instability	Translocations	Amplifications	Deletions
CLL	-	-	-	?	+
NHL	-	-	+	+	+
MM	±	-	+	+	+

During most stages of the disease, the genome of these neoplasms is relatively stable and is not affected by the generalized random instability typical of many solid tumors, particularly those of epithelial origin (Johansson et al. 1996). Mature B cell malignancies are also rarely associated with microsatellite instability, the hallmark of molecular defects in DNA mismatch repair genes observed in some hereditary cancer predisposition syndromes as well as in most sporadic tumor types (Gamberi et al. 1997). The genome of NHL, CLL, and MM is characterized by few, sometimes single, non-random chromosomal abnormalities. In NHL and MM, these abnormalities include specific chromosome amplifications and deletions as well as reciprocal chromosomal translocations. Intriguingly, chromosomal translocations are virtually absent in CLL, suggesting that the mechanisms leading to genomic instability may be different in this disease.

With the exception of CLL, the hallmark of B cell malignancies is the presence of specific chromosomal translocations which are often specifically associated with specific disease subtypes. The common feature of these translocations is the presence of proto-oncogenes in proximity to the chromosomal recombination sites. At variance with the translocations associated with acute lymphoblastic leukemia (ALL) which often lead to gene fusions, the structure of the proto-oncogene, and in particular its coding domain, is not affected by the translocation in NHL and MM. The pattern of expression of the proto-oncogene is altered as a consequence of the juxtaposition of heterologous regulatory sequences derived from the partner chromosome (transcriptional deregulation).

Most of the most common chromosomal translocations associated with NHL have been analyzed at the molecular level, while those associated with MM appear more heterogeneous and much less is known about their structural and functional features. Table 2 summarizes the current knowledge regarding the distribution of chromosomal translocations in various NHL subtypes, the respective proto-oncogene involved, their normal function and the mechanism of alteration (see Gaidano and Dalla-Favera 1997 for a detailed review). This chapter will focus on briefly reviewing current knowledge about the BCL-6 gene which is involved in chromosomal translocations in diffuse large cell lymphoma (DLCL) and is a key regulator of the formation of germinal centers (GC), the structure from which most NHL appear to derive.

Table 2. Chromosomal translocations, target genes and their function in NHL.

Tumor[a]	Chromosomal Translocation	Proto-Oncogene	Proto-Oncogene Function	Mechanism of Alteration
LPL	t(9;?)(p13;?)[b]	*PAX*-5	Transcription factor	Transcriptional deregulation
MCL	t(11;14)(q13;q32)	*BCL*-1	Cell cycle regulator	Transcriptional deregulation
FL	t(14;18)(q32;q11)	*BCL*-2	Anti-apoptosis	Transcriptional deregulation
DLCL	t(3;?)(q27;?)[b]	*BCL*-6	Transcription factor	Transcriptional deregulation
BL	t(8;14)(q24;q32)[c]	c-*MYC*	Transcription factor	Transcriptional deregulation
ALCL	t(2;5)(p23;q35)	*NPM/ALK*	Nucleolar phosphoprotein /Tyrosine kinase	Fusion protein
CTCL	der(10)(q24)	*LYT*-10	Transcription factor	Truncation/deregulation

a: MCL, mantle cell lymphoma; FL, follicular lymphoma; DLCL, diffuse large cell lymphoma; BL, Burkitt's lymphoma; LPL, lymphoplasmacytoid lymphoma; ALCL, anaplastic large cell lymphoma; CTCL, cutaneous T-cell lymphoma. b: question marks indicate that alternative partner chromosomes can be involved in different cases. c: variant translocations are not listed.

The BCL-6 Protein: a POZ/Zinc-Finger Transcriptional Repressor

The BCL-6 gene encodes a 95kd nuclear phosphoprotein belonging to the POZ/Zinc finger (ZF) family of transcription factors (Fig. 1). It contains six *Kruppel*-type C-terminal ZF motifs which have been shown to recognize specific DNA sequences *in vitro* (Chang et al., 1996; Seyfert et al., 1996), and a N-terminal POZ, a protein-protein interaction motif shared by various ZF molecules motif (Albagli et al., 1995). BCL-6 functions as a potent transcriptional repressor of genes containing its DNA binding site. This function requires DNA binding by the ZF and a transrepression domain which includes the POZ (Deweindt et al., 1995; Chang et al., 1996; Seyfert et al., 1996). The central portion of the protein contains multiple MAPK phosphorylation sites embedded in PEST motifs involved in controlling BCL-6 stability (Niu et al. 1998; see below).

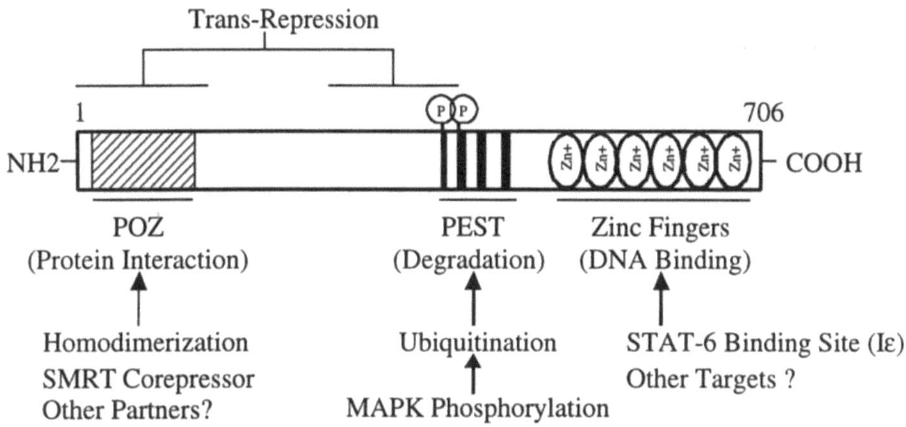

Fig. 1. Schematic representation of the BCL-6 protein and its functional domains.

BCL-6 is Required for Germinal-Center Formation

BCL-6 is an important regulator of lymphoid development and function. In the B cell lineage, the BCL-6 protein is found only in B cells within germinal centers (GC), but not in pre-B cells or in differentiated progenies such as plasma cells. In the T lineage, BCL-6 protein is detectable in cortical thymocytes and in $CD4^+$ T cells within GC as well as scattered in the perifollicular area (Cattoretti et al., 1995; Allman et al., 1996). Mice deficient in BCL-6 display normal B cell, T cell and lymphoid organ development, but have a selective defect in T cell-dependent antibody responses due to the inability of follicular B cells to proliferate and form germinal centers (GC) (Dent et al., 1997; Ye et al., 1997). In addition, BCL-6-deficient mice develop an inflammatory response in multiple organs characterized by infiltrations of eosinophils and IgE-bearing B lymphocytes typical of a Th2-mediated inflammatory response. These phenotypes may be explained by the ability of BCL-6 to bind the STAT-6 DNA binding site and repress transcription activated by STAT-6, the main nuclear effector of IL-4 signaling (Dent, et al., 1997; Ye et al. 1997).

Regulation of BCL-6 Expression

The pattern of expression of BCL-6 induction in GC and its downregulation in post-GC cells suggest that its expression may be regulated by signals important for GC development and differentiation. There is no knowledge about the signals that induce BCL-6 expression, as most stimuli involved in GC formation are not sufficient to induce BCL-6 in naïve B cells *in vitro*. However, some of the signaling pathways capable of down-regulating BCL-6 have been identified. In an *in vitro* system involving anti-μ treatment of the Ramos B cell line, we have demonstrated that antigen-receptor activation leads to BCL-6 phosphorylation by mitogen-activated protein kinase (MAPK). Phosphorylation, in turn, targets BCL-6 for rapid degradation by the ubiquitin/proteasome pathway (Niu et al. 1998). More recently, we have shown that, in the same system, signaling by CD40 or by the CD40 functional homolog EBV-LMP1 also leads to BCL-6 downregulation at least in part at the transcriptional level (unpublished results). BCL-6, in turn, modulates IL-4 signaling via modulation of STAT-6 induced transcription. Thus, BCL-6 may represent a transcriptional switch integrating various signals critical for GC development (Fig. 2). However, the timing of these signals and their combined effect on BCL-6 expression remains to be determined.

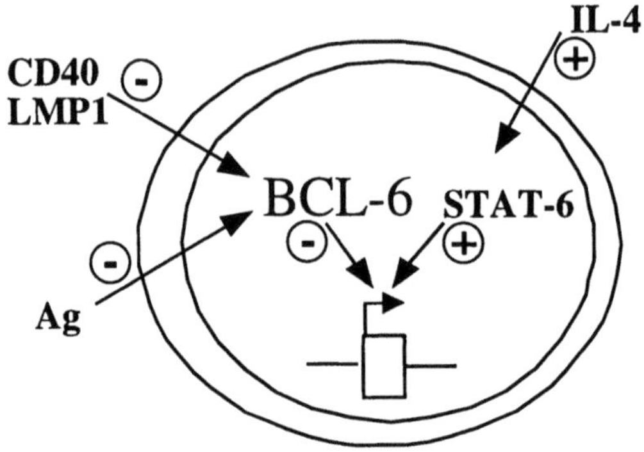

Fig.2. Schematic representation of the signaling pathways regulating and regulated by BCL-6

Alterations of the BCL-6 Gene in NHL

The *BCL-6* proto-oncogene was identified by virtue of its involvement in chromosomal translocations in diffuse large cell lymphoma (DLCL), the most common form of non-Hodgkin lymphoma (NHL) (Ye at al.1993; Kerckaert et al. 1993; Baron et al. 1993; Miki et al. 1994). Subsequent studies have demonstrated that rearrangements of the *BCL-6* gene can be found in ~35% of DLCL and in a minority (5-10%) of follicular lymphoma (FL) (Fig. 3) (LoCoco et al. 1994). These rearrangements juxtapose heterologous promoters, derived from other chromosomes, to the *BCL-6* coding domain (Ye et al. 1995). The common denominator of these promoters is their broader pattern of activity in the B cell lineage, and in particular their persistence activity in post-GC cells such as immunoblast and plasma cells (Chen et al. 1998). Thus, when juxtaposed to the BCL-6 coding domain, these promoters alter the GC-specific pattern of BCL-6 expression and, in particular, prevent its downregulation associated with post GC differentiation. The persistent expression of BCl-6 may contribute to lymphomagenesis by blocking B cell differentiation within GC. This model awaits demonstration in transgenic mice expressing BCL-6 under the control of heterologous promoters.

Hypermutation of the BCL-6 Promoter Region in Normal B Cells and NHL

While in 35% of diffuse large cell lymphomas (DLCL) and 5-10% follicular lymphomas (FL) the BCL-6 gene is structurally altered by chromosomal translocations (LoCoco et al. 1994), mutations of its 5' non-coding region were frequently found in DLCL and FL in the absence of translocations involving this locus (Migliazza et al. 1995) (Fig. 3).

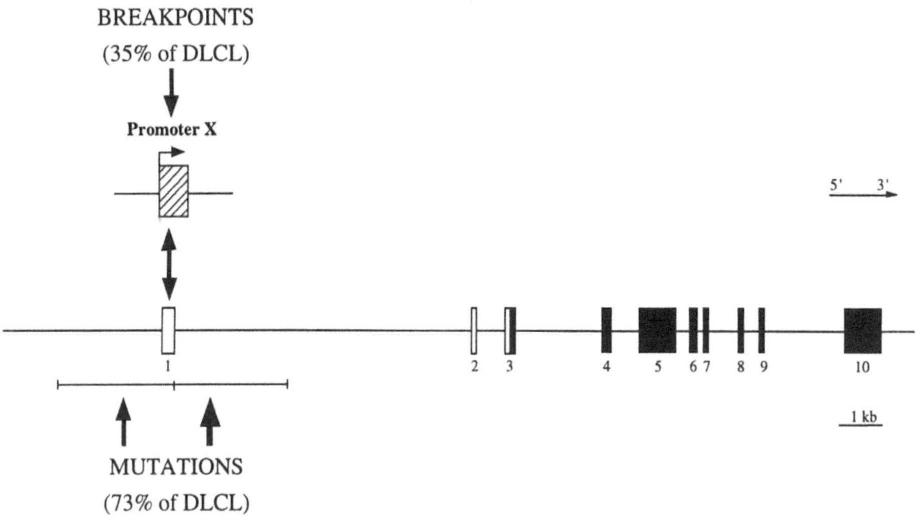

Fig. 3. Position of breakpoints and mutations within the 5' non-coding region of BCL-6

In most tumor cases, mutations were multiple, often biallelic, and clustered in the 5' regulatory sequences at frequencies (7×10^{-4}-1.6×10^{-2}/bp) comparable to that of Ig genes in B cells (Migliazza et al. 1995). In a subsequent analysis, we examined BCL-6 and Ig heavy-chain V (IgV_H) mutations in B cell malignancies representative of various stages of B cell development, including GC, pre- and post-GC stages. BCL-6 mutations, like IgV mutations, were found in GC or post-GC derived tumors including DLCL, FL, BL, and MM. To determine whether BCL-6 mutations represent a tumor-associated misfunction or the effect of the IgV hypermutation process acting on non-Ig genes, we investigated the presence of BCL-6 mutations in normal GC by PCR amplification and sequencing of DNA from single cells (Pasqualucci et al., 1998).

Table 3. . Characteristics of mutations in BCL- 6 and IgVH genes in normal GC cells versus DLCL

	BCL-6		IgV_H	
	Normal GC	DLCL	Normal GC	DLCL
Frequency $\times 10^{-2}$/bp (Range)	0.05 (0-0.4)	0.23 (0-1.6)	5 (0-13)	15.2 (6.3-20.5)
Single bp Substitutions	+	+	+	+
Deletions	+	+	+	-
Transitions/ Transversions	+	+	+	+
Strand Polarity	-	-	+	+
RGYW Bias	+ (0.05)	+ (0.05)	+ (<0.001)	+ (<0.001)

Thirty percent of GC B cells, but not naive B cells, displayed mutations in the 742 bp region within the first intron of BCL-6 (overall frequency: 5 x 10^{-4}/bp) (Table 3) (Pasqualucci et al. 1998; see also Shen et al. 1998). In both normal and transformed cells, the features of BCL-6 mutations closely resembled those displayed by IgV sequences strongly suggesting that they may derive from the same mechanism (Table 3). Thus, these findings indicate that the somatic hypermutation mechanism affecting Ig genes can physiologically target non-Ig sequences. The role of BCL-6 mutations in normal B cells as well as their role in lymphomagenesis remains to be investigated.

References

Albagli O, Dhordain P., Deweindt C. et al. (1995) The BTB/POZ domain: a new protein-protein interaction motif common to DNA- and actin-binding proteins. Cell Growth & Differ. 6:1193-1198.

Allman D, Jain A, Dent A et al. (1996) BCL-6 expression during B-cell activation. Blood 87:5257-5268.

Baron BW, Nucifora G, McCabe N et al. (1993) Identification of the gene associated with the recurring chromosomal translocations t(3;14)(q27;q32) and t(3;22)(q27;q11) in B-cell lymphomas. Proc. Natl. Acad. Sci. U.S.A. 90: 5262-5266.

Cattoretti G, Chang CC, Cechova K, et al. (1995) BCL-6 protein is expressed in germinal-center B cells. Blood 86:45-53.

Chang CC., Ye BH, Chaganti RSK et al. (1996) BCL-6, a POZ/zinc-finger protein, is a sequence-specific transcriptional repressor. Proc. Natl. Acad. Sci. U.S.A. 93: 6947-6952.

Chen W, Iida S, Louie DC et al. (1998) Heterologous promoters fused to BCL-6 by chromosomal translocations affecting band 3q27 cause its deregulated expression during B-cell differentiation. Blood 91: 603-607.

Dent AL, Shaffer AL, Yu X et al. (1997) Control of inflammation, cytokine expression, and germinal center formation by BCL-6. Science 276: 589-592.

Deweindt C, Albagli O, Bernardin F et al. (1995) The LAZ3/BCL6 oncogene encodes a sequence-specific transcriptional inhibitor: a novel function for the BTB/POZ domain as an autonomous repressing domain. Cell Growth & Differ. 6: 1495-503.

Gaidano G, Dalla-Favera R (1997) Molecular biology of Lymphomas. In: Principles and Practice of Oncology, DeVita, VT, Hellman, S., Rosenberg SA (eds) JB Lippincott Co (publ) p. 2131-2145.

Gamberi B, Gaidano G, Parsa N et al. (1997) Microsatellite instability is rare in B-cell Non-Hodgkin's Lymphoma. Blood 89:975-979.

Johansson B, Mertens F, Mitelman F (1996) Primary vs. secondary neoplasia associated chromosomal abnormalities - balanced rearrangements vs. genomic imbalances? Genes Chrom. & Cancer 16: 155-163.

Kerckaert JP, Deweindt C, Tilly H et al. (1993) LAZ3, a novel zinc-finger encoding gene, is disrupted by recurring chromosome 3q27 translocations in human lymphomas. Nature Genetics 5:66-70.

Lo, Coco F, Ye BH, Lista F et al. (1994) Rearrangements of the BCL6 gene in diffuse large cell non-Hodgkin's lymphoma. Blood 83: 1757-1759.

Migliazza A, Martinotti S, Chen S et al. (1995) Frequent somatic hypermutation of the 5' noncoding region of the BCL6 gene in B-cell lymphoma. Proc. Natl. Acad. Sci. U.S.A. 92: 12520-12524.

Miki T, Kawamata N, Hirosawa S and Aoki N (1994) Gene involved in the 3q27 translocation associated with B-cell lymphoma, BCL5, encodes a Kruppel-like zinc-finger protein. Blood 83: 26-32.

Niu H, Ye BH, Dalla-Favera R (1998) Antigen-receptor signaling induces MAP kinase-mediated phosphorylation and degradation of the BCL-6 transcription factor. Genes & Development 12:1953-1961.

Pasqualucci L, Migliazza A, Fracchiolla N et al. (1998) BCL-6 mutations in normal germinal center B cells: Evidence of somatic hypermutation acting outside Ig loci. Proc. Nat. Acad. Sci. USA 95:11816-11821.
Seyfert VL, Allman D, He Y, and Staudt LM (1996) Transcriptional repression by the proto-oncogene BCL-6. Oncogene 12: 2331-2342.
Shen HM., Peters A, Baron B et al. (1998) Mutation of BCL-6 gene in normal B cells by the process of somatic hypermutation of Ig genes. Science 280: 1750-1752.
Ye BH, Cattoretti G, Shen Q et al. (1997) The BCL-6 proto-oncogene controls germinal-centre formation and Th2-type inflammation. Nature Genetics 16: 161-170.
Ye BH, Chaganti S, Chang CC et al. (1995) Chromosomal translocations cause deregulated BCL6 expression by promoter substitution in B cell lymphoma. EMBO J. 14: 6209-6217.
Ye BH, Lista F, Lo Coco F et al. (1993) Alterations of a zinc finger-encoding gene, BCL-6, in diffuse large-cell lymphoma. Science 262: 747-750.

Discussion

George Klein: LMP-1 downregulates BCL-6; LMP-1 has a major responsibility for blast transformation. Is blast transformation directly suppressing BCL-6 expression, even if you induce it with CD40/CD40 ligand interaction? Germinal center memory cells would be activated by an antigen complex. Could that downregulate BCL-6 expression and does the mutation prevent down-regulation? Could this mechanism prevent the normal exit of the B cell from the germinal center?

Riccardo Dalla-Favera: BCL-6 is downregulated by LMP-1, CD40 signaling or by antigen receptor signaling. I cannot make a general statement on the effects of mutations on BCL-6 regulation because the mutations are so numerous and so different in different cases that every mutation has to be studied for its functional significance and that may require a long time. However, we know that some mutations deregulate the basal level of BCL-6 transcription, and we know that promoter substitution by chromosomal translocation prevents BCL-6 downregulation by CD40.

Siegfried Janz: These are interesting data, but could you furnish some additional information on the mutation frequency of BCL-6? Secondly, do you believe that you see targeting by the hypermutation machinery on three different chromosomes, i.e. the heavy chain locus, BCL-6 and myc? These three loci are in different chromosomes. The hypermutation machinery might scan the entire genome and target specific sites to introduce mutations. Alternatively, are you looking at overall, general B cell mutagenesis?

Riccardo Dalla-Favera: Let us start from the last point which is important. We are not looking at overall B cell mutagenesis. We have controls for various transcribed and non-transcribed regions of other genes that do not mutate. Regarding the frequency of cells carrying BCL-6 mutations, we examined around 100 between centroblast and centrocyte. They are all mutated within V regions, while one third of them carry mutations of BCL-6. The frequency of mutation in those mutated cells is approximately 1 order of magnitude lower than immunoglobulin V regions. These data are described in detail in our paper by Pasqualucci et al., and have also been reported by Ursula Storb's group using memory B cells.

Siegfried Janz: You can use those point mutations to establish clonal relationships, of course, and you can look at those mutations as clonotypic markers, if you like. When you compare the mutational specificity among different mutated cells, do you see a clonal relationship, or are these all independent mutations?

Riccardo Dalla-Favera: We have analyzed single cells derived from a whole tonsil. Thus the cells were presumably derived from numerous germinal centers and clonal relationships could not be established. Regarding the use of BCL-6 mutations as markers of germinal center transit, they could be used, but IgV mutations are better for this purpose because they are more frequent and are present in all germinal center B cells.

Stephen Pals: Is BCL-6 also mutated in CD4-positive T cells in the germinal center? Did you check if it is expressed?

Riccardo Dalla-Favera: It is expressed but we did not study whether it is mutated.

Stephen Pals: Concerning the marginal zone lymphomas in the mouse how do they compare to human marginal zone lymphomas? In the human you find, according to the present definition and classifications, marginal zone lymphomas in the MALT and in the lymph nodes. They have a lot of somatic mutations so are mouse tumors also post-germinal center cells?

Sandy Morse: Right. We have not analyzed yet the characteristics of the V regions but we are going to do that. These are all IgM-positive, non-switched, and they do resemble, I think in many ways, the MALT lymphomas. If you look at the mouse MALT, it also has the morphological features of marginal zone lymphoma, and I think that the MALT and also the nodal non-MALT lesions are all marginal zone.

Stephen Pals: But would they be different from the human marginal zone lymphomas which are mutated?

Sandy Morse: No. We don't have the data on mutation yet.

Riccardo Dalla-Favera: Do the marginal zone lymphomas express BCL-6?

Sandy Morse: No, they don't.

Riccardo Dalla-Favera: They don't, so these are different?

Sandy Morse: Yes.

Jacques van Dongen: Can I ask Riccardo about the mutations in BCL-6? Is their distance from the BCL-6 promoter comparable to that observed for IgV genes, i.e. ~1kb?

Riccardo Dalla-Favera: The area of BCL-6 which is most frequently mutated is comparable to the one of the V region in terms of distance from transcription initiation, i.e. it is around 1kb. This is actually the only analogy, together with transcription and transcription in germinal center cells, that we see between the two phenomena.

Una Chen: You have shown that the marginal zone lymphomas in certain strains of mice occur in higher frequency than in other strains of mice, so is it a primary or a secondary effect? Because ecotropic murine leukemia virus is known to induce preT cells to T cell leukemia, so if the cells are sitting in the marginal zone where they have a constant stimulation in this particular area they might have a predisposition to T cell stimulation before they become marginal zone lymphoma. So is it possible to isolate those marginal zone cells, to transfer them either *in vitro* culture or by adoptive transfer into another neutral environment, and compare these cells from different strains of mice to see if it is because of this secondary effect?

Sandy Morse: That is a good point. In the genesis of the tumors I described, chronic antigenic stimulation is perhaps a uniting characteristic. We know in NZB there is no ecotropic virus at all, so the source would have to be something else, perhaps the endogenous xenotropic viruses in NZB. But there are other circumstances where in many old mice this is an unrecognized lesion. It occurs in old B6 mice, it occurs in old BALB/c mice, it occurs in many strains of mice, but it just has not been recognized as being of that particular origin. It was thought of as being lymphoma of the typical old mouse spleen – TOMS is what a number of pathologists used to call it, or a subset of reticulum cell sarcoma type B.

Una Chen: Is it related to the cleanliness of the mouse colony?

Sandy Morse: We are beginning to find that out. Our congenic mice have been in a somewhat dirty environment, and we do not know how much the disease might be environmentally antigen-driven. We are putting them into SPF conditions to find out if that changes the tumor incidence.

Carel van Noesel: Could you speculate on the potential physiological role of BCL-6 mutation in the clonal selection process?

Riccardo Dalla-Favera: I have no idea. It is puzzling that the mutations occur in the promoter of a putative oncogene. I think that we have to accumulate more data on the whole repertoire of mutations in germinal centers, and perhaps compare memory cells and plasma cells to see whether there is any selection.

Mike Potter: Whatever happened to Thelma Dunn's type B reticulum cell sarcoma and what relationship does it have?

Sandy Morse: We have gone back to her slides and what she has is, one of her classic reticulum cells are prominent is clearly marginal zone lymphoma.
Mike Potter: One?
Sandy Morse: We have not been able to find all of her cases. We have some of her cases that are still available, and of those, most of them are marginal zone lymphoma in the old mice.
Jason Cyster: Have you looked to see if other components of the normal marginal zone expand to keep up with the lymphoma cells, like marginal zone macrophages?
Sandy Morse: No, we need to do that.
Michael Reth: We heard that BCL-6 is also regulated by mitogen-activated protein kinase (MAPK) so did you look in any human or mouse lymphoma to see whether the MAPK pathway was deregulated or upregulated?
Riccardo Dalla-Favera: All tumors regardless of whether they have rearranged BCL-6 or not, if they have a germinal center phenotype, express BCL-6. So either that pathway is not active or something is modulating it. We do not know the mechanism.
Sandy Morse: In relation to the question that was asked earlier, do the marginal zone lymphomas express BCL-6? They do express it at very low levels. If you inhibit MAP kinase in human Burkitt lymphoma you see an increase in the levels. So I think what is happening is that our marginal zone tumors have activated this pathway which is responsible for degradation or maybe shortening the half-life of protein, so that they are behaving as a post-germinal center cell.
Garnett Kelsoe: Regarding the MAP-kinase and CD40 pathways, both of which downregulate BCL-6, it is sort of contradictory that injection of anti-CD40 ligand antibody, presumably blocking T-B collaboration in germinal centers, does not prolong germinal center life, but rather shortens its half-life. This would imply an effect opposite to the one that you are seeing *in vitro*.
Riccardo Dalla-Favera: CD40 and B cell receptor signaling are both necessary for germinal center formation, which is associated with BCL-6 induction, and for germinal center exit, which is associated with BCL-6 downregulation. Thus, I agree with you that we have to understand much more about the timing of those signaling events and consider that they may be differentially modulated *in vivo*. The *in vitro* systems are only useful to establish the existence of a certain signaling pathway.
George Klein: Riccardo has indicated that immunoblastic transformation downregulates BCL-6, whereas your data, Sandy, showed a high expression in immunoblastic lymphoma. Is there a species difference?
Sandy Morse: There may well be but I think that there are a number of tumors which express BCL-6 that are immunoblastic and what we have called immunoblastic lymphoma.
Riccardo Dalla-Favera: My view is that it is a problem of classification: what you call immunoblastic lymphoma in mouse is a BCL-6 positive tumor, and thus probably a germinal center-derived tumor. In humans, immunoblastic lymphomas are BCL-6 negative and LMP-1 positive. Thus, I think that it may be a matter of nomenclature. I believe that BCL-6 expression identifies germinal center derivation of the tumor; if there are V region mutations and BCL-6 is off, then it is most likely a post-germinal center tumor. This model fits well with current classifications of human lymphoma..
Heinz Jacobs: Concerning the reinsertion of the pro-virus, did you analyze the insertion sites?
Sandy Morse: We have cloned out about six insertions sites now and we are in the process of examining them to see if they are recurrent and where they might be.
Heinz Jacobs: But you did not check for non-clonal insertion sites?
Sandy Morse: Yes we did, and we did not find them.

ATM and Lymphoid Malignancies; Use of Oriented Peptide Libraries to Identify Novel Substrates of ATM Critical in Downstream Signaling Pathways

G.A. Rathbun[1], Y. Ziv[2], J.H. Lai[3], D. Hill[4], R.H. Abraham[5], Y.Shiloh[2], and L.C. Cantley[3]

[1]Center for Blood Research, Harvard Medical School, USA, [2]Department of Human Genetics, Sackler School of Medicine, Tel Aviv University, Israel, [3]Department of Medicine, Beth Israel Deaconess Hospital, Harvard Medical School, USA, [4]Oncogene Research Products, USA, [5]Department of Pharmacology and Cancer Biology, Duke University, USA

Ataxia telangiectasia (AT) is a rare, autosomal recessive disorder that manifests as a pleiotropic developmental defect with symptoms including a progressive cerebellar ataxia, thymic hypoplasia, variable immunodeficiencies, hypogonadism, and telangiectasias of blood vessels in the eyes, hands and face. Patients with AT show marked radiosensitivity to ionizing radiation, and AT-derived cell lines are defective in G_1S, S and G_2M cell cycle checkpoints. AT patients have a greatly enhanced predisposition for tumor development, particularly lymphoid malignancies (Sedgwick and Boder 1991; Taylor et al. 1998).

The gene responsible for the AT disorder, termed ATM (Ataxia Telangiectasia Mutated) was identified by positional cloning (Savitsky et al. 1995). Based on homology to approximately 300 amino acids in the p110 catalytic domain of PI-3 kinase, ATM is a member of a family of the PI-3 kinase related protein kinases (PIK). This family includes several eukaryotic DNA repair and cell cycle checkpoint proteins, including mammalian ATR (AT-Related), mTOR (Mammalian Target of Rapamycin), DNA-Dependent Protein Kinase catalytic subunit (DNA-PKcs), the recently described TRRAP gene (McMahon et al. 1998), *Drosophila* Mei 41 and the *S. cerevisiae* and *S. pombe* proteins: MEC1, TEL1, Rad3, TOR1 and TOR2. (Hunter 1995; Lehmann and Carr 1995). Analyses of yeast PIK cell cycle checkpoint genes are providing significant insights into the role of these proteins in signaling pathways involved in the cell cycle checkpoint function (Elledge 1996).

Lymphocytes of AT patients are prone to chromosomal instabilities including translocations and inversions generally involving the antigen receptor loci of B and T cells (Taylor et al. 1998). In T cells of AT patients, additional complex aberrations involving chromosomal instabilities are also often present, however, the main group of abnormal chromosomal rearrangements involved T cell receptor (TCR) γ, β and α. Two classes of translocations and inversions have been described (reviewed in Taylor et al. 1998). One such category was an inter-locus event in which a translocation or inversion involved only TCR loci. Peripheral T cells with these rearrangements have been observed to persist as small circulating lymphocytes, and have also been seen in normal patients; these were not associated with malignant transformation.

The second category is defined by non-immune locus translocations and inversions, in which one chromosomal partner containing β or α TCR sequences has rearranged into a site unrelated to antigen receptor genes. This class of chromosomal aberrations is predominantly seen in malignant lymphoid transformants in AT patients. These cells can persist and proliferate in the periphery over a period of years before eventually becoming neoplastic. T cell tumors in AT patients are predominantly CD4+CD8+ double positive (DP) or CD8+CD4- single positive, and the malignant cells can be surface CD3 + or - (Taylor et al. 1998). Mice in which the ATM gene has been disrupted by targeted mutation succumb to thymic tumors that are usually DP, CD3- (Barlow et al. 1996; Xu et al. 1996; Elson et al. 1996).

Anomalous V(D)J rearrangement events have been hypothesized as a mechanistic driving force in certain of the translocations and inversions observed in AT lymphoid cells (Russo et al 1988; Sedgwick and Boder 1991; Kirsch 1994; Taylor et al. 1998). This was based on the observation that recombination signal sequences (RSS) associated with rearranging antigen receptor genes from at least one of the translocating sequences could usually be identified. In some cases, however, the sequences of the partner 'RSS' in non-immune loci were not compelling as true RSSs. The recent *in vitro* characterization of RAG1/RAG2 transposase activity (Hiom et al. 1998; Agrawal et al. 1998) in which a DNA double strand break (DSB), created by RAG1/2 cleavage, can rearrange into sequences unrelated to antigen receptor RSSs, provides a potentially important insight into an additional mechanism for V(D)J recombinase-mediated abnormal chromosomal rearrangements (Hiom et al. 1998).

V(D)J recombination takes place during the early stages of T and B cell development, and is subject to cell cycle control. RAG2 protein is degraded in all stages except G_0/G_1 (Lin and Desiderio 1994), and DNA DSBs adjacent to RSSs in antigen receptor genes undergoing rearrangement in immature T and B cells are predominantly observed in G_0/G_1 (Schlissel et al. 1993). In the same context (under normal circumstances) the transposase activity of RAG1 and 2 could be controlled, for example, through specific cell cycle regulation in which the activity, or opportunity for aberrant rearrangements (see below) is down-regulated or suppressed. A second control would be onset of rapid cell death following an inappropriate transpositional event. ATM may thus play important roles in developing lymphocytes in the context of communicating with signaling pathways that control cell cycle checkpoints critical for normal V(D)J rearrangement as well as pathways involved in lymphoid cell survival versus cell death.

Malignant transformation of lymphoid cells in AT patients likely arises as a consequence of a multi-hit phenomenon, summarized in Fig. 1. In the absence of ATM, one of the earliest hits in differentiating T or B cells would be the developmentally programmed, RAG-mediated DNA DSBs in antigen receptor loci that takes place in normal V(D)J recombination (Hit 1, Fig. 1). Lack of ATM may allow a high proportion of these breaks to persist past G_0/G_1 into later, inappropriate stages of the cell cycle and our preliminary data suggest that this, indeed, may be the case. Persistence of DSBs in later stages of the cell cycle would result in liberation of free recombinogenic DNA ends (i.e., a blunt end with a free 3'-hydroxyl) (Hit 2) and an enhanced potential for anomalous transpositional DNA strand invasion and rearrangement into unrelated loci.

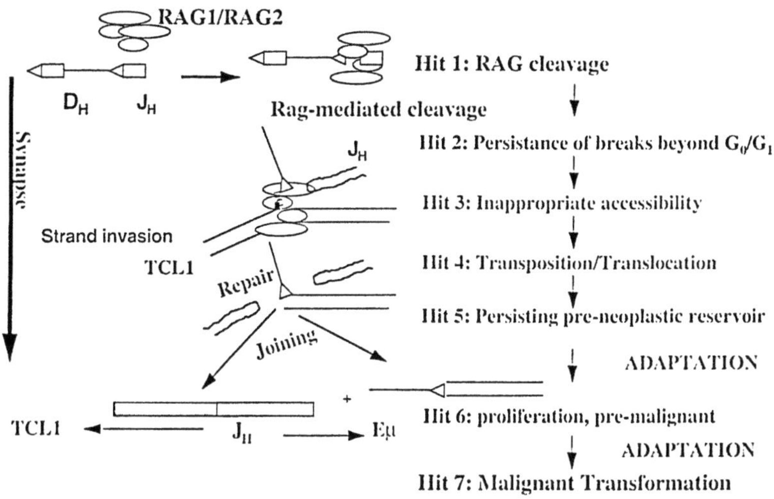

Fig.1. Depiction of potential successive steps that may result in lymphocytic malignancies arising as a consequence of ATM functional loss. The complex containing RAG1 and RAG2 proteins normally recognizes and cleaves at the RSS (triangles) of variable region gene segments (rectangles). Cleavage results in a free 3'-hydroxyl adjacent to the RSS which may then be available for an abnormal transposition event. One of the earliest of the 'hits' eventually leading to lymphoid malignancy may be abnormal persistence of RAG-generated DSB during antigen receptor assembly through late stages of the cell cycle, leading to a RAG-mediated transposition or translocation event into a non-immune locus (e.g., 14q32 or Xq28, containing the related T Cell Leukemia 1 (TCL1) and Mature T Cell Proliferation 1 (MTCP1) genes, respectively - see Taylor et al. (1998), for review, and references therein). The aberrant rearrangement leads to abnormal activation of nearby genes and contributes to maintenance and proliferation of lymphoid cells now prone to neoplastic transformation. See text for further details.

Inappropriate accessibility, also a possible consequence of the AT defect, may render non-immune loci vulnerable to RAG-mediated transposition or canonical V(D)J rearrangement (Hit 3). Ordinarily, this irrelevant locus 'accessibility' to abnormal recombination would be excluded from normal V(D)J recombinase activity by many factors, including cell cycle and lymphoid developmental stage as well as suppression of abnormal RAG transposase activity. Loss of ATM cell cycle checkpoint function may result in presentation of normally protected loci such as TCL1 and MTCP1 (Fig.1) as targets for anomalous recombination events (Hit 4) by a deranged V(D)J assembly process (commonly active over vast distances in antigen receptor loci rearrangements), the latter of which is still ongoing during later, inappropriate stages of the cell cycle.

Selection must operate throughout the time frame required for malignant transformation to take place in AT lymphocytes. On a cellular level, a pre-neoplastic reservoir containing lymphoid cells with abnormal DSB or rearrangements may persist rather than be immediately eliminated by ATM-directed apoptotic pathways (Hit 5). ATM-/- mice contain an abnormally high level of DP, CD3- thymocytes (Barlow et al. 1996; Xu et al. 1996; Elson et al. 1996), suggesting an accumulation of cells present which have failed to produce a functional TCR rearrangement, yet nonetheless persists. A second wave of selection is represented by lymphoid cells with specific chromosomal rearrangements that escape into the periphery. These cells adapt and proliferate, representing a circulating, pre-malignant reservoir (Taylor et al. 1998) (Hit 6). This population, now inherently prone to genomic instabilities, can be maintained in AT patients for several years, and ultimately provide the cell(s) targeted for malignant transformation by a yet unknown additional mutation (Hit 7, Fig. 1).

To understand the critical roles of ATM important for normal development, cell cycle control and prevention of malignancies, a relevant approach is dissection of ATM-directed signaling pathways. Recently, several studies have shown that ATM is a protein kinase, making it highly likely that this activity is intimately associated with signaling functions of ATM (Banin et al. 1998; Canman et al. 1998; Sarkaria et al 1998). Identification of downstream substrates of ATM protein kinase activity should provide important insights into ATM function and the signaling pathways influenced by ATM. In addition, given the early, central importance of ATM in normal development across a wide range of tissues (e.g., immune-related, gonadal and neuronal), characterization of substrates targeted by ATM protein kinase activity may provide novel components for replacement therapy and targets for chemotherapeutic intervention against malignancies.

We therefore assayed degenerate, oriented peptide libraries to identify substrates of ATM protein kinase activity. This method takes advantage of the recognition that protein kinase catalytic clefts generally recognize primary amino acid sequences around a fixed phosphorylation site (Songyang and Cantley 1998). This site usually consists of 9-12 amino acids of substrate sequence which is likely to contact the active site in the catalytic cleft. The advantage of this technology is that theoretically, several billion distinct peptides can be assayed for the presence of optimal motifs in a single given library; typically, four or five degenerate positions are amino and carboxy-terminal to a fixed Ser, Thr or Tyr, the latter of which are phosphorylated by kinase activity (Songyang et al. 1994; 1995; 1996; Songyang and Cantley 1998). Furthermore, the peptide libraries are interrogated without bias. This is an important consideration since ATM plays a crucial role in development of several tissues (Sedgwick and Boder 1991). Therefore, optimal motif(s) selected from a library by ATM protein kinase activity may be present in vastly different sets of proteins from unrelated tissues, each with distinctive functional roles.

The protein kinase, or in some cases, an isolated, protein kinase domain, is generated by recombinant Baculovirus, bacterial GST fusion proteins or assayed in immunoprecipitations. The phosphopeptide products of the kinase reaction with the library are separated from the non-phosphorylated majority through a ferric chloride column and sequenced (Songyang and Cantley 1998). Increasingly mature optimal motifs are successively determined, synthesized and assayed. The selected sequences are analyzed in data base searches, and likeliest substrates may then be analyzed as potential targets, based on the cellular location of the protein kinase and its potential substrates within that region. Additionally, optimal motifs may be utilized to derive information regarding biochemistry of a given protein kinase and, indirectly, active site requirements for substrate interactions.

Baculovirus constructs of the entire ATM protein are inefficiently expressed and the protein products difficult to extract (Ziv et al. 1997; Scott et al 1998). Isolated, baculovirus-generated, Gst-fusions of the isolated protein kinase domain exhibited no activity (data not shown). In contrast, immunoprecipitation of native ATM from cell extracts yielded highly specific, active ATM protein kinase (Fig. 2).

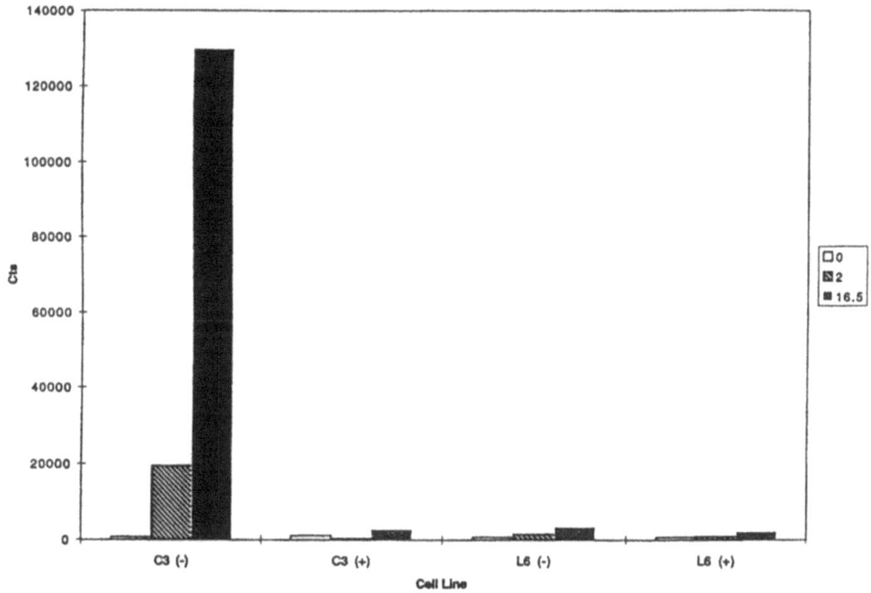

Fig. 2. ATM phosphorylation of a degenerate peptide library with central, fixed serine is specific and inhibited by wortmannin. Immunoprecipitation and protein kinase assays of ATM were performed as described by Sarkaria et al. (1998) and Banin et al (1998). The experiment shown is a representative small scale screen using wild-type C3ABR (C3) and ATM-/- (L6) EBV-transformed human B cell lines, in the presence (+) or absence (-) of 1 μM wortmannin, and assayed for ATM protein kinase activity using as the target, 100μg of the '4S4' library (i.e., containing 4 degenerate positions immediately N and C-terminal to a fixed serine residue). ATM phosphorylation activity of the library at time points 0, 2 and 16.5 hrs is depicted as open, hatched and closed bars. Large scale screens are aimed at phosphorylating approximately 1% of a given library. The phosphorylated peptides are then purified in a succession of columns (see text) and sequenced.

We screened several peptide libraries, including those with Tyr at the fixed position using immunoprecipitated ATM as the source for protein kinase activity. We found that a library with a fixed Ser (the 4S4 library) was highly selected as a target in terms of its phosphorylation by ATM compared to those oriented to Tyr (Fig. 2, data not shown). Significantly, the protein kinase activity of ATM immunoprecipitated from cell extracts of EBV-transformed human peripheral B cell lines was inhibited by a low concentration of wortmannin (Fig. 2). These data are consistent with recent studies showing wortmannin sensitivity of ATM phosphorylation of PHAS-1 and p53 (Banin et al. 1998; Canman et al. 1998; Sarkaria et al. 1998).

Notably, the L6 EBV-transformed human B cell line, in which ATM has a stop mutation at position 35, shows a substantially reduced level of phosphorylation, contrasted to the robust protein kinase activity of ATM in a wild-type, counterpart human B cell line, arguing for an ATM-specific reaction (Fig. 2). Finally, with certain peptide libraries, a significant level of phosphorylation was observed, however, this activity was not inhibited by wortmannin, suggesting that other protein kinases may co-precipitate with ATM. In the future, it may be useful to further investigate these additional kinases. Concerning ATM, a specific inhibitor such as wortmannin, and a kinase-dead mutant, as represented by the L6 cell line, are critical reagents whose lack of activity provide a compelling argument for high specificity of ATM for the 4S4 library. The sequences of the selected peptide substrates, originally defined in the 4S4 library, are currently being refined in successive screens. We are hopeful that novel, downstream substrates of ATM will be identified using the oriented peptide library approach, leading to a clearer understanding of ATM-directed signaling pathways that play important roles in development, cell cycle checkpoints and intervention strategies for treatment of certain malignancies.

We thank Dr. Fritz Melchers for insights and suggestions, Ms. Leslie Nicklin for careful editorial assistance, Dr. Martin Lavin for the C3ABR cell line, and Mr. Ted O'Neill and Ms Alison Dwyer for technical assistance. We are grateful to Dr. JoAnn Sekiguchi for thoughtful comments and criticisms of the manuscript. G.A.R. is supported by NIH GM57018. Due to space limitations we are able to cite only a limited number of references and oversights to published work are unintended.

References Cited:

Agrawal A, Eastman QM, Schatz DG (1998) Transposition mediated by RAG1 and RAG2 and its implication for the evolution of the immune system. Nature 394:744-751

Banin S, Moyal L, Shieh S, Taya Y, Anderson CW, Chessa L Smorodinsky NI, Prives C, Reiss Y, Shiloh Y, Ziv Y (1998) Enhanced phosphorylation of p53 by ATM response to DNA damage. Science 281:1674-1677

Barlow C, Hirotsune S, Paylor R, Liyanage M, Eckhaus M, Collins F, Shiloh Y, Crawley JN, Ried T, Tagle D, Wynshaw-Boris A (1996) Atm-deficient mice: a paradigm of ataxia telangiectasia. Cell 86:159-171

Canman CE, Lim DS, Cimprich KA, Taya Y, Tami K, Sakaguci K, Appella E, Kastan MB, Siliciano JD (1998) Science 281:1677-1679

Elledge SJ (1996). Cell cycle checkpoints: preventing an identity crisis. Science 274:1664-1672

Elson A, Wang Y, Daugherty CJ, Morton CC, Zhou F, Campos-Torres J, Leder P (1996) Pleiotropic defects in ataxia-telangiectasia protein-deficient mice. Proc Natl Acad Sci USA 93:13084-13089

Hiom K, Melek M, Gellert M (1998) DNA transposition by the RAG1 and RAG2 proteins: a possible source of oncogenic traslocations. Cell 94:463-470

Hunter T (1995) When Is a Lipid Kinase Not a Lipid Kinase? When it is a Protein Kinase. Cell 83:1-4

Kirsch IR (1994) V(D)J recombination and ataxia telangiectasia: a review. Int J Radiat Biol 66:S97

Lehmann AR, Carr AM (1995). The ataxia-telangiectasia gene: a link between checkpoint controls, neurodegeneration and cancer. TIG 11:375-377

Lin WC, Desiderio S (1994) Cell cycle regulation of V(D)J recombination-activating protein RAG-2. PNAS 91:2733-2737

McMahon SB, Van Buskirk HA, Dugan KA, Copeland TD, Cole MD (1998) The novel ATM-realted protein TRRAP is an essential cofactor for the c-myc and E2F oncoprotiens. Cell 94:363-374

Russo G, Isobe M, Pegoraro L, Finan J, Nowell P, Croce CM (1988) Molecular analysis of a t(7;14)(q35;32) chromosome translocation in a T cell leukemia of a patient with ataxia telangiectasia. Cell 53:137-144

Sarkaria JN, Tibbetts RS, Busby EC, Kennedy AP, Hill DE, Abraham RT (1998) Inhibition of phosphoinositol 3-kinase related kinases by the radiosensitizing agent wortmannin. Cancer Res 58:4375-82

Savitsky K, Bar-Shira A, Gilad S, Rotman G, Ziv Y, Vanagaite L, Tagle DA, Smith S, Frydman M, Harnik R, Patanjali SR, Simmons A, Clines GA, Sartiel A, Gatti RA, Chessa L, Sanal O, Lavin MF, Jaspers NGJ, Taylor AMR, Arlett CF, Sherman TM, Weissman SM, Lovett M, Collins FS, Shiloh Y (1995) A single Ataxia Telangiectasia Gene with a product similar to PI-3 kinase. Science 268:1749-1753

Schlissel M, Constantinescu A, Morrow T, Baxter M, Peng A (1993) Double-strand signal sequence breaks in V(D)J recombination are blunt, 5'-phosphorylated, RAG-dependent, and cell cycle regulated. Genes Dev 7:2520-2532

Scott SP, Zhang N, Khanna KK, Khromykh A, Hobson K, Watters D, Lavin MF (1998) Cloning and expression of the ataxia-telangiectasia gene in baculovirus. Biochem Biophys Res Commun 245:144-148

Sedgwick PP, Boder E (1991) Ataxia-telangiectasia. In: Hereditary neuropathies and spinocerebellar atrophies. Handbook of Clinical Neurology 60: Series 16 (Vinken, PJ, Btuyn, GW, Klawans, HL and de Jong, JMBV, eds) pp. 347-423

Songyang Z, Blechner S, Hoaglard N, Hoekstra MF, Piwnica-Worms H, Cantley LC (1994) A novel oriented peptide library technique for determining optimal substrates of protein kinases. Current Biology 4:973-982

Songyang Z, Carraway, KL III, Eck MJ, Harrison SC, Feldman RA, Mohammodi M, Schlessinger J, Hubbard SR, Mayer BJ, Cantley LC (1995) Catalytic specificity of protein-tyrosine kinases is critical for selective signaling. Nature 373:536-539

Songyang Z, Lu LP, Kuan Y, Tsai L-H, Filhol O, Cochet C, Soderling TR, Bartleson C, Graves DJ, Hoekstra MF, Blenis J, Hunter T, Cantley LC (1996) A Structural Basis for Substrate Specificities of Protein Ser/Thr-Kinases:Primary Sequence Preferences of Casein Kinase I and II, NIMA, Phosphorylase Kinase, Cam Kinase II, CDK5 and Erk1. Mol Cell Biol 16:6486-6493

Songyang Z, Cantley LC (1998) The use of peptide library for determination of kinase peptide substrates In: Methods in Molecular Biology (Cabilly S, Ed) Humana Press, Inc. Totowa, NJ 87:87-98

Taylor AM, Metcalfe JA, Thick J, Mak YF (1998) Leukemia and Lymphoma in ataxia telangiectasia. Blood 87:423-438

Xu Y, Ashley T, Brainerd EE, Bronson RT, Meyn S, Baltimore D (1996) Targeted disruption of ATM leads to growth retardation, chromosomal fragmentation during meiosis, immune defects, and thymic lymphoma. Genes Dev 10:2411-2422

Ziv Y, Bar-shira A, Pecker I, Russel P, Jorgenson TJ, Tsarfati I, Shiloh Y (1997) Recombinant ATM protein complements the cellular A-T phenotype. Oncogene 15:159-167

Discussion

Dirk Eick: Is the phosphorylation consensus site that you discussed in agreement with the phosphorylation site that has been described in the amino terminus of p53?
Gary Rathbun: Yes it is, absolutely. That was one of the things that makes me optimistic that we will find a number of substrates that are relevant. The data base search was performed with an immature motif, but it has already popped out p53 and a number of other DNA repair proteins.
Katherine Siminovitch: In view of the protein's homology with the p110 component of PI3-kinase, do you know whether ATM has lipid kinase activity?
Gary Rathbun: Dr. Rachel Meyers in Lew Cantley's lab has looked hard and does not see any.
Fritz Melchers: You say that the ATM defect sends the cells automatically either into repair or, if ATM does not work, into apoptosis, so any mutated cell could only be rescued if you inhibited the apoptosis? So, if by some second mutation you induced longevity or block of apoptosis, in that cell...
Gary Rathbun: That is what the translocation may do. For example, there was a recent study in which the MTCP1 gene has been hooked up to a CD2 promoter and put into mice. In the transgenic animals, like humans, the T cell proliferative defect goes over 15 or 16 months, and then you suddenly get transformation. I think that MTCP1 has been localized at the mitochondria, which might involve it in some kind of anti-apoptotic effect.
Riccardo Dalla-Favera: So ATM patients and AT-deficient mice develop T malignancies much more than B?
Gary Rathbun: With respect to human patients, the thinking, I believe, has been a prevalence for T malignancies to develop in AT patients, but I am not sure that this is holding up as the numbers start stacking up. Certainly Malcolm Taylor in the UK has found a prevalence for T cell malignancies. T cell malignancies have been the most well characterized in terms of the lymphoid neoplasias in AT patients.
Riccardo Dalla-Favera: So the question is, where is ATM expressed in the B lineage?
Gary Rathbun: It is constitutively expressed throughout.
Fritz Melchers: Carlo Croce told me that the mutations in the ATM gene are rather frequent in the human population, so many people are actually heterozygous for an ATM mutation. The scenario that could be envisaged is a somatic mutation of the other allele to get homozygous ATM deficiency. This one somatic ATM mutant homozygous cell would be the origin of a neoplastic cell.
Gary Rathbun: I think there is some truth in what you say. There has also been some debate about the number of heterozygous people in the population: it has been estimated to be as high as 1% which is significant. Certainly there are examples of T cell leukemias in non-AT patients that have been analyzed which had developed ATM mutations, usually compound in nature, on both alleles.

MHC-linked Control of Murine SLE

N. Ibnou-Zekri[1], T. J. Vyse[2], S. J. Rozzo[3], M. Iwamoto[1], T. Kobayakawa[4], B. L. Kotzin[3] and S. Izui[1]

[1] Department of Pathology, Centre Médical Universitaire, University of Geneva, 1211 Geneva 4, Switzerland
[2] Rheumatology Section, Imperial College School of Medicine, Hammersmith Campus, London W12 0NN, England
[3] Division of Clinical Immunology, University of Colorado Health Sciences Center, Denver, CO 80262, USA
[4] Department of International Affairs and Tropical Medicine, Tokyo Women's Medical University, Tokyo, Japan

Introduction

Systemic lupus erythematosus (SLE) is a disorder of generalized autoimmunity characterized by the formation of a variety of autoantibodies and subsequent development of severe glomerulonephritis [1]. It is now well established that SLE is under some form of polygenic control, in which several genetic factors independently contribute to the overall susceptibility and progression of the disease. Studies suggest that heterogeneous combinations of multiple disease-associated genes operate in a threshold manner to generate the disease [2-4]. Among such genetic factors, the importance of the genes encoded within or closely linked to the MHC locus has been shown. However, it has not yet been determined whether the development of lupus-like disease is predominantly mediated by MHC class II genes and which other genes within MHC may contribute to this effect.

Association of H-$2^{d/z}$ Heterozygosity with Murine SLE

One of the best-studied models of human SLE is the (NZB x NZW)F_1 hybrid, whose females spontaneously develop high titers of IgG autoantibodies and succumb to glomerulonephritis before one year of age. Studies in backcross and F_2 intercross mice as well as H-2 congenic mice have consistently demonstrated a strong association of the H-$2^{d/z}$ heterozygosity (vs H-$2^{d/d}$ or H-$2^{z/z}$) with the development of the disease, indicating the co-dominant contribution from each strain (H-2^d from NZB and H-2^z from NZW) [3, 5, 6]. Recent analysis of (C57BL.H-2^z x NZB)F_1 x NZB and (NZW x BALB/c)F_1 x NZW backcross mice has additionally supported the importance of H-$2^{d/z}$ heterozygous expression in the development of SLE [7, 8]. Since the development of SLE is dependent on $CD4^+$ T-cells and blocked by treatment with anti-I-A antibodies, it has been proposed that mixed-haplotype class II molecules produced by heterozygous pairing of an α-chain from one haplotype with a β-chain from the other might play a critical role in the development of SLE.

This hypothesis has been recently tested by determining whether A^z or E^z transgene expression could lead to the accelerated development of SLE in (C57BL x NZB)F1 x NZB backcross mice, since the transgene expression should result in the generation of mixed-haplotype I-A ($A\alpha^zA\beta^d$ and $A\alpha^dA\beta^z$) or I-E ($E\alpha^zE\beta^d$ and $E\alpha^dE\beta^z$) heterodimers in these backcross mice. Although a subset of the H-$2^{d/d}$ homozygous backcross mice produce high levels of IgG autoantibodies and develop severe glomerulonephritis, the inheritance of neither transgene is linked to the accelerated development of the disease [9, 10]. Our results, together with a recent report showing the lack of disease-enhancing effect of an $A\beta^z$ transgene in H-$2^{d/d}$ homozygous (NZB x NZW.H-2^d)F1 mice [11], argue against the sole contribution from MHC class II genes in the H-$2^{d/z}$ heterozygous effect in (NZB x NZW)F1 hybrid mice, but rather suggest the involvement of separate MHC genes. In this regard, it should be mentioned that the *Tnfa* allele of the NZW strain, associated with reduced production of TNF-α, has been previously proposed as a candidate gene that may underlie the H-2^z contribution to lupus in (NZB x NZW)F1 mice [12]. In addition, one can speculate that polymorphisms within the MHC class III genes, such as complement (*C2* and *C4*) genes, may account for an additional genetic factor contributed by the NZB strain, in view of a well-known association of human lupus with hereditary complement deficiencies and the importance of complement components in the generation of immune responses and the induction of B-cell tolerance.

Contribution of the *Ea* Gene to Murine SLE

Additional evidence that supports the contribution of the MHC to the regulation of murine SLE is that the lupus susceptibility is more closely linked to the H-2^b haplotype than to the H-2^d and H-2^k haplotypes in lupus-prone BXSB and (NZB x BXSB)F1 mice [13-15]. This MHC effect is, however, relative and markedly influenced by other factors in the genetic background of individual lupus-prone mice. This was well documented in (NZB x BXSB)F1 hybrid mice, in which the development of SLE is markedly delayed, but not completely prevented in H-$2^{d/d}$ female hybrids, while the H-$2^{d/d}$ is barely protective in their male counterparts, which are genetically more predisposed to SLE because of the presence of a mutant gene, *Yaa* (Y-linked autoimmune acceleration) [14]. This suggests that a reduced lupus susceptibility associated with the H-2^d and H-2^k haplotypes can be due to the presence of a more disease-protective allele or the absence of a more disease-predisposing allele within or closely linked to the H-2^d and H-2^k gene complexes and that either action of such alleles may be overcome by other predisposing factors present in mice highly susceptible to SLE.

The autoimmune inhibitory effect of the H-2^d and H-2^k haplotypes can be related to the expression of I-E molecules or the *Ea* gene, since mice bearing the H-2^b haplotype fail to express I-E because of a deletion within the promoter region of the *Ea* gene. In fact, recent studies have shown that the development of SLE is almost completely prevented in BXSB (H-2^b) mice homozygous for the Ea^d transgene, as is the case for homozygous H-2^d and H-2^k BXSB mice, and that the expression of two functional *Ea* (transgenic and endogenous) genes in either H-$2^{d/b}$ (NZB x BXSB)F1 or H-$2^{k/b}$ (MRL x BXSB)F1 mice provides protection from SLE at levels comparable to those conferred by the H-$2^{d/d}$ or H-$2^{k/k}$ haplotype [15]. These results indicate that the reduced susceptibility associated with the I-E^+ H-2^d and H-2^k haplotypes (vs the I-E^- H-2^b) is largely, if not all, contributed by the *Ea* gene, and not by the genes encoding the I-A molecules or other genes within the MHC.

It should be stressed that the development of SLE in H-$2^{b/d}$ or H-$2^{b/k}$ heterozygous BXSB and (NZB x BXSB)F1 mice is not accelerated, but rather slightly delayed, as compared with their H-$2^{b/b}$ homozygous mice [13, 14]. Therefore, the expression of the *Ea* gene at higher levels present in homozygous mice may be necessary to exhibit a maximal autoimmune inhibitory effect in lupus-prone mice, consistent with only a marginal protection observed in BXSB mice expressing the Ea^d transgene at the heterozygous level [15, 16]. Such a gene dosage effect could explain the linkage of an increased lupus susceptibility to several H-2 heterozygosities, which are also I-E heterozygous, in different genetic crosses: H-$2^{b/z}$ vs H-$2^{z/z}$ in (C57BL x NZM)F1 x NZM and NZW x (NZW x BXSB)F1 backcross mice [2, 17], H-$2^{q/d}$ vs H-$2^{d/d}$ in (SWR x NZB)F1 x NZB backcross mice [18] and H-$2^{b/d}$ vs H-$2^{d/d}$ in (C57BL x NZB)F1 and NZB backcross mice [9, 10]. If this model is correct, different *Ea* genes may exert very different effects on disease susceptibility, since the introduction of the Ea^z transgene in (C57BL x NZB)F1 x NZB backcross mice showed no effect on the development of autoantibody production [9, 10].

Our studies also indicate that the level of protection associated with the expression of the Ea^d transgene markedly differs among lupus-prone mice studied, and is apparently dependent on their overall susceptibilities to SLE. This may be related to the presence or absence of specific disease-associated alleles present in different lupus-prone strains [2-4]. (NZB x BXSB)F1 and (NZW x BXSB)F1 mice are more genetically susceptible to SLE than (MRL x BXSB)F1 mice, followed by BXSB mice, as documented by the development of a lethal SLE in (NZB x BXSB)F1 and (NZW x BXSB)F1 females, but not in (MRL x BXSB)F1 and BXSB females, and by a higher level of autoantibody production in (MRL x BXSB)F1 females than in BXSB females [19]. Accordingly, the level of the Ea^d transgene-mediated protection in these four different lupus-prone mice - the highest in BXSB, intermediate in (MRL x BXSB)F1 and the lowest in (NZB x BXSB)F1 and (NZW x BXSB)F1 - inversely correlates with their genetic susceptibilities to severe disease [16, 20, 21]. This idea is also consistent with the finding that as compared with their female hybrids, the autoimmune inhibitory effect of the *Ea*^{d} transgene is less prominent in (NZB x BXSB)F1 male mice bearing the *Yaa* mutation, which dramatically enhances the frequency and severity of the disease [21].

It should be emphasized that the protection conferred by the *Ea*^{d} transgene is dependent on its level of expression, but not on that of whole I-E molecules on the surface of B cells [16, 21]. This has been best shown in (NZB x BXSB)F1 hybrids expressing three different levels of the transgene, in which the protection of SLE is well correlated with the level of the transgene expression, despite comparative levels of cell surface I-E expression in these mice [21]. Notably, the absence of any feature of immune deficiency in these transgenic mice excludes the possibility that the prevention of the autoimmune disease results from a functional defect in B cells secondary to overexpression of the transgene.

The precise mechanisms responsible for the *Ea* gene (and transgene)-mediated protection of SLE remain to be elucidated. Previous studies showed the selective production of autoantibodies by non-transgenic B cells in transgenic and non-transgenic double bone marrow chimeras, indicating that B cells, and not T cells, are the major cellular site of the transgene effect on the suppression of autoimmune responses [20]. In addition, the transgene expression reduces selectively IgG, but not IgM, anti-DNA autoantibody production [21]. Thus, it can be speculated that the transgene expression in B cells may modulate the presentation of autoantigen-derived peptides, thereby interfering with an efficient interaction between autoreactive T and B cells. The presentation of pathogenic self-peptides by I-A molecules could be diminished as a result of increased formation of I-E α-chain-derived peptides displaying a high affinity for the I-A molecule [16, 20, 21]. This idea was supported by our recent in vitro studies, which have shown that the capacity of the transgenic B cells to activate T helper cells by presenting I-A-restricted peptides of foreign antigens was substantially diminished (unpublished results). An additional possibility is that the modulation of pathogenic self-peptide presentation by I-A molecules resulted from the induction or increased expression of mixed-haplotype I-E molecules, such as an $E\alpha^dE\beta^b$ mixed-haplotype heterodimer, as observed in BXSB and (NZB x BXSB)F1 mice bearing the *Ea*^{d} transgene [20, 21]. The mixed-haplotype I-E molecules, as a consequence of capturing autoantigenic peptides, may interfere or compete with the presentation of pathogenic determinants of autoantigens by I-A molecules [23]. Finally, the excessive expression of the transgene, leading either to the quantitative and qualitative changes in I-E expression or to the diminishment of densities of I-A molecules presenting autoantigenic peptides, may cause the immune deviation of TH responses. We have recently shown that the progression of murine lupus nephritis is associated with the activation of TH1 cells, which is accompanied by the increased production of IgG2a and IgG3 autoantibodies [24, 25]. The IgG2a isotype having a higher affinity to type III Fcγ receptors than other IgG isotypes can be highly nephritogenic by promoting Fcγ

receptor-mediated inflammatory responses, as suggested recently [26]. In addition, autoantibodies of the IgG3 isotype could be especially nephritogenic, because of a cryoglobulin activity associated with the γ3 constant region [27, 28].

Conclusion

The MHC class II *Ea* gene apparently contributes to the reduced susceptibility to SLE by suppressing autoimmune responses in mice. However, the *Ea* gene is not the only gene encoded within the MHC region that determines susceptibility to murine SLE. Studies in New Zealand mice have clearly demonstrated that IgG autoantibody production and the development of lupus nephritis are associated with H-$2^{d/z}$ heterozygosity. This contribution from MHC genes appears to be mostly independent of the expression of the *Ea* gene, and involve genes other than the classical immune response genes. Accordingly, the MHC region likely encodes more than one lupus-associated gene, which may contribute to the development of SLE by acting at various levels of the disease process.

Acknowledgements. This work was supported by a grant from the Swiss National Foundation for Scientific Research, by a grant AR37070 from the National Institute of Health, USA, and by a grant from the Ministry of Health and Welfare, Japan.

References

1. Kotzin BL (1996) Systemic lupus erythematosus. Cell 85:303-306
2. Morel L, Rudofsky UH, Longmate JA, Schiffenbauer J, Wakeland EK (1994) Polygenic control of susceptibility to murine systemic lupus erythematosus. Immunity 1:219-229
3. Kono DH, Burlingame RW, Owens DG, Kuramochi A, Balderas RS, Balomenos D, Theofilopoulos AN (1994) Lupus susceptibility loci in New Zealand mice. Proc Natl Acad Sci USA 91:10168-10172
4. Drake CG, Rozzo SJ, Hirschfeld HF, Smarnworawong NP, Palmer E, Kotzin BL (1995) Analysis of the New Zealand Black contribution to lupus-like renal disease. Multiple genes that operate in a threshold manner. J Immunol 154:2441-2447
5. Hirose S, Ueda G, Noguchi K, Okada T, Sekigawa I, Sato H, Shirai T (1986) Requirement of H-2 heterozygosity for autoimmunity in (NZB x NZW)F1 hybrid mice. Eur J Immunol 16:1631-1633
6. Kotzin BL, Palmer E (1987) The contribution of NZW genes to lupus-like disease in (NZB x NZW)F1 mice. J Exp Med 165:1237-1251
7. Rozzo SJ, Vyse TJ, Drake CG, Kotzin BL (1996) Effect of genetic background on the contribution of New Zealand Black loci to autoimmune lupus nephritis. Proc Natl Acad Sci USA 93:15164-15168
8. Vyse TJ, Morel L, Tanner FJ, Wakeland EK, Kotzin BL (1996) Backcross analysis of genes linked to autoantibody production in New Zealand White mice. J Immunol 157:2719-2727
9. Vyse TJ, Rozzo SJ, Drake CG, Appel VB, Lemeur M, Izui S, Palmer E, Kotzin BL (1998) Contribution of $E\alpha^z$ and $E\beta^z$ MHC genes to lupus susceptibility in New Zealand mice. J

Immunol 160:2757-2766
10. Rozzo SJ, Vyse TJ, David CS, Palmer E, Izui S, Kotzin BL (1999) Analysis of class II MHC genes in the contribution of *H2z* to lupus susceptibility in New Zealand mice. J Immunol, in press.
11. Nishimura H, Ishikawa S, Nozawa S, Awaji M, Saito J, Abe M, Gotoh Y, Tokushima M, Kimoto M, Tsurui H, Hirose S, Shirai T (1996) Effects of transgenic mixed-haplotype major histocompatibility complex class II molecules $A\alpha^{d}A\beta^{z}$ on autoimmune disease in New Zealand mice. Int Immunol 8:967-976
12. Jacob CO, Fronek Z, Lewis GD, Koo M, Hansen JA, McDevitt HO (1990) Heritable major histocompatibility complex class II-associated differences in production of tumor necrosis factor. Proc Natl Acad Sci USA 87:1233-1237
13. Merino R, Fossati L, Lacour M, Lemoine R, Higaki M, Izui S (1992) H-2-linked control of the *Yaa* gene-induced acceleration of lupus-like autoimmune disease in BXSB mice. Eur J Immunol 22:295-299
14. Merino R, Iwamoto M, Gershwin ME, Izui S (1994) The *Yaa* gene abrogates the major histocompatibility complex association of murine lupus in (NZB x BXSB)F_1 hybrid mice. J Clin Invest 94:521-525
15. Ibnou-Zekri N, Iwamoto M, Fossati L, McConahey PJ, Izui S (1997) Role of the major histocompatibility complex class II *Ea* gene in lupus susceptibility in mice. Proc Natl Acad Sci USA 94:14654-14659
16. Iwamoto M, Ibnou-Zekri N, Araki K, Izui S (1996) Prevention of murine lupus by an I-E α chain transgene: Protective role of I-E α chain-derived peptides with a high affinity to $I\text{-}A^{b}$ molecules. Eur J Immunol 26:307-314
17. Ida A, Hirose S, Hamano Y, Kodera S, Jiang Y, Abe M, Zhang D, Nishimura H, Shirai T (1998) Multigenic control of lupus-associated antiphospholipid syndrome in a model of (NZW x BXSB)F_1 mice. Eur J Immunol 28:2694-2703
18. Ghatak S, Sainis K, Owen FL, Datta SK (1987) T-cell-receptor β- and I-Aβ-chain genes of normal SWR mice are linked with the development of lupus nephritis in NZB x SWR crosses. Proc Natl Acad Sci USA 84:6850-6853
19. Fossati L, Iwamoto M, Merino R, Izui S (1995) Selective accelerating effect of the *Yaa* gene on immune responses against self and foreign antigens. Eur J Immunol 25:166-173
20. Merino R, Iwamoto M, Fossati L, Muniesa P, Araki K, Takahashi S, Huarte J, Yamamura K-I, Vassalli J-D, Izui S (1993) Prevention of systemic lupus erythematosus in autoimmune BXSB mice by a transgene encoding I-E α chain. J Exp Med 178:1189-1197
21. Iwamoto M, Ibnou-Zekri N, Kobayakawa T, Izui S (1998) Effect of genetic background on *Ea^{d}* transgene-mediated protection from murine lupus. J Autoimmunity 11:241-248
22. Rudensky AY, Preston-Hurlburt P, Hong SC, Barlow A, Janeway Jr CA (1991) Sequence analysis of peptides bound to MHC class II molecules. Nature 353:622-627
23. Deng H, Apple R, Clare-Salzler M, Trembleau S, Mathis D, Adorini L, Sercarz E (1993) Determinant capture as a possible mechanism of protection afforded by major histocompatibility complex class II molecules in autoimmune disease. J Exp Med 178:1675-1680
24. Takahashi S, Fossati L, Iwamoto M, Merino R, Motta R, Kobayakawa T, Izui S (1996) Imbalance towards Th1 predominance is associated with acceleration of lupus-like autoimmune syndrome in MRL mice. J Clin Invest 97:1597-1604
25. Santiago ML, Fossati L, Jacquet C, Müller W, Izui S, Reininger L (1997) Interleukin-4 protects against a genetically linked lupus-like autoimmune syndrome. J Exp Med 185:65-70
26. Clynes R, Dumitru C, Ravetch JV (1998) Uncoupling of immune complex formation and kidney damage in autoimmune glomerulonephritis. Science 279:1052-1054
27. Berney T, Fulpius T, Shibata T, Reininger L, Van Snick J, Shan H, Weigert M, Marshak-Rothstein A, Izui S (1992) Selective pathogenicity of murine rheumatoid factors of the cryoprecipitable IgG3 subclass. Int Immunol 4:93-99
28. Fulpius T, Spertini F, Reininger L, Izui S (1993) Immunoglobulin heavy chain constant region determines the pathogenicity and the antigen-binding activity of rheumatoid factor. Proc Natl Acad Sci USA 90:2345-2349

Discussion

Edward Wakeland: In your model of the alpha suppression in the case of the NZB x W model, both of those haplotypes actually express an I-E molecule and yet still you can see the association with heterozygosity. How does that fit in to the way you are looking at the role of the I-E molecule?

Shozo Izui: As suggested by the studies on A^z and E^z transgenic mice, the H-2$^{d/z}$ heterozygous effect observed in NZB x W F1 hybrids does not apparently involve the MHC class II genes themselves, but genes other than the classical immune responses genes. Since H-2^d, H-2^z and H-2$^{d/z}$ mice are homozygous for the *Ea* gene, it is clear that the H-2$^{d/z}$ heterozygous effect is likely to be independent of the suppressive effect of the *Ea* gene. However, the group of Dr Shirai has shown the enhanced development of lupus in NZB x W mice expressing I-E at a heterozygous level, as compared with conventional NZB x W mice. This supports an autoimmune suppressive effect of the *Ea* gene.

Edward Wakeland: I know that Hugh McDevitt some years ago discussed the fact that when he made transgenic mice he found rather profound effects on the B cell lineage, dependent upon individual strains. Have you looked at the B cell lineage in your transgenics?

Shozo Izui: We looked very carefully at the development of B cells and their immunological functions in our *Ea* transgenic mice. However, there is no particular deficiency of B cells in the presence of the transgene. So I don't think that the prevention of lupus results from a possible functional defect in B cells due to overexpression of the transgene.

The Adaptor Protein SLP-65/BLNK Controls the Calcium Response in Activated B Cells

B. Wollscheid, J. Wienands and M. Reth

Department of Molecular Immunology, Biology III, University Freiburg and Max-Planck-Institute for Immunobiology, Stübeweg 51, 79108 Freiburg, Germany

Introduction

The B cell antigen receptor (BCR) complex consists of the membrane-bound immunoglobulin molecule (mIg) and the Ig-α/Ig-β heterodimer involved in antigen-binding and signal transduction, respectively (DeFranco 1997; Kurosaki 1997; Reth and Wienands 1997). In the absence of antigen the Ig-α and Ig-β cytoplasmic tails are non-phosphorylated, but during BCR activation, Ig-α and Ig-β become phosphorylated (Gold *et al.* 1991) on the tyrosines of the Immunoreceptor Tyrosine-Based Activation Motif (ITAM) (Reth 1989; Thomas 1995). To transduce signals, the resting BCR should be connected to intracellular effector elements. How the non-phosphorylated Ig-α/Ig-β cytoplasmic tails are connected to intracellular signaling molecules is not yet clear. In co-precipitation studies, using total cellular lysates, an association between Ig-α/Ig-β and the N-terminal part of the Src-family kinase Lyn was found (Yamanashi *et al.* 1991; Clark *et al.* 1994; Pleiman *et al.* 1994). However, recent genetic data from Lyn knock-out mice do not support the notion that the Src-family kinase Lyn is the first and an essential signal-transducing element of the BCR (Chan *et al.* 1998; Hibbs *et al.* 1995)

In our biochemical studies, we failed to co-purify any intracellular signaling molecules together with the BCR complex from cellular lysates using a panel of different detergents (Schamel and Reth, unpublished). The failure to detect (new) BCR-associated proteins suggested to us that the binding between the receptor and its transducing elements is of low affinity and not stable in the detergent lysate. The postulated low affinity receptor/transducer interaction seems reasonable if one assumes that the transition between a resting and an activated BCR requires changes in the binding and composition of intracellular BCR-associated proteins. To identify early transducing elements of the BCR we therefore used a different approach. In a time course experiment, we studied the kinetics of phosphorylation of different protein tyrosine kinase (PTK) substrate proteins which became phosphorylated following BCR engagement (Kim *et al.* 1993) or upon exposure of the B cells to the phosphotyrosine phosphatase (PTP) inhibitor pervanadate (Wienands *et al.* 1996). We reasoned that the most rapidly phosphorylated PTK substrates are the ones which are most proximal in the BCR-induced signaling cascade. The purification of these proteins led to the discovery of the new B cell-specific adaptor protein, called SLP-65/BLNK.

Identification of early PTK Substrates

PTK substrate phosphorylation can be induced in BCR-positive transfectants of J558L in two different ways. These are either the engagement of the BCR by the antigen NIP_{12}-BSA or the exposure of cells to the PTP inhibitor pervanadate. Pervanadate induces a more robust protein phosphorylation than BCR triggering, but in both cases the same PTK substrate protein became phosphorylated as monitored by two-dimensional gel electrophoresis (Wollscheid 1999). For the purification of PTK substrate proteins we stimulated $2x10^{10}$ J558Lμm3 cells with pervanadate. After lysis of the cells, the PTK substrate proteins were affinity purified with anti-phosphotyrosine antibodies coupled to sepharose beads and eluted with phenyl phosphate. Subsequently, proteins were concentrated and size-separated by preparative SDS-PAGE. Coomassie blue-stained protein bands were excised from the gel and digested with the protease Lys-C. The obtained peptides were fractionated via HPLC and sequenced. With this approach we identified the phosphoproteins pp80, pp70 and pp55 as being the hematopoietic-specific protein HS-1, the heat shock protein HSC70 and the cytoskeleton adaptor protein SH3P7, respectively (Wollscheid 1999; Larbolette *et al.* 1999). We were particularly interested in the identity of a 65 kDa protein (pp65), as it is the most rapidly phosphorylated substrate after engagement of the BCR or after exposure of cells to pervanadate (Wienands *et al.* 1996). Furthermore, the pp65 phosphorylation was strictly dependent on BCR expression (Wienands *et al.* 1996; Zhang *et al.* 1998)

Characterisation of SLP-65

We obtained sequences of eight different pp65 peptides. Using this information, we isolated the complete pp65 cDNA (Wienands *et al.* 1998). The deduced protein sequence shows that pp65 is a 457 amino acid long adaptor protein with a C-terminal SH2 domain. This SH2 domain shows the closest sequence similarity to that of the T cell adaptor protein SLP-76 (SH2-containing lymphocyte adaptor protein of 76 kDa) (Jackman *et al.* 1995). Although the overall sequence identity between SLP-76 and the p65 protein is only 33%, both proteins exhibit a similar composition of structural elements (Figure 1). We therefore concluded that pp65 is the B cell analogue of SLP-76 and thus called it SLP-65 for SH2-containing lymphocyte adaptor protein of 65 kDa. The same protein was also identified in Andrew Chan's Laboratory in mouse and human B cell lines and called BLNK

(Fu *et al.* 1998). According to its sequence, SLP-65 is a very basic protein with a pI of 8.5. This theoretical value matched the pI we obtained for p65 by NEPHGE gel electrophoresis (Wollscheid *et al* 1999). At its N-terminus SLP-65 bears a high content of positively charged amino acids whose function is at present unknown. This region is followed by a mostly negatively charged sequence containing 5 tyrosines which are potential PTK targets and which all have the consensus sequence YxxP. Following phosphorylation the sites can interact with SH2 domains of proteins like Vav (Onodera *et al.* 1996). The consensus phosphorylation motifs are followed by a mostly positively charged and proline-rich sequence. Here several consensus binding sites for SH3 domains are found (Mayer and Eck 1995). This area is also most likely interacting with the adaptor protein Grb2, which we found constitutively associated with SLP-65. Finally, at its C-terminus, SLP-65 carries an SH2 domain. In summary, SLP-65 is a protein which can mediate the contact of multiple binding partners. This can be a constitutive interaction, involving SH3 domain binding. Once tyrosine phosphorylated, SLP-65 may interact with several other SH2-containing proteins. Furthermore, the C-terminal, the SH2-domain of SLP-65, can bind to yet unknown tyrosine-phosphorylated proteins. In our biochemical studies we found a constitutive interaction of SLP-65 with the adaptor protein Grb2 and Vav, the latter functioning as a GDP/GTP exchange factor for the small G-protein Rho. Other SLP-65/BLNK-associated proteins, identified in Dr. Chan's lab, are PLC-γ and the adaptor protein Nck. This lab also provides evidence that SLP-65 is phosphorylated by the PTK Syk (Fu *et al.* 1998).

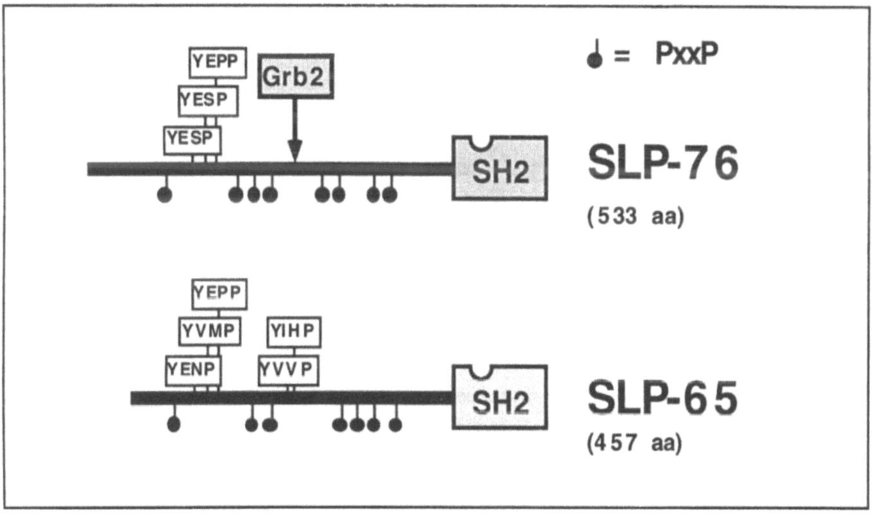

Fig. 1: Comparison of the overall structure of the adaptor proteins SLP-76 and SLP-65, expressed dominantly in T and B cells, respectively. The position of the tyrosine phosphorylation sites YxxP and of the potential SH3 domain binding sites (black circles) are indicated. An arrow shows the position of the Grb2 binding site in SLP-76.

Role of Adaptor Proteins in Receptor Signal Transduction

To determine the function of the SLP-65 adaptor protein it will be important to generate mutant B cell lines and mice deficient for SLP-65 gene expression. Experiments in these directions are underway. In a first attempt to demonstrate a functional role of SLP-65 in signal transduction from the BCR, we overexpressed an HA-tagged version of this protein in the B lymphoma line K46. The expression of HA-SLP-65 in two transfectants of K46 was confirmed by Western blotting using anti-SLP-65 antibodies (Figure 2). We used a Flow Cytometer to monitor the calcium mobilisation in transfected K46 cells following cross-linking of their BCR by anti-immunoglobulin antibodies. Under the chosen experimental conditions, the K46 parental line shows only a minor calcium response, whereas the two SLP-65 transfectants have a drastically augmented calcium response (Figure 2).

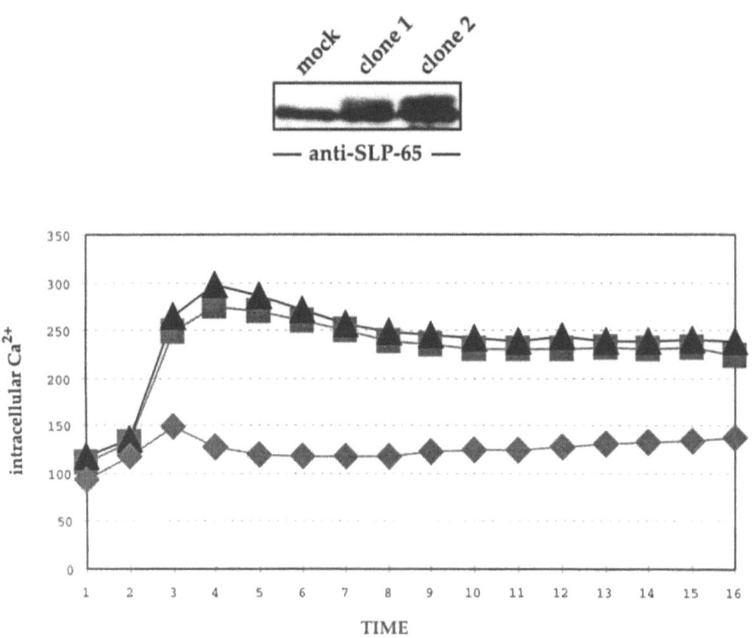

Fig. 2: Overexpression of an HA-tagged version of SLP-65 in K46 leads to increased Ca^{2+} influx upon BCR crosslinking. Expression of SLP-65 analysed by anti-SLP-65 immunoblotting (upper part) and calcium response analysed in a Flow Cytometer (lower part) in wild type K46 cells (rhombus) and two HA-SLP-65 transfectants, (clone 1, (square) and clone 2 (triangle)). Measured values are representing the ratio of calcium ions in time gates of 20 sec after cell stimulation.

These data indicate that SLP-65 plays an important role in signal transduction from the BCR by controlling the release of intracellular calcium, an essential event during B-lymphocyte activation. SLP-65 seems to organize and to bring together key signaling elements in the calcium response in activated B cells like PLC-γ and Syk (Takata *et al.* 1994; Takata and Kurosaki 1996). How SLP-65 is coupled to the BCR, either directly or indirectly, is not yet clear. Our studies of the J558L parental line and Ig transfectants of these cells show that the BCR is required for the phosphorylation of SLP-65 (Wienands *et al.* 1996). We have used a hormone-regulated Cre enzyme to express the BCR in an inducible manner on the surface of J558L cells (Zhang *et al.* 1998). By monitoring PTK phosphorylation during BCR induction we could demonstrate that Syk and SLP-65 phosphorylation is strictly dependent on BCR expression. These data suggest that Syk and its substrate SLP-65 are organized by the BCR but the molecular details of this interaction remain to be identified. The identification of adaptor proteins acting immediately downstream of the antigen receptor of T and B cells is in line with recent studies of other types of receptors on mammalian (Tezuka *et al.* 1998) and insect (Raabe *et al.* 1996) cells, demonstrating that the receptor/adaptor organisation is an evolutionary conserved scheme in the transduction and processing of intracellular signals.

References

Chan VW, Lowell CA, DeFranco AL (1998) Defective negative regulation of antigen receptor signaling in Lyn-deficient B lymphocytes. Curr Biol 8:545-553

Clark MR, Johnson SA, Cambier JC (1994) Analysis of Ig-alpha-tyrosine kinase interaction reveals two levels of binding specificity and tyrosine phosphorylated Ig-alpha stimulation of Fyn activity. EMBO J 13:1911-1919

DeFranco AL (1997) The complexity of signaling pathways activated by the BCR. Curr Opin Immunol 9:296-308

Fu C, Turck CW, Kurosaki T, Chan AC (1998) BLNK: A central linker protein in B cell activation. Immunity 9:93-103

Gold MR, Matsuuchi L, Kelly RB, DeFranco AL (1991) Tyrosine phosphorylation of components of the B-cell antigen receptors following receptor crosslinking. Proc Natl Acad Sci USA 88:3436-3440

Hibbs ML, Tarlinton DM, Armes J, Grail D, Hodgson G, Maglitto R, Stacker SA, Dunn AR (1995) Multiple defects in the immune system of Lyn-deficient mice, culminating in auto immune disease. Cell 83:301-311

Jackman JK, Motto DG, Sun Q, Tanemoto M, Turck CW, Peltz GA, Koretzky GA, Findell PR (1995) Molecular cloning of SLP-76, a 76-kDa tyrosine phosphoprotein associated with Grb2 in T cells. J Biol Chem 270:7029-7032

Kim KM, Alber G, Weiser P, Reth M (1993) Signalling function of the B-cell antigen receptors. Immunol Rev 132:125-146

Kurosaki T (1997) Molecular mechanisms in B cell antigen receptor signaling. Curr. Opin Immunol 9:309-318

Larbolette O, Wollscheid B, Schweikert J, Nielsen PJ, Wienands J (1999) SH3P7 is a cytoskeleton adaptor protein and is coupled to signal transduction from lymhocyte antigen receptors. Mol Cell Biol 19:*in press*

Mayer BJ, Eck MJ (1995) Minding your p's and q's. Curr Biol 4:364-367

Onodera H, Motto DG, Koretzky GA, Rothstein DM (1996) Differential regulation of activation-induced tyrosine phosphorylation and recruitment of SLP-76 to Vav by distinct isoforms of the CD45 protein-tyrosine phosphatase. J Biol Chem 271:22225-22230

Pleiman CM, Abrams C, Gauen LT, Bedzyk W, Jongstra J, Shaw AS, Cambier JC (1994) Distinct p53/56lyn and p59fyn domains associate with nonphosphorylated and phosphorylated Ig-alpha. Proc Natl Acad Sci USA 91:4268-4272

Raabe T, Riesgo-Escovar J, Liu X, Bausenwein BS, Deak P, Maroy P, Hafen E (1996) DOS, a novel pleckstrin homology domain-containing protein required for signal transduction between sevenless and Ras1 in Drosophila. Cell 85:911-920

Reth M (1989) Antigen receptor tail clue. Nature 338:383

Reth M, Wienands J (1997) Initiation and processing of signals from the B cell antigen receptor. Ann Rev Immunol 15:453-479

Takata M, Kurosaki T (1996) A role for Bruton's tyrosine kinase in B cell antigen receptor-mediated activation of phospholipase C-gamma 2. J Exp Med 184:31-40

Takata M, Sabe H, Hata A, Inazu T, Homma Y, Nukada T, Yamamura H, Kurosaki T (1994) Tyrosine kinases Lyn and Syk regulate B cell receptor-coupled Ca^{2+} mobilization through distinct pathways. Embo J 13:1341-1349

Tezuka T, Yoshida Y, Fukada T, Ohtani T, Yamanaka Y, Nishida K, Nakajima K, Hibi M, Hirano T (1998) Gab1 acts as an adaptor molecule linking the cytokine receptor gp130 to ERK mitogen-activated protein kinase. Mol Cell Biol 18:4109-4117

Thomas ML (1995) Of ITAMs and ITIMs: Turning On and Off the B Cell Antigen Receptor. J Exp Med 181:1953-1956

Wienands J, Larbolette O, Reth M (1996) Evidence for a preformed transducer complex organized by the B cell antigen receptor. Proc Natl Acad Sci USA 93:7865-7870

Wienands J, Schweikert J, Wollscheid B, Jumaa H, Nielsen PJ, Reth M (1998) SLP-65: A new signaling component in B lymphocytes which requires expression of the antigen receptor for phosphorylation. J Exp Med 188:791-794

Wollscheid B, Reth M, Wienands J (1999) Characterization of the B cell-specific adaptor SLP-65 and other protein tyrosine kinase substrates by two-dimensional gel electrophoresis. Immunol Lett *in press*

Yamanashi Y, Kakiuchi T, Mizuguchi J, Yamamoto T, Toyoshima K (1991) Association of B cell antigen receptor with protein tyrosine kinase Lyn. Science 251:192-194

Zhang Y, Wienands J, Zuern C, Reth M (1998) Induction of the antigen receptor expression on B lymphocytes results in rapid competence for signaling of SLP-65 and Syk. EMBO J 17:7304-7310

Discussion

Katherine Siminovitch: Do you think your new protein SLP-65 is directly associated with the Ig-α/Ig-β heterodimer or only through its association with Syk?

Michael Reth: So far we can co-purify Ig α only from total cellular lysates together with SLP-65, so we don't yet know whether it is a direct or an indirect interaction. We have many GST-Ig-α fusion proteins at hand and we only have to get the right fusion protein for SLP-65 to test this interaction in more detail.

Katherine Siminovitch: You suggest that BTK does not phosphorylate SLP-65, but that SLP-65 is a substrate for Syk. Is this conclusion consistent with the fact that BTK binds SLP-65?

Michael Reth: The Syk experiment was done in Drs Chan and Kurosaki's labs where they transfected SLP-65/BLNK into DT40 cells which have knockouts of either Lyn, Syk or BTK. The adaptor protein was phosphorylated in all cells, except in the Syk knockout. We are repeating this experiment *in vitro* as we have produced these kinases in the Baculovirus system.

Hans-Reimer Rodewald: Do you see a different distribution of SLP-65 in the cell after expression of surface Ig?

Michael Reth: We know that SLP-65 is also in the cell line which does not have the B cell receptor. We want to find out if there is a change in the localization upon BCR expression. We are trying to purify and analyze this protein from the different cells, and we use GFP fusion proteins.

Dirk Eick: Do you see variation of tyrosine phosphorylation during B cell development? If you look at pre-B cells, B cells, plasma cells, can you validate the experiment?

Michael Reth: Pervanadate is a very drastic drug: when you use it for B-lymphoma cells you see more proteins phosphorylated than in myeloma cells, because they express more receptors and maybe also kinases. If you use normal B cells you also see many phosphoproteins. In myeloma cells the tyrosine phosphorylation is reduced and the phosphorylation of most substrate proteins are dependent on BCR expression. The reason for this is probably that myeloma cells have lost many other surface proteins. In other cell types you do not see a drastic difference of tyrosine phosphorylation between BCR positive and negative cells exposed to pervanadate.

Dirk Eick: Was this analysis done with anti-phosphotyrosine Western blots?

Michael Reth: Yes.

Jason Cyster: Do you have any data on levels of SLP-65 expression in different stages of B cell maturation?

Michael Reth: We have only looked in myeloma, B-lymphoma and Abelson cell lines so far and they all seem to express SLP-65 at the same level.

Kazuo Ohnishi: Does engagement of the BCR also promote tyrosine phosphorylation of SLP-65?

Michael Reth: Yes, when one cross-links the BCR you get the same substrate proteins phosphorylated than after exposure of cells to pervanadate. However, SLP-65 phosphorylation is not so prominent in normal B cells than in myeloma cells. That shows that phosphorylation of SLP-65 is more tightly regulated in normal B cells, as you would expect.

Mike Potter: We have Kishimoto's IL-6 transgenic mouse and it is a remarkable mouse because it accumulates large numbers of plasma cells in the peripheral lymph nodes and you can isolate many millions of pure plasma cells from one mouse. It would be interesting to compare these plasma cells, which are very close to normal, with the J558L plasmacytoma cells to find out what is being expressed on them. Theoretically they should be just exactly like the tumors but maybe they are not.

Michael Reth: I think that myeloma cells are very heterogeneous and we see that in our culture where we have all kinds of variants. But it would be interesting to know whether they also have a program to switch off CD20, CD22, CD19 and CD 45. Did you look for any of these markers?

Mike Potter: No.

Involvement of the SHP-1 Tyrosine Phosphatase in Regulating B Lymphocyte Antigen Receptor Signaling, Proliferation and Transformation

K.A. Siminovitch, A.-M. Lamhonwah, A.-K. Somani, R. Cardiff,[1] and G.B Mills[2]
From the Departments of Medicine, Immunology and Molecular & Medical Genetics, University of Toronto and the Samuel Lunenfeld Research Institute, Mount Sinai Hospital, Room 656A, 600 University Avenue, Toronto, Ontario, M5G 1X5, Canada; [1]Department of Pathology, School of Medicine, University of California at Davis, Davis, California, 95616 and [2]Molecular Oncology, Division of Medicine, The University of Texas, MD Anderson Cancer Center, Houston, Texas 77030, USA

Introduction

The SHP-1 tyrosine phosphatase is a cytosolic protein tyrosine phosphatase (PTP) distinguished by its predominant expression in haemopoietic cells and the presence of two tandemly-located SH2 domains [1,2]. A pivotal role for this PTP in regulating lymphoid cell proliferation and growth was initially revealed by the discovery that loss-of-function mutations in the gene encoding SHP-1 are responsible for the severe systemic autoimmunity and inflammation observed in mice homozygous for the motheaten (*me*) or viable motheaten (*me*^{v}) mutations [3, 4]. These animals manifest multiple myeloid/macrophage and lymphoid cell defects, the latter of which include overexpansion of the normally minor B-1 cell population in the periphery and consequent hypergammaglobulinia, autoantibody production and immune complex deposition [5, 6].

The profile of B cell defects observed in the context of SHP-1 deficiency is highly suggestive of an inhibitory role for SHP-1 in relation to B cell growth and activation. This possibility has now been confirmed by many lines of evidence which identify SHP-1 as a downregulator of growth-promoting cascades not only in B cells, but also in many other haemopoietic cell lineages [7-10]. In B lymphocytes, SHP-1 effects on cell behaviour have been particularly well-studied in relation to elucidating the mechanisms coupling B cell antigen receptor (BCR) engagement to cell response. As outlined below, the results of these studies, many of which have capitalized on the availability of SHP-1-deficient motheaten mice, have revealed SHP-1 effects on BCR signaling to be mediated by a very broad range of molecular interactions and to impact not only on the transmission of growth stimulatory signals, but also upon the biochemical events underlying B cell transformation.

SHP-1 Effects on BCR Signaling

Tyrosine phosphorylation of the BCR heterodimeric Igα/β chains is key to the signal transducing capacity of this receptor and is dependent upon the actions of Src-family cytosolic protein tyrosine kinases (PTKs) which become rapidly activated following BCR engagement [11, 12]. Of particular importance in this regard is the phosphorylation of two tyrosine residues mapping within a conserved motif (designated Immunoreceptor Tyrosine-based Activation Motif or ITAM) present in the cytosolic regions of Igα, Igβ and numerous other signal transducing receptors [13, 14]. Once phosphorylated, the Igα/β ITAMs interact with Syk, resulting in Syk activation, recruitment of secondary signaling molecules and induction of a myriad of downstream molecular interactions which coordinate signal transduction to the nucleus [12].

Just as the activation of selected PTKs and other signaling effectors creates a biochemical circuitry to promote BCR signaling, maintenance of cellular homeostasis predictably requires a molecular framework for attenuating or terminating signal relay to the nucleus. Such an inhibitory role would be anticipated to be subserved, at least in part, by protein tyrosine phosphatases, the activities of which can negate PTK effects by counter-modulating the same substrates or, alternatively, different targets within the same activation cascade. This hypothesized potential for PTPs to negatively regulate growth promoting signaling cascades is, in fact, exemplified in B cells by the properties of the SHP-1 tyrosine phosphatase. Thus, for example, the lack of SHP-1 activity in *me* and me^v B cells is associated with marked enhancement in the induction of proliferation, intracellular calcium mobilization and mitogen activated protein kinase activation following BCR ligation [15-17]. Similarly, SHP-1 deficient *me* B cells expressing an anti-hen egg lysozyme (HEL) immunoglobulin transgene have been shown to be hyperresponsive to HEL exposure, the latter inducing in the SHP-1-deficient bone marrow deletion of B cells normally rendered anergic in this context [16]. Together these observations identify a major role for SHP-1 in suppressing BCR signaling activity and suggest that SHP-1 inhibitory effects on the BCR increase the signaling threshold required for coupling this receptor to not only proliferation, but also other cell responses, such as clonal deletion.

The capacity of SHP-1 to downregulate BCR signaling has been linked to SHP-1 interactions with a number of signaling elements and to the SHP-1 activity expressed in both unstimulated and BCR-stimulated cells. In resting B cells, for example, SHP-1 has been shown to interact with the BCR and dephosphorylate the Igα/β components of the receptor complex [17]. The mechanism for this association, which does not appear to be mediated by an SH2 domain-phosphotyrosine interaction, is unclear, but the localization of SHP-1 within the resting BCR complex suggests that SHP-1 activity provides a means to maintaining the Igα/β components in a tyrosine dephosphorylated state prior to antigenic stimulation.

In contrast to its BCR association in resting B cells, SHP-1 is no longer detectable in BCR complexes following ligation of the antigen receptor [17]. Instead SHP-1 interacts with a number of cell surface accessory molecules which are also implicated in the negative modulation of BCR signaling. As illustrated in Figure 1, these include, for example, the FcγRIIB, CD22 and the paired Ig-like receptor, PIR-B [18-21]. Each of these latter receptors undergoes tyrosine phosphorylation upon BCR ligation and each has been shown to inhibit BCR-triggered increases in intracellular calcium concentration, the FcγRIIB and CD22 receptors inhibiting calcium influx and PIR-B inhibiting intracellular calcium release upon co-crosslinking with the BCR [21-23]. SHP-1 has been shown to interact with the cytosolic domains of these receptors by binding of its SH-2 domains with a phosphotyrosine embedded in a specific sequence (I/V-X-pY-X-X-L) designated as an Immunoreceptor Tyrosine-based Inhibitory Motif (ITIM) [18, 20, 21, 24]. Phosphorylated ITIMs interact with at least two phosphatases in addition to SHP-1, the structurally similar SHP-2 tyrosine phosphatase and the inositol 5 phosphatase, SHIP [24, 25]. Thus, for example, the FcγRIIB phosphorylated ITIM interacts with SHIP as well as SHP-1 and the SHP-1 binding phosphorylated ITIMs of the PIR-B protein also interact with SHP-2 [21, 26]. SHP-1 has also recently been shown to interact with the ITIM motifs contained in another BCR co-modulator, the

CD72 transmembrane protein [27]. The functions of CD72 are not well defined, but this protein has been implicated in B cell development and, depending on the stage of cell development, in the induction of either proliferation or cell death following BCR cross-linking [28-30]. The relevance of SHP-1, however, to CD72-mediated BCR modulation remains to be determined. Similarly, the extent to which the BCR inhibitory behaviour of any of the ITIM-containing co-receptors is influenced by SHP-1 per se or, alternatively, by the coordinate activities of SHP-1, SHP-2 and/or SHIP, is currently unclear. While resolving these issues requires further investigation, the available data suggest that a very significant component of SHP-1 negative effects on BCR signaling is attributable to its interaction with at least some of the BCR inhibitory co-receptors.

Figure 1. Mechanisms by which SHP-1 modulates BCR signaling

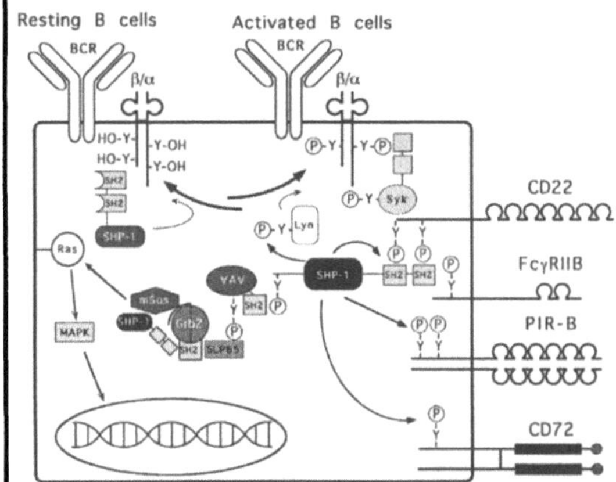

Legend: Mechanisms by which SHP-1 modulates BCR signaling. SHP-1 associates with the BCR in resting B cells, but after BCR engagement interacts with several phosphorylated inhibitory coreceptors and cytosolic effectors such as Vav, Grb2 and Lyn.

In addition to BCR co-receptors, a number of cytosolic effectors involved in BCR signaling also interact with SHP-1. As shown in Figure 1, these include the Lyn PTK, which our group has shown not only associates with SHP-1 via an SH2 domain-phosphotyrosine interaction, but is subject to SHP-1-mediated downregulation by dephosphorylation of tyrosine 505 within the kinase domain (Somani et al., manuscript in preparation). SHP-1 has also been shown to bind but not dephosphorylate Grb2 and Vav, an observation which suggests that SHP-1 may target other Vav and/or Grb2-associated proteins and thereby downregulate BCR-triggered signaling events downstream of Ras and potentially Rho GTPase activation [32]. In view of data identifying the Vav/Grb2-binding Slp76 adaptor protein as a SHP-1 substrate in T cells [7, 36], the B cell homologue of Slp76 (Slp65) represents one potential Vav/Grb2-associated effector in B cells [33] likely to be targeted by SHP-1 and relevant to SHP-1 negative modulation of BCR signaling. While this possibility and identification of the full range of SHP-1 substrates in B cells requires further investigation, the available data indicate SHP-1 effects on BCR signaling function to be consistently inhibitory, to be realized through a diversity of mechanisms and molecular interactions, and to translate to the suppression of the spectrum of biological outcomes potentially triggered by BCR engagement.

Association of SHP-1 Deficiency with B Lymphomagenesis

While mice heterozygous for the *me* or *me*^{v} mutations appear phenotypically normal at young ages, we have observed these mice to be unusually susceptible to B cell lymphomas over time. The tumors involve a multiplicity of tissues, most often occurring in the spleen, liver, lungs, lymph nodes and salivary glands. As illustrated by the immunohistochemical data shown in Figure 2, the lymphoma cells express membrane immunoglobulin, MHC class II, B220 and CD5 (not shown) on the cell surface and therefore appear to arise from the B-1 lineage and to phenotypically as well as morphologically resemble the subset of human non-Hodgkin's lymphomas encompassing mantle cell lymphoma and small lymphocytic lymphoma. These tumors develop in 40% of *me*^{v} heterozygous mice by the age of two years and cannot be ascribed to genetic background per se, as lymphomas develop in only 15% of similarly-aged congenic (i.e. C57BL6) wild-type mice and also in C3HeBFeJ motheaten heterozygous mice housed in the same facility. Most significantly, results of both immunohistochemical (Fig. 2) and immunoblotting analyses (Fig. 3A) indicate expression of SHP-1 to be either undetectable or markedly reduced in the lymphoma cells compared to lymphoid cells from healthy *me*^{v} heterozygous mice. Expression of SHP-1 transcript also appears to be reduced in these cells (Fig. 3B), a finding which links the lack of SHP-1 protein to a defect in expression of the SHP-1 gene. Whether this defect reflects a mutation, an alteration in promoter region methylation status or some other genetic modification remains to be determined.

Figure 2. Immunostaining of malignant lymphoma in liver of *me*^{v}/+ mouse

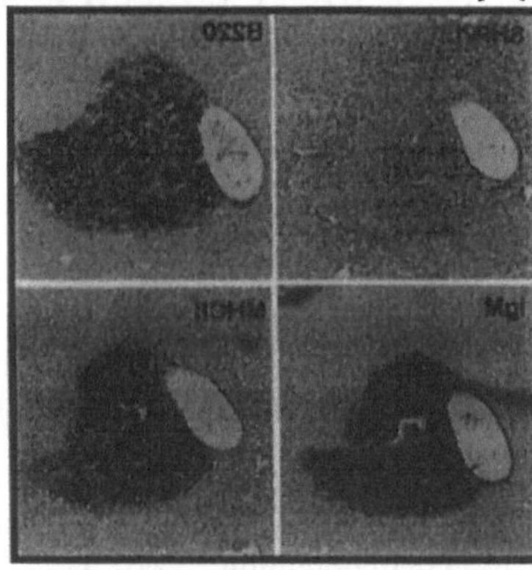

Legend: Low power photomicrograph of an *me*^{v}/+ lymphoma. Immunohistochemical analysis reveals expression of the B cell lineage- associated antigens (sIgM, B220, MHC class II), but lack of SHP-1 expression

However, the available data revealing these murine lymphomas to be associated with inactivation of the SHP-1 gene raise the possibility that SHP-1 functions as a tumor suppressor in B lineage cells. This hypothesis is further supported by the localization of the human SHP-1 gene to 12p12-p13, a chromosomal region that is deleted/translocated in about 10% of childhood acute lymphoblastic leukemias [34]. When considered in conjunction with SHP-1 inhibitory effects on BCR-driven mitogenesis, these data strongly suggest that SHP-1 represents a B cell tumor suppressor, the functional deactivation of which promotes malignant transformation of B-1 and possibly other B lineage cells.

Figure 3. Immunoblot analysis showing loss or reduction of SHP-1 expression in me^v/+ lymphomas

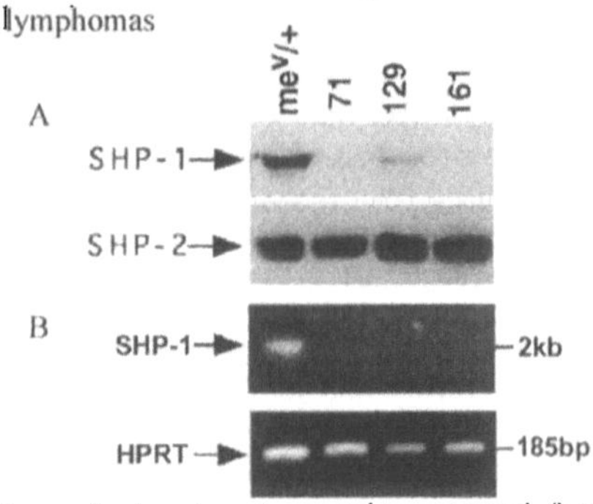

Legend: A. Lysate proteins prepared from *me*^{v} heterozygote (*me*^{v}/+) spleen and the lymphomatous tissues of *me*^{v}/+ mice 71, 129 and 161 were immunoblotted with anti-SHP-1 antibody and the blots then stripped and reprobed with anti-SHP-2 antibody to confirm equal loading.
B. Total RNA from *me*^{v}/+ spleen and from splenic lymphomas of *me*^{v} /+ mice 71, 129 and 161 was subjected to RT-PCR using oligoprimers for amplification of the full-length SHP-1 gene and a 185 bp segment of the HPRT gene.

The association of SHP-1 deficiency with transformation and, by extension, growth dysregulation of B-1 lymphoid cells is consistent with available data linking the development of B-1 cells to stimulatory signals evoked by autoantigenic exposure during B cell ontogeny. Such data include, for example, the demonstration of reduced B-1 cell development in mice genetically ablated for signaling effectors, such as Btk, Vav and CD19, which positively influence BCR signaling [35-37]. Similarly, differences in the degree to which B-1 cells develop in mice lacking SHP-1 versus CD45, PTPs with the opposite effects on BCR signaling, highlight the pivotal role for BCR signal relay in promoting differentiation of these cells [17]. Thus the development of B-1 lymphomas in association with loss of SHP-1 activity is not unexpected and might be envisioned as a logical consequence of dysregulated BCR signaling.

Concluding Remarks

The SHP-1 tyrosine phosphatase is now recognized as a critical element in regulation of the BCR signaling pathways evoking B cell activation and proliferation. The inhibitory effects of SHP-1 on such pathways, together with the association between SHP-1-deficiency and B cell lymphomagenesis, provide compelling evidence that SHP-1 also subserves a tumor suppressor function in these cells. This conclusion is consistent with the capacity for selected PTPs to suppress the transforming effects of specific oncogenes and of PTP inhibitors to induce or facilitate the transformation of cultured cells [38, 39]. Together these observations suggest important roles for PTPs in suppression not only of cell growth, but also transformation. Characterization of the roles for SHP-1 in B lymphomagenesis therefore provides a unique opportunity to delineate the biochemical events linking PTP signal modulatory functions to transformation and to define the molecular interactions which give rise to B-1 lineage lymphomas.

Acknowledgements

This work was supported by grants from the Medical Research Council of Canada and National Cancer Institute of Canada (to K.A.S.) and the National Institutes of Health (CA74247 to G.B.M). Katherine A. Siminovitch is a Research Scientist of the Arthritis Society of Canada and Ally-Khan Somani is the recipient of a Steve Fonyo NCIC Studentship award.

References

1. Shen SH, Bastien L, Posner PI, Chretien P. (1991). A protein tyrosine phosphatase with sequence similarity to the SH2 domain of the protein-tyrosine kinases. Nature 352: 736-739.
2. Yi T, Cleveland JL, Ihle JN (1992). Protein tyrosine phosphatase containing SH2 domains. Characterization, preferential expression in hemopoietic cells, and localization to human chromosome 12p12-13. Mol Cell Biol 12: 836-846.
3. Kozlowski M, Mlinaric-Rascan I, Feng G-S, Shen R, Pawson T, Siminovitch KA. (1993). Expression and catalytic activity of the tyrosine phosphatase PTP1C is severely impaired in motheaten and viable motheaten mice. J Exp Med 178: 2157-2163.

4. Tsui HW, Siminovitch KA, deSouza L, Tsui FW. (1993). Motheaten and viable motheaten mice have mutations in the hemopoietic cell phosphatase gene. Nature Genet 4: 124-129.
5. Sidman CL, Shultz LD, Unanue ER. (1978) The mouse mutant "motheaten". I. Development of lymphocyte populations. J Immunol 121: 2392-2398.
6. Sidman CL, Shultz LD, Hardy RR, Hayakawa K, Herzenberg LA. (1986) Production of immunoglobulin isotypes by Ly-1 + B cells in viable motheaten and normal mice. Since 232: 1423-1425.
7. Pani G, Fischer KD, Mlinaric-Rascan I, Siminovitch KA. (1996). Signaling capacity of the T cell antigen receptor is negatively regulated by the PTP1C tyrosine phosphatase. J Exp Med 184: 839-852.
8. Chen HE, Chang S, Trub T, Neel BG. (1996). Regulation of colony-stimulating factor 1 receptor signaling by the SH2 domain-containing tyrosine phosphatases SHPTP1. Mol Cell Biol 16: 3685-3697.
9. Paulson RF, Vesely S, Siminovitch KA, Bernstein A. (1996). Signaling by the W/Kit receptor tyrosine kinase is negatively regulated in vivo by the protein tyrosine phosphatase Shp1. Nature Genet 13: 309-315.
10. Klingmuller U, Lorenz U, Cantley L, Neel B, Lodish H. (1995). Specific recruitment of SH-PTP1 to the erythropoietin receptor causes inactivation of JAK2 and termination of proliferative signals. Cell 80: 729-738.
11. De Franco AL. (1993). Signaling pathways activated by protein tyrosine phosphorylation in lymphocytes. Curr Biol 6: 364-371.
12. Cambier JC, Pleiman CM, Clark MR (1994). Signal transduction by the B cell antigen receptor and its coreceptors. Annu Rev. Immunol 12: 457-486.
13. Weiss A (1993). T-cell antigen receptor signal transduction – a tale of tails and cytoplasmic protein-tyrosine kinases. Cell 73: 209-212.
14. Reth M. (1995). The B cell antigen receptor complex and coreceptors. Immunol Tod 16:310-313.
15. Pani G, Kozlowski M, Cambier JC, Mills GB, Siminovitch KA (1995). Identification of the tyrosine phosphates PYP1C as a B cell antigen receptor-associated protein involved in the regulation of B cell signaling. J Exp Med 181: 2077-2084.
16. Cyster JG, Goodnow CC. (1995). Protein tyrosine phosphatase 1C negatively regulates antigen receptor signaling in B lymphocytes and determines thresholds for negative selection. Immunity 2: 1- 20.
17. Pani G, Siminovitch KA, Paige CJ. (1997). The motheaten mutation rescues B cell signaling and development in CD45-deficient mice. J Exp Med 186: 581-588.
18. D'Ambrosio D, Hippen KL, Minskoff SA, Mellman F, Pani G, Siminovitch KA, Cambier JC. (1995). Recruitment and activation of PTP1C in negative regulation of antigen receptor signaling by Fc gamma RIIB1. Science 268:293-297.
19. Lankester AC, van Schijn del GMW, van Lier RAW. (1995). Haemopoietic cell phosphatase is recruited to CD22 following B cell antigen receptor ligation. J. Biol. Chem. 270: 20305-20308.
20. Doody GM, Justement LB, Delibrias CC, Matthews RJ, Lin J, Thomas ML, Fearon DT (1995). A role in B cell activation for CD22 and the protein tyrosine phosphatase SHP. Science. 169: 242-244.
21. Bléry M, Kubagawa H, Chen C-C, Vély F, Cooper MD, Vivier E. (1997). The paired Ig-like receptor PIT-B is an inhibitory receptor that recruits the protein-tyrosine phosphtase SHP-1. Proc Natl Acad Sci USA 95: 2446-2451.
22. Nitschke L, Carsetti R, Ocker B, Kohler G, Lamers MC. (1997). CD22 is a negative regulator of B cell receptor signaling. Curr Biol 7:133-143
23. Ono M, Bolland S, Tempst P, Ravetch JV. (1996). Role of the inositol phosphatase SHIP in negative regulation of the immune system by the receptor Fc(gamma)RIIB. Nature 383: 263-265.

24. Cambier JC. (1997). Inhibitory receptors abound? Proc Natl Acad Sci USA 94: 5993-5995.
25. Scharenberg A, Kinet J. (1996). The emerging field of receptor-mediated inhibitory signaling: SHP or SHIP? Cell 87: 961-964.
26. Ono M, Okada H, Bolland S, Yanagi S, Kurosaki T, Ravetch JV. (1997). Deletion of SHIP or SHP-1 reveals two distinct pathways for inhibitory signaling. Cell 90: 293-301.
27. Adachi T, Flaswinkel H, Yakura H, Reth M, Tsubata T. (1998). The B cell surface protein CD72 recruits the tyrosine phosphatase SHP-1 upon tyrosine phosphorylation. J Immunol 160: 4662-4665.
28. Gordon J. (1994). B cell signaling via the c-Type lectins CD23 and CD72. Immunol Today 15: 411-417.
29. Nomura T, Han H, Howard MC, Yagita H, Yakura H, Honjo T, Tsubata T. (1996). Antigen receptor-mediated with dextran sulfate and is defective in autoimmunity-prone mice. Inter Immunol 8: 867-875.
30. Ying H, Healy JI, Goodnow CC, Parnes JR (1998). Regulation of mouse CD72 gene expression during B lymphocyte development. J. Immunol 161: 4760-4767.
31. Kon-Kozlowski M, Pani G, Pawson T, Siminovitch KA. (1996). The tyrosine phosphatase PTP1C associates with Vav, Grb2 and mSos1 in hematopoietic cells. J Biol Chem 271: 3856-3862.
32. Binstadt BA, Billadeau DD, Jevremovic D, Williams BL, Fang N, Yi T, Koretzky GA, Abraham RT, Leibson PJ. (1998). Slp-76 is a direct substrate of SHP-1 recruited to killer cell inhibitory receptors. J Biol Chem 273: 27518-27523.
33. Wienands J, Schweikert J, Wollscheid B, Jumaa H, Nielsen PJ, Reth M (1998). Slp-65: a new signaling component in B lymphocytes which requires expression of the antigen receptor for phosphorylation. J Exp Med 188: 791-795.
34. Raimondi SC, Williams DL, Callihan T, Peiper S, Rivera GK, Murphy SB. (1986). Nonrandom involvment of the 12p12 breakpoint in chromosome abnormalities of childhood acute lymphoblastic leukemia. Blood 68: 69-75.
35. Thomas JD, Sideras P, Edward Smith CI, Vorechovsky I, Chapman V, Paul WE. (1993). Colocalization of X-linked agammaglobulinemia and X-linked immunodeficiency genes. Science 261: 355-358.
36. Tarakhovsky A, Turner M, Schaal S, Mee PJ, Duddy LP, Rajewsky K, Tybulewicz LJ. (1995). Defective antigen receptor-mediated proliferation of B and T cells in the absence of Vav. Nature 374: 467-477.
37. Richert RC, Rajewsky K, Roes J. (1995). Impairment of T cell-dependent B cell responses and B-1 cell development in CD19-deficient mice. Nature 376: 352-355.
38. Brown-Shimer S, Johnson KA, Hill DE, Bruskin AM. (1992). Effect of protein tyrosine phosphatase 1B expression on transformation by the human neu oncogene. Cancer Res 52: 478-482.
39. Karland JK. (1985). Transformation of cells by an inhibitor of phosphatases acting on phosphotyrosine in proteins. Cell 41: 707-717.

Discussion

Jim Kenny: Do the viable motheaten mice which develop lymphomas show the typical MOTT cells that come up in the motheaten animals?
Katherine Siminovitch: You are right, the homozygous motheaten and viable motheaten animals do manifest MOTT cells. However, these are not the cells constituting the lymphoma.
Jim Kenny: Is the loss of SHP-1 in motheaten homozygous mice accompanied by that same kind of transformation?
Katherine Siminovitch: The tumor cells might be expected to resemble the SHP-1-deficient cells in some but not all ways as motheaten cells develop in the context of SHP-1 deficiency, whereas loss of SHP-1 is an acquired lesion in the tumor cells. Conversely, loss of SHP-1 in motheaten homozygotes probably does predispose to tumors but the mice die too early (3 weeks) to allow for tumor development.
Gary Rathbun: Have you analyzed the tumors that develop in heterozygous animals in relation to chromosomal translocations?
Katherine Siminovitch: I don't know if these tumors show translocations as we haven't looked for cytogenetic lesions.
Heinz Jacobs: What happens if you put a functional SHP back into the tumors?
Katherine Siminovitch: We have tried hard to derive cell lines so that we can do this experiment. But so far we have been unsuccessful.
Siegfried Janz: Did you look at immunoglobulin expression in these tumors?
Katherine Siminovitch: Yes, they express surface IgM.
Sandy Morse: Have you looked at pre-lymphomatous mice to see whether you detect any early lesions?
Katherine Siminovitch: No we haven't looked at pre-lymphomatous mice. We have waited until the animals get tumors and sacrificed them then. However, it would certainly be worthwhile sacrificing some of the "healthy" heterozygote mice to look for those early lesions.
Sandy Morse: We do not have any examples of murine mantle lymphomas in our series, except for tumors we call centrocytic lymphomas, which we find very difficult to say are or not of mantle zone origin in the mouse. But that is all we have seen in our series and even these tumors are extremely rare. So it is a really fascinating situation.
Mike Potter: You showed a great array of proteins, were they all phosphatases?
Katherine Siminovitch: Yes, the number of phosphatases, including tyrosine phosphatases, identified and characterized is steadily increasing.
Mike Potter: According to your findings, these phosphatases are all candidate genes as potential suppressers?
Katherine Siminovitch: Not all of them. Tyrosine phosphatases can act in a paradoxical fashion with respect to regulation of cell growth. For example CD45, which is probably the most extensively studied tyrosine phosphatase in hematopoiesis, has a positive impact on cell growth which contrasts with the growth inhibitory effect of other phosphatases. However, I believe that phosphatases do, in general, represent very good candidates for tumor suppressers. This idea was postulated a long time ago in view of the functional role for tyrosine phosphatases in counter-balancing tyrosine kinase activity.
Mike Potter: It would be a very interesting exercise to find out where the various phosphatases map.
Katherine Siminovitch: Yes, that data would provide valuable information to combine with available gene mapping or cytogenetic data on potential tumor suppressor loci.

Antigen Receptor Signaling Induces Differential Tyrosine Kinase Activation and Population Stability in B-Cell Lymphoma

R.C. Hsueh[1], A.K. Hammill[1], R. Marches[2,3], J.W. Uhr[2,3], and R.H. Scheuermann[1,3]
[1] Department of Pathology, [2]Department of Microbiology, [3]Cancer Immunobiology Center, University of Texas Southwestern Medical Center, Dallas, TX 75235-9072, USA

Introduction

Cancer dormancy is a phenomenon where neoplastic cells exist within a host without progressive growth (1-3). Clinical examples of dormancy in humans can be found in cases of melanoma (4,5), breast carcinoma (6) , and lymphoma [R. Levy personal communication]. To identify potential mechanisms regulating cancer dormancy, a murine lymphoma model has been established. This dormancy model system utilizes a mouse B-cell lymphoma, BCL_1, whose aggressive growth normally leads to rapid splenomegaly, late onset leukemia, and eventual death within 30 days after challenge. However, the development of splenomegaly and subsequent disease can be prevented by immunization of syngeneic recipients with membrane immunoglobulin (mIg) purified from BCL_1 prior to challenge. Seventy percent of immunized animals do not develop tumor by 60 days and in some cases can survive up to 2 years, the lifespan of a normal animal. Dormancy established in these animals is not simply the elimination of BCL_1 by the host immune system because BCL_1 can be specifically detected using polymerase chain reaction and can be isolated using flow cytometry from the spleen of dormant animals. Adoptive transfer of splenocytes from dormant animals to naive recipients results in regrowth of the tumor (7), and is further evidence that BCL_1 cells are present.

The dormancy model was also investigated in SCID mice to determine the potential roles of anti-tumor antibodies in dormancy. Studies using the SCID model system demonstrate that dormancy can be induced in animals that receive an intraperitoneal injection of anti-mIg antibodies prior to injection of BCL_1 (7). Additional studics in SCID mice argue against some traditional immunological effector mechanisms such as ADCC and anti-tumor, NK cell-mediated lysis as major contributors to the establishment and maintenance of dormancy (7). Although T-cells can affect the longevity of dormancy, antibodies are sufficient to inducc dormancy in the SCID model (7). Taken together these results support the hypothesis that antibodies induce dormancy and regulate lymphoma growth by activating signal transduction pathways originating from the antigen receptor.

Results

Cross-linking mIg *In Vitro* Results in Cell Cycle Arrest, Apoptosis, and Signal Transduction

To examine the importance of signaling through mIg in regulating growth of BCL_1, an *in vitro* cell line, BCL_1.3B3, has been established. To determine the changes in growth parameters resulting from cross-linking of mIg, BCL_1.3B3 was incubated with polyclonal anti-Ig antibodies *in vitro* and the membrane permeability and cell cycle status evaluated using flow cytometry. Cross-linking results in a partial cell cycle arrest as indicated by a decrease in the proportion of cells in S, G_2, and M phases of the cell cycle at all doses of anti-Ig antibodies used (Figure 1A). Cross-linking also induces apoptosis in some cells (Figure 1B); however, only high doses of cross-linking antibodies induce apoptosis. This result suggests that the extent of cross-linking in some way controls the balance between growth arrest and cell death.

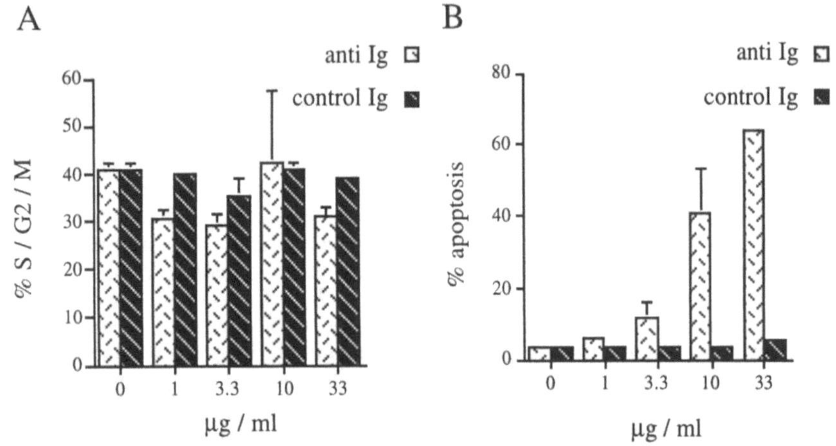

Fig. 1. Anti-Ig antibodies induce cell cycle arrest and apoptosis in BCL_1.3B3. A. Induction of growth arrest by polyclonal anti-Ig antibodies. Cells were plated in duplicate in medium containing polyclonal goat anti-murine IgM (hatched bars) or a goat anti-ovalbumin (striped bars) as indicated. Cells were incubated at 37°C for 24 hours, harvested, and analyzed for membrane permeability by 7-amino-actinomycin D (7AAD) (Molecular Probes) exclusion and DNA content by Hoechst 33342 fluorescence using flow cytometry (8). The percentage of cells in $S/G_2/M$ was determined by gating on viable cells (those that exclude 7AAD) and quantifying cells with a >2n and ≤4n DNA content. B. Induction of apoptosis by polyclonal anti-Ig antibodies. The cells that take up the vital dye 7AAD are scored as apoptotic. The hallmark of apoptosis, DNA fragmentation, is also induced (7).

To demonstrate that the balance between these processes is dependent on the extent of cross-linking, BCL_1.3B3 cells were incubated with monoclonal anti-Ig antibodies or monoclonal antibodies hypercross-linked with a secondary antibody (9). Cells treated with monoclonal antibodies, and therefore having minimal mIg cross-linking, are induced into cell cycle arrest with no accompanying apoptosis. However, hypercross-linking of the monoclonal with a secondary antibody results in both cell cycle arrest and apoptosis (Table I), demonstrating that the degree to which mIg is cross-linked can shift the balance between growth arrest and cell death.

This observation raises many questions regarding the mechanism of negative signaling. Is there a qualitative difference in the signal transduced at low concentration versus high concentration? Are different signal transduction pathways activated, one for cell cycle arrest at low concentrations and one for apoptosis at high concentrations? Is apoptosis dependent on cell cycle arrest; are the two processes linked? Or are they independent of one another; are they separable?

Table I. Effects of cross-linking on induction of CCA and apoptosis in BCL_1.3B3

Degree of cross-linking	Cell Cycle Arrest (CCA)	Apoptosis	Ref.
low polyclonal	++	-	Figure 1
high polyclonal	+	++	Figure 1
monoclonal	++	-	(9)
monoclonal hypercross-linked	+	++	(9)

In a series of experiments designed to identify potential kinases involved in one or both of these processes induced through mIg, the SRC family tyrosine kinase, Lyn, was implicated in the cell cycle arrest response (8). Depletion of the Lyn tyrosine kinase, using Lyn specific antisense oligonucleotides in BCL_1.3B3, resulted in an abrogation of the cell cycle arrest induced through mIg. However, apoptosis remains unaffected in these cells. This result suggests that signaling of cell cycle arrest and apoptosis might involve distinct molecules, and potentially, different pathways.

A second non-receptor cytoplasmic tyrosine kinase, Syk, has been implicated in apoptosis and not cell cycle arrest. The human Burkitt's B-cell lymphoma cell line, Daudi, also exhibits cell cycle arrest and apoptosis after mIg cross-linking. We have stably transfected Daudi with an antisense expression vector targeting Syk mRNA. Stable transfectants that express antisense targeting Syk message exhibit reduced Syk activity as compared with controls (data not shown). In these transfectants, cell cycle arrest is induced as strongly as controls (Figure 2A). However, apoptosis induced through mIg is severely compromised (Figure 2B). This correlation between reduced Syk activity and reduced apoptosis further supports the DT40 experiments which implicate Syk in apoptosis (10). Syk deficient DT40 cells have significantly reduced levels of mIg induced apoptosis as compared to controls. Furthermore Lyn knockout DT40 cells still undergo control levels of apoptosis, supporting the possibility that Lyn and Syk activate separate pathways that result in distinct cellular outcomes. Unfortunately, cell cycle arrest was not examined in these DT40 experiments.

Taken together these data support the following model for the cellular response to antigen receptor signaling. It is likely that at low concentrations of cross-linking antibody, a small mIg cluster forms at the cell surface. This small cluster is sufficient to activate Lyn and cell cycle arrest without significantly activating Syk or inducing apoptosis. Indeed, lower amounts of cross-linking antibody are required for Lyn activation than for Syk activation (Table II). At high concentrations a larger cluster of mIg forms, Syk is activated, and apoptosis is induced. More detailed experimentation is ongoing to examine this model.

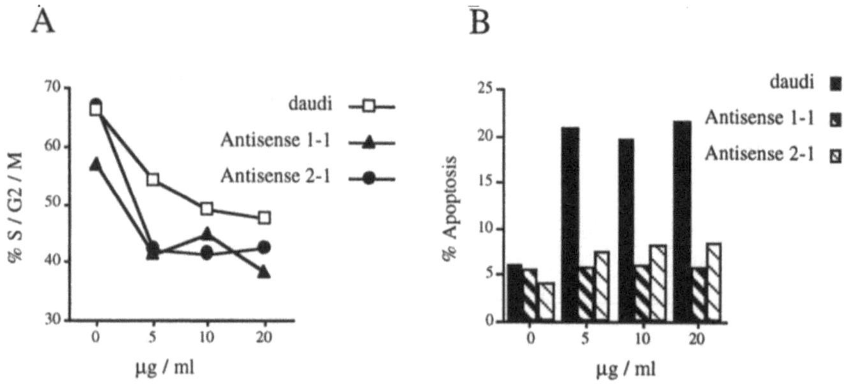

Fig. 2. Antisense targeting Syk mRNA abrogates apoptosis but not cell cycle arrest induced through mIg in Daudi. A. Cell cycle arrest in antisense Syk transfectants. Daudi cells were transfected with an expression construct containing full length human Syk cDNA in the antisense orientation whose expression is driven by the cytomeglovirus promoter. Transfectants were selected in G418 containing medium, and plated in medium containing 0, 5, 10, or 20 µg/ml of anti-human IgM (Chemicon). Cells were incubated at 37°C for 24 hours, harvested, stained with 7AAD and Hoechst 33342, and analyzed by flow cytometry as described in Figure 1. Two antisense transfectants (solid circles and triangles) that demonstrated reduced Syk activity (data not shown) were analyzed and compared to wildtype Daudi (open circle) B. Apoptosis is abrogated. Cells were treated and analyzed as in part A. Antisense Syk transfectants (striped bars) were found to show markedly reduced levels of 7AAD positive cells as compared to wildtype Daudi (solid bars).

Table II. Effects of cross-linking on kinase activation in BCL_1.3B3

Activating antibody	Lyn activity	Syk activity	Ref.
low concentration polyclonal	+	+/-	unpublished
high concentration polyclonal	+	++	unpublished

Antigen Receptor Cross-linking Results in Stable Cell Numbers Over Time

The *in vitro* system used to examine the role of specific molecules involved in cell cycle arrest and apoptosis induced through mIg may be a good reflection of the dormant state of BCL_1 in animals. In dormant animals the total number of BCL_1 cells remains stable and does not change significantly over time (11). Population stability is also observed *in vitro* in that the number of cells in anti-Ig treated cultures remains relatively constant for 12 days (Figure 3), regardless of the starting number of cells. Flow cytometric analysis of these cells suggests that apoptosis and cell cycle progression are ongoing (data not shown). From these results we propose that cell cycle arrest, apoptosis, and cell cycle progression contribute to the stability observed *in vitro* and *in vivo* in dormant animals, and that this balance between cell cycle arrest, apoptosis, and cell cycle progression must be tightly regulated. At present the mechanism controlling this balance is under investigation.

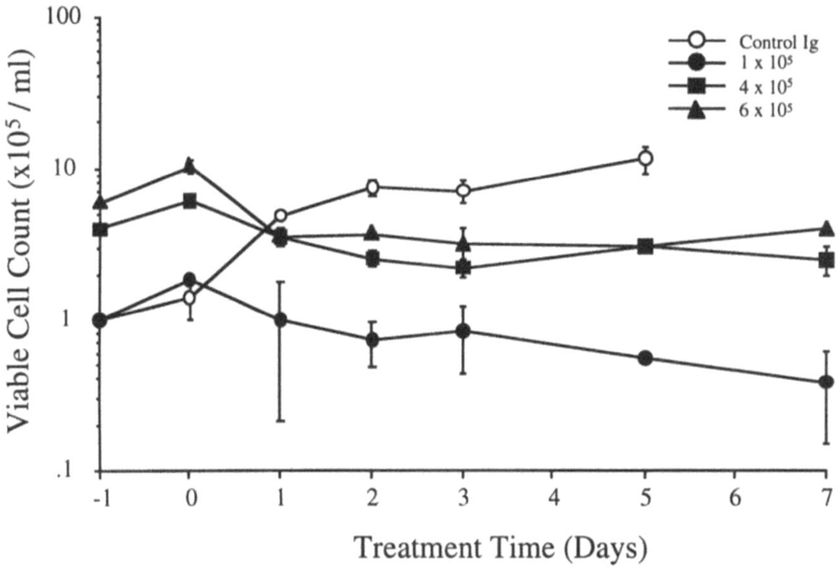

Fig. 3. Numbers of BCL_1.3B3 cells remain constant up to 12 days in culture. Cells were plated in medium for 24 hours at $1x10^5$, $4x10^5$, and $6x10^5$ and then treated with 25 µg/ml of a polyclonal anti-Ig (solid symbols) or a polyclonal, species matched control (open symbols) on day 0. Cells were then harvested, stained with trypan blue, and viable cells counted at the days indicated.

Discussion

The results described here attempt to elucidate cellular processes that cumulatively give rise to tumor dormancy in the murine lymphoma model. We know from the SCID dormancy model that antibodies targeting mIg of BCL_1 are important and sufficient to induce dormancy *in vivo* by stabilizing the numbers of BCL_1 cells within a dormant animal via signal transduction. *In vitro* cross-linking data demonstrates that the population stability we see in culture is most likely the result of a well orchestrated balance of cell cycle arrest, apoptosis, and cell cycle progression. The data summarized and presented here implicate the non-receptor tyrosine kinase, Lyn, in cell cycle arrest and the non-receptor tyrosine kinase, Syk, in apoptosis. From these findings our hypothesis is that the same processes that regulate population stability *in vitro* may also do so *in vivo* in the dormant animal.

Different therapies targeting membrane immunoglobulin have been used in clinical trials with some success (12,13). Anti-idiotype antibodies induce phosphorylation of intracellular proteins in a patient's lymphoma cells and reduce the number of detectable tumor cells (14). This result demonstrates the possible utility of targeting surface receptors and signal transduction as a means of therapy. In light of our results, the efficacy of specific treatments in clinical trials may be related to the ability to efficiently trigger growth inhibition or apoptosis. Furthermore, anti-Ig therapy may be used in conjunction with chemical reagents or antibody to other receptors that activate specific signal transduction pathways. For example, if Syk activation is required to induce apoptosis, then therapeutic reagents that activate Syk might give the most effective result. The fact that Syk is implicated in apoptosis induced through mIg in B-cells from different species suggests that Syk may be a good candidate target. At any rate understanding the underlying mechanisms of dormancy and the mechanisms that lead to cell cycle arrest and apoptosis induction *in vitro* may elucidate new means of treating lymphoma that might be more efficacious and potentially applicable to other cancers.

References

1. Hadfield, G. (1954) The dormant cancer cell. Br Med J 2, 607
2. Wheelock, E. F., Weinhold, K. J., and Levich, J. (1981) The tumor dormant state. Adv Cancer Res 34, 107-40.
3. Yefenof, E., Scheuermann, R. H., ed. (1996) Premalignancy and Tumor Dormancy . Springer-Verlag: Heidelberg, Germany.
4. Callaway, M. P., and Briggs, J. C. (1989) The incidence of late recurrence (greater than 10 years); an analysis of 536 consecutive cases of cutaneous melanoma. Br J Plast Surg 42(1), 46-9.
5. Shaw, H. M., Beattie, C. W., McCarthy, W. H., and Milton, G. W. (1985) Late relapse from cutaneous stage I malignant melanoma. Arch Surg 120(10), 1155-9.
6. Meltzer, A. (1990) Dormancy and breast cancer. J Surg Oncol 43(3), 181-8.
7. Racila, E., Scheuermann, R. H., Picker, L. J., Yefenof, E., Tucker, T., Chang, W., Marches, R., Street, N. E., Vitetta, E. S., and Uhr, J. W. (1995) Tumor dormancy and cell signaling. II. Antibody as an agonist in inducing dormancy of a B cell lymphoma in SCID mice. J Exp Med 181(4), 1539-50.
8. Scheuermann, R. H., Racila, E., Tucker, T., Yefenof, E., Street, N. E., Vitetta, E. S., Picker, L. J., and Uhr, J. W. (1994) Lyn tyrosine kinase signals cell cycle arrest but not apoptosis in B-lineage lymphoma cells. Proc Natl Acad Sci U S A 91(9), 4048-52.
9. Marches, R., Racila, E., Tucker, T. F., Picker, L., Mongini, P., Hsueh, R., Vitetta, E. S., Scheuermann, R. H., and Uhr, J. W. (1995) Tumour dormancy and cell signalling--III: Role of hypercrosslinking of IgM and CD40 on the induction of cell cycle arrest and apoptosis in B lymphoma cells. Ther Immunol 2(3), 125-36.
10. Takata, M., Homma, Y., and Kurosaki, T. (1995) Requirement of phospholipase C-gamma 2 activation in surface immunoglobulin M-induced B cell apoptosis. J Exp Med 182(4), 907-14.
11. Vitetta, E. S., Tucker, T. F., Racila, E., Huang, Y. W., Marches, R., Lane, N., Scheuermann, R. H., Street, N. E., Watanabe, T., and Uhr, J. W. (1997) Tumor dormancy and cell signaling. V. Regrowth of the BCL1 tumor after dormancy is established. Blood 89(12), 4425-36.
12. Vitetta, E. S., Thorpe, P. E., and Uhr, J. W. (1993) Immunotoxins: magic bullets or misguided missiles? Trends Pharmacol Sci 14(5), 148-54.
13. Maloney, D. G., Brown, S., Czerwinski, D. K., Liles, T. M., Hart, S. M., Miller, R. A., and Levy, R. (1992) Monoclonal anti-idiotype antibody therapy of B-cell lymphoma: the addition of a short course of chemotherapy does not interfere with the antitumor effect nor prevent the emergence of idiotype-negative variant cells. Blood 80(6), 1502-10.
14. Vuist, W. M., Levy, R., and Maloney, D. G. (1994) Lymphoma regression induced by monoclonal anti-idiotypic antibodies correlates with their ability to induce Ig signal transduction and is not prevented by tumor expression of high levels of bcl-2 protein. Blood 83(4), 899-906.

Discussion

Isaac Witz: What determines the steady state *in vivo* during tumor dormancy that can last for two years? Do you have antibody synthesis all the time?
Richard Scheuermann: Yes.
Isaac Witz: Is IgM formation unchanged all the time?
Richard Scheuermann: There are serum anti-idiotype antibodies that you can demonstrate in these animals and this is maintained with time. However, I have oversimplified the *in vivo* requirements for dormancy here. We know that T cells and T cell-derived cytokines can have an impact on the longevity of dormancy and on the number of animals that become dormant. So there are definitely other effects. The stroma is probably also playing some kind of role that we have not addressed.
Isaac Witz: If I recall, there is sometimes a spontaneous escape from dormancy. What would be the mechanism for that? Altered antibody synthesis? Effects on angiogenesis?
Richard Scheuermann: Yes. We get escape from dormancy in these animals. Escapees can be divided into two groups. One group is still susceptible to dormancy induction when you put them into new mice, so presumably there has been some change in the original host. The other group is now permanently resistant to dormancy induction. We have started to look to see if we could detect any changes in those escapees, and we have found that some of them have alterations in some of these signal transduction proteins, like Syk and HS1, which is a Lyn target.
Siegfried Janz: What is the tissue site of dormancy? Is it the spleen?
Richard Scheuermann: We can certainly detect lymphoma cells in the spleen, but there is also probably a reservoir in lymph nodes as well.
Siegfried Janz: How does it look? Do you have a small, distinct focus of terminal cells or individual scattered cells?
Richard Scheuermann: In the spleen we see individual scattered cells in the red pulp.
Andreas Radbruch: Do you also find idiotype variants among the escapees?
Richard Scheuermann: Yes, about ten to fifteen percent.
Michael Reth: Did you get any BCR-negative variants in these experiments?
Richard Scheuermann: In the escapees in the animal, we did not get idiotype-negative variants, we got anti-Ig-negative variants. We think that is because we have a polyclonal response to the idiotype, so it is hard to get an Id-negative variant, but about 10-15% were Ig-negative variants. We have not seen that *in vitro*.
Michael Reth: Were these cells surface Ig-negative or completely Ig-negative?
Richard Scheuermann: I am not sure.

Importance of CD44 Variant Isoforms in Mouse Models for Inflammatory Bowel Disease

U. Günthert
Basel Institute for Immunology, Grenzacherstrasse 487, CH-4005 Basel, Switzerland

Introduction

A major part of immune surveillance is controlled by cell surface molecules. Defined changes in the cellular communication are features of haemopoiesis, immune pathology, embryonic development and neoplastic transformation. The transmembrane glycoprotein CD44 and its many isoforms is one of these adhesion molecules (reviewed in Günthert 1996).

Experimental evidence has pointed out the involvement of CD44 isoforms in lymphocyte activation and homing into inflamed tissues, haemopoiesis, tumour dissemination and pattern formation in embryogenesis (as reviewed in Kincade et al. 1997; Lesley et al. 1997; Günthert 1996; Stauder and Günthert 1995; Ruiz et al. 1995; Günthert et al. 1995). This multipurpose nature of CD44 can possibly be explained by the enormous number of isoforms. Although only encoded by one gene, CD44 isoforms represent a large family of molecules which differ in the primary structure. These differences are produced by alternative splicing of at least ten unique exons, encoding extracellular regions out of a total of twenty exons. The function of specific variant isoforms (CD44v) has been a matter of debate for a long time. With the availability of genetically modified mice a clearer picture is emerging now. The purpose of this article is to give an overview on our current knowledge of the role of CD44 isoforms in autoimmune diseases and inflammation, with special emphasis on inflammatory bowel disease.

Inflammatory bowel disease (IBD) is regarded as a dysregulated immune response to components of the normal intestinal flora (reviewed in MacDonald, 1999). In humans, Crohn's disease and ulcerative colitis are most severe chronic inflammations with a devastating presentation. The lamina propria is massively infiltrated by activated lymphocytes, plasma cells and macrophages. The lymphocytes are mostly of T helper 1 subsets (Th1), secreting pro-inflammatory cytokines, such as IL-2 and IFN-γ, whereas the macrophages secrete IL-1, IL-6, IL-8, IL-12 and TNF-α. Activated human and mouse lymphocytes are known to upregulate CD44v isoforms (reviewed in Stauder and Günthert, 1995) and hence we were interested to find out whether CD44v is of importance for the disease process in mouse models for inflammatory bowel disease. Whether the data on mouse models also apply to humans still has to be further analysed. Consistent in the two species is an exaggerated Th1 response in the lamina propria, accompanied by injury of the mucosa.

Mouse Models for Inflammatory Bowel Disease

Our understanding of the human disease has gained enormous progress by the availability of animal models. These include the chemically induced experimental colitis such as the 2,4,6-trinitrobenzene sulfonic acid (TNBS)-induced colitis and the dextran sodium sulfate (DSS)-induced colitis (reviewed in Strober et al. 1997). Furthermore, rather unexpectedly, transgenic mice bearing targeted deletions for TCR-α or -β, MHC class II, IL-2 or IL-10 also develop colitis (for review see Strober and Ehrhardt 1993). In a third model the pivotal role of $CD4^+$ T cells in experimental colitis has been demonstrated: adoptive transfer of $CD4^+CD45RB^{hi}$ ("naive") cells into immunodeficient mice (C.B-17 scid and Rag -/- mice) leads to spontaneous chronic inflammation. Another subset of $CD4^+$ T cells is able to prevent the disease when co-transferred, namely the $CD45RB^{lo}$ ("memory") population (see reviews by Powrie 1995; Mason and Powrie 1998). In the non-inflamed mucosa, subsets of so-called regulatory T cells mediate antigen-specific immunoregulation and thereby prevent inappropriate responses to foreign antigens and to self antigens. Disease in all three models is characterized by a highly polarized Th1 response accompanied by the production of pro-inflammatory cytokines (as reviewed in Ludviksson et al. 1997).

A single rectal application of **TNBS** in susceptible mice (129SV and Balb/c) induces a severe colitis, leading to wasting disease and often death within a short period. This inflammatory reaction is driven by an unbridled Th1 response, caused by a dysregulation of pro-inflammatory and regulatory cytokines. Knowing that certain CD44v isoforms are explicitly involved in lymphocyte activation and can be upregulated by inflammatory cytokines (Mackay et al. 1994), we have asked whether antibodies against variant regions would influence this inflammatory reaction. Application of anti-CD44v7 given at 2 and 24 hours after TNBS treatment, but not of anti-v6 or -v10 antibodies, strongly prevents this experimentally induced colitis (Wittig et al. 1998). Even after the onset of the disease, treatment with anti-v7 antibodies leads to a complete regeneration of the intestine (Wittig et al. 1998). While in mice treated with TNBS alone the lamina propria is strongly infiltrated by leukocytes in 96% of the mice, TNBS plus anti-v7 antibody treated mice show signs of inflammation, but only in the initial phase after TNBS treatment, then in 71% of the mice the intestine recovers completely. The ongoing inflammatory reaction in the control mice is evident by an increased production of IFN-γ, while in the anti-v7 treated mice a slight reduction of IFN-γ is accompanied by a strong increase in the secretion of the anti-inflammatory cytokine IL-10 ten days after TNBS application (Wittig et al. 1998). Thus, anti-CD44v7 may prove to be a very efficient and highly specific therapeutic agent in IBD which could interfere by restraining the unbalanced Th1 reaction.

To further define the role of CD44v6/v7 containing isoforms in colitis, mice bearing a targeted deletion for either exons v6+v7 or v7 alone, without affecting expression of the residual CD44 regions, have been treated with TNBS. Whilst most of the wildtype mice from the same breedings develop severe signs of colitis, mice lacking CD44v6/v7 or CD44v7 containing isoforms show only weak inflammatory reactions shortly after TNBS treatment, then recover completely (Wittig et al. submitted). Analyses of the cytokine pattern of lamina propria cells in CD44v6v7 and CD44v7 k.o. mice treated with TNBS have revealed a strong reduction of inflammatory cytokines/chemokines, such as IL-12, IFN-γ and MIP-1α/β at later stages after treatment, whereas in the wildtype mice these substances continued to be produced at high levels. On the other hand, the anti-inflammatory cytokines, IL-10 and TGF-β, are downregulated in the wildtype mice upon TNBS treatment, these cytokines are still present at late stages in the TNBS treated CD44v k.o. mice (Wittig et al. submitted). The cytokine patterns clearly indicate that the inflammatory reaction in the TNBS treated k.o. mice is downregulated.

The beneficial regulatory role of **IL-10** in mucosal inflammation has been explicitly analysed in the human disease, as well as in animal models (van Deventer et al. 1997, Groux et al. 1997). Consequently, IL-10 deficient mice spontaneously develop a generalized enterocolitis under conventional housing conditions, and the inflammation can be prevented by administration of recombinant IL-10 (Kühn et al., 1993 and reviewed in Rennick et al. 1997). Treatment with IL-10 also ameliorates inflammation in the TNBS-induced colitis (Duchmann et al., 1996), or in the adoptive transfer of $CD4^{+}CD45RB^{hi}$ cells into immunodeficient mice (reviewed by Mason and Powrie 1998). The cause for the intestinal inflammation in IL-10 deficient mice is supposedly the inability to downregulate the production of inflammatory cytokines by macrophages and Th1 cells resulting in an excessive generation and activation of Th1 cells. Treatment with antibodies against the Th1 polarizing cytokines IL-12 or IFN-γ prevents enterocolitis in IL-10 deficient mice; furthermore $CD4^{+}$ T cells from IL-10 -/- mice are able to transfer enterocolitis to Rag -/- mice (reviewed in Rennick et al. 1997).

CD44 variant isoforms are only expressed at the base of the colonic crypts in the non-inflamed intestine (Gotley et al. 1996), therefore we were interested to find out the expression pattern in the inflamed lesions. Lamina propria cells prepared from wildtype mice treated with TNBS or from IL-10 deficient mice express a variety of large CD44v isoforms, mostly including v6 and v7 regions. The expression patterns are very similar to the one observed after activation of human T cells and in high grade non-Hodgkin lymphoma cells (Stauder and Günthert 1995). Comparison of CD44v expression patterns in Th1 and Th2 cells reveals exclusive expression of CD44v6 and v7 containing isoforms in the Th1 subsets, but not in the Th2 cells (Wittig et al. submitted).

An essential role for CD44v6/v7 isoforms in the maintenance of colitis has further been substantiated by crossbreeding the CD44v6/v7 -/- mice with mice carrying a targeted deletion for IL-10. The inability to express CD44v6/v7 containing isoforms in mice lacking IL-10 production (double deficient mice) has attenuated the onset of the intestinal inflammation substantially and furthermore has strongly ameliorated the disease as compared to IL-10 -/- CD44 wildtype mice (Wittig et al. submitted).

From the experiments outlined in this brief overview it is evident that CD44 variant isoforms, namely CD44v7 containing isoforms, are functionally involved in inflammatory processes in experimental colitis. Two different murine models for IBD reveal that the disease cannot only be blocked by anti-CD44v7 specific antibodies, but mice deficient for the expression of CD44v6v7 and CD44v7 containing isoforms are protected against a full-blown disease. In the TNBS induced colitis the k.o. mice only show initial signs of inflammation, then the intestine recovers. The deficiency for v6v7 containing isoforms in IL-10 -/- mice ameliorates the chronic enterocolitis in these colitis-prone mice substantially.

Why and at which stage is the region encoded by CD44v6/v7 important in murine IBD? We know that the inflammatory lesions in the colon are massively infiltrated by activated Th1 cells, which show a specific upregulation of CD44v6v7 containing isoforms (Wittig et al. submitted). This upregulation is specific for Th1 cells, it is not observed on Th2 cells (Wittig et al. submitted). Modulation of the surface of the strongly expanding Th1 cells, which is pivotal for the inflammatory process, could be essential for the interaction with macrophages. In the initial inflammatory reaction the expanding Th1 cells secrete IFN-γ, TNF-α and IL-2 (Figure 1). Mainly the

IFN-γ production stimulates IL-12 secretion by macrophages, accompanied by other inflammatory cytokines. IL-12 plays a central role in establishing a chronic inflammatory disease, because it stimulates in a feedback loop the production of IFN-γ by Th1 cells. The effects we observe by blocking this interaction between Th1 cells and macrophages with CD44v7 specific antibodies or generating Th1 cells which are unable to express CD44v7 could explain why these mice only have an initial inflammatory response, then recover. Another important surface interaction between Th1 cells and macrophages or other antigen presenting cells (APCs) is brought about by the costimulatory molecules CD40L (on Th1 cells) and CD40 (on APCs). Ligation of CD40-CD40L results in an immediate and dramatic increase of CD44H expression on both cell types, the Th1 cells and the APCs (Guo et al. 1996). However, in contrast to what has been published by Guo and colleagues (1996) we observe a strong upregulation of CD44 variant isoforms in addition to CD44H upon CD40-CD40L ligation (unpublished observation). Hence, when CD40-CD40L ligation induces CD44v7 expression on Th1 cells and APCs, CD44v7 molecules may be required for the sustained interaction between Th1 cells and macrophages (Figure 1).

In a healthy environment, immunoregulatory mechanisms suppress the generation of autoreactive T cells. Among the population of $CD4^{+}CD45RB^{lo}$ cells, so-called T regulatory (Tr) cells exist, which secrete TGF-β and IL-10 (Groux et al., 1997). Tr cells, generated from $CD4^{+}$ T cells in the presence of IL-10, can mediate bystander suppression in immunodeficient mice, adoptively transferred with colitis-inducing $CD4^{+}CD45RB^{hi}$ cells (Groux et al., 1997).

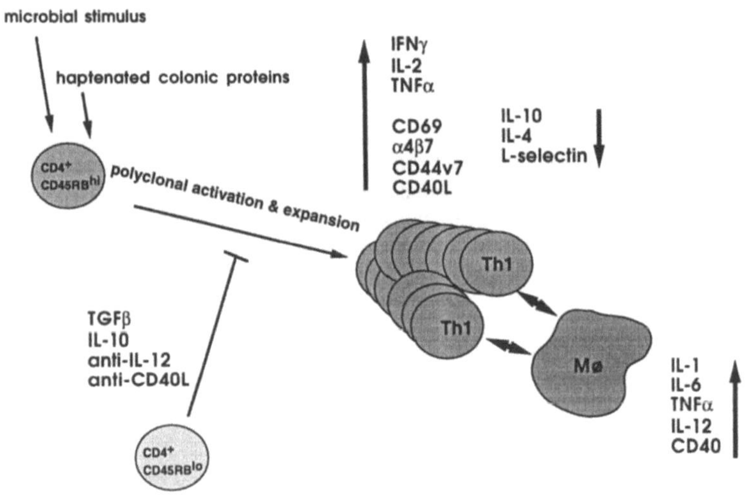

Figure 1: Involvement of CD44v7 in mouse inflammatory bowel disease. Microbial stimuli and/or haptenated colonic proteins lead to a massive expansion of Th1 cells, most likely resulting from the polyclonal activation of $CD4^{+}CD45RB^{hi}$ effector cells. This expansion can be blocked by $CD4^{+}CD45RB^{lo}$ cells (including the Tr regulatory cells), secreting TGF-β and IL-10, or by application of anti-IL-12 or anti-CD40L antibodies (Stüber et al. 1996). Th1 cells secrete IFN-γ, IL-2 and TNF-α and upregulate expression of CD69, α4β7, CD40L and CD44v6v7. L-selectin, IL-10 and IL-4 are downregulated. The interaction with macrophages, predominantly via CD40-CD40L ligation then induces IL-12 production by macrophages which in a feedback loop stimulates further IFN-γ production by Th1 cells, sustaining the inflammatory reaction. Anti-CD44v7 antibodies may block the interaction between Th1 cells and macrophages.

Mouse Models for Other Autoimmune Diseases

Do the above described observations also apply for other Th1 driven autoimmune diseases? **Experimental autoimmune encephalomyelitis** (EAE), an animal model for multiple sclerosis, is a chronic inflammatory autoimmune disease of the central nervous system (CNS) and characterized by demyelination of nerve axons, axonal loss and infiltration of the CNS by mononuclear cells. $CD4^+$ Th1 cells seem to be important for the onset of this inflammatory process as well and consequently, blocking the CD40-CD40L interaction can efficiently cure EAE in mice (Gerritse et al. 1996). CD44 variant isoforms are upregulated in these infiltrates in humans, monkeys and mice (Laman et al. in prep.). Treatment of SJL mice with various anti-CD44 variant mAb at the time of induction of EAE with proteolipid protein (PLP) leads to a substantial amelioration of disease burden pointing out the importance of CD44 variant isoforms in this autoimmune disease as well (Laman et al. 1998).

Further evidence for an essential role of CD44 in autoimmune diseases has been obtained in a murine model for **rheumatoid arthritis** (RA) (Mikecz et al. 1995). Treatment of affected mice with an anti-panCD44 antibody which recognizes all isoforms, completely abrogated tissue oedema, joint stiffness and leukocyte infiltration. Our preliminary data indicate that treatment with anti-CD44v antibodies also leads to a dramatic reduction of disease in the collagen induced RA, again pointing out the significance of the variant CD44 region in this Th1 driven autoimmune disease.

Concluding Remarks

The data obtained with mouse models for autoimmune diseases concerning the involvement of CD44 variant isoforms highlight the apparent importance of CD44v6v7 containing isoforms in inflammatory autoimmune diseases characterized by the infiltration of Th1 lymphocytes. It is tempting to speculate that the data obtained in mouse models may also apply for human Th1 driven autoimmune diseases such as ulcerative colitis, Crohn's disease, multiple sclerosis, rheumatoid arthritis, systemic lupus erythrematosus and insulin-dependent diabetes mellitus. Therapeutic treatment with humanized antibodies or peptides interfering with the CD44v6v7 region in humans may be of major importance in future drug design for treating these widespread chronic diseases.

Acknowledgements

I am grateful to my colleagues Drs. Bianca Wittig and Christoph Schwärzler for their invaluable help, suggestions and thoughtful comments. For critical review of the manuscript I would like to thank Drs. Annegret de Baey and Thomas Harder. The Basel Institute was founded and is supported by F. Hoffmann La Roche, Inc., Basel, Switzerland.

References

Duchmann R, Schmitt E, Knolle P, Meyer zum Büschenfelde KH, Neurath M (1996) Tolerance towards resident intestinal flora in mice is abrogated in experimental colitis and restored by treatment with interleukin-10 or antibodies to interleukin-12. Eur J Immunol 26:934-938

Gerritse K, Laman JD, Noelle RJ, Aruffo A, Ledbetter JA, Boersma WJA, Claassen E (1996) CD40-CD40 ligand interactions in experimental allergic encephalomyelitis and multiple sclerosis. Proc Natl Acad Sci USA 93:2499-2504

Gotley DC, Fawcett J, Walsh MD, Reeder JA, Simmons DL, Antalis TM (1996) Alternatively spliced variants of the cell adhesion molecule CD44 and Tumour progression in colorectal cancer. Br J Cancer 74:342-351

Groux H, O'Garra A, Bigler M, Rouleau M, Antonenko S, de Vries JE, Roncarolo MG (1997) A CD4+ T-cell subset inhibits antigen-specific T-cell responses and prevents colitis. Nature 389:737-742

Günthert U (1996) CD44 in malignant disorders. Current Topics Microbiol Immunol 213-I:271-285

Günthert U, Stauder R, Mayer B, Terpe H-J, Finke L, Friedrichs K (1995) Are CD44 variant isoforms involved in human tumour progression? Cancer Surveys 24:19-42

Guo Y, Wu Y, Shinde S, Sy MS, Aruffo A, Liu Y (1996) Identification of a costimulatory molecule rapidly induced by CD40L as CD44H. J Exp Med 184: 955-961

Kincade PW, Zheng Z, Katoh S, Hanson L (1997) The importance of cellular environment to function of the CD44 matrix receptor. Curr Opin Cell Biol 9: 635-642

Kühn R, Löhler J, Rennick D, Rajewski K, Müller W (1993) Interleukin-10-deficient mice develop chronic enterocolitis. Cell 75:263-274

Laman JD, Maassen CBM, Schellekens MM, Visser L, Kap M, de Jong E, van Puijenbroek M, Stipdonk MJB, van Meurs M, Schwärzler C, Günthert U (1998) Therapy with antibodies against CD40L (CD154) and CD44-variant isoforms reduces experimental autoimmune encephalomyelitis induced by a proteolipid protein peptide. Multiple Sclerosis 4:147-153

Lesley J, Hyman R, English N, Catterall JB, Turner GA (1997) CD44 in inflammation and metastasis. Glycoconj J 14:611-622

Ludviksson BR, Ehrhardt RO, Fuss IJ, Strober W (1997) Mucosal and thymic dysregulation. Role in human intestinal inflammation. Immunologist 5/6:202-209

MacDonald TT (1999) Effector and regulatory lymphoid cells and cytokines in mucosal sites. CTMI 236:113-135

Mackay CR, Terpe H-J, Stauder R, Marston WL, Stark H, Günthert U (1994) Expression and modulation of variant isoforms in humans. J Cell Biol 124:71-82

Mason D, Powrie F (1998) Control of immune pathology by regulatory T cells. Curr Opin Immunol 10:649-655

Mikecz K, Brennan FR, Kim JH, Glant TT (1995) Anti-CD44 treatment abrogates tissue oedema and leukocyte infiltration in murine arthritis. Nature Med 1:558-563

Powrie F (1995) T cells in inflammatory bowel disease: protective and pathogenic roles. Immunity 3:171-174

Rennick DM, Fort MM, Davidson NJ (1997) Studies with IL-10 -/- mice: an overview. J Leukoc Biol 61:389-396

Ruiz P, Schwärzler C, Günthert U (1995) CD44 isoforms during differentiation and development. BioEssays 17:17-24

Stauder R, Günthert U (1995) CD44 isoforms - impact on lymphocyte activation and differentiation. Immunologist 3:78-83

Strober W, Ehrhardt RO (1993) Chronic intestinal inflammation: an unexpected outcome in cytokine or T cell receptor mutant mice. Cell 75: 203-205

Strober W, Kelsall B, Fuss I, Marth T, Ludviksson B, Ehrhardt R, Neurath M (1997) Reciprocal IFN-γ and TGF-β responses regulate the occurrence of mucosal inflammation. Immunol Today 18:61-64

Stüber E, Strober W, Neurath M (1996) Blocking the CD40L-CD40 interaction in vivo specifically prevents the priming of T helper 1 cells through the inhibition of interleukin 12 secretion. J Exp Med 183:693-698

van Deventer SJ, Elson CO, Fedorak RN (1997) Multiple doses of intravenous interleukin 10 in steroid-refractory Crohn's disease. Gastroenterology 113:383-389

Wittig B, Schwärzler C, Föhr N, Günthert U, Zöller M (1998) Curative treatment of an experimentally induced colitis by a CD44 variant v7 specific antibody. J Immunol 161:1069-1073

Discussion

Mike Potter: Can you tell us more about what TNBS does to the colon?
Ursula Günthert: TNBS is a contact-sensitizing allergen which haptenates normal colonic proteins by transferring TNP groups and thereby generates a strong stimulus.
Steven Pals: Can you say more about the mechanism by which CD44 acts. There are papers by Mark Siegelman's group which show that CD44 mediates rolling on hyaluronate-positive vessels at sites of inflammation. Do you think that your knockout somehow interferes with this hyaluronic binding. Of course CD44v6v7 is not a hyaluronate binding domain, but it might be that the hyaluronate binding is complexly inhibited? Did you look in the complete CD44 k.o. of Tak Mak's group?
Ursula Günthert: I do not think that hyaluronic acid is involved because we can specifically block with the anti-CD44v7 antibody, and it has been shown that there are not such big differences between the interaction with hyaluronic acid, whether it is the standard or any of the variant isoforms. Secondly, the Tak Mak CD44 k.o. mice appear to be leaky due to trans-splicing between the standard exons 1 and 4, hence they are still able to generate the variant molecules, but are deficient in hyaluronate binding. Maybe they are a good model for differentiating between ability to bind or not to bind to hyaluronate via CD44.
Steven Pals: This is a very acute disease so is there any role for granulocytes? You say it is a T cell-mediated disease but because it looks like an acute toxic mega-colon-like disease, there should be a massive polynuclear influx as well. What is the role of granulocytes?
Ursula Günthert: We have not analyzed the role of granulocytes. We have, however, analyzed two models for inflammatory bowel disease with a chronic development, namely colitis in the IL-10 k.o. mice and the adoptive transfer of T cells into immunodeficient mice. We crossed the IL-10 k.o. mice onto the CD44v6v7-deficient background. We could show that the onset of the chronic inflammatory disease is greatly attenuated by about 10 to 15 weeks in the double k.o. mice, and although the double k.o. mice developed a prolapse of the colon at later stages, the histology of the colon is almost normal as compared to the IL-10 k.o. mice. In the adoptive transfer model of Fiona Powrie CD45RBhi T cells can induce colitis in immunodeficient mice. The colitis can be blocked by co-transferring CD45RBlo T cells. However, when we co-transfer CD45RBlo cells of the CD44v6v7 k.o. mice, they are unable to block the colitis. We could also show efficient blocking of the disease mediated by CD45RBhi cells by treating the mice with anti-CD44v7 antibodies.
Mike Potter: What are the etiological factors in chronic inflammatory bowel disease that occurs in various species? I am thinking of my favorite cat that I lost last year to this disease. Does helicobacter play a role?
Ursula Günthert: The microenvironment definitely plays a very strong role initially, hence in a germ-free environment the mice do not get colitis.
Frans Kroese: Some people say that maybe breaking tolerance to the micro-flora might be involved, so in respect to that we studied the coating of bacteria with IgA, IgM and IgG on the flora. This shows that patients with inflammatory bowel disease have very high levels of coating on the bacteria, so it might be interesting to study Ig coating on your bacteria: your mice are sitting in their cages so you just have to test some of their fecal samples.
Ursula Günthert: Before we treat the mice with TNBS, we take them out of the SPF unit and put them into the non-SPF for one week.
Sandy Morse: What happens with other inflammatory stimuli, such as croton oil, or with pristane in the belly, or other things like that?
Ursula Günthert: We have not done that yet. I would assume that these inflammatory stimuli also upregulate CD44v.

Reference:

Appelmelk BJ, Faller G, Claeys D, Kirchner T, Vandenbroucke-Grauls CMJE (1998) Bugs on trial: the case of Helicobacter pylori and autoimmunity. Immunol Today 19:296-299

EBNA2 and c-myc in B Cell Immortalization by Epstein-Barr Virus and in the Pathogenesis of Burkitt's Lymphoma

U. Zimber-Strobl, L. Strobl, H. Höfelmayr, B. Kempkes, M. S. Staege, G. Laux, B. Christoph, A. Polack, and G. W. Bornkamm
Institut für Klinische Molekularbiologie und Tumorgenetik, GSF-Forschungszentrum für Umwelt und Gesundheit, Marchioninistr. 25, D-81377 München

Introduction

Epstein-Barr virus (EBV) is a ubiquitous human herpes virus with the unique ability to immortalize primary resting human B lymphocytes. The virus is the causative agent of infectious mononucleosis and is associated with a number of human malignancies including Burkitt's Lymphoma, Nasopharyngeal Carcinoma, Hodgkin's Disease, and Immunoblastic Lymphoma arising in immunocompromized individuals (for review, see Rickinson and Kieff, 1995). The pathogenicity of the virus is closely linked to its immortalizing capacity. Studying the role of EBV in B cell immortalization may thus help to better understand the role of the virus in disease pathogenesis. In EBV immortalized cells only a limited set of viral gene products is expressed including six nuclear (EBNA1, EBNA2, EBNA3A, -3B, -3C and EBNA-LP) and two membrane proteins (LMP1 and LMP2) (for review, see Kieff, 1995). For several reasons EBNA2 plays a pivotal role in B cell immortalization: (i) deletion of the EBNA2 gene leads to the loss of the immortalizing capacity of the virus, (ii) EBNA2, together with EBNA-LP, is the first viral gene expressed in infected B cells, and (iii) EBNA2 is a transcriptional regulator acting as a master switch regulating the expression of a number of cellular genes (e.g. CD21 and CD23) and viral genes involved in B cell immortalization. Amongst the viral genes regulated by EBNA2 are the LMP1 and LMP2 genes and the large transcription unit giving rise to EBNA-LP and EBNA2 as well as the family of EBNA3 proteins. EBNA2 exerts its function as a transcriptional regulator without binding to DNA directly. It is thus of primary importance to elucidate the molecular mechanism of action of EBNA2.

Burkitt's lymphoma is a highly malignant B cell tumor prevalent in areas with tropical climate (central Africa and New Guinea) as well as in HIV positive individuals, and occurs with low incidence in all parts of the world. About 95% of the cases from Africa and New Guinea and about 50% of the cases in HIV seropositives harbor the viral genome, whereas only about 10 to 15% of the other cases are EBV positive. The tumor is, however, invariably characterized by chromosomal translocations juxtaposing the c-myc gene of chromosome 8 to one of the immunoglobulin gene loci on chromosome 2, 14, or 22 leading to very high and unregulated expression of this oncogene. Remarkably, of the viral genes involved in B cell immortalization only EBNA1 is expressed in Burkitt lymphoma cells (so called group I pattern of viral gene expression as opposed to the group III pattern in EBV immortalized cells) (Rickinson and Kieff, 1995).

We have studied the molecular mechanism of action of EBNA2 and have developed a model system in which important features of the pathogenesis of Burkitt's lymphoma can be recapitulated *in vitro*.

EBNA2 binds to EBNA2 response elements through interaction with the cellular protein RBP-Jκ

Studying the LMP2 promoter we have been able to identify an EBNA2 response element (EBNA2RE) and to narrow it down by deletion analysis to 81 bp (-177 to -258) relative to the transcriptional start site of LMP2. Analysis of scanning mutations revealed that a duplicated sequence motif of 11 bp within the EBNA2RE is critical not only for transactivation by EBNA2 but also for binding of a 60 kd cellular protein which tethers EBNA2 to its response element (Zimber-Strobl et al., 1993, 1994) and acts as a repressor in the absence of EBNA2 (Dou et al., 1994; Hsieh and Hayward, 1995). Several groups including ours have purified this protein and identified it as RBP-Jκ, a ubiquitously expressed nuclear protein which is highly conserved in evolution (Henkel et al., 1994; Grossman et al., 1994; Waltzer et al., 1994; Zimber-Strobl et al., 1994). RBP-Jκ is part of the *Notch* signal transduction pathway. *Notch* is a membrane receptor (with four mammalian homologues) involved in asymmetric cell division and cell fate decisions in organisms as diverse as C.elegans, Drosophila and mammals (Artavanis-Tsakonas et al., 1995). As shown in Fig. 1, *Notch* is clipped off the membrane upon binding of its ligands *Delta* or *Serrate* (and the mammalian homologues *Delta* and *Jagged*), translocates to the nucleus, binds to RBP-Jκ, and acts as a transcriptional activator of genes harboring RBP-Jκ binding sites (Schroeter et al., 1998). EBNA2 can thus be regarded as a viral homologue of activated *Notch* (Hsieh et al., 1996).

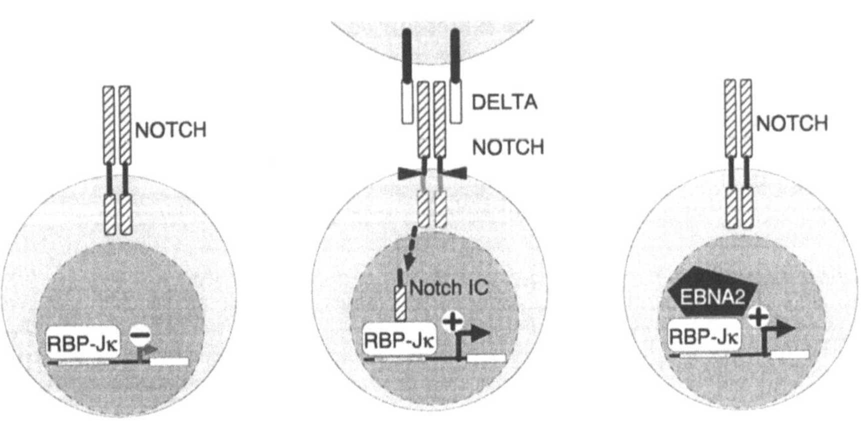

Fig. 1. Schematic representation of the mechanism of action of RBP-Jκ, EBNA2 and the intracellular domain of Notch.

c-myc is a Target of Positive and Igμ a Target of Negative Regulation by EBNA2

Besides the biochemical studies of EBNA2 we were aiming to develop a system in which the contribution of EBNA2 to B cell proliferation could be studied directly.

To this end, we have constructed genes encoding N- and C-terminal fusions of EBNA2 with the hormone binding domain of the estrogen receptor (ER-EBNA2/EBNA2-ER) to render the function of EBNA2 regulatable by estrogen (Picard et al., 1988). These fusion genes were used to complement the defect of the immortalization incompetent, EBNA2 defective P3HR1 virus and to immortalize primary human B lymphocytes with this virus in the presence of estrogen (Kempkes et al., 1995). Lymphoblastoid cell lines (EREB lines) were thus established which proliferate in the presence of estrogen and stop proliferating when estrogen is withdrawn from the growth medium. Arrest of proliferation is reversible in these cells. The cells resume growth after readdition of estrogen and reenter S phase 18 hours after turning on EBNA2 again. The onset of DNA synthesis is preceded by a cascade of events starting with the induction of transcription of the LMP1 and c-myc genes one to two hours after addition of estrogen, followed by induction of transcription of cyclin D2 and cdk4 after about 6 hours and induction of E2F1 and phosphorylation of Rb at about 10 to 12 hours (Kempkes et al., 1995). As opposed to LMP1 and c-myc, Igμ expression is strongly upregulated by withdrawal of estrogen and downregulated to the low initial expression level when hormone is readded to the cells (Jochner et al., 1996, Fig. 2).

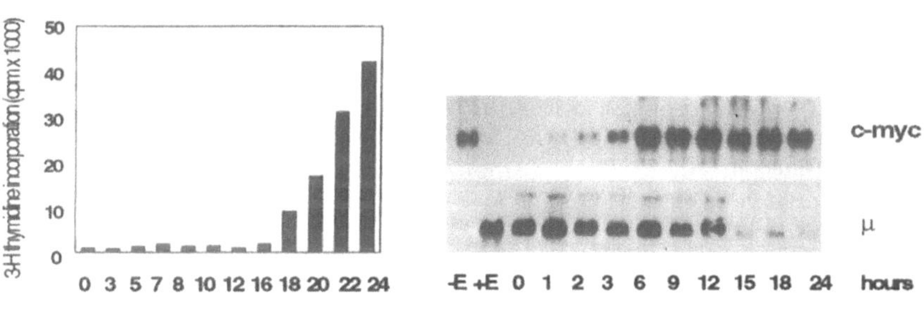

Fig. 2. Induction of DNA synthesis in hormone-deprived EREB cells upon readdition of estrogen is preceded by upregulation of c-myc (left) and downregulation of Igμ expression (right panel).

Constitutive High c-myc but not LMP1 Expression Renders Proliferation of EREB Cells Independent of EBNA2 and its Target Genes

The oncogenic potential of c-myc and LMP1 is very well documented. Since both genes are direct target genes of EBNA2, it was obvious to ask whether constitutive high expression of c-myc or LMP1 would substitute for EBNA2 in the maintenance of proliferation. LMP1 constitutively expressed from the SV40 promoter on an EBV derived episomal vector contributed significantly to survival of EREB cells after estrogen deprivation but failed to promote cell proliferation on its own (Zimber-Strobl et al., 1996). Overexpression of c-myc on an episomal construct mimicking a chromosomal t(2;8) and bringing c-myc expression under the control of the Igκ intron and 3′ enhancers rendered proliferation of the cells, however, independent of EBNA2, LMP1 and other target genes of EBNA2

(Polack et al., 1996). Not only could proliferation of EREB cells be rescued in the absence of estrogen, the cells started moreover to grow as a single cell suspension and adopted the phenotype of Burkitt lymphoma cells *in vivo* (the so called BL group I phenotype). Adhesion (CD54 and CD58) and coactivation molecules (CD80 and CD86) were significantly downregulated as well as activation markers like CD21, CD23, CD39 and CD40, whereas molecules highly expressed on germinal center B cells and not or barely expressed on EBV immortalized cells (CD10 and CD38) were significantly upregulated (Polack et al., 1996 and Fig.3).

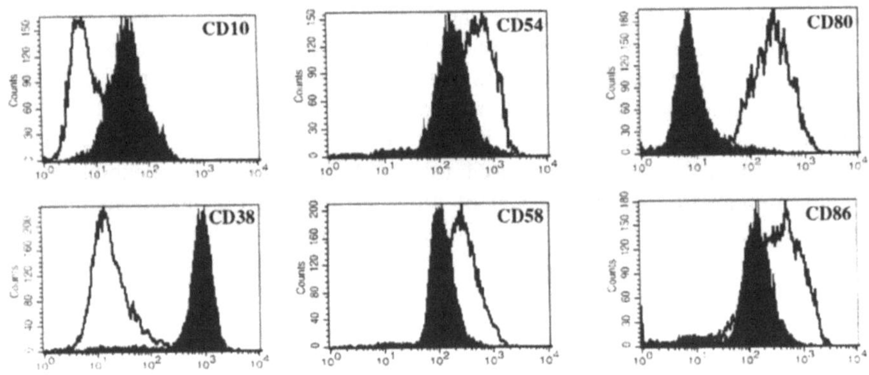

Fig. 3: Markers of germinal center cells (CD10 and CD38) are upregulated, whereas adhesion (CD54 and CD58) and coactivation molecules (CD80 and CD86) are downregulated in hormone-deprived c-myc overexpressing EREB cells (cell line A1, black curves) as compared to parental EREB cells (white curves).

High c-myc Expression in Hormone Deprived EREB Cells Severely Impairs Antigen Processing and Presentation

Masucci and coworkers have shown that Burkitt lymphoma group I cells exhibit selective downregulation of the HLA-A11 allele (Gavioli et al., 1992), low expression of the proteasome components Lmp2 and Lmp7 as well as an altered cleavage specificity of the proteasome for peptides (Frisan et al., 1998). Remarkably, highly c-myc expressing estrogen-deprived EREB cells (the cell line A1) not only exhibit a cell surface phenotype with downregulation of adhesion and coactivation molecules indistinguishable from Burkitt lymphoma group I cells, their proteasomes also show the same subunit composition and enzymatic activity as Burkitt lymphoma cells which are clearly different from that of EBV immortalized lymphoblastoid cells (Frisan et al., 1998). These findings suggest that virtually all cellular functions related to antigen processing, presentation and recognition are severely impaired in c-myc overexpressing hormone-deprived EREB cells in a fashion very similar if not indistinguishable from that of Burkitt lymphoma cells. As expected from the data presented, A1 cells are indeed neither recognized by HLA-restricted antigen-specific T cells nor by allogeneic peripheral blood mononuclear cells in a mixed lymphocyte reaction (Staege et al., manuscript in preparation).

Discussion

We have shown that a number of important features of Burkitt lymphoma cells including growth pattern, cell surface phenotype, antigen processing and presentation can be recapitulated in c-myc overexpressing hormone-deprived EREB cells *in vitro*. Our data indicate that the described properties of Burkitt lymphoma cells do not reflect their origin from germinal center cells. We rather conclude that the phenotype and some of the properties of germinal center cells are imposed onto the cells by high c-myc expression in the absence of expression of genes involved in B cell activation such as EBNA2 and LMP1. A critical step in the natural history of EBV infection is the establishment of *in vivo* latency. Thorley-Lawson and coworkers have shown that EBV persists in the B cell memory compartment and appears to exploit the physiological mechanisms of B cell development to establish latency and thus longevity in resting B cells *in vivo* (Miyashita et al., 1997; Babcock et al., 1998). The establishment of *in vivo* latency requires that the viral proliferation program with EBNA2 as a master switch for the other viral and cellular genes involved in this process be switched off. The mechanism how EBNA2 and the viral proliferation program is switched off, is, however, still totally elusive. The cytokine milieu might be important as suggested by the fact that IL-6 can induce differentiation of the lymphoblastoid cell line CESS associated with switching off the expression of EBNA2 as well as LMP1 (Altmeyer et al., 1997). The mechanism of establishing *in vivo* latency with EBNA2 being switched off is also of prime importance for the development of Burkitt's lymphoma for at least two reasons. First, EBNA2 negatively regulates expression of the IgH locus including a c-myc gene translocated into this locus through chromosomal t(8;14) translocation (Jochner et al., 1996), and secondly, EBNA2 antagonizes the effect of high c-myc expression on antigen processing and presentation (Staege et al., manuscript in preparation). EBNA2 and c-myc thus cooperate only as long as c-myc is expressed at a moderate level as in EBV immortalized cells. Expression of EBNA2 is, however, incompatible with the features of Burkitt lymphoma cells described above which are imposed by high c-myc expression. Understanding the shut-off mechanism of EBNA2 expression *in vivo* is thus crucial not only to understand EBV latency *in vivo* but also to elucidate the pathogenesis of Burkitt's lymphoma.

Acknowledgement

This work was supported by die Deutsche Forschungsgemeinschaft (SFB 217, SFB 1586, Forschergruppe "Multiproteinkomplexe") and EU Biomed 2.

References

Altmeyer A, Simmons RC, Krajewski S, Reed JC, Bornkamm GW, Chen-Kiang S (1997) Reversal of EBV immortalization precedes apoptosis in IL-6-induced human B cell terminal differentiation. Immunity 7: 667-677

Artavanis-Tsakonas S, Matsuno K, Fortini ME (1995) Notch signalling. Science 268: 225-232.

Babcock GJ, Decker LL, Volk M, Thorley-Lawson DA (1998) EBV persistence in memory B cells in vivo. Immunity 9: 395-404

Dou S, Zeng X, Cortes P, Erdjument-Bromage H, Tempst P, Honjo T, Vales LD (1994) The recombination signal sequence-binding protein RBP-2N functions as a transcriptional

repressor. Mol Cell Biol 14: 3310-3319
Frisan T, Levitsky V, Polack A, Masucci M (1998) Phenotype-dependent differences in protea some subunit composition and cleavage specifity in B cell lines. J Immunol. 160: 3281-3289
Gavioli R, De Campos-Lima PO, Kurilla MG, Kieff E, Klein G, Masucci MG (1992) Recogni tion of the Epstein-Barr virus-encoded nuclear antigens EBNA-4 and EBNA-6 by HLA-A11-restricted cytotoxic T lymphocytes: implications for down-regulation of HLA-A11 in Burkitt lymphoma. Proc Natl Acad Sci USA 89: 5862-5866
Grossman SR, Johannsen E, Tong X, Yalamanchili R, Kieff E (1994) The Epstein-Barr virus nuclear antigen 2 transactivator is directed to response elements by the Jκ recombination signal binding protein. Proc Natl Acad Sci USA 91: 7568-7572
Henkel T, Ling PD, Hayward SD, Peterson MG (1994) Mediation of Epstein-Barr virus EBNA2 transactivation by recombination signal-binding protein Jκ. Science 265: 92-95
Hsieh JJ, Hayward SD (1995) Masking of the CBF1/RBP-Jκ transcriptional repression domain by Epstein-Barr virus EBNA2. Science 268: 560-563
Hsieh JJ, Henkel T, Salmon P, Robey E, Peterson MG, Hayward SD (1996) Truncated Mammalian Notch1 activates CBF1/RBPJk-repressed genes by a mechanism resembling that of Epstein-Barr virus EBNA2. Mol Cell Biol 16: 952-959
Jochner N, Eick D, Zimber-Strobl U, Pawlita M, Bornkamm GW, Kempkes B (1996) Epstein-Barr virus nuclear antigen 2 is a transcriptional suppressor of the immunoglobulin μ gene: implications for the expression of the translocated c-myc gene in Burkitt's lymphoma cells. EMBO J 15: 375-382
Kempkes B, Spitkovsky D, Jansen-Dürr P, Ellwart JW, Kremmer E, Delecluse HJ, Rottenberger C, Bornkamm GW, Hammerschmidt W (1995) B-cell proliferation and induction of early G_1-regulation proteins by Epstein-Barr virus mutants conditional for EBNA2. EMBO J 14: 88-96
Kieff E (1995) Epstein-Barr virus and its replication. In: Fields: Virology, Lippincott Raven Publishers, Philadelphia, New York
Laux G, Adam B, Strobl LJ, Moreau-Gachelin F (1994) The Spi-1/PU.1 and Spi-B ets family transcription factors and the recombination signal binding protein RBP-Jκ interact with an Epstein-Barr virus nuclear antigen 2 responsive cis-element. EMBO J 13: 5624-5632
Miyashita EM, Yang B, Babcock GJ, Thorley-Lawson DA (1997) Identification of the site of Epstein-Barr virus persistence in vivo as a resting B cell. J Virol 71: 4882-4891
Picard D, Salser SJ, Yamamoto KR (1988) A movable and regulable inactivation function within the steroid binding domain of the glucocorticoid receptor. Cell 54: 1073-1080
Polack A, Hörtnagel K, Pajic A, Christoph B, Baier B, Falk M, Mautner J, Geltinger C, Bornkamm GW, Kempkes B (1996) c-myc activation renders proliferation of Epstein-Barr virus (EBV)-transformed cells independent of EBV nuclear antigen 2 and latent membrane protein 1. Proc Natl Acad Sci USA 93: 10411-10416
Rickinson AB, Kieff E (1995) Epstein Barr-virus and ist replication. In: Fields: Virology, Lippincott-Raven Publishers, Philadelphia, New York
Schroeter EH, Kisslinger JA, Kopan R (1998) Notch-1 signalling requires ligand-induced proteolytic release of intracellular domain. Nature 393: 382-386
Waltzer L, Logeat F, Brou C, Israel A, Sergeant A, Manet E (1994) The human Jκ recombination signal sequence binding protein (RBP-Jκ) targets the Epstein-Barr virus EBNA2 protein to its DNA responsive elements. EMBO J 13: 5633-5638
Zimber-Strobl U, Kremmer E, Grässer F, Marschall G, Laux G, Bornkamm GW (1993) The Epstein-Barr virus nuclear antigen 2 interacts with an EBNA2 responsive cis-element of the terminal protein 1 gene promoter. EMBO J 12: 167-175
Zimber-Strobl U, Strobl LJ, Meitinger C, Hinrichs R, Sakai T, Furukawa T, Honjo T, Bornkamm GW (1994) Epstein-Barr virus nuclear antigen 2 exerts ist transactivating function through interaction with recombination signal binding protein RBP-Jκ, the homologue of Drosophila Suppressor of Hairless. EMBO J 13: 4973-4982
Zimber-Strobl U, Kempkes B, Marschall G, Zeidler R, Van Kooten C, Banchereau J, Bornkamm GW, Hammerschmidt W (1996) Epstein-Barr virus latent membrane protein (LMP1) is not sufficient to maintain proliferation of B cells but both it and activated CD40 can prolong their survival. EMBO J 15: 7070-7078

Discussion

Richard Scheuermann: Do the LCL cell lines express EBNA2?
Georg Bornkamm: Yes, otherwise they would not grow.
Richard Scheuermann: Right, so then they upregulate myc but would that not turn them into a Burkitt cell line?
Georg Bornkamm: No, the level of myc upregulation is low as in a conventional lymphoblastoid cell line. It has low myc levels and you need a combination of other genes in order to drive proliferation. To induce a Burkitt-like phenotype, you have to drive myc really high.
Michael Carroll: Do the myc-transfected cells express FAS?
Georg Bornkamm: The LCLs do, but in the myc transfectants FAS is downregulated, along with the other T cell activation markers.

V

Myeloma, Plasmacytomas and Related Subjects

The Control of Proliferation, Survival and Apoptosis in Human Multiple Myeloma Cells *in vitro*

K. Nilsson, P. Georgii-Hemming, H. Spets and H. Jernberg-Wiklund
Laboratory of Tumor Biology, Department of Genetics and Pathology, University of Uppsala, S-751 85 Uppsala, Sweden.

Introduction

The biology of human multiple myeloma (MM) was poorly understood until recently. Only when IL-6 had been identified as an important growth factor for MM cells has it been possible to establish cell lines and to maintain fresh MM biopsy cells *in vitro* for weeks-months (Kawano et al 1988, Klein et al 1990, Nilsson et al 1990). This has allowed controlled *in vitro* studies of various aspects of the genotype and phenotype of MM cells during the 1990s. Some features are characteristic for MM cells. They include a restriction of the growth of MM cells almost exclusively to the bone marrow, chromosomal heterogeneity within and between individual MM clones, genetic instability, the presence at a high frequency of a translocation to the immunoglobulin (Ig) heavy chain or Ig light chain locus, a high and deregulated expression of c-Myc, a high expression of Bcl-2 and often a dependence of IL-6 and/or IGF-I as growth and survival factors. A common characteristic of MM cells both *in vitro* and *in vivo* is also that they proliferate slowly. At the population level the doubling time is often several days as a result of a long generation time (usually exceeding 36 hrs) and a high apoptotic rate. The first MM cell line established in our laboratory was in 1970 (Nilsson et al 1970). During the following decades additional MM lines were established (Nilsson, 1992) and a selected panel of lines, consisting also of MM cell lines established elsewhere, have been instrumental in studies on the control of growth and apoptosis during the last few years. The study at various levels of *in vitro* passages of two pairs of MM cell lines (Jernberg et al 1992a, Scibienski et al 1992) has given some insight in the progression of cultured MM clones with respect to genotypic and phenotypic properties. This paper summarizes some of these studies with the aim of presenting a hypothetical view on how certain genes in the tumor cells, and paracrine cytokines, interact to balance the growth and apoptosis in MM in favour of growth. The evolution *in vitro* seems to be such that MM cells with capacity for faster growth and less propensity for apoptosis are selected. Such MM cells develop *in vitro,* and most likely also *in vivo,* as a consequence of the ongoing genomic rearrangements that are the result of the genomic instability typical of MM.

Evolution of Enotypic and Phenotypic Properties During Long-term *in vitro* Culture

Studies on the evolution of several phenotypic characteristics and of the status and expression of selected genes controlling proliferation and apoptosis, i.e. c-Myc, Bcl-2, Rb, Ras, and p53, have been performed in some of our MM cell lines during long-term growth *in vitro*. (Nilsson 1977, Jernberg et al 1987, Nilsson 1994). The cell lines were examined during the process of establishment (a few - several months), during early passages (1-2 years) and during late passages (3-several years). Most MM clones are dependent on feeder cells (bone marrow derived stromal cells or human skin fibroblasts or glial cells) during early passages. Without a close contact with the feeder cells the MM cells will die. The signals involved to stimulate survival and growth seem to be cell-cell contacts, cell-extracellular matrix interactions and paracrine cytokines, primarily IL-6 (Jernberg et al 1991, Scibienski et al 1992, Van Riet et al 1997). During the phase of establishment MM cells grow very slowly, and the frequency of apoptotic cells is usually high. The few MM cell lines tested for tumorigenicity subcutaneously in nude mice have failed to form tumors. During the early passages MM lines can be observed to lose the dependence on direct contacts with the feeder cells but many lines retain the dependence on paracrine growth factor stimulation, i.e. IL-6. Such lines can be grown in non-stirred suspension cultures with supernatants from feeder cells as a source of IL-6. Most MM cell lines will increase their growth rate and decrease the apoptotic fraction of cells during long term *in vitro* culture. This improved growth and decreased apoptosis *in vitro* have also been found to correlate with the acquisition of the capacity to form tumors in nude mice and may thus be regarded as a progression towards a more malignant phenotype. In late passages most MM cell lines have become independent of IL-6 as a paracrine growth factor - in rare cases (the U-266 cell line) this appears to be the result of the development of an autocrine IL-6 loop (Jernberg-Wiklund et al 1992a). However, as will be discussed below, MM cell lines are very heterogeneous with respect to IL-6 dependence.

Table 1. Steps in the progression of human multiple myeloma cell lines *in vitro*

Characteristic	Newly explanted	Early passage	Late passage
Stromal cell dependence	+	+	-
IL-6 dependence	+	+/-	-/+
IGF-I dependence	+	+/-	-/+
Growth rate	Very slow	Slow	Rapid
Tumorigenicity	-	-	+
Apoptosis	High	Moderate	Low
Oncogene expression			
c-Myc	+	+/++	++
Bcl-2	+	+/++	+
Rb	+	+	-/+

The expression of c-Myc is generally high but variable in MM cells (Jernberg-Wiklund 1992b). In the U-266 the expression of Myc (L-Myc) increased with time in continuous culture, and this may be a general phenomenon in MM cell lines. Also the Bcl-2 expression is high in MM cell lines (Pettersson et al 1992). In the U-266 cell line the Bcl-2 expression decreased during long-term passage *in vitro*. In the U-266 the observed evolution of the cell line towards improved growth and survival thus correlates with an increase in c-Myc expression, a decrease in Bcl-2 expression and the development of an autocrine IL-6 loop. It is also notable that the Rb gene has been deleted on both alleles in late passage U-266 cells and that p53 is mutated (Corradini et al 1994, Nilsson 1994). This, and the observed increased frequency of mutations in Ras and p53, and Rb deletions in biopsies MM cells from patients with advanced disease (Hallek et al 1998), suggest that both *in vitro* and *in vivo* cells are selected within the genetically unstable MM clones which have deregulated c-Myc expression and mutations/deletions in other genes controlling proliferation and apoptosis. Taken together (Table 1) this might suggest that c-Myc and Bcl-2 are deregulated early during the evolution of MM while the Rb deletions and the Ras and p53 mutations are changes that reflect the Darwinistic selection mechanisms which occur later during the tumor progression.

IL-6 as a Growth and Survival Factor in Multiple Myeloma Cell Lines

MM cells interact with non-neoplastic cells in the bone marrow microenvironment. The nature of these contacts is not fully clear. However, several cell types seem to interact with MM cells by cell-cell contacts and by paracrine cytokine loops. Fig 1. summarizes our own and some studies of other groups on some of these interactions.

IL-6 seems to be a major paracrine growth and survival factor for MM cells, at least *in vitro* (Klein et al 1989). However, only a fraction of MM cell lines and MM biopsy cells requires IL-6 for growth and survival, as already pointed out. Among MM lines the heterogeneity is extensive (Jernberg et al 1991, Nilsson 1994, Spets et al 1997). MM cell lines depending on exogenous IL-6 can be classified into three groups - lines dependent on IL-6 for survival and growth, lines in which IL-6 is primarily a factor stimulating proliferation and lines dependent on IL-6 for survival but not growth. The IL-6 MM cell lines independent of exogenous IL-6 can be categorized into completely IL-6 independent cell lines, which are the majority, and lines in which an autocrine IL-6 loop is operating. Under serum-free conditions IL-6 usually is a growth and survival factor for IL-6 dependent MM cells lines but in one cell line (U-266) IL-6 may enhance apoptosis.

Whether this heterogeneity of MM cell lines and MM biopsy cells *in vitro* with respect to response to IL-6 mirrors the situation for MM cells in the bone marrow environment of the patients is not clear. Some recent studies (Westendorf et al 1994, Sati et al 1998) suggest that the cytokine network *in vivo*, as expected, is different from that *in vitro*, e.g. induced autocrine IL-6 loops in MM cells may be more frequent than hitherto assumed.

IGF-I as a Growth and Survival Factor in Multiple Myeloma Cell Lines

As depicted in Fig. 1 IGF-I is produced in the bone marrow microenvironment by several cell types, e.g. stromal cells, osteoblasts and osteoclasts. This, and the fact that IGF-I can inhibit c-Myc induced apoptosis in murine fibroblasts as shown by Harrington et al (1994), prompted us to investigate whether IGF-I might play a role in the control of proliferation/apoptosis in MM cells, known to express a possibly deregulated c-Myc at a high level.

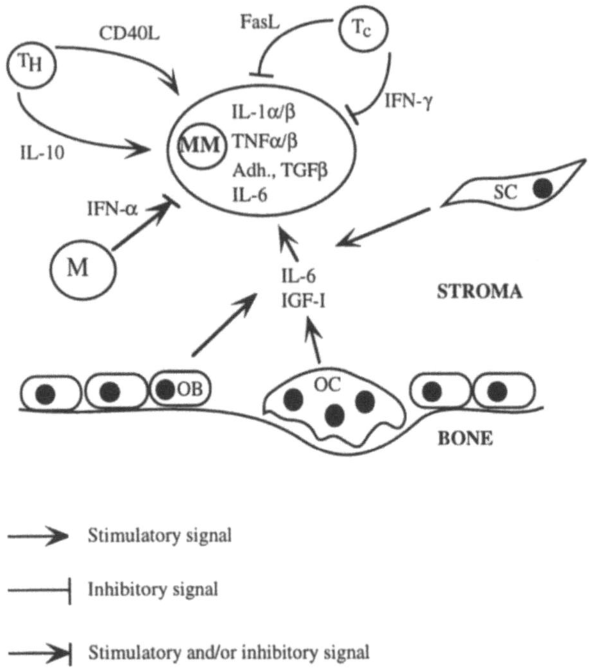

Fig 1. Interactions of MM with non-neoplastic cells of the bone marrow microenvironment. Results from other groups suggest that IL-1α/β, TNFα/β, IL-6 and some other cytokines and/or cell-cell contacts may mediate the activation of cells in the bone marrow. Data from our group suggest that MM cells may produce TGFβ1 that may activate cells of the bone marrow microenvironment. The activation leads to an increased production of factors, e.g. IL-6, IGF-I, IFN-α, IFN-γ, FasL, CD40L and IL-10, that regulate the growth and survival of MM cells. TH, T-helper lymphocytes. Tc, T-cytotoxic lymphocytes. M, macrophages. SC, other stromal cell. OB, osteoblast. OC, osteoclast.

Using a panel of three MM cell lines (EJM, Karpas 707 and LP-1), selected on the basis of their feeder cell and IL-6 independency, we first demonstrated that all lines expressed both IGF-I receptor (IGF-IR) and IGF-I mRNA and protein (Georgii-Hemming et al 1996). The expression of IGF-I and its receptor varied between the cell lines. Two cell lines (LP-1 and Karpas 707) responded in a dose-dependent manner to the stimulation of exogenous IGF-I by an increased growth and survival. The anti-apoptotic effect was strongest in the Karpas 707 cells. The possibility of autocrine IGF-I stimulation was examined by incubating LP-1 and Karpas 707 cells with an IGF-IR blocking antibody in the culture medium. In both cell lines proliferation was inhibited and viability was decreased. Also in IL-6 dependent MM cell lines the proliferation was found to be inhibited and apoptosis to be induced by the anti-IGF-IR antibody. This corroborated with the finding of Jelinek et al (1997) that IL-6 and IGF-I act synergistically to promote growth in MM cell lines. Recent experiments have shown that the mitogenic effect IGF-I is comparatively weak but that the anti-apoptotic effect in MM cells is strong. It can thus be concluded that an autocrine IGF-I loop may contribute to stimulate growth and survival in some MM cell lines.

In fresh, B-B4 antibody selected MM biopsy cells IGF-I and IL-6 individually, and synergistically, increased survival when such cells were explanted *in vitro*. However, as in the cell lines the response was heterogeneous. All samples of purified MM biopsy cells expressed the IGF-IR. The function of IGF-I as a paracrine and autocrine survival and growth factor for MM cells *in vivo* has not yet been examined.

In a set of experiments using octreotide, a somatostatin analogue known to be active *in vivo* to inhibit the effect of IGF-I by different mechanisms, the importance of IGF-I stimulation for growth and survival of MM cells was indirectly studied in MM cell lines and B-B4 selected cells (Georgii-Hemming et al 1999). MM cells were found to express somatostatin receptors. After exposure to octreotide the growth of both IL-6 dependent and IL-6 independent MM cell lines was inhibited by 25-45%. In 3/8 cell lines and in biopsy MM cells a weak induction of apoptosis was also found. The results thus demonstrate a new way of inhibiting the growth and decreasing the survival of MM cells - activation of somatostatin receptor signaling. The mechanism by which this inhibition is induced is not known in MM cells.

As mentioned MM cells express high levels of Bcl-2 (Pettersson et al 1992). The level of expression is comparable to that in cultured B-lymphoma cells carrying a translocation of Bcl-2, t(14:18). In one cell line U-266-1970 there is a fourfold amplification of Bcl-2. It is therefore possible that Bcl-2 protein and other proteins of the Bcl-2 family may act to increase the threshold for induction of apoptosis in MM cells, perhaps in order to balance the apoptotic effect of the highly expressed c-Myc. Such anti-apoptotic proteins, i.e. Bcl-2, Mcl-1 and Bcl-xL and the pro-apoptotic Bax protein, have been shown to be regulated by cytokines, e.g. IL-6 (Spets et al, unpublished data). To examine whether IGF-I might regulate the sensitivity to apoptosis by increasing the resistance to apoptotic stimuli we examined the influence of IGF-IR mediated signaling on two well-known apoptotic pathways - dexamethasone and Fas activation-induced apoptosis (Georgii-Hemming et al to be published). Using the Karpas 707 and LP-1 cell lines, previously demonstrated to respond to IGF-I (Georgii-Hemming et al 1996), we have demonstrated that IGF-I inhibits the dexamethasone-induced apoptosis completely (Karpas 707) or partially (LP-1) while apoptosis induced by Fas-activation was essentially unaffected. Anti-IGF-IR antibodies on the other hand potentiated the apoptosis-inducing effect of both dexamethasone and Fas-activation. Taken together the data suggest that IGF-IR signaling interferes with the execution of dexamethasone and Fas-activation induced apoptosis in MM cells.

Interferon-γ (IFN-γ) and Interferon-α (IFN-α) can Regulate CD95 (Fas/Apo-1) Induced Death in Multiple Myeloma Cell Lines

MM cells may express Fas antigen but only in a few cases will the cells respond to Fas-activation by apoptosis (Hata et al 1995, Shima et al 1995, Westendorf et al 1995). As IFN-γ and IFN-α are known to regulate growth and apoptosis in MM (Idestrom et al 1979, Ludwig et al 1983, Einhorn and Strander 1984, Brenning et al 1985, Jernberg et al 1991, Jourdan et al 1991. Portier et al 1993), and since IFNs in other cell systems have been suggested to activate the Fas-mediated apoptosis (Nagata and Golstein 1995, Selleri et al 1997) we examined whether IFNs may make MM cells sensitive to Fas-mediated apoptosis (Spets et al 1998).

Three cell lines, one IL-6 independent (U-266-1984) and two IL-6 dependent (U-266-1970 and U-1958), were selected for these studies. In all cell lines both IFN-α and IFN-γ sensitized the cells to Fas-induced apoptosis. Using the U-266-1984 cell lines the antiproliferative effect and the apoptosis sensitizing effect of the IFN-γ could be dissociated. As expected (Jernberg et al 1991) IFN-γ did not inhibit growth in U-266-1984 cells but IFN-γ treatment lead to an upregulation of their Fas antigen expression and to induction of sensitivity to Fas-mediated apoptosis. The mechanisms by which the sensitivity to Fas-mediated apoptosis is induced in MM cells is presently not known. Increase in Fas antigen expression, suggested to explain the apoptosis sensitizing effect of IFNs in other cell types, was found only in one of the three examined cell lines, and the expression of some genes regulating apoptosis (Bcl-2 and Bax) was unaltered. However, activation of Fas-mediated apoptosis seems to be a novel mechanism by which IFNs can inhibit MM cells *in vitro* and possibly also *in vivo*.

Balanced Regulation of Proliferation and Apoptosis - a Summary

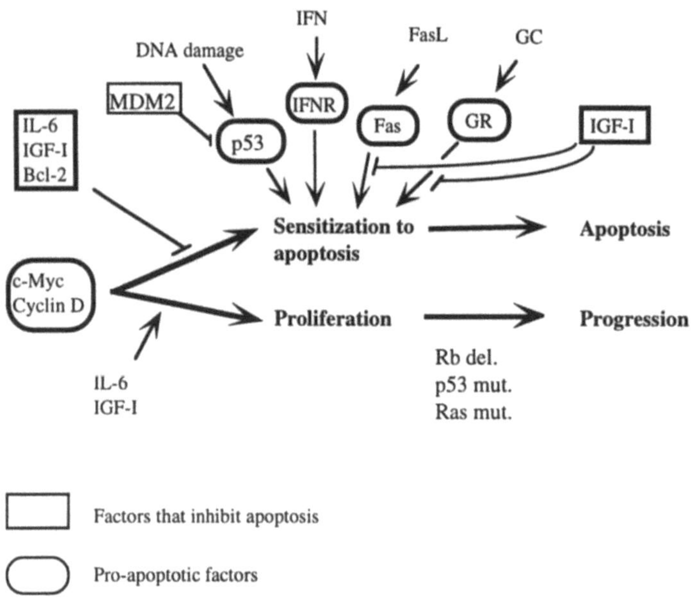

Fig. 2. A tentative model of the regulation of growth and survival in MM. A genetic alteration and/or overexpression of c-Myc and/or cyclin D may be early events in the development of MM, leading to increased proliferation and increased sensitivity to apoptotic signals. The MM cells are dependent on survival factors such as IL-6, IGF-I and Bcl-2 which inhibit apoptosis. The transformed cells are probably more sensitive to apoptotic signals e.g. IFNs, FasL and glucocorticoids than normal cells providing a therapeutic window of opportunity. During the progression the tumor accumulates additional genetic aberrations e.g. Rb deletions, p53 mutations and Ras mutations which may make the MM cells gradually less dependent on paracrine signals for growth and survival. The sensitivity to apoptosis is also decreased which probably contributes to the development of resistance to cytotoxic drugs. GC, glucocorticoid. GR, glucocorticoid receptor.

Our data seem to suggest a dynamic interaction between the intracellular signals that control growth and differentiation and that the selection process during long-term *in vitro* cultivation favours the selection of cells with a higher capacity for proliferation and a decreased propensity for apoptosis.

Fig 2. presents a hypothetical model for the regulation of growth and differentiation in MM cells which is adopted from a general model recently proposed for the interactions between oncogenes and death signals by Evan and Littlewood (1998).

Acknowledgements

The work summarized in this overview was supported by grants from the Swedish Cancer Society and the Hans von Kantzow Foundation.

References

Brenning G, Ahre A, Nilsson K (1985) Correlation between *in vitro* and *in vivo* sensitivity to human leucocyte interferon in patients with multiple myeloma. Scand J Haematol 35:543-549

Corradini P, Inghirami G, Astolfi M, Ladetto M, Voena C, Ballerini P, Gu W, Nilsson K, Knowles DM, Boccadoro M, et al (1994) Inactivation of tumor suppressor genes, p53 and Rb1, in plasma cell dyscrasias. Leukemia 5:758-767

Einhorn S, Strander H (1984) Studies with interferon-alpha in human tumors. Med Oncol Tumor Pharmacother 1:97-99

Evan G, Littlewood T (1998) A matter of life and cell death. Science 281:1317-22

Georgii-Hemming P, Strömberg T, Janson ET, Stridsberg M, Jernberg Wiklund H, Nilsson K (1999) The somatostatin analogue octreotide inhibits growth of IL-6 dependent and IL-6 independent human multiple myeloma cell lines. Blood, in press.

Georgii-Hemming P, Wiklund HJ, Ljunggren O, Nilsson K (1996) Insulin-like growth factor I is a growth and survival factor in human multiple myeloma cell lines. Blood 88:2250-2258

Hallek M, Leif Bergsagel P, Anderson KC (1998) Multiple myeloma: increasing evidence for a multistep transformation process. Blood 91:3-21

Harrington EA, Bennett MR, Fanidi A, Evan GI (1994) c-Myc-induced apoptosis in fibroblasts is inhibited by specific cytokines. EMBO J 13:3286-3295

Hata H, Matsuzaki H, Takeya M, Yoshida M, Sonoki T, Nagasaki A, Kuribayashi N, Kawano F, Takatsuki K (1995) Expression of Fas/Apo-1 (CD95) and apoptosis in tumor cells from patients with plasma cell disorders. Blood 86:1939-1945

Idestrom K, Cantell K, Killander D, Nilsson K, Strander H, Willems J (1979) Interferon therapy in multiple myeloma. Acta Med Scand 205:149-154

Jelinek DF, Witzig TE, Arendt BK (1997) A role for insulin-like growth factor in the regulation of IL-6-responsivehuman myeloma cell line growth. J Immunol 159:487-496

Jernberg H, Pettersson M, Kishimoto T, Nilsson K (1991) Heterogeneity in response to interleukin 6 (IL-6), expression of IL-6 and IL-6 receptor mRNA in a panel of established human multiple myeloma cell lines. Leukemia 5:255-265

Jernberg H, Zech L, Nilsson K (1987) Cytogenetic studies on human myeloma cell lines. Int J Cancer 40:811-817

Jernberg-Wiklund H, Pettersson M, Carlsson M, Nilsson K (1992a) Increase in interleukin 6 (IL-6) and IL-6 receptor expression in a human multiple myeloma cell line, U-266, during long-term in vitro culture and the development of a possible autocrine IL-6 loop. Leukemia 6:310-318

Jernberg-Wiklund H, Pettersson M, Larsson LG, Anton R, Nilsson K (1992b) Expression of myc-family genes in established human multiple myeloma cell lines: L-myc but not c-myc gene expression in the U-266 myeloma cell line. Int J Cancer 51:116-123

Jourdan M, Zhang XG, Portier M, Boiron JM, Bataille R, Klein B (1991) IFN-alpha induces autocrine production of IL-6 in myeloma cell lines. J Immunol 147:4402-4407

Kawano M, Hirano T, Matsuda T, Taga T, Horii Y, Iwato K, Asaoku H, Tang B, Tanabe O, Tanaka H, Kuramota A, Kishimoto T (1988) Nature 332:83-85

Klein B, Zhang XG, Jourdan M, Boiron JM, Portier M, Lu ZY, Wijdenes J, Brochier J, Bataille R (1990) Interleukin-6 is the central tumor growth factor in vitro and in vivo in multiple myeloma.Eur Cytokine Netw :193-201

Klein B, Zhang XG, Jourdan M, Content J, Houssiau F, Aarden L, Piechaczyk M, Bataille R (1989) Paracrine rather than autocrine regulation of myeloma-cell growth anddifferentiation by interleukin-6. Blood 73:517-526

Ludwig CU, Durie BG, Salmon SE, Moon TE (1983) Tumor growth stimulation in vitro by interferons. Eur J Cancer Clin Oncol 19:1625-1632

Nagata S, Golstein P (1995) The Fas death factor. Science 267:1449-1456

Nilsson K (1977) Established cell lines as tools in the study of human lymphoma and myeloma cell characteristics. Hamatol Bluttransfus 20:253-264

Nilsson K (1992) Human B-lymphoid cell lines. Hum Cell 5:25-41

Nilsson K (1994) The control of growth in human multiple myeloma cell lines. In Multiple Myeloma and related Disorders, B Barlogie, F Dammacco. Eds. (Rome, Italy:Ares-Serono Symposia Publications) pp 83-92

Nilsson K, Bennich H, Johansson SG, Ponten J (1970) Established immunoglobulin producing myeloma (IgE) and lymphoblastoid (IgG) cell lines from an IgE myeloma patient. Clin Exp Immunol 7:477-489

Nilsson K, Jernberg H, Pettersson M (1990) IL-6 as a growth factor for human multiple myeloma cells--a short overview. Curr Top Microbiol Immunol 166:3-12

Pettersson M, Jernberg-Wiklund H, Larsson LG, Sundstrom C, Givol I, Tsujimoto Y, Nilsson K (1992 Expression of the bcl-2 gene in human multiple myeloma cell lines and normalplasma cells. Blood 79:495-502

Portier M, Zhang XG, Caron E, Lu ZY, Bataille R, Klein B (1993) gamma-Interferon in multiple myeloma: inhibition of interleukin-6 (IL-6)-dependent myeloma cell growth and downregulation of IL-6-receptor expression in vitro. Blood 81:3076-3082

Sati HI, Apperley JF, Greaves M, Lawry J, Gooding R, Russell RG, Croucher PI (1998) Interleukin-6 is expressed by plasma cells from patients with multiple myeloma and monoclonal gammopathy of undetermined significance. Br J Haematol 101:287-295

Scibienski RJ, Paglieroni T, Caggiano V, Lemongello D, Gumerlock PH, Mackenzie MR (1992) Factors affecting the in vitro evolution of a myeloma cell line. Leukemia 6:940-947

Selleri C, Sato T, Del Vecchio L, Luciano L, Barrett AJ, Rotoli B, Young NS, Maciejewski JP (1997) Involvement of Fas-mediated apoptosis in the inhibitory effects of interferon-alpha in chronic myelogenous leukemia. Blood 89:957-964

Shima Y, Nishimoto N, Ogata A, Fujii Y, Yishisaki K, Kishimoto T (1995) Myeloma cells express Fas antigen/Apo-1 (CD95) but only some are sensistive to anti-Fas antibody resulting in apoptosis. Blood 85:757-764

Spets H, Georgii-Hemming P, Siljason J, Nilsson K, Jernberg-Wiklund H (1998) Fas/APO-1 (CD95)-mediated apoptosis is activated by interferon-gamma and interferon- in interleukin-6 (IL-6)-dependent and IL-6-independent multiplemyeloma cell lines. Blood 92:2914-2923

Spets H, Jernberg-Wiklund H, Sambade C, Soderberg O, Nilsson K (1997) The effects on growth and survival of IL-6 can be dissociated in theU-266-1970/U-266-1984 and HL407E/HL407L human multiple myeloma cell lines. Br J Haematol 98:126-133

Van Riet I, De Greef C, Aharchi F, Woischwill C, De Waele M, Bakkus M, Lacor P, Schots R, Van Camp B (1997) Establishment and characterization of a human stroma-dependent myeloma cell line (MM5.1) and its stroma-independent variant (MM5.2). Leukemia 11:284-293

Westendorf JJ, Ahmann GJ, Armitage RJ, Spriggs MK, Lust JA, Greipp PR, Katzmann JA, Jelinek DF(1994) CD40 expression in malignant plasma cells. Role in stimulation of autocrineIL-6 secretion by a human myeloma cell line. J Immunol 152:117-128

Westendorf JJ, Lammert JM, Jelinek DF (1995) Expression and function of Fas (APO-1/CD95) in patient myeloma cells and myeloma cell lines. Blood 85:3566-3576

Discussion

Dirk Eick: Have you tested whether B-14R, B-16, is upregulated when you bring myelomas in cell culture?
Kenneth Nilsson: No.
Isaac Witz: You talked about the induction by myeloma cells of IL-6 secretion by osteoblasts. Was the factor that induced the IL-6 secretion identified? Secondly, are there any other features besides proliferation or resistance to apoptosis which characterize the malignancy phenotype of myeloma cells, such as invasion? Can you tell us more about the factors that control them?
Kenneth Nilsson: To the first one, with respect to the interaction between osteoblasts, we think that the most important factor is TGF-beta 1. It has been reported that IL-1 and TNF-alpha and TNF-beta would be operative, but we cannot repeat that. So we think it might be TGF-beta 1 but probably it is also something else. This is a very complex regulation. With respect to other important biological features of myeloma, it is obvious that we know very little. It is essentially a very heterogeneous disease biologically, so one would have to make such a question more precise, in asking what is the situation in plasma cell leukemia, or plateau-phase myeloma?, etc. The background for this is probably that myeloma is so genetically aberrant. With respect to complex genetic changes it is the most epithelial cancer-like tumor within the hemopoietic system. So I do not think I should hypothesize too much.
George Klein: In the days when Janos Sümegi worked with us, we found that three out of four plasma cell leukemias had myc amplification. Has this been pursued further and is that a characteristic of plasma cell leukemia? There is obviously no human tumor which is analogous to mouse plasmacytoma, perhaps because there is no BALB/c-like human, but are there mouse tumors which are analogous to multiple myeloma tumors?
Kenneth Nilsson: To the latter, I think the tumor that may be closest to the human is the mouse model of Jiri Radl. This is a mouse tumor which homes to the bone marrow. It develops spontaneously in mice at old age. With respect to differences in myc expression in plasma cell leukemia and non-plasma cell leukemia, this has not been studied to any great extent. But there are reports from at least four different laboratories now, agreeing that myc is highly expressed and that it is deregulated. In about 20% there are explanations for that. For instance Carlo Croce's group observed that about 10% had mutations in the MLVI-4 locus downstream of c-myc, and mutations in the 5' untranslated region have also been demonstrated. But translocations per se are rare.
Michael Reth: Are myelomas in culture producing IL-6 and IGF-1?
Kenneth Nilsson: IL-6 is produced very rarely. In the U-266 cell line where it is best examined as an autocrine loop, it was not present in early passage. The autocrine IL-6 production is possibly something that the cell has used to improve its growth and survival. IL-6 is a growth factor for myeloma. We have found IGF-1 to be more strongly expressed during early passage, so it may be a factor that most myelomas use during the early part of the tumor progression, and in one instance we have seen an autocrine loop. But it is difficult to see the wood for the trees in myeloma, because there are such an enormous number of trees and bushes, and difficulties. I think it is due to its terribly complex genetic alterations.

Activation Molecules on Human Myeloma Cells

B. Klein[1], X.Y. Li[1], Z.Y. Lu[1], M. Jourdan[1], K. Tarte[1], J. Brochier[1], E. Claret[2], J. Wijdenes[2] and J.F. Rossi[1]

1 : INSERM U475, 99 Rue Puech Villa, 34194 Montpellier, France.
2 : Diaclone, 1 Bd Flemming, 25020 Besançon, France
Email: **klein@montp.inserm.fr**

Interleukin-6 is a Necessary but not a Sufficient Survival and Proliferation Factor for Primary Myeloma Cells from Patients with Chronic Disease

IL-6 is now recognized as a major survival and proliferation factor for murine and human malignant plasma cells (Klein *et al* 1995; Lattanzio *et al* 1997). This is especially true for patients with terminal multiple myeloma and extramedullary proliferation. In these patients, we and others have shown the possibility to reproducibly obtain cell lines whose survival and proliferation are dependent on addition of exogenous IL-6, and more generally of cytokines of the IL-6 family (Zhang *et al* 1994; Westendorf *et al* 1996; Jernberg *et al* 1987). Using these cell lines, cytokines other than IL-6 were recognized as myeloma cell survival or proliferation factors, namely interferon-alpha (Ferlin-Bezombes *et al* 1998), tumor necrosis factor (Jourdan *et al* 1999), insulin growth factor (Georgii-Hemming *et al* 1996; Jelinek *et al* 1997) or hepatocyte growth factor (Borset *et al* 1996).
In patients with chronic disease and a medullary involvement, primary myeloma cells survive and slightly proliferate when cultured for several days together with bone marrow stromal cells. IL-6 is highly produced in these cultures by stromal cells (Portier *et al* 1991) and controls the slight proliferation of myeloma cells since anti-IL-6 antibodies inhibit it (Klein *et al* 1989).
However, IL-6 alone is not sufficient to trigger the survival of primary myeloma cells from patients with chronic disease. Indeed, when these primary myeloma cells were highly purified, 60-80% of myeloma cells died by apoptosis within 2 days of culture (Fig. 1).
IL-6 could reduce apoptosis but did not support a long-term survival. Other myeloma cell survival factors (interferon-alpha or tumor necrosis factor-alpha) independent of IL-6 also reduced the apoptosis but did not support long term survival. Thus bone marrow stromal cells provide critical signals that support the survival of primary myeloma cells together with IL-6. In patients with extramedullary proliferation, additional mutations should have occurred in tumoral cells, making it possible for myeloma cells to survive and proliferate with IL-6 alone.

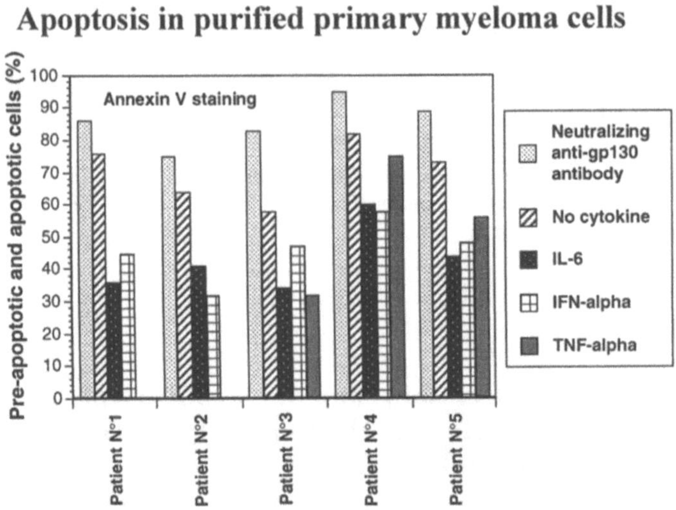

Fig. 1: Apoptosis in primary myeloma cells. Bone marrow cells were harvested from 5 patients with chronic myeloma. Myeloma cells were purified from bone marrow mononuclear cells using the MI15 anti-syndecan-1 mAb and MACS magnetic microbeads. Purified myeloma cells were cultured for 2 days at a cell concentration of 5 x 10^5 cells/ml in RPMI 1640 culture medium and 10% of fetal calf serum (FCS) with no cytokine, 10 µg/ml of neutralizing anti-gp130 mAb (Gu *et al* 1996), 3 ng/ml of IL-6, 100 U/ml of IFN-α2b or 100 U/ml of TNFα. At the end of the culture, the percentage of apoptotic cells was determined by staining with annexin V and FACS analysis.

Activation and Adhesion Molecules on Myeloma Cells

As illustrated in Fig. 2, malignant plasma cells fail to express most of the B cell activation molecules : CD19, CD20, CD21, B cell receptor, B7-1. They express CD40 molecules, a weak density of B7-2 and a very large density of CD38. Unlike B cells, myeloma cells express CD28 molecules and syndecan-1. We looked to see whether these activation or adhesion molecules were functional on myeloma cells and could provide costimulatory survival and proliferation signals.

Myeloma CD28 Molecules

Myeloma cell lines express a similar density of CD28 molecules as found on T cells (Zhang *et al* 1994). The myeloma CD28 was functional in terms of binding to B7-1 and recruitment of P85 subunit of the PI-3 kinase upon activation (Zhang *et al* 1998). However, using IL-6 dependent cell lines, we failed to find that activation of myeloma CD28 promoted an increased survival, proliferation, induction of activation markers or induction of cytokine production in myeloma cells. CD28 is also expressed on primary myeloma cells from 41% patients with myeloma, mainly patients with active disease (Robillard *et al* 1998). However, using agonist mAb to CD28, we failed to improve the survival of purified primary myeloma cells when cultured alone or with IL-6 (Zhang *et al* 1998). Thus, the myeloma CD28 is likely an important activation molecule on tumoral cells but it is not able to replace the survival signal provided by stromal cells to primary myeloma cells from patients with chronic disease.

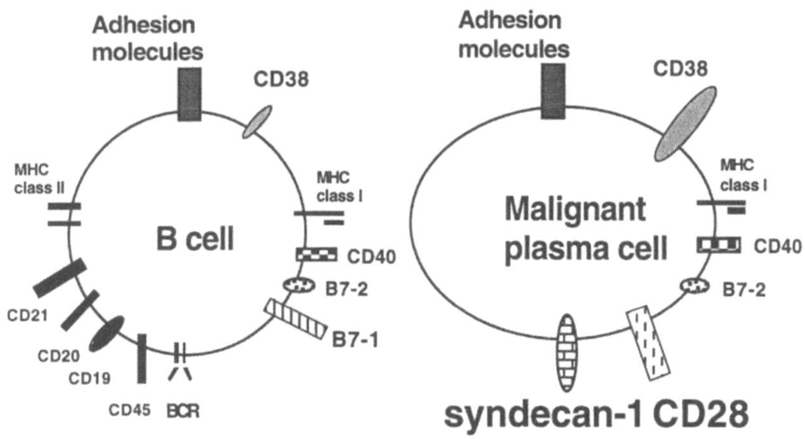

Fig. 2: Activation and adhesion molecules on human myeloma cells.

Myeloma CD40 Molecules

Myeloma cells express a similar density of CD40 molecules as normal B cells (Pellat Deceunynck *et al* 1994). Challenging results have been reported concerning the functions of myeloma CD40. Some groups have shown that an activation of myeloma CD40 resulted in an autocrine production of IL-6 and proliferation (Westendorf *et al* 1994; Urashima *et al* 1995). One group has reported an inhibitory role of myeloma CD40 activation (Bergamo *et al* 1997). Regarding the induction of B7 molecules and immunogenicity, we found that an activation of myeloma CD40 by CD40-ligand transfected cells failed to induce B7-1 expression on myeloma cells (10 patients and six cell lines) and to confer immunogenicity on these cells (unpublished results). We also found no survival effect of CD40 activation on either primary myeloma cells or myeloma cell lines. However, we found an increase in the densities of Fas and CD54 molecules on all myeloma cell samples studied indicating some functions of CD40 activation (unpublished results). As CD40 is a critical activation molecule for B cells, we could not exclude that it plays a role for triggering the survival of primary myeloma cells in conjunction with IL-6.

Syndecan-1 on Human Myeloma Cells

Syndecan-1 is a proteoglycan that is expressed by simple and stratified epithelia, fibroblasts, stratified keratinocytes, endothelial cells (Wijdenes *et al* 1997). In murine B lymphopoiesis, it is specifically expressed on pre B and plasma cells. Several monoclonal antibodies specific to human myeloma cells were subsequently recognized as anti-syndecan-1 antibodies (Wijdenes *et al* 1996; Horvathova *et al* 1995). Its expression on human pre B cells is not formally proven. Syndecan-1 bears heparan and sometimes chondroitin sulfates. Five putative glycoaminoglycan attachment sites are located in the ectodomain and a protease cleavage site is located at its C-terminus. Syndecan-1 is an adhesion molecule to collagen type I and fibronectin. Like heparin, syndecan-1 binds several proteins, and in particular, the fibroblast growth factor (Carey, 1997). Membrane syndecan-1 can be cleaved by proteases, thrombin or epidermal growth factor (Subramanian *et al* 1997). Soluble syndecan-1 is also able to bind FGF and may behave as an agonist or an antagonist of FGF depending on the level of poorly sulfated domains in heparan sulfate chains (Kato *et al* 1998). The role of syndecan-1 in B cell differentiation and, especially, in multiple myeloma is poorly known. It is an adhesion molecule of myeloma cells to collagen type 1 (Ridley *et al* 1993). More recently, soluble syndecan-1 has been shown to inhibit myeloma cell proliferation by unknown mechanisms (Dhodapkar *et al* 1998).

It was not clear whether membrane syndecan-1 was present on all primary myeloma cells and myeloma cell lines. Recently, we have shown that all viable myeloma cells highly express syndecan-1 but that this expression is rapidly lost on apoptotic cells (Jourdan *et al* 1998). This is documented in Fig. 3.

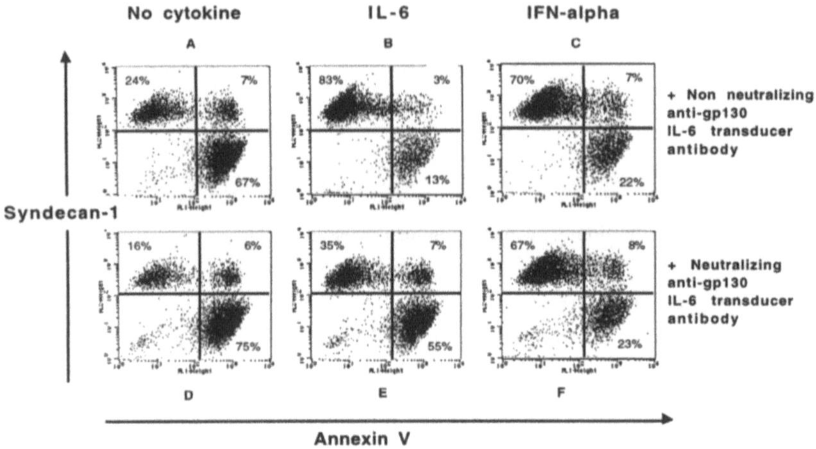

Fig. 3: Myeloma cells from the XG-6 cell lines were cultured 3 days with either no cytokine (A,D), 1 ng/ml of IL-6 (B,E) or 100 U/ml of IFN-alpha (C,F) with 150 μg/ml of a non neutralizing anti-gp130 IL-6 transducer mAb (A,B,C) or a neutralizing one (D,E,F). At the end of the cultures, myeloma cells were first labeled with MI-15 anti-syndecan-1 mAb and PE-GAMIG, then with FITC-annexin V. The fluorescence profiles were determined with a FACScan apparatus. The percentages of cells in each quadrant are indicated.

Membrane syndecan-1 on IL-6-dependent myeloma cells rapidly disappears on apoptotic cells upon removal of IL-6. IL-6 or IFN-α can prevent the loss of syndecan-1. Soluble syndecan-1 is produced by myeloma cells. This production is inhibited by low doses of cycloheximide that did not induce a major myeloma cell apoptosis. There was no correlation between the membrane density of syndecan-1 and the rate of soluble syndecan-1 production with some cell lines producing virtually no soluble syndecan-1. This suggests that the production of soluble syndecan-1 is regulated by presently unknown mechanisms. Using an ELISA detecting soluble syndecan-1, we found increased levels of soluble syndecan-1 in plasma from patients with myeloma compared to those of age-related healthy subjects. The median value was 369 U/ml in myeloma patients versus 35 U/ml in healthy subjects. Finally, we found that soluble syndecan-1 is a powerful prognostic factor in patients with newly diagnosed myeloma (Fig. 4). The mean survival was 24 months in patients with plasma syndecan-1 > 369 U/ml compared to 48 months for patients with plasma syndecan-1 < 369 U/ml. As soluble syndecan-1 may be either an agonist or an antagonist molecule depending on the level of poorly sulfated domains in heparan sulfate chains, the function of circulating syndecan-1 in patients with multiple myeloma needs to be studied. Syndecan-1 might play an important role in the myeloma physiopathology, namely as a receptor for heparin-binding growth factors. FGF could be an important molecule because t(4;14) translocations involving FGR3 gene and immunoglobulin genes are found in 20% of the patients with myeloma (Chesi *et al* 1997). In addition, mutations leading to a constitutive activation of this receptor are also found in some myeloma samples (Chesi *et al* 1997). IGF could be another interesting growth factor because it is an important myeloma cell survival and growth factor independent of IL-6 (Georgii-Hemming *et al* 1996; Jelinek *et al* 1997). High rate of plasma IGF circulate bound to IGF-binding proteins (IGF-BP) and heparan sulfate can bind and dissociate IGF/IGF-BP complexes leading to free IGF release (Arai *et al* 1994).

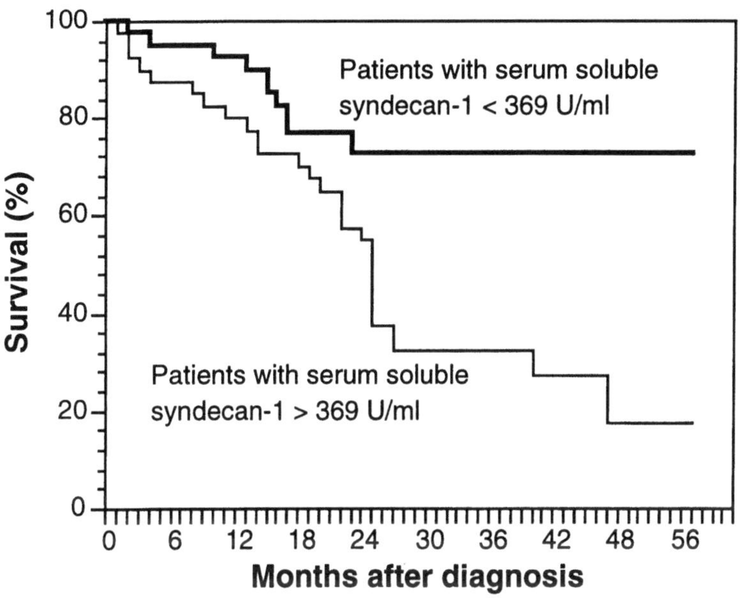

Fig. 4: Prognostic value of plasma soluble syndecan-1 of patients with multiple myeloma. Plasma from 42 patients with MM at diagnosis were collected and frozen. The concentration of plasma soluble syndecan-1 was measured using an ELISA. The median plasma concentration was 369 U/ml in myeloma patients and 35 U/ml in age-related healthy individuals. Patients with plasma soluble syndecan-1 > 369 U/ml had a decreased survival duration ($p < 0.001$) compared to patients with plasma syndecan-1 <369 U/ml.

Conclusion

If IL-6 is a necessary proliferation factor for primary myeloma cells, additional signals produced by stromal cells are required to promote the survival of primary myeloma cells from patients with chronic disease. We have reviewed our recent data showing that two functional activation molecules present on myeloma cells, CD28 and CD40, are not able to provide the survival signals exerted by stromal cells. Membrane syndecan-1 might be an important molecule in the myeloma biology, in particular as a receptor for fibroblast growth factor and eventually of insulin growth factor. Finally, stromal cells may provide other unidentified signals that are critical for myeloma cell survival in conjunction with IL-6.

References

Arai, T, Parker, A, Busby, W,Jr, Clemmons, DR (1994) Heparin, heparan sulfate, and dermatan sulfate regulate formation of the insulin-like growth factor-I and insulin-like growth factor-binding protein complexes. *J Biol Chem*, 269, 20388-20393

Bergamo, A, Bataille, R, Pellat-Deceunynck, C (1997) CD40 and CD95 induce programmed cell death in the human myeloma cell line XG2. *Br J Haematol*, 97, 652-655

Borset, M, Hjorth-Hansen, H, Seidel, C, Sundan, A, Waage, A (1996) Hepatocyte growth factor and its receptor c-met in multiple myeloma. *Blood*, 88, 3998-4004

Carey, DJ (1997) Syndecans: multifunctional cell-surface co-receptors. *Biochem J*, 327, 1-16

Chesi, M, Nardini, E, Brents, LA, Schrock, E, Ried, T, Kuehl, WM, Bergsagel, PL (1997) Frequent translocation t(4;14)(p16.3;q32.3) in multiple myeloma is associated with increased expression and activating mutations of fibroblast growth factor receptor 3. *Nat Genet*, 16, 260-264

Dhodapkar, MV, Abe, E, Theus, A, Lacy, M, Langford, JK, Barlogie, B, Sanderson, RD (1998) Syndecan-1 Is a Multifunctional Regulator of Myeloma Pathobiology: Control of Tumor Cell Survival, Growth, and Bone Cell Differentiation. *Blood*, 91, 2679-2688

Ferlin-Bezombes, M, Jourdan, M, Liautard, J, Brochier, J, Rossi, JF, Klein, B (1998) IFN-alpha is a survival factor for human myeloma cells and reduces dexamethasone-induced apoptosis [In Process Citation]. *J Immunol*, 161, 2692-2699

Georgii-Hemming P, Wiklund, HJ, Ljunggren O, Nilsson, K (1996) Insulin-like growth factor I is a growth and survival factor in human multiple myeloma cell lines. *Blood*, 88, 2250-2258

Gu, ZJ, Wijdenes, J, Zhang, XG, Hallet, MM, Clement, C, Klein, B (1996) Anti-gp130 transducer monoclonal antibodies specifically inhibiting ciliary neurotrophic factor, interleukin-6, interleukin-11, leukemia inhibitory factor or oncostatin M. *J Immunol Methods*, 190, 21-27

Horvathova, M, Gaillard, JP, Liautard, J, Duperray, C, Lavabre-Bertrand, T, Bourquard, P, Rossi, JF, Klein, B, Brochier, J (1995) Identification of novel and specific antigens of human plasma cells by mAb. *Leucocyte Typing V* p.713 Oxford University Press, London

Jelinek, DF, Witzig, TE, Arendt, BK (1997) A role for insulin-like growth factor in the regulation of IL-6- responsive human myeloma cell line growth. *J Immunol*, 159, 487-496

Jernberg, H, Nilsson, K, Zech, L, Lutz, D, Nowotny, H, Scheirer, W (1987) Etablishment and phenotypic characterization of three human myeloma cell lines (U-1957, U-1958, and U-1996). *Blood*, 69, 1605

Jourdan, M, Ferlin, M, Legouffe, E, Horvathova, M, Liautard, J, Rossi, JF, Wijdenes, J, Brochier, J, Klein, B (1998) The myeloma cell antigen syndecan-1 is lost by apoptotic myeloma cells. *Br J Haematol*, 100, 637-646

Jourdan M, Tarte K, Legouffe E, Brochier, J, Rossi, JF Klein, B (1999) Tumor necrosis factor is a survival and proliferation factor for human myeloma cells. *Eur Cytokine Netw*, (In Press)

Kato, M, Wang, H, Kainulainen, V, Fitzgerald, ML, Ledbetter, S, Ornitz, DM, Bernfield, M (1998) Physiological degradation converts the soluble syndecan-1 ectodomain from an inhibitor to a potent activator of FGF-2. *Nat Med*, 4, 691-697

Klein, B, Zhang, XG, Jourdan, M, Content, J, Houssiau, F, Aarden, L, Piechaczyk, M, Bataille, R (1989) Paracrine rather than autocrine regulation of myeloma-cell growth and differentiation by interleukin-6. *Blood*, 73, 517-526

Klein, B, Zhang, XG, Lu, ZY, Bataille, R (1995) Interleukin-6 in human multiple myeloma. *Blood*, 85, 863-872

Lattanzio, G, Libert, C, Aquilina, M, Cappelletti, M, Ciliberto, G, Musiani, P, Poli, V (1997) Defective development of pristane-oil-induced plasmacytomas in interleukin-6-deficient BALB/c mice. *Am J Pathol*, 151, 689-696

Pellat Deceunynck, C, Bataille, R, Robillard, N, Harousseau, JL, Rapp, MJ, Juge Morineau, N, Wijdenes, J, Amiot, M (1994) Expression of CD28 and CD40 in human myeloma cells: a comparative study with normal plasma cells. *Blood*, 84, 2597-2603

Portier, M, Rajzbaum, G, Zhang, XG, Attal, M, Rusalen, C, Wijdenes, J, Mannoni, P, Maraninchi, D, Piechaczyk, M, Bataille, R, Klein, B (1991) In vivo interleukin-6 gene expression in the tumoral environment in multiple myeloma. *Eur J Immunol*, 21, 1759-1762

Ridley RC, Xiao H, Hata, H, Woodliff, J, Epstein, J, Sanderson, RD (1993) Expression of syndecan regulates human myeloma plasma cell adhesion to type I collagen. *Blood*, 81, 767-774

Robillard, N, Jego, G, Pellat-Deceunynck, C, Pineau, D, Puthier, D, Mellerin, MP, Barille, S, Rapp, MJ, Harousseau, JL, Amiot, M, Bataille, R (1998) CD28, a marker associated with tumoral expansion in multiple myeloma. *Clin Cancer Res*, 4, 1521-1526

Subramanian SV, Fitzgerald ML, Bernfield, M (1997) Regulated shedding of syndecan-1 and -4 ectodomains by thrombin and growth factor receptor activation. *J Biol Chem*, 272, 14713-14720

Urashima, M, Chauhan, D, Uchiyama, H, Freeman, GJ, Anderson, KC (1995) CD40 ligand triggered interleukin-6 secretion in multiple myeloma. *Blood*, 85, 1903-1912

Westendorf JJ, Ahmann GJ, Armitage, RJ, Spriggs, MK, Lust, JA, Greipp, PR, Katzmann, JA, Jelinek, DF (1994) CD40 Expression in Malignant Plasma Cells - Role in Stimulation of Autocrine IL-6 Secretion by a Human Myeloma Cell Line. *J Immunol*, 152, 117-128

Westendorf, JJ, Ahmann, GJ, Greipp, PR, Witzig, TE, Lust, JA, Jelinek, DF (1996) Establishment and characterization of three myeloma cell lines that demonstrate variable cytokine responses and abilities to produce autocrine interleukin-6. *Leukemia*, 10, 866-876

Wijdenes, J, Vooijs, WC, Clement, C, Post, J, Morard, F, VIta, N, Laurent, P, Sun, RX, Klein, B, Dore, JM (1996) A plasmocyte selective monoclonal antibody (B-B4) recognizes syndecan-1. *Br J Haematol*, 94, 318-323

Wijdenes, J, Clement, C, Klein, B, Dore, JM (1997) CD138 (syndecan-1) worhshop panel report. *Leucocyte Typing VI* (ed. by T Kishimoto, H Kikutani, AEGK Von dem Borne, S.M Goyert, DY Mason, M Miyasaka, L Moretta, K Okumura, S Shaw, TA Springer, K Sugamura and H Zola), p.249 Garland Publishing, New York, London

Zhang, XG, Gaillard, JP, Robillard, N, Lu, ZY, Gu, ZJ, Jourdan, M, Boiron, JM, Bataille, R, Klein, B (1994) Reproducible obtaining of human myeloma cell lines as a model for tumor stem cell study in human multiple myeloma. *Blood*, 83, 3654-3663

Zhang XG, Olive D, Devos J, Rebouissou C, Ghiotto-Ragueneau M, Ferlin M, Klein B (1998) Malignant plasma cell lines express a functional CD28 molecule. *Leukemia*, 12, 610-618

Discussion

Federico Caligaris-Cappio: Does the stimulation of CD40 and CD28 interfere with the apoptotic program of the plasma cells?

Bernard Klein: No, we used purified primary myeloma cells from patients with medullary disease and we could not restore the survival, either alone or in the presence of IL-6.

Bart Barlogie: We have worked with Sir Ralph Sanderson on syndecan for quite some time and Madhav Dhodapkar reported that soluble syndecan causes apoptosis of cell lines and primary cells, and seems to stimulate osteoblasts and inactivate osteoclasts. So all this collective experience indicates it is a favorable feature if you look at cell lines that have been transfected: syndecan positive and negative transfectants had very different behavior in the mouse, where the ones that were transfected had less of a spread, certainly in terms of extra-medullary disease presentation compared to syndecan-negative ones. So it is an interesting story.

Bernard Klein: Yes, but you know that soluble syndecan-1 may have either an antagonist or agonist function depending on the enzymes able to cleave the poorly sulfated domains in heparan sulfate chains. These enzymes could be present in the inflammatory tumoral sites.

Riccardo Dalla-Favera: Do increased titers of soluble syndecan-1 reflect higher tumor mass or increase secretion?

Bernard Klein: Plasma levels of soluble syndecan-1 are correlated with those of b2-microglobulin that reflect the tumor mass.

Riccardo Dalla-Favera: So you are not only saying that some myeloma cells secrete more, or shed more, it is just the number of cells?

Bernard Klein: This is an interesting point. We have now 15 different myeloma cell lines that express variable densities of membrane syndecan-1. Some cell lines that express a low density could produce a high level of circulating syndecan-1 and vice versa. It is interesting to understand the mechanisms.

Peritoneal B-1 Cells Switch *in vivo* to IgA and these IgA Antibodies can bind to Bacteria of the Normal Intestinal Microflora

F. G.M. Kroese and N. A. Bos
Department of Histology and Cell Biology, University of Groningen, Oostersingel 69/1, 9713 EZ Groningen, The Netherlands

Introduction

A prominent feature of the mucosal immune system is formed by IgA secreting cells located in the lamina propria, immediately beneath the epithelium. In the intestine of the mouse at least 15 million cells secrete IgA into the surrounding connective tissue [1]. Subsequently, secretory IgA is transported across the single layer of epithelial cells and pumped into the gut lumen. Here, IgA can bind to food antigens and to the numerous microorganisms (in humans about 10^{11} bacteria per gram colon contents!). This interaction may help to prevent invasion and infection of the body with microbes, e.g. by preventing binding to the mucus layer and the epithelial cells ('immune exclusion').

The vast majority of IgA secreting cells in the gut are thought to be short-lived with a half-life of approximately 5 days [2]. This implies that many IgA secreting cells are replaced by precursor cells every day. There is accumulating evidence that in addition to conventional (B-2) cells from Peyer's patches also B-1 cells, located in the peritoneal cavity, may serve as an important source for IgA secreting cells at mucosal sites (for reviews see e.g. [3, 4]). This evidence is largely based upon transfer experiments with irradiated or otherwise B cell depleted mice and analysis of genetically altered (e.g. transgenic mice) or immune deficient mice (e.g. CBA/N). Despite this potential role of B-1 cell to participate in mucosal IgA production, little is known about the relative contribution of B-1 cells to the pool of IgA secreting cells in normal, unmanipulated mice. Furthermore, another key issue is whether B-1 cell derived IgA differs in function from IgA derived from Peyer's patch B-2 cells. In this paper we provide some data that address these points by showing that: i) peritoneal IgM^+ B-1 cells can undergo class switching towards IgA *in vivo* in normal, untreated mice, ii) T cells in the peritoneal cavity may provide cytokines that might be involved in isotype switching and development of plasma cells, iii) B-1 cell derived IgA binds to a variety of bacteria of the normal intestinal flora *in vivo* and *in vitro* and iv) B-1 cell derived IgA can influence the composition of the gut flora.

Class Switching of B-1 Cells in Normal, Untreated Mice

An early sign of class switching of IgM^+ B cells to IgA expression is the presence of germline $C\alpha$ mRNA transcripts [5]. These germline transcripts start 5' of an $I\alpha$ exon, proceed through the switch region and terminate downstream of the $C\alpha$ exon. The germline IgA transcript is formed after splicing of the $I\alpha$ exon. Germline transcripts precede the actual isotype switching, although their exact role in this process is not clear. To examine the ability of peritoneal B-1 cells from normal, untreated BALB/c mice to switch *in vivo* to IgA we performed RT-PCR analysis for germline Cα mRNA and full-length IgA mRNA transcripts on FACS sorted peritoneal B cell subsets [6]. We found that germline transcripts and full-length IgA transcripts could be detected in peritoneal B-1 cells but not (or very little) in peritoneal conventional B cells (B-2). Furthermore, we demonstrated that both the germline Cα transcripts and full-length IgA transcripts were largely confined to the $CD5^-$ B-1 subset (so-called B-1b) cells) and were almost absent from the $CD5^+$ B-1a cell subset. Germline transcripts are only present during the early phase of isotype switching. Thus, the observation that we could detect germline Cα transcripts among peritoneal B-1 cells not only shows that B-1 cells can and do switch *in vivo*, but also that this switching might be initiated inside the peritoneal cavity.

Cytokine Production by Peritoneal T Cells

Isotype switching and subsequent differentiation to IgA secreting plasma cells is regulated by a variety of cytokines including IL-5, IL-6 and TGFβ, produced by Th cells. T cells might also be involved in B-1 cell responses [7]. Taki *et al.* provided some evidence that T cells might be involved in IgA production by B-1 cells [8]. They showed that SCID mice repopulated with both (unprimed) T cells and B-1 cells have 10-fold higher serum IgA levels compared to SCID mice injected with B-1 cells only. IL-5 is an important cytokine for the development of IgA secreting cells. This cytokine appears also to play a significant role in IgA production by peritoneal B-1 cells [9-11]. Bao *et al.* have recently shown, using IL-5 deficient mice, that B-1 cell derived, but not B-2 cell derived IgA, is IL-5 dependent [12]. Furthermore the majority of B-1 cells in normal and even in germfree mice express the IL-5R [10]. In view of the potential role of T cells and cytokines in isotype switching and differentiation of B-1 cells we analyzed the phenotype and cytokine profile of peritoneal T cells, using multiparameter (up to 10 colors and 12 parameters) flow-cytometry [FGM Kroese *et al.*, manuscript in preparation]. Peritoneal washout cells from normal, untreated BAB/25 mice contain only relatively few T cells (~2.5% of all peritoneal cells). Strikingly, most (50-70%) $TCR\alpha\beta^+CD4^+$ peritoneal T cells express high levels of CD11a and CD44. This phenotype is typical for activated T cells [13]. By contrast, only 10-15% of splenic $TCR\alpha\beta^+CD4^+$ T cells have this profile. Within the $TCR\alpha\beta^+CD4^+$ T cell subset in the peritoneal cavity there are approximately 10 times more IFNγ, IL-4, IL-5, and IL-10 and 2.5 times more IL-2 and IL-6 producing cells, compared to their splenic counterpart. For example, 30% of the peritoneal $TCR\alpha\beta^+CD4^+$ T cells produce IFNγ, 4% produce IL-4 and 2% produce IL-5. Thus, the peritoneal cavity harbors relatively high numbers of activated T cells producing a variety of cytokines. The finding that peritoneal cavity T cells, but not splenic T cells, produce IL-5 supports the hypothesis that peritoneal T cells might be involved in local differentiation to IgA producing B-1 cells.

Binding of B-1 Cell Derived IgA to the Normal Intestinal Microflora

B-1 cells are known to produce IgM antibodies which are largely directed to micro-organism(-related) antigens [14]. To study the specificity of IgA antibodies they produce, we generated a panel of eight IgA producing hybridomas from B-1-cells [15]. All eight IgA monoclonal antibodies (IgA mAbs) have been shown to bind to

Table 1. Percentage of staining of anaerobic monocultured bacteria by IgA monoclonal antibodies

Species / IgA mAb	2B4	3G8	1B5	2F7	2D 11	1F6	3C 10	3C6
Bacteroides distasonis	0-10 %	0-10 %	0-10 %	0-10 %	0-10 %	0-10 %	0-10 %	0-10 %
Bacteroides eggerthii	10-20 %	0-10 %	0-10 %	0-10 %	0-10 %	0-10 %	0-10 %	0-10 %
Bacteroides fragilis	20-40 %	10-20 %	0-10 %	10-20 %	10-20 %	0-10 %	10-20 %	20-40 %
Bacteroides thetaiotaomicron	20-40 %	0-10 %	0-10 %	20-40 %	10-20 %	0-10 %	10-20 %	0-10 %
Bacteroides vulgatus	0-10 %	0-10 %	0-10 %	0-10 %	0-10 %	0-10 %	0-10 %	0-10 %
Clostridium butyricum	0-10 %	0-10 %	0-10 %	0-10 %	0-10 %	0-10 %	0-10 %	0-10 %
Clostridium indolis	0-10 %	0-10 %	0-10 %	0-10 %	0-10 %	0-10 %	0-10 %	0-10 %
Clostridium innocuum	0-10 %	0-10 %	0-10 %	0-10 %	0-10 %	0-10 %	0-10 %	0-10 %
Clostridium maleno	0-10 %	0-10 %	0-10 %	0-10 %	0-10 %	0-10 %	0-10 %	0-10 %
Clostridium nexile	0-10 %	0-10 %	0-10 %	0-10 %	0-10 %	0-10 %	0-10 %	0-10 %
Clostridium paraputrificum	10-20 %	0-10 %	0-10 %	20-40 %	10-20 %	0-10 %	10-20 %	0-10 %
C. perferingens (mouse)	0-10 %	0-10 %	0-10 %	0-10 %	0-10 %	0-10 %	0-10 %	0-10 %
C. perferingens (human)	40-60 %	0-10 %	60-100 %	60-100 %	0-10 %	0-10 %	60-100 %	60-100 %
Eubacterium cylindroides	0-10 %	0-10 %	0-10 %	0-10 %	0-10 %	0-10 %	0-10 %	0-10 %
Eubacterium ruminantium	0-10 %	0-10 %	0-10 %	0-10 %	0-10 %	0-10 %	0-10 %	0-10 %
Fusobacterium mortiferum	0-10 %	0-10 %	0-10 %	0-10 %	0-10 %	0-10 %	0-10 %	0-10 %
Fusobacterium vanium	0-10 %	0-10 %	0-10 %	0-10 %	0-10 %	0-10 %	0-10 %	0-10 %
Lactobacillus acidophilus	0-10 %	0-10 %	0-10 %	0-10 %	0-10 %	0-10 %	0-10 %	0-10 %
Morganella morganii	0-10 %	10-20 %	0-10 %	60-100 %	20-40 %	0-10 %	10-20 %	0-10 %
Peptostreptococcus anaerobius	60-100 %	20-40 %	10-20 %	60-100 %	0-10 %	10-20 %	20-40 %	10-20 %
P. asaccharolyticus	0-10 %	0-10 %	0-10 %	0-10 %	0-10 %	0-10 %	0-10 %	0-10 %
Peptostreptococcus productus	60-100 %	10-20 %	0-10 %	10-20 %	0-10 %	0-10 %	0-10 %	0-10 %
Proprionibacter acnes	0-10 %	0-10 %	0-10 %	0-10 %	0-10 %	0-10 %	0-10 %	0-10 %

0-10 % = ☐ 10-20 % = ☐ 20-40 % = ☐ 40-60 % = ☐ 60-100 % = ☐

Cultured anaerobic bacterial strains were incubated with IgA mAbs and, after washing, stained with goat-anti-mouse IgA~FITC and analyzed by flow cytometry. Numbers represent percentages of coated bacteria after substraction of the signal obtained with the second step reagent alone.

fecal bacteria. To define the specificity of the B-1 cell derived IgA mAbs, they were tested on a panel of mostly anaerobic monocultured bacteria. Table 1 shows that each of our IgA mAbs has a unique, but sometimes overlapping, broad specificity towards bacterial antigens. Most of the anaerobic bacteria used in our panel are known to be common inhabitants of the intestinal tract. Many monocultured bacteria regularly showed low percentages of staining by different IgA mAbs, although some (*Morganella morganii, Clostridium perfringens, Peptostreptococcus anaerobius and Peptostreptococcus productus*) showed staining by one or more IgA monoclonals in percentages above 40%. Because the reactivity pattern of each of the IgA mAbs with this panel of bacteria was different, we conclude that the variable regions of the IgA molecules are (at least partly) involved in this binding.We cannot, however, exclude the possibility that there is some binding mediated by superantigens or Fc receptors.

The low percentages of staining of the monocultured bacteria by the IgA mAbs suggest that the recognized epitopes are only available on part of the bacterial populations. Alternatively, such interactions can be of relative low affinity, resulting in significant loss of signal during our washing procedures. It is known that B-1 cells can produce IgM of relative low affinity [14]. If IgA derived from B-1 cells has similar properties, this could explain the low, but nevertheless clearly visible staining by the IgA mAbs. Recently, in human secretions natural, polyreactive IgA with similar properties has been described [16].

Effect of B-1 Derived IgA Administration on the Composition of the Microflora

The effects of IgA on the indigenous flora is unknown. Removal of IgA by gene disruption of Ig gene expression does not lead to obvious changes in composition of the indigenous gut flora in mice with a limited complex flora [17]. In normal mice a large number of the normal gut bacteria are coated with IgA, varying from 30% in fecal samples up to 90% in small intestinal samples [18]. Also in humans about 50% of the fecal bacteria are normally coated with IgA [19]. Reconstitution of SCID mice with B-1 cells (PerC cells) results in coating of fecal bacteria with IgA starting two weeks after transfer [18]. This indicates that B-1 derived IgA also can bind to bacteria of the gut flora *in vivo*. To test if B-1 cell derived IgA monoclonal antibodies can influence the composition of the normal gut flora, we have introduced a B-1 cell derived IgA-producing hybridoma as "back-pack" tumor in SCID mice and evaluated the composition of the flora. Changes in gut flora where observed by their ability to be coated with the monoclonal IgA antibody. Figure 1 shows that there is an increase in the percentage of IgA coated fecal bacteria within two weeks, after which a plateau of approximately 30-35% is reached. By determining the amount of gut bacteria that are *in vivo* coated with the injected IgA monoclonal antibody 1B5 we could provide evidence that the normal

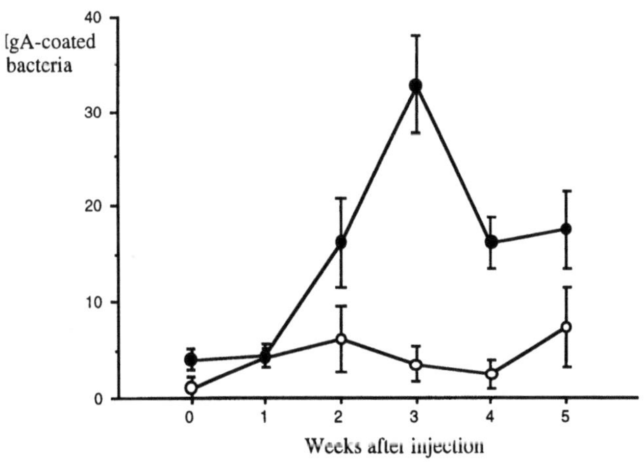

Fig. 1. Fecal samples from SCID mice after injection of 10^6 IgA producing hybridoma cells (1B5) closed symbols or PBS (open symbols) were analyzed by flow cytometry for IgA coated bacteria after incubation with a rat anti-mouse IgA mAb (71.14), followed by goat anti-rat-Ig~FITC. Numbers represent percentages of coated bacteria after subtraction of the signal obtained by goat anti-rat-Ig~FITC alone.

gut flora has changed after *in vivo* treatment with the monoclonal IgA antibodies. Since 1B5 normally only stains about 5% of the bacterial population of untreated SCID mice [15], the increase of IgA-coated bacteria observed in the faeces can most likely be explained by changes in the composition of the gut flora. Recently we have confirmed the alterations in the composition of the gut flora after *in vivo* treatment with IgA monoclonal antibodies by *in situ* hybridization with probes specific for 16S rRNA variations among different groups of intestinal bacteria [NA Bos *et al.*, submitted].

After intraperitoneal injection of other members of the B-1 cell derived IgA hybridoma panel in SCID mice, similar changes in the IgA coating of the fecal bacteria were observed with even percentages up to 90% of the population being coated with the injected monoclonal IgA antibodies [20].

We realize that the amount of monoclonal IgA used in these experiments by far exceeds the normal amount present of such an antibody, but it is to our knowledge the first positive evidence that B-1 cell derived IgA reactive with indigenous gut bacteria can influence the composition of the gut flora. Although the mode of action of IgA reactive with indigenous bacteria and the impact of such regulation under normal physiological conditions still needs to be determined, the possibilities to use these IgA molecules to interfere with the gut ecosystem are challenging.

Conclusions

Culminating evidence by us and others show that B-1 cells appear to be an important source for mucosal IgA production. The microenvironment of the peritoneal cavity is very unique, not only by the presence of relatively high numbers of B-1 cells but, as we have shown here, also because most peritoneal T cells have an activated phenotype. The finding that germline $C\alpha$ transcripts are found among B-1 cells and that peritoneal T cells produce IL-5 support the idea that this unique microenvironment supports local switching and differentiation of B-1 cells to IgA production. This is also reflected by the fact that, in susceptible mouse strains, intraperitoneal injection with pristane leads to a high incidence of peritoneal plasmacytomas that preferentially secrete IgA [21]. However, the molecular and cellular events that lead to B-1 derived IgA producing cells in the gut remain puzzling. Thus, in addition to conventional B cells derived from Peyer's patches, also B-1 cells contribute to the pool of IgA secreting cells in the intestinal mucosa.

The effector functions of secretory IgA in the gut lumen are still unclear. Passive transfer of monoclonal IgA reactive with pathogenic bacteria such as *Salmonella typhymorium* and *Vibrio cholera* by a 'back-pack' tumor of IgA producing hybridoma cells, results in protection against infection with these pathogenic bacteria and exclusion of these bacteria from the gut [22, 23]. Michetti *et al.*, suggested that prevention of attachment of the bacteria to the gut wall ('immune exclusion') is the possible protection mechanism of this IgA [24].

In the colon of normal mice 30% of the (anaerobic) bacteria are coated with IgA [18]. Despite this coating, these commensal bacteria remain in the gut lumen. This seems to be in contradiction with the above-mentioned experiments by Michetti *et al.*. We like to speculate here that differences in affinities (or specificities) of antibodies could explain this notion. B-1 cell derived IgA mAb's usually bind with only a fraction of the monocultured anaerobic bacteria (see Table 1), which might reflect low affinity interaction of these IgA antibodies with bacteria. *In vivo*, this may lead to partial clearance of a certain bacterial species and thus an ineffective 'immune exclusion'. As a consequence, a dynamic equilibrium is reached in which commensal bacteria are able to maintain themselves within the gastro-intestinal tract despite this IgA coating. This is in accordance with experiments whereby germfree mice are monoassociated with the commensal bacteria *Morganella morganii* [25]. In these experiments, IgA production is initially observed in the Peyer's patches, resolving the initial translocation of these bacteria to internal organs, which is followed by a continuous IgA production in the lamina propria of the small intestine resulting in a dynamic equilibrium with a stable number of *Morganella morganii* within the gut.

In conclusion, IgA produced by the two B cell lineages might exert different effects *in vivo* on bacteria present in the intestinal lumen. Low affinity IgA antibodies derived from B-1 cells could thus play a role in maintaining a stable microflora, whereas high affinity antibodies (originating from conventional B cells located in Peyer's patches) could result in 'immune exclusion'. Future experiments will aim to test this hypothesis.

References

1. Van der Heijden PJ, Stok W, and Bianchi ATJ. (1987). Contribution of immunoglobulin-secreting cells in the murine small intestine to the 'background' immunoglobulin production. Immunology 62:551-555.
2. Mattioli C, and Tomasi T. (1973). The life span of IgA plasma cells from the mouse intestine. J Exp Med 138:452-460.
3. Kroese FGM, Cebra JJ, Van der Cammen MJF, Kantor AB, and Bos NA. (1995). Contribution of B-1 cells to intestinal IgA production in the mouse. Methods 8:37-43.
4. Kroese FGM, Kantor AB, and Herzenberg LA. (1994). The role of B-1 cells (Ly-1 B cells) in mucosal immune responses. In: Ogra PL, Lamm ME, McGhee JR, Mestecky J, Strober W, Bienenstock J (Eds) Handbook of Mucosal Immunology. Academic Press, Inc. San Diego. pp 217-224..
5. Lebman DA, Nomura DY, Coffman RL, and Lee FL. (1990). Molecular characterization of germline immunoglobulin A transcript produced during transforming growth factor type β-induced isotype switching. Proc Natl Acad Sci USA 87:3962-3966.
6. De Waard R, Dammers PM, Tung JW, Kantor AB, Wilshire JA, Bos NA, Herzenberg LA, and Kroese FGM. (1998). Presence of germline and full-length IgA mRNA transcripts among peritoneal B-1 cells. Dev Immunol 6:81-87.
7. Vogel LA, and Metzger DW. (1995). Approaches for the study of T-cell influences on B1-cell function. Methods 8:61-69.
8. Taki S, Schmitt M, Tarlington D, Förster I, and Rajewsky K. (1992). T cell-dependent antibody production by Ly-1 B cells. Ann N Y Acad Sci 651:328-335.
9. Wetzel GD. (1990). Interleukin 5 regulation of peritoneal B-cell proliferation and antibody secretion. Scand. J. Immunol. 31:91-101
10. Hitoshi Y, Yamaguchi N, Tominaga A, and Takatsu K. (1992). Coexpression of CD5 and IL-5 receptor on peritoneal B cells. Ann N Y Acad Sci 651:261-263
11. Takatsu K, Kariyone A, Kouro T, Kikuchi Y, Hitoshi Y, and Takaki S. (1995). Interleukin-5 receptor and CD5-positive B cells. Methods 8:45-59.
12. Bao S, Beagley KW, Murray AM, Caristo V, Matthaei KI, Young G, and Husband AJ. (1998). Intestinal IgA plasma cells of the B1 lineage are IL-5 dependent. Immunology 94:181-188.
13. Baumgarth N, Egerton M, and Kelso A. (1997). Activated T cells from draining lymph nodes and effector site differ in their responses to TCR stimulation. J Immunol 159:1182-1191.
14. Hardy RR, and Hayakawa K. (1992). Developmental origins, specificities and immunoglobulin gene biases of murine Ly-1 B cells. Int Rev Immunol 8:189-207.
15. Bos NA, Bun JCAM, Popma SH, Cebra ER, Deenen GJ, Cammen MJFvd, Kroese FGM, and Cebra JJ. (1996). Monoclonal Immunoglobulin A derived from peritoneal B cells is encoded by both germ line and somatically mutated VH genes and reactive with commensal bacteria. Inf Immun 64:616-623.
16. Quan CP, Berneman A, Pires R, Avrameas S, and Bouvet JP. (1997). Natural polyreactive

secretory immunoglobulin A autoantibodies as a possible barrier to infection in humans. Inf Immun 65:3997-4004.
17. Marcotte H, and Lavoie MC. (1996). No apparent influence of immuno-globulins on indigenous oral and intestinal microbiota of mice. Inf Immun 64:4694-4699.
18. Kroese FGM, De Waard R, and Bos NA. (1996). B1 cells and their reactivity with the murine intestinal microflora. Sem Immunol 8:11-18.
19. Van der Waaij LA, Limburg PC, Mesander G, and Van der Waaij D. (1996). In vivo IgA coating of anaerobic bacteria in human faeces. Gut 38:348-354.
20. Bos NA, Rijsemus AN, Van de Werf M, Schut F, and Welling GW. 1997. Usage of 16S rRNA in situ hybridisation to study bacterial population dynamics in host-flora interactions. In: Hashimoto K, Sakakibara B, Tazume S, Shimizu K (Ed) Germfree life and its ramifications. XII ISG Publishing Committee, Shiozawa, pp 231-235.
21. Potter M, and Wiener F. (1992). Plasmacytomagenesis in mice: a model of neoplastic development dependent upon chromosomal translocations. Carcinogenesis 13:1681-1697.
22. Michetti P, Mahan MJ, Slauch JM, Mekalanos JJ, and Neutra MR. (1992). Monoclonal secretory immunoglobulin A protects mice against oral challlenge with the invasive pathogen *Salmonella typhimurium*. Inf Immun 60:1786-1792.
23. Apter FM, Lenger WI, Finkelstein RA, Mekalanos JJ, and Neutra MR. (1993). Monoclonal immunoglobulin a antibodies directed against cholera toxin prevent the toxin-induced chloride secretory response and block toxin binding to intestinal epithelial cells in vitro. Inf Immun 61:5271-5278.
24. Michetti P, Porta N, Mahan MJ, Slauch JM, Mekalanos JJ, Blum AL, Kraehenbuhl J, and Neutra MR. (1994). Monoclonal immunoglobulin A prevents adherence and invasion of polarized epithelial cell monolayers by *Salmonella typhimurium*. Gastroenterology 107:915-923.
25. Shroff KE, Meslin K, and Cebra JJ. (1995). Commensal enteric bacteria engender a self-limiting humoral mucosal immune response while permanently colonizing the gut. Inf Immun 63:3904-3913.

Discussion

Fritz Melchers: How do SCID mice or RAG2 knockout mice actually manage the bacterial flora?
Frans Kroese: This is a very important question. Apparently IgA is not needed for the flora itself, but you can alter the flora.
Sandy Morse: You took a look at IgA germline transcripts, and did you look at other classes to see these things?
Frans Kroese: No, we have to do that.
Sandy Morse: Because it could be that you are saying that IgA is there.
Frans Kroese: I think IgE might be very important, too. We have to check that.
Sandy Morse: Secondly, this could be the devil's advocate, as the other side of the whole B-1 story is as Henry Wortis argues that if you contact any cell with a polyvalent antigen, such as a bacterial antigen, you are going to induce CD5. So I could argue that what you have in the peritoneum are cells which are CD5-expressing because they have seen bacterial antigen, and you give me the same readout by saying that they make antibodies to bacteria.
Frans Kroese: I did not want to speak about a lineage issue, but the major argument against Henry Wortis is of course that if you take an irradiated mouse and give it back bone marrow, you never get back any CD5-positive cells.
Sandy Morse: I disagree with that. I have reconstituted lots of mice and I cannot get it!
Frans Kroese: Sure, that is why I did not want to go into lineage.
Una Chen: I am asking an artistic question. If you have ten different pigments and you put them together, it is black. If you have ten different fluorescent colors, and you put them together, it is white. The question is, if you have a condition where ten cytokines are all expressing in one single cell, what kind of color do you get?
Frans Kroese: That is a very difficult question to answer.
Andreas Radbruch: Why did you not test TGFβ expression in the T cells, because it is the only responsive cytokine able to induce the IgA antibody class switch?
Frans Kroese: To be honest, I failed to conjugate the antibody the week before I left!
Riccardo Dalla-Favera: Are the variable regions mutated or germline?
Frans Kroese: Of these eight antibodies, two of them were germline and eight were mutated.
Riccardo Dalla-Favera: Where do you think they mutate?
Frans Kroese: Of the six that were mutated, two of them appeared to be really the result of antigen-driven selection.
Ulf Klein: But in mouse not all V genes are known.
Frans Kroese: No, that is the major problem: For two of them we are sure, for some of them we are not completely sure. But two of them were real germline, and one of them was directed against dextran.

Inhibition of Pristane-Induced Peritoneal Plasmacytoma Formation

M. Potter and L. Kutkat
Laboratory of Genetics, National Cancer Institute, National Institutes of Health, Bethesda, MD 20892, USA

Unraveling the pathogenetic natural history of the PCT has proven to be complex and to involve several factors. The inducing agents, though chemically and physically different, are not obviously genotoxic, and it is reasonable to assume they exert their effects by slowly and persistently inducing a chronic inflammatory process. The nature of this chronic inflammation varies with the inducing agent. The genetic vulnerability of BALB/c B cells, however, is the important underlying factor in peritoneal plasmacytomagenesis (PCTGEN). It is the response of these cells to the unusual peritoneal environment that determines progression to neoplasia. Remarkably, despite both genetic susceptibility and acquisition of a myc-activating chromosomal translocation, other factors can interfere with plasma cell tumor formation. This paper will review the various methods for inhibiting PCTGEN and attempt to sketch models to show their interrelationship to the process of PCT development. These inhibitions include the refractoriness of pristane injected specific pathogen free (SPF) raised BALB/cAn, IL-6 deficient and BALB/c.CBA/N (Xid) mice; the inhibition of PCTGEN by indomethacin and the reduction of PCT development in conventionally raised BALB/c mice.

Plasmacytomas (PCTs) are induced in high frequency in genetically susceptible strains of mice, e.g., BALB/cAn (B/C) [1] and BALB/cAn.DBA/2-Idh1-Pep3 (C.D2-I/P). Induction is initiated by introducing poorly metabolized materials (paraffin oils [1], plastic objects [2], silicone gels [3]) into the peritoneal space. These materials cause the formation of various kinds of chronic inflammatory tissues on peritoneal surfaces where the PCTs develop. The best studied material is the paraffin oil pristane (2,6,10,14-tetramethylpentadecane). This is given in 3 doses of 0.2-0.5 ml each on days 0, 60 and 120. Pristane injected into the peritoneal space disperses into innumerable oil droplets of variable sizes. Peritoneal macrophages and neutrophils surround these oil droplets and the complexes adhere to peritoneal surfaces. There then ensues a prolonged interaction at the interface between the oil and surrounding cells which at first is inflammatory but much later becomes inactive with the deposition of hyaline like material in locations occupied by the oil. Developing PCTs in the form of multiple focal proliferations of plasma cells can be found in oil granuloma tissue sections of some mice from day 75 on [4]. The first PCTs develop after 120 days and are detected by finding atypical plasma cells in the peritoneal fluid using Wright-Giemsa stained cytofuge preparations. 10^5 or more atypical plasma cells per field from primary hosts are transplantable in pristane conditioned hosts. The mean latent periods are around 180 days for C.D2-I/P and 220 days for B/C. The incidence of PCTs in susceptible hosts is between 50% (for B/C) and 70% for C.D2-I/P. Karyotypic analysis of these PCTs has revealed that 95% of them carry reciprocal translocations T(12;15) or T(6:15) (see [5]). These illegitimate recombinations deregulate the transcription of c-myc [6,7].

Inhibitions with B Cell Developmental Implications

SPF

When conventionally reared (CV) BALB/cAnPt mice were rederived in SPF conditions, they became refractory to PCT induction by pristane, developing an incidence of only 5% PCTs [8]. These mice do not colonize their GI tracts as neonates nor as adults with the same large number of microbial species as do conventional mice. As adults SPF mice are maintained in isolation from other mice and are fed sterile water and autoclaved mouse pellets.

During fetal and neonatal life B cells with $sIgM^{hi}$, $sIgD^{lo}$, $B220^{lo}$ and $CD5^{+/-}$ phenotype are the prevailing B cells, known as B-1 cells in the mouse. These cells are exposed primarily to autoantigens in fetal life and microbial antigens during the colonization of the gastrointestinal tract in neonatal life [9]. At around 40 days of age the *de novo* generation of B cells with these phenotypes virtually ceases [10]. B-1 cells are continuously replenished from $V_HD_HJ_H$ and V_LJ_L rearranged self renewing precursors [11,12,10]. Depletion of B-1 cells during the neonatal period creates life-long immune defects (see [10]).

A dramatic example of the effects of the SPF status is the work of Murakami *et al.* [13,14] who utilized a transgenic mouse carrying genes for an autoantibody to mouse red blood cells (auto-Ab Tg). The auto-Ab Tg mice have very few conventional B cells and are mostly populated by B-1 cells that have escaped elimination and which can survive in protected peritoneal microenvironments. They found that when the auto-Ab TG mice are raised in conventional conditions, about 50% of them develop hemolytic anemia (HA); but when the mice were rederived as SPF or germ free (GF), none of the mice developed HA [13]. They also showed that when 100 μg LPS was directly introduced into the GI tract of SPF or germ free autoAb-TG mice, 25% of them developed HA [15]. They proposed that microorganisms in the GI tract or LPS can activate peritoneal B-1 cells [13]. Possible explanations for how the SPF state renders susceptible BALB/cAn mice refractory to pristane PCT induction is through antigenic deprivation. In the neonatal period this may limit the B-1 repertoire in adult mice. It may reduce antigenic and mitogenic B cell signals required for maintenance and proliferation.

Xid

We have recently found that BALB/cAn.CBA/N$^{xid/xid}$ mice (i.e., BALB/c mice carrying the X linked immunodeficency gene, Btk^{xid}) are resistant to PCT induction by pristane (submitted for publication). The basic immunological defects in Xid mice, most of which were originally described in CBA/N but probably also characterize C.CBA/N as well, are an inability to respond to type 2 thymus independent (TI-2) antigens [16,17] and a profound reduction in B-1 lymphocytes [12]. The product of the xid gene is Bruton's agammaglobulinemia tyrosine kinase (Btk) a kinase that is activated in B cells by cross-linking sIgM receptors (BCR). Btk plays an important role in signal transduction from BCR crosslinking leading to DNA synthesis and completion of the cell cycle in B cells [18,19]. This is particularly critical in B cells whose Igs bind to type 2 thymus independent antigens [20]. Antigens that crosslink BCRs have repetitive similar epitopes often on polysaccharide backbones. B-1 lymphocytes with defective Btk^{xid} alleles that are stimulated by TI-2 antigens fail to complete the cell cycle and are probably eliminated by apoptosis [18,19], and this could possibly explain the basis for the deficiency in B-1 cells.

Despite these defects Xid mice can be successfully raised and maintained in conventional conditions. When, however, Xid mice are challenged by potential pathogens such as *Salmonella typhimurium* [21] or *Streptococcus pneumoniae* [22], they are hypersusceptible to the lethal effects of these organisms. Other defects in conventional bone marrow derived B-lymphocytes (B-2 cells) have been found in Xid mice. These mice develop poor primary responses to some thymus dependent antigens but are able to generate secondary responses that are comparable to those in wild type mice [23]. Proof, then, that B-1 cells are the precursors of PCTs must await reconstitution experiments.

The ubiquity of TI-2 antigens in the internal and external environments of the mouse makes it possible for those B cells capable of responding to these antigens to be continuously and intermittently stimulated. If a memory-like state exists in B-1 cells, the life of individual clones could be greatly extended by repeated exposure to these ubiquitous antigens. In autoimmune mice, e.g., NZB or (NZW x NZB)F1, it has been possible to demonstrate clonal longevity by successive marker mutations resulting in somatic hypermutations [24]. Similar patterns have been found in rheumatoid synovial membranes [25] and in salivary glands from Sjogren syndrome patients [26]. The latter two examples are of particular relevance because the B cells are proliferating in extra lymphoid sites. Essentially, cells with one oncogenic mutation [e.g., the myc-activating T(12;15) translocation in PCTGEN] proliferate, and their progeny undergo secondary changes. It is postulated that clonal longevity in cells responding to TI-2 antigens could alternatively accumulate genetic changes, i.e., mutations or possibly epigenetic changes that modify their genomes in such a way that they begin to proliferate without control (neoplastic phenotypes). Evidence for unusual clonal expansions has been observed in NZB mice as so-called B-CLL like clones [27]. But even in non-autoimmune mice such as C57BL/6 selected B cell clones expand with age [28]. Thus, it becomes possible in wild type (non Xid) hosts for B cell clones to be extended by re-encounters with the same antigens. Should oncogenic changes such as the myc activating T(12;15) translocations occur in one of these long lived clones, this may further immortalize the clone and make it a candidate for further progression to more autonomous growth.

Summary

Both the SPF and Xid findings may affect B cell responses to TI-2 antigens (Fig. 1). Reducing the exposure to antigens during the neonatal period in SPF mice and also throughout adult life may effectively limit the sustained devlopment of these B cell clones. A possible explanation for how the Xid mutation renders BALB/c mice resistant to PCT induction is that these mice cannot respond properly to T1-2 antigens and, hence, do not develop clones that can be continuously stimulated to undergo proliferation by these abiquitous antigens. This either reduces this B cell population or results in a failure to activate the B cells that are the most prone to become PCTs.

Inhibition by NSAIDS

Indomethacin

In 1965 Takakura and Hollander inhibited mineral oil induced PCTGEN by daily injections of cortisol [29]. Subsequently, our laboratory began studying the non-steroidal antiinflammatory (NSAID) agent indomethacin (Indo) and found that continuous administration in the drinking water for 200 to 300 days profoundly and sometimes completely inhibited the development of plasma cell tumors [30,2]. Indo does not inhibit the growth and transplantability of primary PCTs, therefore it is an inhibitor of PCT development. When Indo treatment is delayed for 25 or 50 days after the first injection of pristane, there is a striking but not complete reduction in the number of PCTs from 70% to 15-18%, suggesting that by 25 days some B cells have become refractory to Indo in the 25 day interval (Fig. 2). Thus, Indo appears to affect the early development of the PCT, probably by its effects on the B-lymphocyte precursors and not by inhibiting the proliferation of established tumor cells. Also, Indo does not appear to be associated with a lack of detectable T(12;15) translocations [2].

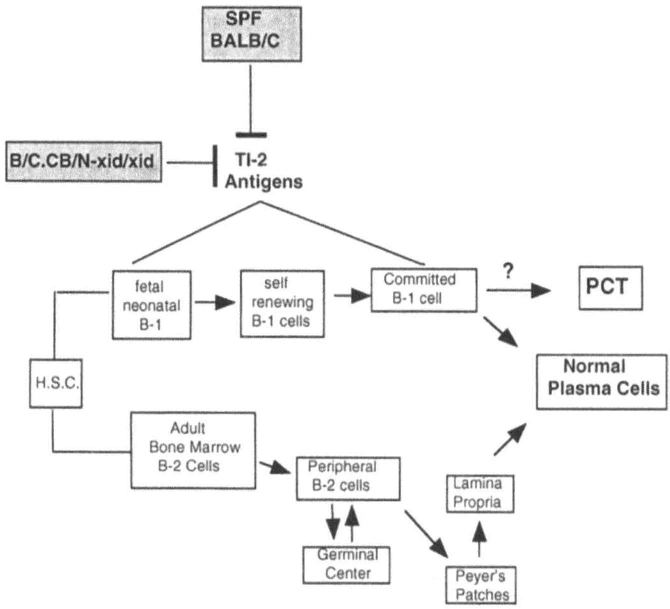

Fig 1. Scheme showing the development of B cells from hematopoietic stem cells. During fetal and neontal life B cells responding to autoantigens and ubiquitous microbial antigens undergo development. When the mice become adults the clones arising in fetal and neonatal life are self renewed from V_L/V_H differentiated stem cells in the periphery. The HSCs in bone marrow continuously supply continuosly supply the that adult organism. It is postulated here that PCTs arise B-1 populations because these B cell clones are long lived because of repeated antigenic stimulation from ubiquitous antigens and hence can acculumlate oncogenic mutations.

The mechanism of indomethacin inhibition of PCTGEN has not been determined. There are several different possible explanations relevant to the PCT system. The prevailing concept of Indo action has been until recently that its primary pharmacological effect results from the inactivation of prostaglandin synthase activity [i.e., cyclooxygenases 1 and 2 (COX-1,COX-2)] and the subsequent loss of their synthetic products the prostaglandins: PGE_2, PGD_2, PGI_2, PGF_{2a} and TXA2. COX-1 is constitutively expressed in many cell types, while COX-2 is induced in selective cell types such as macrophages by various agents and conditions (see [31] for review). PGE_2 secretion by B lymphocytes is not well established, and B cells appear to produce only minimal amounts of PGs as compared with macrophages [32]. Thus, exogenous prostaglandins, i.e., those produced by accessory cells such as macrophages and fibroblasts, appear to be the principle sources for lymphocytes.

Indo is an inhibitor of both COX-1 and COX-2. At *in vitro* concentrations close to the levels obtained pharmacologically (around 10 to 20 μM) Indo completely inhibits COX-1, but only 20% of COX-2. These values change quantitatively with different assay systems [33,31]. The oil granuloma contains a great abundance of macrophages which are known to secrete PGs [34]. PGE_2 is, however, biologically

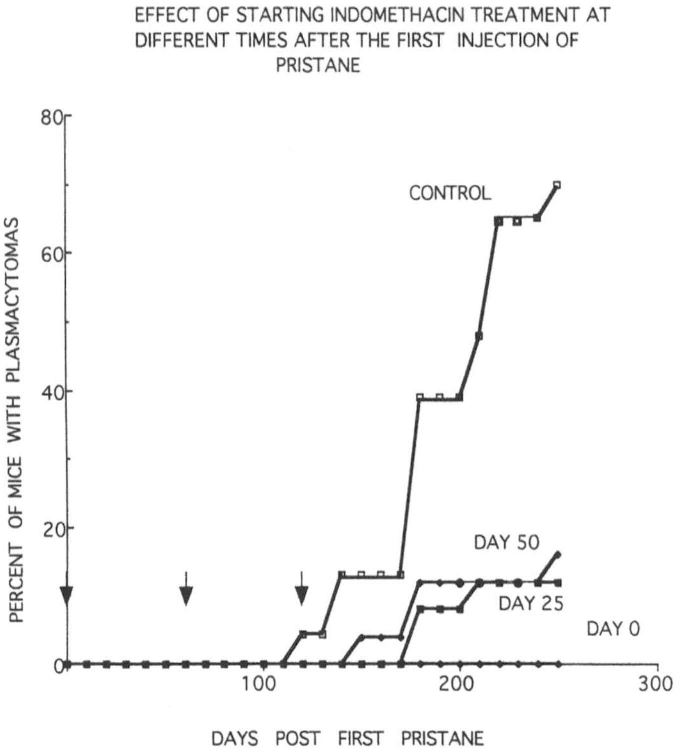

Fig2. Plasmacytoma induction experiment. Three pristane doses of 0.2 , 0.5 and 0.5 ml were given on days 0 ,60 and 120 respectively (arrows). Indomethacin was administered in the drinking water at 20μg/ml beginning on days 0,25 or 50.

active in B lymphocytes which possess PGE_2 receptors (EP1, EP2, EP3 and EP4 receptors) but responses of B cells vary with the state of maturity and differentiation [35]. The binding of PGE_2 to EP receptors initiates a signal that leads to activation of adenylyl cyclase and the formation of cAMP [36]. Elevation of the cAMP levels inhibits B cell activation [37]. These findings in general make it difficult to explain the role of PGE_2 as a growth factor or even as a maintenance factor for B lymphocytes (see discussion in [2] for references).

There is gathering evidence in non-B cell types that NSAIDS may not act in the conventional way by inhibiting prostaglandin synthesis. Recent findings in colonocytes have suggested a direct action of indomethacin and other related NSAIDs on target cells that may be cyclooxygenase independent [38,39,40]. In some of these experiments indomethacin activates an intracellular steroid-like receptor PPAR-γ [41,42,43]. The concentration of Indo that achieves these effects is considerably higher than that required for COX inhibition [41]. Supporting evidence for a COX independent mechanism comes from studies with other structurally related NSAIDs. Sulindac sulfone, which is an oxidative metabolite of sulindac (structurally similar to indomethacin), does not inhibit COX-1 or 2 [44] but nonetheless inhibits azoxymethane-induced colon carcinogenesis in rats. Further, sulindac sulfone induces apoptosis in human colon carcinoma cells [45]. Several COX inhibitors, including indomethacin, induce apoptosis in human colon carcinoma cells *in vitro* that lack COX-1 and 2 [46]. Thus, the possibility must be entertained that indomethacin could be acting on B lymphocytes by a COX independent mechanism and not by eliminating the synthesis of inflammatory prostanoids such as PGE_2. It will be of great interest to explore these pathways and determine if Indo could directly lead to the selective elimination of B cells that are the precursors of the PCTs.

IL-6

Indo could act indirectly by inhibiting the formation of cytokines in accessory cells. There is evidence that PGE_2 can induce IL-6 expression in peritoneal macrophages [34]. It could be argued then that limiting the local availability of IL-6 by lowering the PGE_2 levels would generate a microenvironment in the peritoneum that would not be conducive to plasma cell survival. In these experiments Indo reduced the level of COX-2 mRNA and strongly inhibited PGE_2 formation. Two studies now show that pristane induction of PCTs is strongly, if not completely, inhibited in BALB/c IL-6 defective mice [47,48]. Further, it should be noted here that PPAR-γ agonists, one of which is Indo, can inhibit inflammatory cytokine formation including IL-6 in macrophages [43,38]. Thus, IL-6 suppression by indirectly reducing PGE_2 or the direct suppression of macrophage cytokine formation by Indo is at present the most viable explanation for how Indo works in PCTGEN.

Summary

While the mechanism of how Indo inhibits PCTGEN is not established (Fig. 3), several hypothetical explanations provide new potential experimental approaches. Indo may block production of cytokines such as IL-6 in accessory cells that are critical for B cell growth, viability and maturation, or it may directly target B cells via PPAR-γ receptors. The latter mode of action is described in other cell types but not yet defined in B cells.

Conclusions

The process of PCTGEN in genetically susceptible strains of mice (BALB/cAn or C.D2-I/P) that is set in motion by the i.p. injections of pristane can be inhibited by different means. Adapting and rearing BALB/cAn mice under SPF conditions causes a drastic reduction of PCTs from 50% to 5%. Although the mechanism of this inhibition is not established, it appears to be due to a decreased exposure to antigens and microbial mitogens beginning in the neonatal period and extending throughout

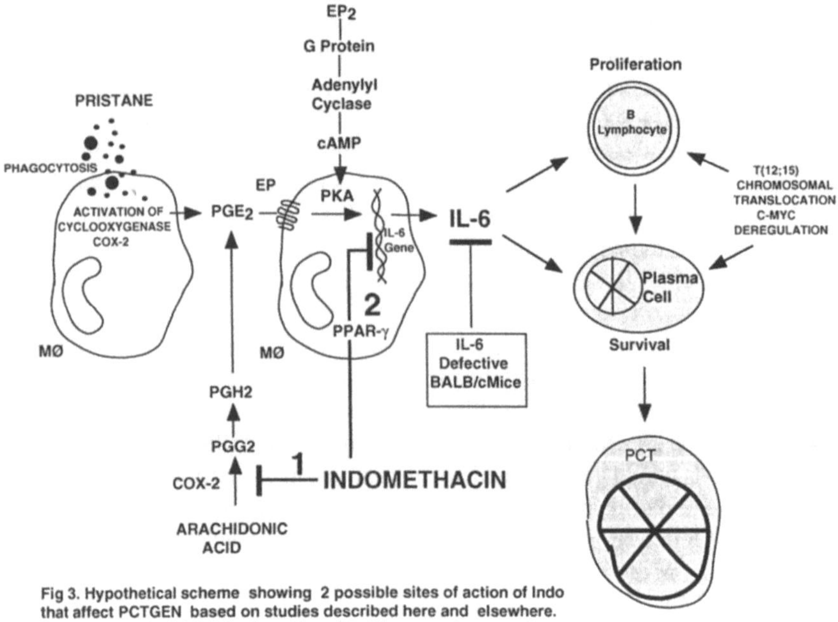

Fig 3. Hypothetical scheme showing 2 possible sites of action of Indo that affect PCTGEN based on studies described here and elsewhere. These appear to inhibit the formation of IL-6 in macrophages and fibroblasts either through inhibiting prostaglandin synthesis or blocking IL-6 synthesis by stimulating PPAR-γ . BALB/c IL-6 defective mice fail to develop PCTS. See text for refs

life. This probably results in a failure to stimulate and maintain B cells and results in a loss of B cells in total B cell number and clonal expansion. The resistance of BALB/c.CBA/N$^{xix/xid}$ to PCT induction may be due to a loss or failure of B cells that respond to ubiquitous TI-2 antigens of microbial and autogenous origin. In both the SPF Xid mice it may be very difficult for potentially responding B cell clones to expand and be restimulated by the same or related antigens. In BALB/c-IL-6 defective mice, as described by others, an essential growth and maturation factor that is apparently made by accessory cells, again can result in B cell clones with limited capability for clonal expansion. The mechanism of indomethacin inhibition is not yet defined but may be mediated in accessory cells (macrophages, fibroblasts) that are sources of growth factors (e.g., IL-6) that are required for maximal B cell maintenance and proliferation. Changes in common environmental conditions, diet and cage bedding appear also to be modulating factors. However, these remain to be substantiated.

References

1. Potter M, Wax JS (1983) Peritoneal plasmacytomagenesis in mice: comparison of different pristane dose regimens. J Natl Cancer Inst 71:391-395
2. Potter M, Wax J, Jones GM (1997) Indomethacin is a potent inhibitor of pristane and plastic disc induced plasmacytomagenesis in a hypersusceptible BALB/c congenic strain. Blood 90:260-269
3. Potter M, Morrison S, Wiener F, Miller FW (1994) Induction of plasmacytomas with silicone gel in genetically susceptible strains of mice. J Natl Cancer Inst 86:1058-1065
4. Potter M, Mushinski EB, Wax JS, Hartley J, Mock BA (1994) Identification of two genes on chromosome 4 that determine resistance to plasmacytoma induction in mice. Cancer Res 54:969-975
5. Potter M, Wiener F (1992) Plasmacytomagenesis in mice: model of neoplastic development dependent upon chromosomal translocations. Carcinogenesis 13:1681-1697
6. Mushinski JF (1988) c-myc oncogene activation and chromosomal translocation in BALB/c plasmacytomas. In: Klein G (ed) Cellular Oncogene Activation. Marcel Dekker, New York, pp 181-222
7. Cory S (1986) Activation of cellular oncogenes in hemopoietic cells by chromosome translocation. Adv Cancer Res 47:189-211
8. Byrd LG, McDonald AH, Gold LG, Potter M (1991) Specific pathogen-free BALB/cAn mice are refractory to plasmacytoma induction by pristane. J Immunol 147:3632-3637
9. Kroese FG, de Waard R, Bos NA (1996) B-1 cells and their reactivity with the murine intestinal microflora. Semin Immunol 8:11-18
10. Kantor AB, Stall AM, Adams S, Watanabe K, Herzenberg LA (1995) De novo development and self-replenishment of B cells. Int Immunol 7:55-68.
11. Hayakawa K, Hardy RR, Stall AM, Herzenberg LA (1986) Immunoglobulin-bearing B cells reconstitute and maintain the murine Ly-1 B cell lineage. Eur J Immunol 16:1313-1316
12. Hayakawa K, Hardy RR, Parks DR, Herzenberg LA (1983) The "Ly-1 B" cell subpopulation in normal immunodefective, and autoimmune mice. J Exp Med 157:202-218
13. Murakami M, Nakajma K, Yamazaki K, Muraguchi T, Serikawa T, Honjo T (1997) Effects of breeding environments on generation and activation of autoreactive B-1 cells in anti-red blood cell autoantibody transgenic mice. J Exp Med 185:791-794
14. Murakami M (1996) Anti-red blood cell autoantibody transgenic mice: murine model of autoimmune hemolytic anemia. Semin Immunol 8:3-9
15. Murakami M, Tsubata T, Shinkura R, Nisitani S, Okamoto M, Yoshioka H, Usui T, Miyawaki S, Honjo T (1994) Oral administration of lipopolysaccharides activates B-1 cells in the peritoneal cavity and lamina propria of the gut and induces autoimmune symptoms in an autoantibody transgenic mouse. J Exp Med 180:111-121
16. Scher I (1982) CBA/N immune defective mice; evidence for the failure of a B cell subpopulation to be expressed. Immunol Rev 64:117-136
17. Mosier DE, Scher I, Paul WE (1976) In vitro responses of CBA/N mice: spleen cells of mice with an X- linked defect that precludes immune responses to several thymus- independent antigens can respond to TNP-lipopolysaccharide. J Immunol 117:1363-1369
18. Satterthwaite AB, Li Z, Witte O (1998) Btk function in B cell development and response. Semin Immunol 10:309-316
19. Brorson K, Brunswick M, Ezhevsky S, Wei DG, Berg R, Scott D, Stein KE (1997) xid affects events leading to B cell cycle entry. J Immunol 159:135-143
20. Bondada S, Garg M (1994) Thymus-independent antigens. In: Handbook of B and T Lymphocytes. Academic Press, pp 343-370
21. O'Brien AD, Scher I, Campbell GH, MacDermott RP, Formal SB (1979) Susceptibility of CBA/N mice to infection with Salmonella typhimurium: influence of the X-linked gene controlling B lymphocyte function. J Immunol 123:720-724

22. Briles DE (1986) Genetic control of the susceptibility to pneumococcal infection. Curr Top Microbiol Immunol 124:103-120
23. Ridderstad A, Nossal GT, Tarlinton DM (1996) The xid mutation diminishes memory B cell generation but does not affect somatic hypermutation and selection. J Immunol 157:3357-3365
24. Shlomchik MJ, Marshak-Rothstein A, Wolfowicz CB, Rothstein TL, Weigert MG (1987) The role of clonal selection and somatic mutation in autoimmunity. Nature 328:895-911
25. Schroder AE, Greiner A, Seyfert C, Berek C (1996) Differentiation of B cells in the nonlymphoid tissue of the synovial membrane of patients with rheumatoid arthritis. Proc Natl Acad Sci USA 93:221-225
26. Stott DI, Hiepe F, Hummel M, Steinhauser G, Berek C (1998) Antigen-driven clonal proliferation of B cells within the target tissue of an autoimmune disease. The salivary glands of patients with Sjogren's syndrome. J Clin Invest 102:938-946
27. Stall AM (1988) Ly-1 B-cell clones similar to human chronic lymphocytic leukemias routinely develop in older normal mice and young autoimmune (New Zealand Black-related) animals. Proc Natl Acad Sci U S A 85:7312-7316
28. LeMaoult J, Delassus S, Dyall R, Nikolic-Zugic J, Kourilsky P, Weksler ME (1997) Clonal expansions of B lymphocytes in old mice. J Immunol 159:3866-3874
29. Takakura K, Mason WB, Hollander VP (1966) Studies on the pathogenesis of plasma cell tumors. I. Effect of cortisol on development of plasma cell tumors. Cancer Res 26:596-599
30. Potter M, Wax JS, Anderson AO, Nordan RP (1985) Inhibition of plasmacytoma development in BALB/c mice by indomethacin. J Exp Med 161:996-1012
31. Taketo MM (1998) Cyclooxygenase-2 inhibitors in tumorigenesis (part I). J Natl Cancer Inst 90:1529-1536
32. Calder PC (1996) Can n-3 polyunsaturated fatty acids be used as immunomodulatory agents? Biochem Soc Trans 24:211-220
33. Meade EA, Smith WL, DeWitt DL (1993) Differential inhibition of prostaglandin endoperoxide synthase (cyclooxygenase) isozymes by aspirin and other non-steroidal anti-inflammatory drugs. J Biol Chem 268:6610-6614
34. Hinson RM, Williams JA, Shacter E (1996) Elevated interleukin 6 is induced by prostaglandin E2 in a murine model of inflammation: possible role of cyclooxygenase-2. Proc Natl Acad Sci USA 93:4885-4890
35. Fedyk ER, Ripper JM, Brown DM, Phipps RP (1996) A molecular analysis of PGE receptor (EP) expression on normal and transformed B lymphocytes: coexpression of EP1, EP2, EP3beta and EP4. Mol Immunol 33:33-45
36. Phipps RP, Lee D, Schad V, Warner GL (1989) E-series prostaglandins are potent growth inhibitors for some B lymphomas. Eur J Immunol 19:996-1001
37. Roper RL, Ludlow JW, Phipps RP (1994) Prostaglandin E2 inhibits B lymphocyte activation by a cAMP-dependent mechanism: PGE-inducible regulatory proteins. Cell Immunol 154:296-308
38. Simmons DL, Madsen ML, Robertson PM (1997) COX-2 and apoptosis: NSAIDs as effectors of programmed cell death. In: Vane J, Botting J (ed) Selective COX-2 Inhibitors. Dordrecht, Kluver Academic, pp 55-65
39. Shiff SJ, Rigas B (1997) Nonsteroidal anti-inflammatory drugs and colorectal cancer: evolving concepts of their chemopreventive actions. Gastroenterology 113:1992-1998
40. Abramson SB, Weissmann G (1989) The mechanisms of action of nonsteroidal antiinflammatory drugs. Arthritis Rheum 32:1-9
41. Lehmann JM, Lenhard JM, Oliver BB, Ringold GM, Kliewer SA (1997) Peroxisome proliferator-activated receptors alpha and gamma are activated by indomethacin and other non-steroidal anti- inflammatory drugs. J Biol Chem 272:3406-3410
42. Ricote M, Li AC, Willson TM, Kelly CJ, Glass CK (1998) The peroxisome proliferator-activated receptor-gamma is a negative regulator of macrophage activation. Nature 391:79-82
43. Jiang C, Ting AT, Seed B (1998) PPAR-gamma agonists inhibit production of monocyte inflammatory cytokines. Nature 391:82-86

44. Piazza GA, Alberts DS, Hixson LJ, Paranka NS, Li H, Finn T, Bogert C, Guillen JM, Brendel K, Gross PH, Sperl G, Ritchie J, Burt RW, Ellsworth L, Ahnen DJ, Pamukcu R (1997) Sulindac sulfone inhibits azoxymethane-induced colon carcinogenesis in rats without reducing prostaglandin levels. Cancer Res 57:2909-2915
45. Piazza GA, Rahm AL, Krutzsch M, Sperl G, Paranka NS, Gross PH, Brendel K, Burt RW, Alberts DS, Pamukcu R (1995) Antineoplastic drugs sulindac sulfide and sulfone inhibit cell growth by inducing apoptosis. Cancer Res 55:3110-3116
46. Hanif R, Pittas A, Feng Y, Koutsos MI, Qiao L, Staiano-Coico L, Shiff SI, Rigas B (1996) Effects of nonsteroidal anti-inflammatory drugs on proliferation and on induction of apoptosis in colon cancer cells by a prostaglandin-independent pathway. Biochem Pharmacol 52:237-245
47. Hilbert DM (1995) Interleukin 6 is essential for in vivo development of B lineage neoplasms. J Exp Med 182:243-248
48. Lattanzio G, Libert C, Aquilina M, Cappelletti M, Ciliberto G, Musiani P, Poli V (1997) Defective development of pristane-oil-induced plasmacytomas in interleukin-6-deficient BALB/c mice [see comments]. Am J Pathol 151:689-696

Discussion

Kenneth Nilsson: So you postulate antigen-driven development, at least in the beginning?
Mike Potter: Yes, I do not know how to control this step but I am hoping that it can be done.
Fritz Melchers: Since the $BTK^{-/-}$ mouse is normal in T cell-dependent stimulation, for instance induced by anti-CD40 and IL-4, would you postulate that your plasmacytomas derive from T cell-independent stimulation?
Mike Potter: Yes, I think they would have to depend upon these special antigens and that the reason why these B cells became tumor is because of what they make.
Michael Carroll: I would like to comment: coreceptor-deficient mice have a limited number of B-1 cells in the peritoneum. In those that are there we have looked at, the repertoire seems to be skewed and missing PtC-specific B-1 cells, so at least it supports the idea that complement might be involved in the amplification scheme that you pointed out.
Mike Potter: I think that is a fabulous approach and I am more than eager to work with you on that.
Katherine Siminovitch: I am not sure that you can attribute the results to the B-1 cell population *per se*. Your findings may merely reflect the fact that BTK is missing.
Mike Potter: I guess you are alluding to the possibility that BTK has more pleiotropic effects on B cells than just the effects in the so-called B-1 population.
Katherine Siminovitch: The presence or absence of BTK activity is going to change the strength of signal evoked by antigen receptor ligation. In other words, since signaling strength appears to be relevant to the production of B-1 cells, the absence of B-1 cells in these mice probably reflects a phenotypic manifestation of the fact that lack of BTK activity reduces the signaling capacity of the antigen receptor. The important variable is impaired signaling, not whether the cell is a B-1 cell.
Fritz Melchers: Many of your tumors produce IgA. I like your whole proposal because of studies that we did about 8 years ago transplanting preB-I cells into SCID mice which showed that transplantation yielded only B cells in SCID mice, and only IgM and IgA, but not IgG production. IgA production was found to be about one-third of the level of normal, without the apparent presence of T cells. So there is T cell-independent induction to IgA switching and production of plasma cells in the lamina propria. The question is whether you find a lot of somatic mutations in your tumors. Can you say something about somatic mutations in the IgA tumors?
Mike Potter: No, I can't, because I cannot prove the neoplastic plasma cells were derived from B-1 cells.

The Role of p16^{INK4a} (*Cdkn2a*) in Mouse Plasma Cell Tumors

Shuling Zhang and Beverly A. Mock
Laboratory of Genetics, DBS, 37 Convent Dr., Bldg. 37, Rm 2B-08, NCI, NIH, Bethesda, MD 20892-4255, USA

Mouse plasma cell tumors (PCT) arise in BALB/cAn and NZB mice due to a protracted series of events culminating in tumor incidences of 60 and 30%, respectively, over a period of 220-360 days[1,2]. These incidences are due to both genetic and environmental factors. During the past several years, we have documented that at least two genes, *Pctr1* and *Pctr2*, on the distal half of mouse Chr 4 play a determining role in the susceptibility of BALB/cAn mice to PCT formation [3-6]. Additional congenic strain analyses are in support of a third locus, *Pctr3*, also residing on Chr 4 between *Pctr1* and *Pctr2*.

Recently, we documented that the *Cdkn2a* locus, coding for two separate proteins, p16^{INK4a} and p19^{ARF}, is a good candidate for the plasmacytoma susceptibility/resistance gene, *Pctr1*[6]. In these studies we demonstrated that BALB/c mice are almost unique in their *Cdkn2a* sequence, with substitutions noted in both exon1α and exon 2. The exon1α variant affects the p16^{INK4a} locus only; however, the exon 2 variant would affect both p16 and p19 proteins. We were able to show that p16 proteins engineered to contain the BALB/c variant of either exon1α, exon 2, or both variants were defective in their ability to inhibit Rb phosphorylation in *in vitro* kinase assays. In contrast, wild-type p16, present in our tumor-resistant strain DBA/2N, could effectively inhibit Rb phosphorylation[6].

The importance of the *Cdkn2a* locus in cancer is underscored by its involvement in the two most important tumor suppressor pathways involved in cancer, namely both the Rb and p53 pathways. Both p16^{INK4a} and p19^{ARF}, two alternative proteins coded for by the *Cdkn2a* locus play an important role in progression of cells through the cell cycle. When p16 binds to the cyclin dependent kinases 4 and 6, it inhibits Rb phosphorylation which in turn, induces G1 phase arrest. When p19^{ARF} binds to Mdm2, it stabilizes and activates p53 by preventing Mdm2 from inhibiting p53 function. The direct consequences of these actions are not well documented; however, it has also been shown that when p19^{ARF} is overexpressed in cell lines, this can lead to growth arrest at both the G1 and G2/M phases of the cell cycle[7]. A growing list of tumors have been shown to incur loss of function mutations in p16 either by deletion or methylation and silencing of expression; data are still being accumulated for p19^{ARF}.

Point mutations or single base change allelic variants of p16 have also been implicated in inherited cancers such as melanoma [8]. Frequently mutant p16 proteins have failed to bind Cdk4; however, there have also been cases documented where mutant p16 proteins still bind to Cdk4, yet they have reduced activity for inhibition of Rb phosphorylation[9]. In the current studies, we set about to examine whether Cdk4 binds to BALB/c and DBA/2 p16 proteins equally. In addition, we determined the status of methylation in several early generation plasma cell tumors induced in (BALB/cAn x C57BL/6N)F1 hybrid mice.

BALB/c Allelic Variants of p16 bind Cdk4 less well than DBA/2N, wild-type p16

To examine whether BALB/c p16 binds CDK4, we prepared lysates containing ^{35}S-methionine labeled cyclin D2/CDK4 from Sf9 cells that had been co-transfected with baculoviruses containing cyclin D2 and the cyclin dependent kinase, CDK4. Aliquots of these lysates were incubated with mutant (BALB/c allelic variants) and wild-type (DBA/2N allelic variant) GST-p16 fusion proteins. The bound complexes were recovered with glutathione sepharose beads, released by boiling in SDS buffer and resolved on 12% SDS PAGE gels. Gels were exposed to autoradiography for 3-10 days and densitometric analyses were performed on a PhosphoImager.

Wild-type (DBA/2) and the BALB/c-derived variants A134C and G232A, as well as the double 'mutant' A134C + G232A, of p16 were all found to bind CDK4 (Fig. 1). Densitometry confirmed that the BALB/c allelic variants of p16 did not bind as well as wild-type p16 proteins.

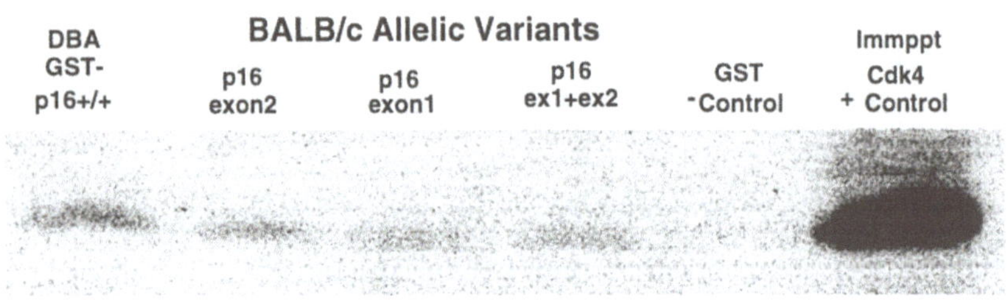

Fig. 1. In vitro binding assay for Cdk4-p16. ^{35}S-methionine labeled cyclin D2/CDK4 were incubated with mutant (BALB/c variants) and wild-type (DBA/2 variants) GST-p16 fusion proteins. The BALB/c allelic variants of p16 bound CDK4 less well than the wild-type DBA/2 variant.

These data support the possibility that inefficient binding of BALB/c p16 to Cdk4 contributes to the inability of BALB/cAn p16 protein to inhibit Rb phosphorylation. In a number of systems, mutant p16 frequently fails to bind to CDK4; however, some of the mutations that moderately reduced the binding activity severely affected the kinase-inhibitory activity of p16[9].

P16 is Methylated in Mouse Plasma Cell Tumors

Northern blot analysis of p16 indicated that the majority of mouse plasma cell tumors do not express exon1α (p16^{INK4a}) transcripts, despite the fact that p16 can be obtained by RT-PCR; in contrast, p16^{INK4a} is expressed in genomic tissues (kidney, spleen, and enriched populations of plasma cells purified from IL6 transgenic mice)[6].

The predominant mechanism of p16 inactivation in tumors has been through homozygous deletion. Kamb et al. cloned p16 by determining the minimal region of overlap of deletions observed in a large series of tumor cell lines[10]. We sought to determine whether allele-specific (DBA) loss was a common feature in F1 hybrid tumors. We examined 16 (BALB/cAn x C57BL/6)F1 and 2 (BALB/cAn X DBA/2N)F1 hybrid tumors induced with pristane alone, as well as, 40 (BALB/cAn x DBA/2N)F1 (ras-myc induced) tumors, and 40 (BALB/cAn x DBA/2N)F1 (abl-myc induced) tumors for loss of heterozygosity at the p16 locus. Only one (BALB/cAn x C57BL/6N)F1 hybrid tumor exhibited LOH at p16; this tumor has always shown a loss of BALB/c alleles of all markers examined on Chr 4. These data indicate that loss of p16 expression by deletion is not the predominant mechanism of inactivation in mouse plasmacytomas.

The second most common mechanism of p16 inactivation in tumors is by methylation. The exon 1 coding sequences of p16 reside within CpG islands and the exon 2 regions are 83% homologous and also constitute CpG islands[11]. CpG islands are usually unmethylated in normal somatic cells. A large number of human tumors have been shown to experience widespread hypermethylation of the p16 gene. De novo 5' CpG island hypermethylation has been found to be associated with transcriptional silencing of the p16 gene[12].

Our efforts were concentrated on determining whether methylation of Hpa II sites within the p16 gene were a common feature of plasmacytomas or not. DNAs from the 16 tumors induced by pristane, as well as, spleen controls from the CxB6F1 hybrid mice were digested with MspI and the methylation sensitive enzyme, HpaII. Southern blot analyses of p16 were performed and 25% (4/16) of the tumors showed evidence of methylation at HpaII sites. As a follow-up we have also examined specific sites of methylation in the promoter, as well as, exon 1 and exon 2 in over 100 primary tumors from a series of backcross mice and 20 cell lines; differences in the amount of methylation within the promoter, exon 1 and exon 2 sequences were observed (data not shown).

Klangby and coworkers[13] have shown that exon 1 sequences of p16 are methylated in 90% of 19 Burkitt's lymphoma (BL) cell lines. Furthermore, no p16 protein was detected in any of the BL lines that were methylated. In contrast, they showed that only 1 of 6 lymphoblastoid cell lines exhibited methylation in p16 exon 1 sequences.

Conclusion

Loss of p16 function is likely to be an important factor contributing to the susceptibility of BALB/c mice for developing plasma cell tumors. (1) The *Cdkn2a* locus encoding both $p16^{INK4a}$ and $p19^{ARF}$ was mapped within the 6 cM interval harboring the *Pctr1* tumor susceptibility locus. (2) BALB/cAn and ABP/Le mice carry a unique allele of p16 among inbred strains of mice. This observation suggests that ABP/Le mice might also represent a model strain for the study of plasma cell tumorigenesis. (3) BALB/c p16 protein is inefficient in its binding to the cyclin dependent kinase, Cdk4 in *in vitro* assays. (4) Furthermore, BALB/cAn p16 proteins do not inhibit Rb phosphorylation in *in vitro* kinase assays. (5) Additional point mutations in the third ankyrin repeat region of the p16 locus have been observed in three well-established plasmacytoma cell lines. (6) Both primary and established tissue culture plasmacytomas have exhibited p16 methylation, suggesting the possibility for further silencing of any residual p16 activity. (7) Induction studies in $p16^{exon2}$ knock-out mice [14] are underway and one mouse has already been diagnosed with a plasma cell tumor at 60 days post pristane; this is vastly accelerated when compared to normal mean latency periods of 220 days.

As such, the *Cdkn2a* locus encodes one or possibly two proteins which could be candidates for the tumor susceptibility/ resistance locus, *Pctr1*. Our work has focused on the role of the $p16^{INK4a}$ protein which interacts with Rb to suppress tumorigenesis, but we have also initiated a series of studies to evaluate the $p19^{ARF}$ protein which is intimately associated with the p53 pathway. By virtue of the fact that substitutions found in BALB/c *Cdkn2a* sequences could affect either $p16^{INK4a}$ (A134C) or $p19^{ARF}$ (G232A), it could be the case that the *Pctr1* phenotype is controlled by both proteins; these two proteins encoded by one locus affect the two most significant pathways, Rb and p53, involved in cell cycle control and cancer.

Loss of *Cdkn2a* function in BALB/c mice could place plasma cells in a permissive state for unchecked proliferation. Rb may become hyperphosphorylated by Cdk4/Cdk6 in the absence of $p16^{INK4a}$; thereby, allowing the release of E2f and continued cycling of plasma cells. This prolonged state of proliferation, or perhaps, a reduction in apoptosis could keep cells around long enough to sustain further somatic mutation and increase their metastatic potential.

Acknowledgements

We wish to thank Edward S. Ramsay, Val Bliskovsky, Wendy DuBois and Michael Potter for their support and contributions to these projects.

References

1. Morse III HC Hartley JW and Potter M (1980) In: Potter, M. (ed.) Progress in Myeloma. Elsevier North Holland, Inc., Amsterdam, pp. 263-279
2. Potter M (1984) Genetics of susceptibility to plasmacytoma development in BALB/c mice. Cancer Surveys 3: 247-264

3. Mock BA Krall MA and Dosik JK (1993) Genetic mapping of tumor susceptibility genes involved in mouse plasmacytomagenesis. Proc. Natl. Acad. Sci. USA 90: 9499-9503
4. Potter M Mushinski EB Wax JS Hartley J and Mock B (1994) Two genes on Chromosome 4 determine resistance to plasmacytoma induction in mice. Cancer Research 54: 969-975
5. Mock BA Hartley J Le Tissier P Wax JS and Potter M (1997) The plasmacytoma resistance gene, *Pctr2*, delays the onset of tumorigenesis and resides in the telomeric region of Chromosome 4. Blood 90: 4092-4098
6. Zhang S Ramsay ES and Mock BA (1998) *Cdkn2a*, the cyclin dependent kinase inhibitor encoding $p16^{INK4a}$ and $p19^{ARF}$ is a candidate for the plasmacytoma susceptibility locus, *Pctr1*. Proc. Natl. Acad. Sci. USA 95: 2429-2434
7. Quelle DE Cheng M Ashmun RA and Sherr CJ (1997) Cancer-associated mutations at the INK4a locus cancel cell cycle arrest by p16INK4a but not by the alternative reading frame protein p19ARF. Proc Natl Acad Sci USA 94: 669-673
8. Ranade K et al. (1995) Mutations associated with familial melanoma impair p16INK4a function. Nature Genetics 10: 114-116
9. Yang R Serrano M Slater J Leung E and Koeffler HP (1996) Analysis of p16INK4a and its interaction with CDK4. Biochemical and Biophysical Research Communications 218: 254-259
10. Kamb A et al. (1994) A cell cycle regulator potentially involved in genesis of many tumor types. Science 264: 436-440
11. Gonzalez-Zulueta M Bender CM Yang AS TuDung N Beart RW Tornout JMV and Jones PA (1995) Methylation of the 5' Cpg island of the p16/Cdkn2 tumor suppressor gene in normal and transformed human tissues correlates with gene silencing. Cancer Research 55: 4531-4535
12. Merlo A Herman JG Mao L Lee DJ Gabrielson E Burger PC Baylin SB and Sidransky D (1995) 5' Cpg island methylation is associated with transcriptional silencing of the tumour suppressor p16/CDKN2/Mts1 in human cancers. Nature Medicine 1: 686-692
13. Klangby U Okan I Magnusson KP Wendland M Lind P and Wiman KG (1998) p16/INK4a and p15/INK4b gene methylation and absence of p16/INK4a mRNA and protein expression in Burkitt's lymphoma. Blood 91: 1-9
14. Serrano M Lee H-W Chin L Cordon-Cardo C Beach D and DePinho RA (1996) Role of the INK4a locus in tumor suppression and cell mortality. Cell 85: 27-37

Discussion

George Klein: It is a wonderful study and probably the furthest progress in this long-standing but very difficult field. Did you show a segregating cross between susceptible and resistant mice?
Beverly Mock: Yes, it is a BALB/DBA backcross. Only 50% of BALB/c mice develop tumors, and in F1 hybrids, 2% develop tumors. In the backcross progeny only about 12% develop tumors; you would expect at least 25% for a single gene trait. So this is a complex genetic trait and we know already from the congenic strain analysis that there are three separate genes on Chr 4. We have localized the *Pctr2* locus to a 1 cM segment on the distal end of Chr 4; we have been isolating BAC clones and ESTs from this region. In the third region we have found a translocation in a cell line, so we are hoping to clone the breakpoint as a start point for identifying a dysregulated locus.
George Klein: Would you not say that if your MPC resistant strain, where you have knocked out p16 and p19R, becomes susceptible to plasmacytomas, then you have probably identified the most important two genes?
Beverly Mock: I don't know. The LOD score in the backcross progeny is highest at a locus residing between *Pctr1* and *Pctr2*; therefore, this locus could be the most important. Obviously, I think p16 is important and one of the interesting questions about p16 is "What is driving the selection for it to be shut-off ?" In BALB/c you already have a defective allele, yet it has some activity. There are additional mutations in tumors in the third ankyrin repeat. Exons 1 and 2 are methylated in tumors. We have also found sequence variants in the p16 promoter; so there could also be differences in transcription factors binding the promoter.
Riccardo Dalla-Favera: What do you define as a trait for genetic analysis?
Beverly Mock: It is the end-stage tumor phenotype.
Riccardo Dalla-Favera: So it could still be a single gene trait if predisposition is the trait?
Beverly Mock: No. Three separate regions of DBA Chr 4 have been introgressively backcrossed onto a BALB/c background. Each of these mouse strains show a reduced susceptibility to tumor formation. In addition, we have created congenics which carry DBA/2 alleles in between these intervals and they are susceptible to tumor induction.
Riccardo Dalla-Favera: In mice that develop tumors, what is the p16 makeup of those tumors allelically?
Beverly Mock: They are likely to carry the BALB/cAn allele of p16.
Riccardo Dalla-Favera: No, I am talking about the tumor versus the germline of that given mouse.
Beverly Mock: I have not sequenced all the backcross tumors, but most of them will have the BALB/c allelic variant; they may also have additional mutations.
Richard Scheuermann: Does the polymorphism affect the p19 coding region as well?
Beverly Mock: The exon 2 variant would, but the exon 1 variant would not.
Richard Scheuermann: It is an amino acid change?
Beverly Mock: Yes. Dawn Quelle showed in her work that exon 2 is not as important for p19 function. This would argue that the exon 1 variant may be the most important variant, functionally. The exon 1 variant is a histidine to proline change, which is a fairly major change compared to the exon 2 variant which changes from a valine to isoleucine.

Transgenic Shuttle Vector Assays for Assessing Oxidative B-cell Mutagenesis *in vivo*

K. Felix, K. Kelliher, G.-W. Bornkamm[1] and S. Janz

Laboratory of Genetics, Division of Basic Sciences, NCI, NIH, Bethesda, MD, USA

[1] Institute for Clinical Molecular Biology and Tumor Genetics, GSF, Munich, Germany

Abstract

The recent development of transgenic mutagenicity assays provides new opportunities for evaluating mutagenic processes *in vivo*. To assess mutant frequencies in tissue B cells, we decided to take advantage of two such assays that utilize the transgenic shuttle vectors, λLIZ and pUR288. Our main interest in this research is to test two basic premises of inflammation-induced plasmacytoma development in genetically susceptible BALB/c mice; i.e., the possibility that plasmacytoma precursor cells may become targets of phagocyte-mediated oxidative mutagenesis *in situ* and the prospect that plasmacytoma susceptibility/resistance genes may contribute to these phenotypes by enhancing/reducing oxidative mutagenesis in B cells. Based on our preliminary experience with the λLIZ and pUR288 transgenic *in vivo* mutagenicity tests, we propose to employ these assays as broadly applicable tools for assessing overall mutagenesis during normal and aberrant (malignant) B-cell development. Furthermore, transgenic shuttle vector assays appear to lend themselves as ideal methods to associate general B-cell mutagenesis with the peculiar, B cell-typical somatic hypermutation processes that target the V(D)J gene segment, the proto-oncogene *bcl-6* and perhaps other, still unknown loci.

Methods

Phage λ-based Assay Using the Shuttle Vector, λLIZ

The principal utility of the transgenic shuttle vector, λLIZ, lies in the ability to transfer a suitable target gene for mutagenesis from the mouse to a convenient E. coli detection system, in which mutant rates can be determined readily and mutation spectra analyzed with great ease. The λLIZ mutagenicity system is commercially available as Big Blue *In vivo* Mutagenesis assay® that was developed by Stratagene (La Jolla, CA). In principal, the assay can be utilized for quantitating mutant

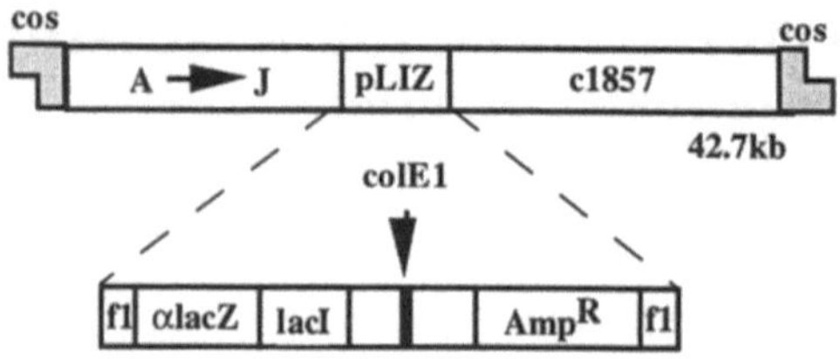

Fig. 1. Shuttle vector λLIZ

frequencies in all tissue types and cells derived therefrom, including B lymphocytes and their progenitors/descendants [3,14,15,19]. The λLIZ shuttle vector (Fig. 1) has been designed to permit the expression; i.e., the de-repression, of a β-galactosidase reporter gene (α*lacZ*) in α-complementing E. coli whenever an inactivating mutation in the *lacI* gene occurs. Gene *lacI* encodes the physiological *lacZ* repressor; i.e., the LacI protein that blocks in its tetrameric form the transcription of gene, *lacZ*. The λLIZ shuttle vector includes in addition to the target gene of mutagenesis, *lacI*, and the reporter gene of mutagenesis, α*lacZ*, plasmid maintenance sequences, the colE1 origin of replication and the ampicillin resistance gene, which permit both target gene recovery and mutant screening as the convenient plasmid, pLIZ (Fig. 1), rather than the less convenient λ phage. The performance of the λLIZ-based mutagenicity assay is illustrated in Fig. 2. It entails the preparation of high molecular weight genomic DNA from the tissue sample or cell preparation, the recovery of the λLIZ transgenes from the genomic DNA as infectious phages (which is accomplished by a phage packaging reaction utilizing the paired cos sites of the prophage indicated in Fig. 1), the infection of restriction deficient E. coli K12 SCS-8 cells with the recovered phage, the plating of the infected bacterial cells in top agarose containing X-gal (a substrate for β-galactosidase), and the enumeration of β-galactosidase-expressing blue mutant plaques after a suitable incubation period at 37° C. Mutant frequencies, the final result of the assay, can be calculated by determining the ratio of blue mutant ($LacI^-$) plaques to colorless non-mutant ($LacI^+$) plaques. To identify the nature of individual mutations in the *lacI* target gene, mutant plaques can be scored, verified by replating and finally analyzed at the molecular level, which is most commonly done by DNA sequencing.

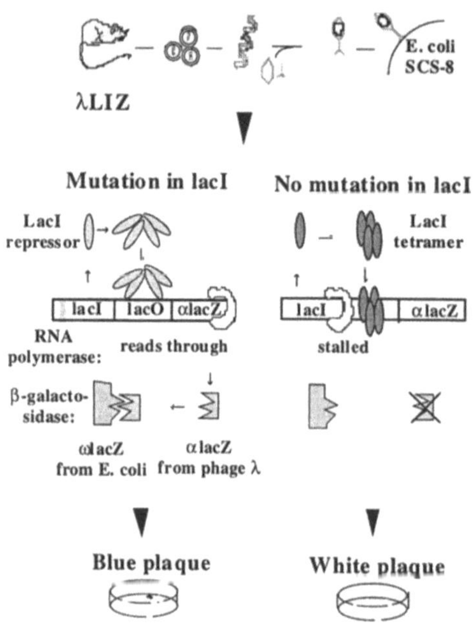

Fig. 2: Principle of the λLIZ-based mutagenicity assay

Plasmid-based Assay Employing the Shuttle Vector, pUR288

To complement the phage λ-based mutagenicity assay with a second, independent assay that relies on a plasmid-derived shuttle vector instead of a phage λ vector, we implemented a system that was developed by Michael Boerrigter and Jan Vijg and utilizes a bacterial *lacZ* gene integrated as 10-copy transgenic concatamers into mouse chromosomes 3 and 4 [1]. In the plasmid assay, gene *lacZ* functions as both the target and reporter gene of mutagenesis. In addition to the *lacZ* gene, the plasmid, pUR288 (Fig. 3), contains the LacI binding site, *lacO*, the recognition site for the cap binding protein (CAP), an origin of replication (ori) and an ampicillin resistance gene (Amp). The principle of the mutagenesis assay is illustrated in Fig. 4. Plasmids containing gene *lacZ* are excised from genomic DNA by restriction with HindIII and then separated from total genomic DNA with the help of a LacI repressor/β-galactosidase fusion protein that has been coupled to magnetic beads. After elution from the beads, which is achieved by the addition of IPTG, and circularization of the linear fragments at the HindIII sites by ligation with T4 ligase, the plasmids are electroporated into E. coli C *lacZ*$^-$, *galE*$^-$ that is deficient in β-galactosidase (*galZ*$^-$), galactose-intolerant due to the absence of galactose epimerase (*galE*$^-$), and restriction negative to prevent the degradation of incoming methylated plasmid DNA. The mutation in gene, *galE*, allows for the positive selection of *lacZ* mutants in medium containing the lactose analog, Phe-gal (phenyl β-D-galactoside). Phe-gal, X-gal and lactose are all substrates of β-galactosidase. The positive selection of *lacZ*$^-$ cells in Phe-gal is made possible by the ability of *lacZ*$^+$, wildtype cells to cleave the non-toxic Phe-gal, thereby releasing galactose that is toxic to *galE*$^-$ cells. Thus, *lacZ*$^+$ cells (on the *galE*$^-$ background) commit suicide in the presence of Phe-gal, whereas *lacZ*$^-$ cells (on the *galE*$^-$ background) are permitted to grow due to their inability to metabolize Phe-gal and generate galactose. A small aliquot; i.e., usually 2 μl out of 2 ml of a suspension of pUR288-transfected E. coli, is plated on a titer plate that has been supplemented with X-gal to determine the rescue efficiency of the plasmid. The presence of X-gal results in a blue halo around growing colonies of LacZ$^+$ wildtype clones. LacZ$^-$ mutants are not counted on the X-gal plate, but this is irrelevant because of their low prevalence on the order of 10^{-5} to 10^{-4}. The remaining 1,998 μl of the E. coli

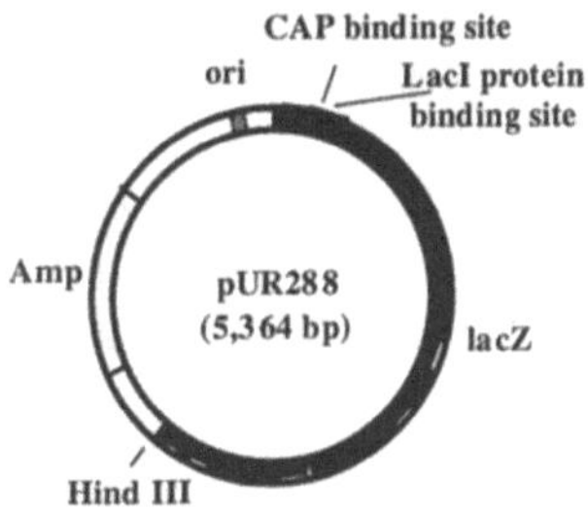

Fig. 3. Shuttle vector pUR288

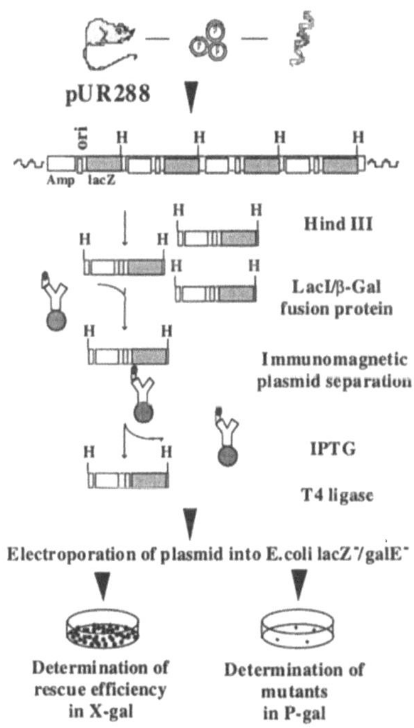

Fig. 4. Principle of the pUR288-based mutagenicity assay

suspension are plated on a single Phe-gal plate to select for and enumerate mutants. Mutant clones emerge as small red colonies in the presence of a tetrazolium salt that has been added for the improved visibility of the sometimes tiny colonies. The mutant frequency is calculated as the ratio of mutants to non-mutants; i.e., the number of colonies enumerated on the selective Phe-gal plate to the number of colonies (x 1000) determined on the X-gal titer plate. To further characterize the mutational spectrum, mutant colonies can be picked from the Phe-gal plate and used as templates in long-distance PCR reactions in which the entire *lacZ* gene is amplified for subsequent restriction fragment analysis and/or DNA sequencing.

Results and Discussion

Phagocyte-Mediated Oxidative Mutagenesis in B Lymphoblasts

We have used both the λLIZ and the pUR288 mutagenicity assay to test the hypothesis that the close proximity to inflammatory phagocytes provides a potentially harmful and mutagenic environment for B cells. In earlier experiments, we had shown that pristane-elicited, phorbol ester-activated phagocytes can induce high levels of DNA damage in co-incubated, LPS stimulated splenic B lymphoblasts [9,16]. DNA damage was inflicted by phagocytes undergoing the oxidative burst; i.e., an inducible metabolic response that is dependent on the activity of the membrane-bound enzyme, NADPH oxidase, and results in the release of millimolar amounts of reactive oxygen species into the extracellular milieu. The B-cell damage and its repair were measured as DNA single and double strand breakage as well as unscheduled DNA synthesis, an assay for the so-called long-patch nucleotide excision repair. More recently, we used the λLIZ mutagenesis assay to quantitate the *lacI* mutant levels in proliferating B cells exposed to PMA-stimulated phagocytes performing the oxidative burst [6]. In ongoing unpublished studies, we employ the pUR288 assay and the gene-targeted phagocytes that are deficient in NADPH oxidase activity due to a mutation in one of its component genes, $p47^{phox}$ [8] to prove formally that reactive oxygen is the critical mutagenic effector mecha-

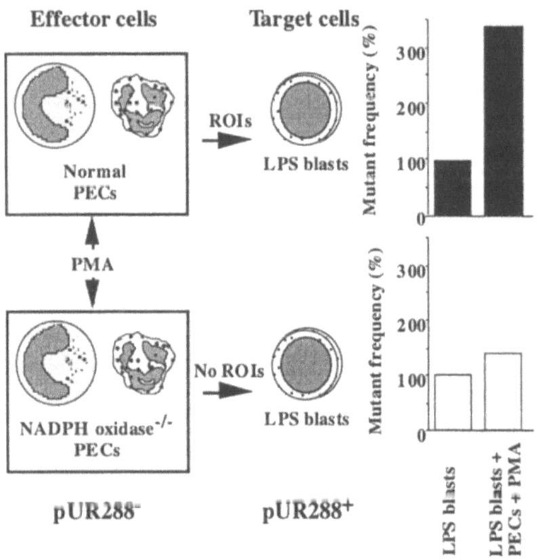

Fig. 5. Phagocyte-mediated oxidative mutagenesis in B cells

nism of inflammatory cells. A typical result is illustrated in Fig. 5, which shows in the upper panel that PMA-stimulated peritoneal exudate cells (PECs) obtained from normal mice with a functional NADPH oxidase are capable of inducing mutagenesis in coincubated LPS blasts. PECs, which consist mainly of macrophages and neutrophils, do not contain the shuttle plasmid, pUR288, whereas LPS blasts do harbor it. Mutagenesis is therefore measured exclusively in the target B cells and is not distorted by the self-inflicted DNA damage that is known to take place in the effector cells, PECs. After exposure to normal PECs, the mutant levels in B cells were found to be elevated approximately 3.5-fold with respect to the background control. In contrast, PMA-stimulated NADPH oxidase null PECs obtained from mice with a targeted deletion in the $p47^{phox}$ gene were unable to mutagenize the co-cultured B cells (see the lower panel in Fig. 5). This result suggests strongly that inflammatory phagocytes can damage the DNA in bystander B cells by oxidative mechanisms.

λLIZ Versus pUR288: What is the Benefit of Using Two Systems?

Based on the experiments described above and additional studies not reported here [4,5,7], we feel that both the phage λ vector, λLIZ, and the plasmid vector, pUR288, are useful for determining the mutant rates in lymphoid tissues as well as partially enriched or highly purified B-cell populations derived thereof. It is important to emphasize that both mutagenesis systems are thought to reflect accurately the mutation rate in the genome [17,18]. In both systems, the shuttle vectors for mutagenesis reside as irrelevant passengers in the genome. Mutations in their target genes, *lacI* and *lacZ*, are neutral; i.e., neither beneficial nor damaging to the cell in which they occur. The passivity of the shuttle vectors becomes plausible when one considers that the genes *lacI* and *lacZ* are presumably not transcribed because of the lack of mammalian promoters and polyadenylation sites. Furthermore, it is likely that both transgenic concatamers are heavily methylated at their integration sites on chromosomes 3 and 4, although this has been shown only for the λLIZ transgene [2]. The λLIZ and pUR288 assays seem to offer therefore ideal indicator systems with which general mutagenesis can be evaluated in the absence of any selective pressure of the mutated gene. Additional motivation for employing the transgenic shuttle vectors for measuring mutant rates *in vivo* can be found in recent reports stating that mutations in reporter genes are remarkably similar to mutation profiles observed in endogenous genes [11], such as the *hprt* gene in lymphocytes [10,12] and the proto-oncogenes Ha-*ras* and *Apc* [13]. However, some important differences that distinguish the λLIZ-based assay from the pUR288-based assay need to be considered when choosing one of them for a mutagenesis project. For example, the phage-based assay, which detects primarily point mutations, frameshifts and small deletions amounting to less than 20 nucleotides, fails to detect larger deletions that range from several hundred base pairs to a couple of kilobase pairs. Larger deletions, the hallmark mutations of oxidative mutagens (clastogens), can be detected readily with the plasmid-based system. In addition, there are important practical differences between both assays. The λLIZ assay requires at least 20 μg of high-quality, high molecular weight genomic DNA, while the pUR288 assay is much less demanding in this regard and, therefore, more likely to be conducive for mutation studies in rare cell populations. The λLIZ assay does not employ a positive selection system for mutants, which renders it more labor intensive than the plasmid assay that permits the positive selection of mutants. The clear strength of the phage-based assay is the ease with which mutational spectra can be analyzed at the DNA sequence level. The approximately 1 kb long target gene of the λLIZ assay, *lacI*, is 3-fold smaller than the target gene of the plasmid assay, *lacZ*, which greatly facilitates sequence analysis. What is more, the data base of known mutations in gene *lacI* is huge and much larger than for gene *lacZ*. This greatly accelerates the identification of the type of mutational assault the B cells have been subjected to; e.g., oxidative versus alkylating DNA damage. In summary, we believe that both the λLIZ- and the pUR288-based assay will have a unique place in the evaluation of B-cell mutagenesis *in vivo*. They may also be instrumental for the comparison of general mutagenesis in the overall genome with the intriguing, yet poorly defined somatic hypermutation processes that target the V(D)J region and the *bcl-6* gene in B cells.

References

1. Boerrigter ME, Dolle ME, Martus HJ, Gossen JA, Vijg J (1995) Plasmid-based transgenic mouse model for studying *in vivo* mutations. Nature 377:657-659
2. Cosentino L, Heddle JA (1996) A test for neutrality of mutations of the *lacZ* transgene. Environ Mol Mutagen 28:313-316
3. Dycaico MJ, Provost GS, Kretz PL, Ransom SL, Moores JC, Short JM (1994) The use of shuttle vectors for mutation analysis in transgenic mice and rats. Mutat Res 307:461-478
4. Felix K, Kelliher K, Bornkamm GW, Janz S (1998) Association of elevated mutagenesis in the spleen with genetic susceptibility to induced plasmacytoma development in mice. Cancer Res 58:1616-1619
5. Felix K, Lin S, Bornkamm GW, Janz S (1998) Tetravinyl-tetramethylcyclo-tetrasiloxane (tetravinyl D4) is a mutagen in Rat2λlacI fibroblasts. Carcinogenesis 19:315-320
6. Felix K, Lin S, Bornkamm GW, Janz S (1997) Elevated mutant frequencies in gene *lacI* in splenic lipopolysaccharide blasts after exposure to activated phagocytes *in vitro*. Eur J Immunol 27:2160-2164
7. Felix K, Potter M, Bornkamm GW, Janz S (1997) *In vitro* mutagenicity of the plasmacytomagenic agent pristane (2,6,10,14-tetramethylpentadecane). Cancer Lett 113:71-76
8. Jackson SH, Gallin JI, Holland SM (1995) The *p47^phox^* mouse knock-out model of chronic granulomatous disease. J Exp Med 182:751-758
9. Janz S, Shacter E (1993) Activated murine neutrophils induce unscheduled DNA synthesis in B lymphocytes. Mutat Res 293:173-186
10. Manjanatha MG, Shelton SD, Aidoo A, Lyn-Cook LE, Casciano DA (1998) Comparison of *in vivo* mutagenesis in the endogenous *Hprt* gene and the *lacI* transgene of Big Blue$^{(R)}$ rats treated with 7, 12-dimethylbenz[a]anthracene. Mutat Res 401:165-178
11. Mientjes EJ, Hochleitner K, Luiten-Schuite A, van Delft JH, Thomale J, Berends F, Rajewsky MF, Lohman PH, Baan RA (1996) Formation and persistence of O^6-ethylguanine in genomic and transgene DNA in liver and brain of lambda(lacZ) transgenic mice treated with N-ethyl-N-nitrosourea. Carcinogenesis 17:2449-2454
12. Mittelstaedt RA, Manjanatha MG, Shelton SD, Lyn-Cook LE, Chen JB, Aidoo A,

Casciano DA, Heflich RH (1998) Comparison of the types of mutations induced by 7,12-dimethylbenz[a]anthracene in the *lacI* and *hprt* genes of Big Blue rats. Environ Mol Mutagen 31:149-156
13. Okonogi H, Ushijima T, Zhang XB, Heddle JA, Suzuki T, Sofuni T, Felton JS, Tucker JD, Sugimura T, Nagao M (1997) Agreement of mutational characteristics of heterocyclic amines in *lacI* of the Big Blue mouse with those in tumor related genes in rodents. Carcinogenesis 18:745-748
14. Provost GS, Kretz PL, Hamner RT, Matthews CD, Rogers BJ, Lundberg KS, Dycaico MJ, Short JM (1993) Transgenic systems for *in vivo* mutation analysis. Mutat Res 288:133-149
15. Rogers BJ, Provost GS, Young RR, Putman DL, Short JM (1995) Intralaboratory optimization and standardization of mutant screening conditions used for a lambda/*lacI* transgenic mouse mutagenesis assay (I). Mutat Res 327:57-66
16. Shacter E, Lopez RL, Beecham EJ, Janz S (1990) DNA damage induced by phorbol ester-stimulated neutrophils is augmented by extracellular cofactors. Role of histidine and metals. J Biol Chem 265:6693-6699
17. Tao KS, Urlando C, Heddle JA (1993) Comparison of somatic mutation in a transgenic versus host locus. Proc Natl Acad Sci U S A 90:10681-10685
18. Vijg J, Dolle ME, Martus HJ, Boerrigter ME (1997) Transgenic mouse models for studying mutations *in vivo*: applications in aging research. Mech Ageing Dev 99:257-271
19. Young RR, Rogers BJ, Provost GS, Short JM, Putman DL (1995) Interlaboratory comparison: liver spontaneous mutant frequency from lambda/*lacI* transgenic mice (Big Blue) (II). Mutat Res 327:67-73

Discussion

Isaac Witz: Was there mutagenesis in the mice which ultimately at 220 days did not develop plasmacytomas?
Siegfried Janz: The experiment was terminated on day 280 after the first injection of pristane. The mice that developed tumors by day 280 post-pristane and the mice that remained tumor-free by this time were characterized by very similar levels of mutagenesis in lymphoid tissues.
Isaac Witz: Would the same type of mutagenesis also be observed in mice grown under pathogen free conditions?
Siegfried Janz: One reason for setting up the mutagenesis systems in our laboratory was to study the relationship between the environmental factors that are known to affect the onset and incidence of plasmacytoma development, on the one hand, and the levels of B-cell mutagenesis *in vivo*, on the other. To look at mutant frequencies in SPF mice would be quite interesting, because SPF conditions have been reported to reduce dramatically the incidence of pristane-induced peritoneal plasmacytomas in BALB/c mice. It is conceivable that the mutant rates in the SPF animals are lower, but we have not demonstrated that.
Fritz Melchers: Have you ever tried to test the rates of mutagenesis not just in whole spleen or whole brain, but made a more guided effort to see whether there are differences in rates of mutations in different cells, like in cells of germinal centers?
Siegfried Janz: You brought up a very important issue. Thus far, we have just determined the mutant rates in whole lymphoid tissues, e.g. in spleens and mesenteric lymph nodes. No attempt has been made yet to look at the various cell lineages residing in these tissues one by one. However, in future experiments we want to accomplish that by working with purified B cells after fractionation by FACS, MACS, or other suitable methods. It is our ultimate goal in this research to determine the mutant frequencies in all major subpopulations of B cells, e.g. pre-B cells, germinal center B cells, and plasma cells.
Riccardo Dalla-Favera: When you constructed your backgrounds you made a series of choices. First, you decided not to control the integration site, so you will go randomly, and second you did not want it transcribed, and therefore you wanted it hypermethylated. I wonder why you chose to do that.
Siegfried Janz: I did not mean to mislead you into believing that the transgenic mouse strains that are so useful for evaluating mutagenesis *in vivo* were created in our laboratory. The phage λ-based assay, λLIZ, was developed by Stratagene and is commercially available as the so-called Big Blue *in vivo* mutagenesis assay™. The plasmid-based assay, pUR288, was devised by Michael Boerrigter in Jan Vijg's laboratory. It has also been made available recently to the scientific community as a product (i. e. the mice and the assay kit) that is distributed by a start-up company in Georgia named "Levens". With respect to the nature and the status of the target genes for mutagenesis, it should be stressed that in both shuttle vector-based systems, λLIZ and pUR288, the target genes, *lacI* and *lacZ*, are of bacterial origin. The target genes are passive passengers that are not transcribed, but are hypermethylated at their random integration sites in Chrs 3 and 4. It is understandable that this situation could raise some concern as to how representative the reporter genes are for endogenous loci, since the latter are partly transcribed and partly not. At present, the answer to this problem is not entirely clear, but a number of published reports in the mutagenicity literature suggest that the mutant frequencies determined with the assistance of the transgenic shuttle vectors do reflect authentically the mutant levels in the overall genome. In other words, the mutation rates in endogenous genes and reporter genes have been shown to be very similar in most cases. This observation has added a lot of creditability to the λLIZ and pUR288 assays.
Riccardo Dalla-Favera: When you do the pristane experiment with or without BSO can you conclude that there is a genetic control of the effect of mutagenesis, or is there a genetic control of a cellular response of the inflammation that determines mutagenesis?
Siegfried Janz: Excellent point. Both the λLIZ and pUR288 assay provide sort of a snapshot of mutagenesis that reveals how many mutant cells are present in a particular tissue at a particular point in time. Not more and not less. The assays do not permit us to draw conclusions on the

mechanism(s) of mutagenesis. For example, they are not very helpful to decide whether elevated mutant rates were caused by the increased production of mutants or the diminished elimination of mutants. The difficulty of discerning the mechanism of mutagenesis is also underscored by your comment on the genetic control of mutagenesis. You state correctly that the observed elevations in mutant levels in BALB/c B cells could have been caused by the genetic preponderance of these cells to undergo mutagenesis or, alternatively, by the unique, genetically determined potency of inflammatory cells to inflict DNA damage and mutagenesis in neighboring B cells. More experiments need to be performed and additional methods need to be recruited to distinguish between the two possibilities.

Sandy Morse: I know with regard to Fritz' question that you have not had the chance to do numerous subset analyses, but at least in the mice that got plasmacytomas did you compare the plasmacytoma, for instance with spleen, for the levels of mutation that you are seeing in the tumors?

Siegfried Janz: It could be very informative to compare the mutant levels in the spleens (and other lymphoid tissues) with those in plasmacytomas. Plasmacytomas, like many other fully transformed and malignant tumors, are thought to be characterized by increased genomic instability. Since elevations in general mutagenesis, as detected by the λLIZ and pUR288 assays, may be a consequence of genomic instability, it is reasonable to predict that lacI and lacZ mutant levels may be higher in plasmacytoma cells than in normal B lymphocytes and plasma cells.

Michael Carroll: What about other mediators of inflammation such as nitric oxide?

Siegfried Janz: There is no question that both nitrosative stress and oxidative stress are potent effectors of DNA damage and mutagenesis in mammalian cells. In our studies we have been focusing on reactive oxygen intermediates as the mutagenic principle. To better appreciate the role of reactive oxygen species *in vivo*, we have made use of mouse mutants that are either deficient in producing active oxygen or compromised in their antioxidative defense. An example for the former is the p47phox nullizygous mouse developed by Steven Holland at the NIH; an example for the latter is the glucose-6-phosphate dehydrogenase partial-loss-of-function mouse developed by Walter Pretsch in Germany. I agree with you that other mouse mutant strains have been generated that should permit us to study the mutagenic potential of nitric oxide and related radicals *in vivo*. Thank you for suggesting this interesting experiment.

Plasmacytoma Induction in Specific Pathogen-Free (SPF) *bcl-2* Transgenic BALB/c Mice

S. Silva and G. Klein
Microbiology and Tumor Biology Center, Karolinska Institutet, Box 280, S-171 77 Stockholm, Sweden.

Summary

Germ-free (GF) and specific pathogen free (SPF) BALB/c mice are refractory to plasmacytoma induction by pristane (McIntire and Princler, 1969, Byrd *et al* 1991). It was therefore suggested that MPC development may depend on antigenic stimulation. If so, it may conceivably act by preventing the apoptotic elimination of tumor precursor cells. We have tested this idea by elevating the apoptotic threshold by the introduction of a *bcl-2* transgene. We have found that MPCs could be induced by pristane oil in transgene carrying SPF mice. An $E\mu$ activated *bcl-2* transgene was introduced into SPF BALB/c mice. The mice were used after two backcrosses (BC-2). Pristane oil treatment was started at 4 to 6 weeks of age (3 x 0.3 ml via i. p. at monthly intervals). For each transgene carrier a transgene negative littermate was used as control. Fifteen of 24 (63 %) transgene carriers developed plasmacytomas after latency periods between 67 and 146 days (X = 112 $\pm$ 30 days) after the first pristane injection. Five additional transgene carriers developed lymphoma (3 cases) or mixed MPC and lymphoma (2 cases). In contrast, no tumors developed in 16 transgene negative littermates that were kept >300 days under observation. Karyotyping showed that 10/15 (66 %) of the MPCs carried a T(12;15) translocation, 4/15 (27 %) carried both T(12;15) and T(6;15) translocations in the same metaphase plate, and 1/15 (7 %) was translocation free. A T(12;15) translocation was also detected in one of the 2 mice with mixed tumor type. Pristane treated *bcl-2* transgenic C57Bl/6 mice remained tumor free, although T(12;15) translocation carrying cells were found in the peritoneal fluid of 4/20 mice 176 days after pristane.

Introduction

Plasmacytomas can be induced in BALB/c and NZB mice by the i.p. implantation of solid plastics, silicon gel or non-metabolizable paraffin oils like pristane (reviewed by Potter and Wiener, 1992). A chronic B-lymphocyte rich inflammatory granuloma (OG) precedes tumor development (Osmond *et al* 1990).

The earliest preneoplastic lesions appear as focal proliferations of plasma cells. Virtually all MPCs carry chromosomal translocations of the *Ig/myc* type. Translocation carrying cells have been detected by PCR in preneoplastic lesions already 30 days after pristane injection (Janz *et al* 1993). They were also found in the OG of pristane treated MPC-resistant DBA/2 mice, but less frequent than in BALB/c (Müller *et al* 1996). Earlier, we have selected a highly MPC susceptible BALB/c subline (BALB/cM2/22) from the relatively resistant BALB/cJ strain. Untreated females of the BALB/cM2/22 strain developed some spontaneous plasmacytomas (Silva *et al* 1997). This showed that treatment with the potentially karyotoxic pristane was not essential to generate *Ig/myc* translocations.

McIntire and Princler (1969) reported that germ-free BALB/c mice, developed only a very low incidence (6 %) of MPC after pristane treatment. It was suggested that antigenic stimuli may provide important cofactors required for MPC development (Byrd *et al* 1991). They may act triggering anti-apoptotic signals that may counteract the apoptotic elimination of translocation carrying cells. If so, raising the apoptotic threshold e. g. by a *bcl-2* transgene may have a similar effect. We have therefore examined whether BALB/c mice kept under SPF conditions would reacquire susceptibility to MPC induction by pristane after the introduction of an *Eμ-bcl-2* transgene. We have found that this was the case.

Material and Methods

Eμ-bcl-2 Transgenic Mice

The *bcl-2* transgene was originally produced on (C57BL/6JWehi x SJL/JWehi)F2 background and has been further introduced in the C57BL/6 strain (Strasser *et al* 1990, 1991). The transgene is preferentially expressed in the B-cell lineage since it is under the influence of the IgH enhancer (*Eμ*) and a SV40 lymphoid promoter (Strasser *et al* 1990). A couple of mice from the C57BL/6-*Eμ-bcl-2-22* line (kindly provided by Dr A Harris, Walter & Eliza Hall Institute, Melbourne, Australia) were used to introduce the transgene into our MPC susceptible BALB/cM2/22 line (Silva *et al* 1997) by serially mating heterozygous transgenic descendants with normal BALB/cM2/22 mice.

SPF-Mouse Colony

Our SPF-mouse colony was established by the transfer of fertilized eggs (4-16 cell stage) from sacrificed donors into pseudopregnant (C57Bl/6 x CBA)F1 recipient females obtained from isolator rearing (see: http://www.cbt.ki.se/meg...#Pathogen de-contamination, for more details). After weaning, all descendants, alternatively the surrogate mothers, were health monitored and serologically screened i.e. for antibodies against MHV, Sendai and Ectromelia virus. After two SPF-generations, two randomly chosen 3-4 week old mice, were sacrificed and tested to confirm their specific pathogen free status.

Transgene Typing

The presence of the transgene was assessed by PCR amplification of genomic DNA extracted from peripheral blood (Winberg G 1991). The amplified sequences corresponded to the SV40 early region promoter of the lymphoyd expression vector carrying the transgene (Rosembaum *et al* 1990).

Plasmacytoma Induction

Four to 6 weeks old mice were divided into tg carriers and tg negatives. Both groups received 0.3 ml pristane i.p. 3 times at monthly intervals. After 30 days from the first injection, the mice were weekly palpated to detect enlargement of the spleen and lymph nodes and for the accumulation of ascites. Cytofuge smears were prepared from peritoneal cells recovered from each mouse that developed ascites. The morphological examination and diagnosis followed the criteria described elsewhere (Silva *et al* 1991).

Cytogenetic Studies

Peritoneal fluid collected from ascites-carrying mice and cell suspension prepared from enlarged organs of sacrificed mice were used to prepare chromosomes following standard methods. Metaphase plates were trypsin-Giemsa banded and the magnified prints from high quality plates from each mouse were used for karyotype analysis. Chromosome identification followed the recomendations of the Committee on Standard Genetic Nomenclature for Mice (1972).

Results

MPC Development in Treated *Bcl-2/C* Mice

Among 40 mice from the second and third backcross generation, 24 were transgene positive and 16 negative. Table 1 shows the tumor incidence after pristane treatment. Only the transgene carrying mice developed plasmacytomas and lymphomas after an observation period of >300 days. Fifteen of 24 mice developed PCs, two had mixtures of lymphoma and plasmacytoma cells and three only lymphomas. Both types of tumors started to develop about 70 days after the first pristane injection (Fig 1). All 16 tg negatives remained tumor free after >300 days of observation.

Cytogenetics

All 15 MPCs and one of the mixed tumors were karyotyped (Table 2). Ten of 15 carried a T(12;15) translocation, four had double translocations T(12;15) and T(6;15) in the same metaphase plate, and one was translocation free. A T(12;15) translocation was also detected in one of the 2 mice with a mixed tumor type. The lymphomas were translocation free and showed only minor numerical changes.

Table 1. Tumor incidence after pristane treatment of SPF-*bcl-2* transgene BALB/c mice.

TRANSGENE	Treated § mice	TUMOR TYPE# *MPC (%)*	*Ly (%)*	*Mixture (%)*
Carriers	**24**	**15 *(63 %)***	**3 *(13%)***	**2 *(8 %)***
Negative	**16**	**0**	**0**	**0**

§ 3 x 0.3 ml pristane i.p. at monthly intervals
# *MPC* = plasmacytoma, *Ly* = lymphoma, *Mixture* = Ly + MPC

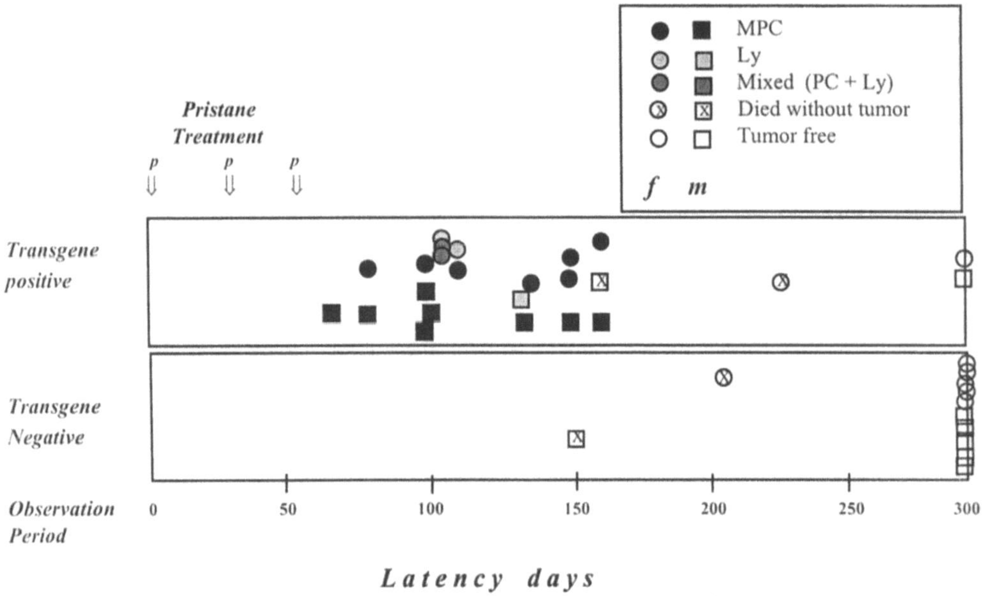

Fig. 1. Tumor development and latency following pristane treatment. Transgene positive mice were found to carry plasmacytoma cells already after 67 days of the first pristane injection. All the 16 transgene negatives remained tumor free. (*f* = female, *m* = male)

Table 2. Cytogenetic findings

Tumor type	**CHROMOSOMAL CHANGES**	
	Numerical	**Structural**
PLASMACYTOMAS		
TEPCBcl-2/C - 3		**T(12;15)**
TEPCBcl-2/C - 4	**-11 -13**	**T(12;15)**
TEPCBcl-2/C - 7		**T(12;15)**
TEPCBcl-2/C - 11		**T(12;15), T(6;15), T(11;12)**
TEPCBcl-2/C - 12	**+9 +10 +17 +19**	**T(12;15)**
TEPCBcl-2/C - 13	**+13 +16 +18**	**T(12;15), T(6;15), M(15+)**
TEPCBcl-2/C - 14	**-7 -12**	**(Tr- free)**
TEPCBcl-2/C - 16		**T(12;15)**
TEPCBcl-2/C - 17	**Tetraploid M**	**T(12;15)**
TEPCBcl-2/C - 18	**-9 -11 -16**	**T(12;15), T(6;15)**
TEPCBcl-2/C - 20		**T(12;15)**
TEPCBcl-2/C - 21		**T(12;15)**
TEPCBcl-2/C - 22		**T(12;15)**
TEPCBcl-2/C - 23		**T(12;15), T(6;15)**
TEPCBcl-2/C - 24		**T(12;15)**
MIXED MPC + Lymphoma cells		
TELPCBcl-2/C - 5	**Tetraploid**	**T(12;15)**

M = marker

Discussion

McIntire and Princler reported in 1969 that only 6 % of germ-free BALB/c mice, developed plasmacytomas after pristane treatment compared to conventionally raised controls. More recently, Byrd *et al* (1991) showed that more than 95 % of BALB/c mice bred in specific pathogen free (SPF) conditions, were refractory to MPC induction by pristane compared to BALB/c mice housed in conventional conditions.

SPF and GF mice are relatively deprived of antigen stimulation and they have very few activated T and B cells (Baur *et al* 1963, Crabbe *et al* 1970). This was taken to indicate that MPC development requires exogenous antigenic stimulation.

B-cells are programmed to died by apoptosis unless activated within a limited time (Lu and Osmond, 1997, Osmond *et al* 1990). Antigen stimulation may prevent the apoptotic elimination of translocation carrying cells. If so, an increased apoptotic threshold may lead to MPC development, also may reestablish the MPC susceptibility of BALB/c mice kept under SPF conditions. To test this hypothesis, we have introduced the *Eμ-bcl-2* transgene, known to prolong the survival of B-cells at all stages of differentiation (McDonnell and Korsmeyer 1991, Strasser *et al* 1990), into our SPF BALB/c mice. We have found that more than 80 % of pristane treated transgenic but none of the transgene negative littermates developed plasmacytomas or lymphomas.

We have previously found that a combination of pristane and Abelson virus treatment increases the relative proportion of tumors with variant translocations. This may be due to the anti-apoptotic effect of v-*abl*. We have therefore examined whether a *bcl-2* transgene may have a similar effect. This was not the case as none of the MPCs carried a variant translocation alone. Unexpectedly, four tumors carried double translocations, a variant T(6;15) and a typical T(12;15). Primary tumors with double translocations have not been described before.

C57BL/6 mice are resistant to MPC induction by pristane. Untreated *Eμ-bcl-2/C57BL/6* developed lymphomas or plasmacytomas at a 10-15 % incidence and with a long latency period. The *bcl-2/6* MPCs had a rearranged *myc* gene (Strasser *et al* 1993). We have explored whether pristane treatment of *bcl-2/6* mice can increase the incidence of peritoneal plasmacytomas compared to untreated *bcl-2/6* transgenic. So far no plasmacytomas have been detected in pristane treated *bcl-2/6* mice kept >300 days under observation (data not shown). The cytogenetic analyzis of peritoneal cells recovered from 20 mice after 176 days revealed the presence of T(12;15) translocations in 4 mice that remained tumor free under observation periods of >300 days. This shows that a combination of translocation activated *myc* gene and a *bcl-2* transgene is not sufficient for MPC development in C57Bl/6 mice.

References

Baur H, Horowitz RE, Levenson SM and Popper H (1963) The response of the lymphatic tissue to the microbial flora. Studies on germfree mice. Am J Pathol 42: 471 - 479.

Byrd LG, McDonald AH, Gold LG and Potter M (1991) Specific pathogen-free BALB/cAn mice are refractory to plasmacytoma induction by pristane. J Immunol 147: 3632 - 3637.

Committee on Standard Genetic Nomenclature for Mice (1972) Standard karyotype of the mouse Mus musculus. J Hered 63: 69 - 72.

Crabbe PA, Nash DR, Bazin H, Eyssen H and Heremans JF (1970) Immunohistochemical observations on lymphoid tissues from conventional and germ-free mice. Lab. Invest. 22: 448 - 453.

Janz S, Müller J, Shaughnessy J and Potter M (1993) Detection of recombinations between c-*myc* and immunoglobulin switch α in murine plasma cell tumors and preneoplastic lesions by polymerase chain reaction . PNAS (USA) 90: 7361 - 7365.

Lu L and Osmond D. (1997) Apoptosis during B lymphopoiesis in mouse bone marrow. J Immunol 158(11): 5136 - 5145.

McDonnell TJ and Korsmeyer SJ (1991) Progression from lymphoid hyperplasia to high-grade malignant lymphoma in mice transgenic for the t(14;18). Nature 349: 254 - 256.

McIntire KR and Princler GL (1969) Prolonged adjuvant stimulation in germ-free BALB/c mice development of plasma cell neoplasia. Immunol 17: 481 - 485.

Müller JR, Jones GM, Potter M and Janz S (1996) Detection of immunoglobulin/c-*myc* recombinations in mice that are resistant to plasmacytoma induction. Cancer Res 56:419-423.

Osmond DG, Priddle S and Rico-Vargas S (1990) Proliferation of B cell precursors in bone marrow of pristane-conditioned and malaria-infected mice: implications for B cell oncogenesis. CTMI 166: 149 - 157.

Potter M and Wiener F (1992) Plasmacytomagenesis in mice: model of neoplastic development dependent upon chromosomal translocations. Carcinogenesis 13:1681-1697.

Rosenbaum H, Webb E, Adams JM, Cory S and Harris AW (1989) N-*myc* transgene promotes B lymphoid proliferation, elicits lymphomas and reveals cross-regulation with c-*myc* EMBO J 8: 749 - 755.

Silva S, Wang Y, Babonits M, Imreh S, Wiener F and Klein G (1997) Spontaneous development of plasmacytomas in a selected subline of BALB/cJ mice. Eur J Cancer 33(3): 479 - 485.

Silva S, Sugiyama H, Babonits M, Wiener F and Klein G (1991) Differential susceptibility of BALB/c and DBA/2 cells to plasmacytoma induction in reciprocal chimeras. Int J Cancer 49: 224 - 228.

Strasser A., Harris AW, Vaux DL, Webb E, Bath ML, Adams JM and Cory S (1990) Abnormalities of the immune system induced by dysregulated *bcl-2* expression in transgenic mice. CTMI 166: 175 - 181.

Strasser A, Whittingham S, Vaux DL, Bath ML, Adams JM, Cory S and Harris AW (1991) Enforced *BCL-2* expression in B-lymphoid cells prolongs antibody responses and elicits autoimmnune disease. PNAS 88: 8661 - 8665.

Strasser A, Harris AW and Cory S (1993) Eμ-*bcl-2* transgene facilitates spontaneous transformation of early pre-B and immunoglobulin-secreting cells but not T cells. Oncogene 8: 1 - 9.

Winberg G (1991) A rapid method for preparing DNA from blood, suited for PCR screening of transgenes in mice. PCR Methods and Applications, Cold Spring Harbor Laboratory Press, 1: 72 - 74.

Acknowledgements

This work was supported by a grant from the Swedish Cancer Society.

Discussion

Georg Bornkamm: Is a gene dosage effect involved?

Santiago Silva: No, my interpretation is that there is a mechanism that is going wrong and allows translocations, probably the immunoglobulin gene somatic RAG1 or RAG2, but this is speculation as I don't know for sure. But there are indications that this mechanism is continuously going on even after the first translocation, so it is not freezing this process in one step.

Michael Reth: But the last case you showed was a tumor, wasn't it?

Santiago Silva: Yes, from a primary tumor carrying Tg mouse, but we have also observed this phenomenon in MPC cell lines.

Siegfried Janz: Did you also observe T(6;15) translocations in the C57BL/6.bcl-2 mice that harbored translocations T(12;15)?

Santiago Silva: Not alone, but in one case we observed both translocations in one mouse.

Richard Scheuermann: Do you have any idea what percent of cells are carrying the translocation?

Santiago Silva: No. Now I am trying to do the statistics because it is apparently polyclonal. Some of the cells carry one translocation, others two. We are now trying to figure out by immunoglobulin germline analysis whether they have a mono- or oligoclonal derivation.

Beverly Mock: With regard to your BCL2 transgenic experiments in BALB/c, do you think that is a transgenic effect or could it be a background genetic effect?

Santiago Silva: Since BCL2 is not required in conventional conditions to induce plasmacytoma, we assume that BCL2 is doing nothing else but recover the B cell from apoptosis.

Induction of B Cell Autoimmunity by Pristane

H. B. Richards, M. Satoh, V. M. Shaheen, H. Yoshida, and W. H. Reeves*
Departments of Medicine and Microbiology/Immunology, Thurston Arthritis Research Center and UNC Lineberger Comprehensive Cancer Center, University of North Carolina, Chapel Hill, NC 27599-7280, USA

Plasmacytomas are induced in BALB/cAn and certain other strains of mice after intraperitoneal injection of 2, 6, 10, 14 tetramethylpentadecane (pristane) (1). The pathogenesis of these tumors remains incompletely understood despite intensive study. Chromosomal translocations involving the immunoglobulin and c-myc loci are generated and may be important for malignant transformation. Production of IL-6 and prostaglandin intermediates within the peritoneal oil granulomas developing in pristane-treated mice also appears to play a critical role. Indomethacin inhibits both IL-6 production and the development of plasmacytomas (2,3). The lack of plasmacytoma development in IL-6 knockout mice further underscores the importance of this cytokine in the neoplastic process (4). The reduced frequency of plasmacytomas in specific pathogen free (SPF) vs. conventionally housed mice (5) argues that antigenic stimulation also may contribute to the pathogenesis of these plasma cell tumors.

Although there is not proof that antigenic stimulation is involved in plasmacytoma development in mice, certain human B cell neoplasms, such as follicular lymphoma and Burkitt's lymphoma, show clear evidence of antigen drive (6,7). In some cases, clonal selection of B cell neoplasms may be driven by autoantigens (8). The potential link between B cell autoimmunity and neoplasia also is supported by the induction of autoantibodies characteristic of systemic lupus erythematosus (SLE) in BALB/c and other strains of mice by pristane (9,10). The present studies further explore the relationship between B cell neoplasia and autoantibody production.

Materials and Methods

Animals

Female BALB/cByJ, BALB/cAn, and BALB/cAn IL-6 -/- mice were housed under pathogen-free conditions in barrier cages. At 3 mo. of age mice received a single 0.5 ml intraperitoneal (i.p.) injection of pristane (Sigma Chemical Co.) or phosphate buffered saline (PBS). Sera were collected from the tail vein before injection, at 2 or 3 weeks, and monthly thereafter. Some mice were treated with indomethacin (Sigma, 20 µg/ml in the drinking water) as described (2).

Immunoglobulin Levels

Total levels of IgG1, 2a, 2b, 3, IgA, and IgM were measured by sandwich ELISA as described (11). Isotype standards (murine myeloma proteins, Southern Biotechnology) were used for standard curve fitting.

* This work was supported by research grants AR44731, AR30701, and AR7416 from the United States Public Health Service. Dr. Richards is an Arthritis Foundation Postdoctoral Fellow.

Autoantibody Assays

Anti-dsDNA antibodies were measured by the *Crithidia luciliae* kinetoplast staining assay at a serum dilution of 1:20 as described (12). Second antibody was 1:40 FITC-conjugated goat anti-mouse IgG (Southern Biotechnology). Sera from an anti-dsDNA positive 5 month old female MRL/*lpr* mouse and from an untreated BALB/c mouse served as positive and negative controls, respectively.

Sera from pristane- and PBS-treated mice were tested by ELISA for various autoantibodies at a 1:500 dilution (12). Anti-nRNP/Sm antibodies were detected using purified U1 snRNPs as antigen and alkaline phosphatase-conjugated goat anti-mouse IgG (γ chain-specific, 1:1000 dilution) as second antibody. IgG anti-chromatin antibodies were measured using chicken chromatin as antigen. Anti-ssDNA and -dsDNA antibodies were measured using heat-denatured or S1 nuclease-treated calf thymus DNA, respectively, as antigens.

Results and Discussion

Induction of Autoantibodies by Pristane

Within several weeks of injecting 0.5 ml pristane i.p., BALB/cByJ and other strains of mice develop IgM anti-ssDNA and histone autoantibodies (10). IgG anti-nRNP/Sm and -Su autoantibodies are produced by about half of the mice starting at 8-12 weeks (9,10). Titers are comparable to, or higher than, those seen in murine (MRL/*lpr*) or human lupus. These autoantibodies are readily detectable by immunoprecipitation of radiolabeled antigens from cell extracts (9). IgG anti-ssDNA antibodies appear later (12). Anti-dsDNA antibodies also develop in BALB/cAn and BALB/cJ mice starting at 7-8 months (12) and can be detected by *Crithidia luciliae* kinetoplast staining (Fig. 1). High levels of anti-chromatin antibodies, approaching those in MRL/*lpr* mice, also develop.

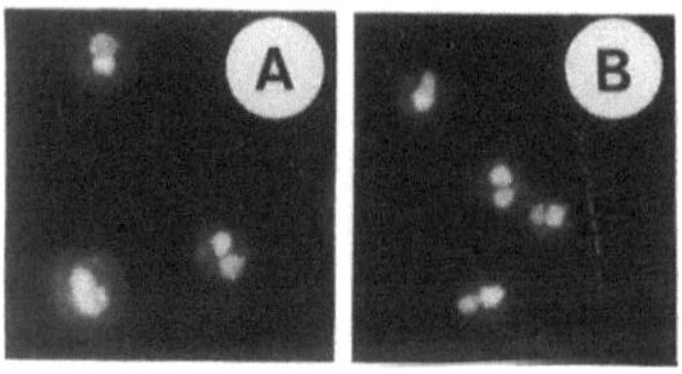

Fig. 1. *Crithidia luciliae* kinetoplast staining. Serum from a pristane-treated BALB/cAn mouse (A) and an anti-dsDNA antibody positive MRL/lpr mouse (B) were diluted 1:20 and used in the *Crithidia luciliae* kinetoplast staining assay. Autoantibody binding was detected using FITC-conjugated goat anti-mouse IgG antibodies (1:40 dilution).

Susceptibility to Autoantibody Induction

BALB/cAn and other sublines of BALB/c mice, with the exception of BALB/cJ, are susceptible to plasmacytoma induction by pristane (13). In contrast, all BALB/c sublines appear susceptible to the induction of autoantibodies, as do other strains of mice that are resistant to plasmacytoma induction. However, there are differences among strains in the types of autoantibodies generated (Table 1). For example, BALB/cByJ produced high levels of IgM anti-ssDNA and histone antibodies, but little or no IgG, whereas both BALB/cAn and BALB/cJ produced IgG anti-ssDNA and IgG anti-chromatin autoantibodies. IgG anti-dsDNA antibody production also appears restricted to BALB/cAn and BALB/cJ (Table 1). IgG anti-nRNP/Sm and Su autoantibodies are produced at high titers by all three BALB/c sublines, but are unusual in SJL mice.

Immunoprecipitation of ribonuclease-treated U1 snRNPs revealed that the response in BALB/cByJ mice is directed primarily against nRNP determinants (polypeptides 70K, A, and C), whereas certain other strains developed a more prominent anti-Sm response.

Table 1. Susceptibility of pristane-treated mice to autoimmunity and plasmacytomas

Strain	Plasmacytoma	IgM ssDNA	IgG ssDNA	IgG dsDNA	IgG Chromatin	IgG nRNP/Sm
BALB/cAn	S	S	S	S	S	S
BALB/cByJ	n.a.	S	R*	R*	R*	S
BALB/cJ	R	S	S	S	S	S
BALB/c IL-6 -/-	R	n.a.	R	R	R	S
BALB/c *nu/nu*	R	S	R**	R	R**	R
SJL	R	R	S	R	n.a.	R
C57BL/6	R	S	S	R	R**	S

*S, susceptible; R, resistant; * data available only up to 6 months; ** spontaneous production of autoantibody occurs but is not increased by pristane treatment; n.a., not available*

Role of Oil Granulomas in the Induction of Autoimmunity

Intraperitoneal injection of pristane in BALB/cAn mice induces a foreign body-like inflammatory response accompanied by macrophage activation, T cell recruitment and cytokine production (3,14). The inflammatory cells organize into lipogranulomas (15), within which plasmacytomas develop. Human ingestion of mineral oil also leads to the development of lipogranulomas (16). It has been suggested that local production of IL-6 promotes plasmacytoma development (4,17,18). It was of interest to investigate the role of IL-6 in the development of pristane-induced autoimmunity because of the proposed role of this cytokine in other autoimmune processes (19,20).

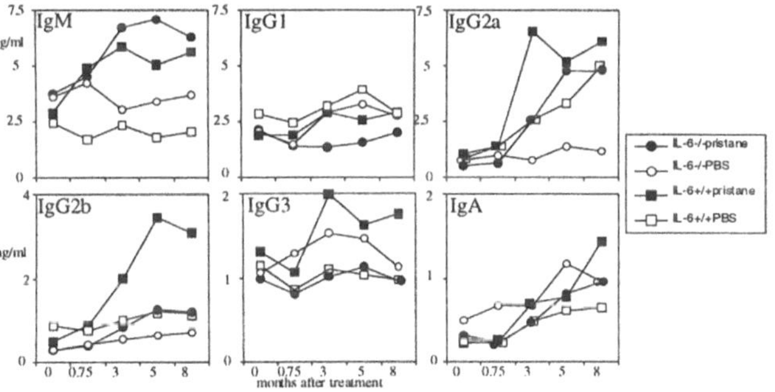

Fig. 2. Total Ig levels. Sera from IL-6 -/- or +/+ BALB/cAn mice before treatment and at 0.75, 3, 5 and 8 months after treatment were analyzed by ELISA for total IgM, IgG1, IgG2a, IgG2b, IgG3, and IgA. Means levels of each isotype (mg/ml) at each time point are shown.

IL-6 Effects on the Induction of Hypergammaglobulinemia by Pristane

Along with autoantibody production, pristane induces a striking polyclonal hypergammaglobulinemia in BALB/c mice (11). To examine the role of IL-6 in hypergammaglobulinemia, IL-6 deficient and intact BALB/cAn mice were treated with pristane or PBS and total Ig levels were determined by ELISA (Fig. 2). Increased total IgM was apparent at 3 weeks in pristane-treated IL-6 +/+ as well as IL-6 -/- mice, but not in PBS-treated controls. IgG2a, IgG2b, and IgG3 levels increased markedly from 1 to 3 months after pristane treatment both in IL-6 +/+ and -/- mice. In general, the increase was less dramatic in the IL-6 -/- group than in the +/+ mice, especially in the case of IgG2b. The difference between total IgG2a levels of the two groups was not large, however. IgG2a is the predominant isotype of the anti-nRNP/Sm, -Su, -dsDNA and -chromatin autoantibodies induced by pristane (10,12). In view of the modest effect of IL-6 deficiency on total IgG2a levels, we examined whether autoantibodies of this isotype were induced by pristane in IL-6 -/- mice.

A Subset of Autoantibodies is IL-6 Dependent

IL-6 deficient (-/-) and intact (+/+) BALB/cAn mice were treated with pristane or PBS and autoantibody production was evaluated by ELISA (anti-nRNP/Sm) or *Crithidia luciliae* kinetoplast staining (anti-dsDNA). Pristane induced IgG anti-nRNP/Sm antibodies in 58% of IL-6 +/+ mice vs. 46% of IL-6 -/- mice (Fig. 3). Despite similar frequencies, the levels were considerably lower in the IL-6 -/- group. A similar trend was observed for IgG anti-Su autoantibodies (12). The lower levels of autoantibodies in IL-6 -/- mice are not surprising, in view of the role of IL-6 as a B cell maturation factor. Unexpectedly, however, pristane-treated IL-6 -/- mice had no detectable IgG anti-dsDNA antibodies, whereas this specificity was produced by 38% of pristane-treated IL-6 +/+ controls at titers up to ≥1:640 by Crithidia assay. Anti-dsDNA activity also was not detectable by ELISA, nor were IgG anti-ssDNA or -chromatin autoantibodies detectable by ELISA (12). Finally, aged IL-6 +/+ BALB/cAn mice developed low levels of IgG anti-chromatin autoantibodies spontaneously, whereas aged IL-6 -/- mice did not.

We conclude that both spontaneous and pristane-induced production of autoantibodies against epitopes of chromatin is strictly IL-6 dependent. In contrast, anti-nRNP/Sm and Su autoantibodies are not produced spontaneously but can be induced by pristane in IL-6 -/- mice. The data suggest that different pathways may be involved in the induction of autoimmunity to different subsets of self-antigens. This may be relevant to the observation that in human SLE, anti-dsDNA antibodies are produced transiently during periods of disease activity, whereas anti-nRNP/Sm autoantibodies are produced at nearly constant levels over extended periods of time and are not good markers of disease activity.

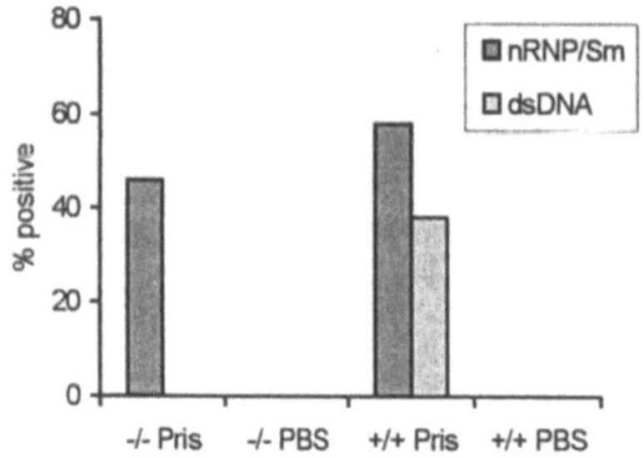

Fig. 3. Frequencies of anti-nRNP/Sm and anti-dsDNA antibodies in BALB/cAn mice. IL-6 -/- and IL-6 +/+ mice were treated with pristane (-/-, n = 28; +/+, n = 26) or PBS (n = 10 per group). Eight months later, sera were tested at 1:500 (ELISA) for anti-nRNP/Sm autoantibodies, or at 1:20 (*Crithidia luciliae* kinetoplast staining assay) for anti-dsDNA antibodies.

Effect of Indomethacin on Autoimmunity

Some oil-induced murine plasmacytomas exhibit specificity for nucleic acid antigens, including ssDNA and RNA (21). The induction of these tumors is highly IL-6 dependent. Administration of indomethacin to pristane-treated BALB/cAn mice greatly inhibits production of IL-6 in the peritoneal cavity (3) as well as the influx of CD4+ T cells (14), and dramatically reduces the incidence of plasmacytomas. In contrast, it does not prevent either peritoneal inflammation or granuloma formation (2) and has a modest effect, at best, on the development of arthritis in pristane-treated BALB/cAn or DBA/1 mice (14,22). Similarly, the induction of rheumatoid factor is unaffected by indomethacin treatment (22). As shown in Table 2, treatment with indomethacin (20 μg/ml in the drinking water) had little or no effect on the frequency of induction of anti-nRNP/Sm or -Su autoantibodies. Similarly, there was little effect on IgG anti-ssDNA or -chromatin autoantibody production (not shown). For unclear reasons, 5/11 of the indomethacin plus pristane-treated mice died despite receiving a dose of the drug reported to be non-toxic (2).

Table 2. Effect of indomethacin on pristane-induced autoimmunity in BALB/cByJ mice

Treatment (n)	Indomethacin	nRNP/Sm	Su	Mortality
Pristane (20)	(-)	55%	45%	5%
Pristane (11)	(+)	71%*	57%*	46%
PBS (20)	(-)	0	0	0

* *surviving mice only; 5/11 mice died of unknown causes before 2 months*

Conclusions

Although SLE is thought to be primarily a genetic disease, pristane can induce a systemic autoimmune disorder with many of the features of lupus in strains of mice not generally considered to be autoimmune-prone. Pristane-treated mice develop autoantibodies characteristic of SLE along with immune complex-mediated glomerulonephritis and erosive arthritis. A subset of autoantibodies induced by pristane (anti-ssDNA, -dsDNA, -chromatin), is absent in IL-6 -/- BALB/cAn mice, whereas another subset (anti-nRNP/Sm, -Su) is produced at comparable frequency in IL-6 -/- vs. +/+ mice. These data raise the possibility that autoantibodies against chromatin/DNA may be produced by a different subset of B cells than anti-nRNP/Sm and -Su autoantibodies. Further support for this idea comes from the fact that certain mineral oils induce IgM anti-ssDNA but not IgG anti-nRNP/Sm or Su antibodies (M Satoh, et al., submitted). IL-6 overproduction also has been implicated in human autoimmunity. For instance, IL-6 secreting atrial myxomas are associated with antinuclear antibody production and autoimmune disease (19), and IL-6 may play a role in immune complex-mediated renal disease (23).

The strong IL-6 dependence of both plasmacytomas and autoimmunity warrants comment. There is increasing evidence that some B cell neoplasms are antigen-stimulated (6,7), sometimes by self-antigens (8). Moreover, oil-induced plasmacytomas in mice that produce autoantibodies with anti-DNA and/or -RNA activity have been reported (21). Despite the fact that not all strains of mice susceptible to the induction of autoimmunity by pristane are susceptible to plasmacytoma induction, it is possible that the IL-6 dependent anti-DNA/chromatin autoantibodies are produced by a B cell subset susceptible to pristane-induced malignant transformation. Conversely, anti-nRNP/Sm and -Su autoantibodies may be produced by a B cell subset that is resistant to transformation. Further studies of the B cell subsets involved in pristane-induced neoplasia and autoantibody production and comparisons of Ig V-gene usage may help to better define the relationship, if any, between B cell neoplasia and autoimmunity.

References

1. Anderson PN, Potter M (1969) Induction of plasma cell tumours in BALB/c mice with 2,6,10,14-tetramethylpentadecane (pristane). Nature (Lond) 222:994-995

2. Potter M, Wax JS, Anderson AO, Nordan RP (1985) Inhibition of plasmacytoma development in BALB/c mice by indomethacin. J Exp Med 161:996-1012
3. Shacter E, Arzadon GK, Williams J (1992) Elevation of interleukin-6 in response to a chronic inflammatory stimulus in mice: inhibition by indomethacin. Blood 80:194-202
4. Hilbert DM, Kopf M, Mock BA, Kohler G, Rudikoff S (1995) Interleukin 6 is essential for in vivo development of B lineage neoplasms. J Exp Med 182:243-248
5. Byrd LG, McDonald AH, Gold LG, Potter M (1991) Specific pathogen-free BALB/cAn mice are refractory to plasmacytoma induction by pristane. J Immunol 147:3632-3637
6. Zelenetz AD, Chen TT, Levy R (1992) Clonal expansion in follicular lymphoma occurs subsequent to antigenic selection. J Exp Med 176:1137-1148
7. Jain R, Roncella S, Hashimoto S, Carbone A, deCelle PF, Foa R, Ferrarini M, Chiorazzi N (1994) A potential role for antigen selection in the clonal evolution of Burkitt's lymphoma. J Immunol 153:45-52
8. Friedman DF, Cho EA, Goldman J, Carmack CE, Besa EC, Hardy RR, Silberstein LE (1991) The role of clonal selection in the pathogenesis of an autoreactive human B cell lymphoma. J Exp Med 174:525-537
9. Satoh M, Reeves WH (1994) Induction of lupus-associated autoantibodies in BALB/c mice by intraperitoneal injection of pristane. J Exp Med 180:2341-2346
10. Satoh M, Kumar A, Kanwar YS, Reeves WH (1995) Antinuclear antibody production and immune complex glomerulonephritis in BALB/c mice treated with pristane. Proc Natl Acad Sci USA 92:10934-10938x
11. Hamilton KJ, Satoh M, Swartz J, Richards HB, Reeves WH (1998) Influence of microbial stimulation on hypergammaglobulinemia and autoantibody production in pristane-induced lupus. Clin Immunol Immunopathol 86:271-279
12. Richards HB, Satoh M, Shaw M, Libert C, Poli V, Reeves WH (1998) IL-6 dependence of anti-DNA antibody production: evidence for two pathways of autoantibody formation in pristane-induced lupus. J Exp Med 188:985-990
13. Potter M, Wax JS (1981) Genetics of susceptibility to pristane-induced plasmacytomas in BALB/cAn: Reduced susceptibility in BALB/cJ with a brief description of pristane-induced arthritis. J Immunol 127:1591-1595
14. McDonald AH, Degrassi A (1993) Pristane induces an indomethacin inhibitable inflammatory influx of CD4+ T cells and IFN-gamma production in plasmacytoma-susceptible BALB/cAnPt mice. Cell Immunol 146:157-170
15. Potter M, MacCardle RC (1964) Histology of developing plasma cell neoplasia induced by mineral oil in BALB/c mice. J Natl Cancer Inst 33:497-515
16. Dincsoy HP, Weesner RE, MacGee J (1982) Lipogranulomas in non-fatty human livers: a mineral oil induced environmental disease. Am J Clin Pathol 78:35-41
17. Vink A, Coulie P, Warnier G, Renauld JC, Stevens M, Donckers D, Van Snick J (1990) Mouse plasmacytoma growth in vivo: enhancement by interleukin 6 (IL-6) and inhibition by antibodies directed against IL-6 or its receptor. J Exp Med 172:997-1000
18. Lattanzio G, Libert C, Aquilina M, Cappelletti M, Ciliberto G, Musiani P, Poli V (1997) Defective development of pristane-oil induced plasmacytomas in interleukin-6-deficient BALB/c mice. Am J Pathol 151:689-696
19. Jourdan M, Bataille R, Seguin J, Zhang XG, Chaptal PA, Klein B (1990) Constitutive production of interleukin-6 and immunologic features in cardiac myxomas. Arthritis Rheum 33:398-402
20. Hirano T, Taga T, Yasukawa K, Nakajima K, Nakano N, Takatsuki F, Shimizu M, Murashima A, Tsunasawa S, Sakiyama F, Kishimoto T (1987) Human B-cell differentiation factor defined by an anti-peptide antibody and its possible role in autoantibody production. Proc Natl Acad Sci USA 84:228-231
21. Schubert D, Roman A, Cohn M (1970) Anti-nucleic acid specificities of mouse myeloma immunoglobulins. Nature (Lond) 225:154-158
22. Nishikaku F, Aono S, Koga Y (1994) Protective effects of D-penicillamine and a thiazole derivative, SM-8849, on pristane-induced arthritis in mice. Int J Immunopharmac 16:91-100
23. Horii Y, Muraguchi A, Iwano M, Matsuda T, Hirayama T, Yamada H, Fujii Y, Dohi K, Ishikawa H, Ohmoto Y, Yoshizaki K, Hirano T, Kishimoto T (1989) Involvement of IL-6 in mesangial proliferative glomerulonephritis. J Immunol 143:3949-3955

Discussion

Michael Carroll: In the IL-6-deficient mice have you looked at other inducers of inflammation to see if the inflammation is impaired or slightly impaired in the pristane-treated animals?
Westley Reeves: In work that Valeria Poli has done it is known that there are deficient inflammatory responses to a number of other substances including turpentine. Interestingly, inflammation elicited by LPS is similar in wild type and IL-6-deficient mice. [Fattori et al. (1994) Defective inflammatory response in interleukin 6-deficient mice. J Exp Med 180:1243-1250]
Michael Carroll: So you might conclude that, at least for induction of anti-single stranded DNA antibody, you need a more robust inflammatory response?
Westley Reeves: Yes, very possibly. For the responses in the peritoneal cavity I believe that the number of the granulomas that stud the inside of the peritoneal cavity is reduced in IL-6-deficient mice, so that is more or less consistent with what you are saying.
Shozo Izui: Is the anti-DNA response also T cell-dependent?
Westley Reeves: Yes, the anti-Sm, RNP, Su and chromatin responses are T cell-dependent, as well. The only antibody response that is not T cell-dependent in this model, or doesn't appear to be T cell-dependent, is the very early IgM anti-single stranded DNA response occurring at 2 weeks. All of the responses appearing at 2-4 months or later are T cell-dependent, since they cannot be induced in BALB/c nude mice.

Cytokine Network Imbalances in Plasmacytoma-Regressor Mice

O. Sagi-Assif[1], D. Douer[2], and I.P. Witz[1]
[1] Dept. of Cell Research and Immunology, George S. Wise Faculty of Life Sciences, Tel Aviv University, Tel Aviv, Israel; [2] Dept. of Medicine, Division of Hematology, Norris Comprehensive Cancer Center, University of Southern California, Los Angeles, CA, USA.

Introduction

It is generally accepted that secondary malignancies, mainly leukemia, are iatrogenic diseases brought about by various anti-cancer treatment modalities such as chemotherapy with alkylating agents, topoisomerase II inhibitors or by radiotherapy (1-4). The exposure to these treatment modalities is associated with various chromosomal aberrations such as chromosomal breaks, gene rearrangements or translocations (5-7). Two of the most frequent genetic changes in secondary, drug induced leukemias are translocation breakpoints of the MLL (HRX) and the AML1 genes (8-9).

Although the mutagenic and leukomogenic effects of the above mentioned anti-cancer treatment regimens (and additional ones not mentioned above) are well established, the contribution of cofactors derived either from the primary malignancy or originating in the host, to the generation and pathogenesis of secondary leukemia, are much less recognized (1,3).

The hypothesis concerning the involvement of cofactors derived from the primary tumor and/or from the host in the development and progression of secondary leukemia is based on several, mostly indirect arguments. For example, there is a relatively high frequency of secondary leukemia in untreated multiple myeloma patients (1), and myelodysplastic syndrome and acute leukemia occurs more frequently in patients with certain types of primary malignancies than in patients with other malignancies treated with the same chemotherapeutic modality (10-11). Another indication for the involvement of host-derived cofactors in the development of secondary leukemia is the 8-fold higher frequency of secondary leukemia in splenectomized Hodgkin's disease patients treated with combined modality therapy than in patients treated only with chemotherapy (12).

One may hypothesize that chemotherapy with carcinogenic agents indeed transforms target cells but that cofactors derived either from the first tumor or from the patient himself, contribute, possibly by conditioning the host, to the development of secondary leukemia.

In previous studies we set out to segregate the contribution of carcinogenic chemotherapy from that of cofactors derived from the primary tumor and/or from the host, to the formation of secondary malignancies.

We developed a mouse model that made it possible to compare the late effects of curative doses of melphalan on MOPC-315 plasmacytoma-bearing mice to the effects of the same dose of melphalan on normal mice (13). We confirmed the reports of other investigators that damage was caused to hematopoietic progenitors by the drug *per se*. However, most of the melphalan-induced effects in non-tumor bearers renormalized after a period of 1-2 months following the termination of the melphalan treatment. In contrast, plasmacytoma-regressor mice (PRM), though seemingly cured of the tumor by melphalan, presented persistent abnormalities which were not evident, or much less so, in otherwise normal mice treated with the same drug. The main findings were that the PRM, which showed no signs of plasmacytoma relapse or any other overt malignancy, had an increased mortality risk, and showed signs of cachexia.

The fact that PRM did not present with any overt leukemia prompted us to investigate whether such mice harbored preleukemic cells which do not progress to leukemia. To test this possibility we utilized an approach to detect preleukemic cells (14). Adoptive transfer of splenocytes originating in PRM to preirradiated but otherwise untreated syngeneic recipients resulted in the development of overt leukemia in a certain fraction of such recipients (15). The presence of leukemia in the primary recipient mice was ascertained by blood counts as well as by spleen histology. Furthermore, splenocytes from the irradiated primary recipients adoptively transferred to non-irradiated secondary recipients caused leukemia formation in 100% of the secondary recipients. Sex-chromosome analysis of the leukemic cells in the irradiated primary recipients clearly showed that they originated in the PRM donors. Melphalan-treated normal mice serving as control did not harbor preleukemic cells. Two leukemic lines were established from leukemias developing in the secondary recipients and both expressed surface markers of hematopoietic progenitor cells as well as markers of T cells (15).

We wished to establish if PRM had abnormalities which could contribute to the development of preleukemia in such mice. Melphalan-treated non-tumor bearer mice (M) or untreated mice (C) served as controls (16). Histopathological examination indicated that the spleen of PRM showed extramedullary hematopoiesis and myeloid-granulocytic hyperplasia (16). Spleens of M controls showed similar abnormalities but to a much lesser extent. Flow cytometric analysis of cellular surface markers of PRM splenocytes indicated a high number of large MAC-1- and GR-1-positive cells compared to splenocytes of both control groups. These large cells also expressed Fcγ receptors, stained positively with non-specific esterase and adhered to plastic dishes; a certain percentage expressed MAC-2 and MAC-3 antigens. The number of CD4-positive T cells and of B cells was reduced, and IL-2 secretion from splenic T cells was suppressed. Circulating levels of TNFα were higher in PRM than in control mice.

Since some or most of the above abnormalities, as well as the preleukemia appearing in PRM may have been facilitated by imbalanced cytokine networks we set out to establish if such imbalances do exist in PRM. Indeed, and as reported above, PRM-derived splenocytes show a suppressed ability to secrete IL-2 and PRM have increased levels of circulating TNF-α as compared to controls.

The results reported below are part of a comprehensive study to establish the nature and magnitude of imbalanced cytokine networks in PRM.

Results

The Secretion of and Response to Myeloid Stimulatory Factors by PRM Splenocytes

In view of the myeloproliferation occurring in PRM, we assayed the ability of splenocytes originating from PRM to secrete factors which stimulate CFU-GM colony formation by normal bone marrow cells. Figure 1 shows that PRM splenocytes indeed secreted CSF for myeloid cells. Splenocytes from M controls or from normal age matched mice induced a significantly lower number of CFU-GM colonies from normal bone marrow cells.

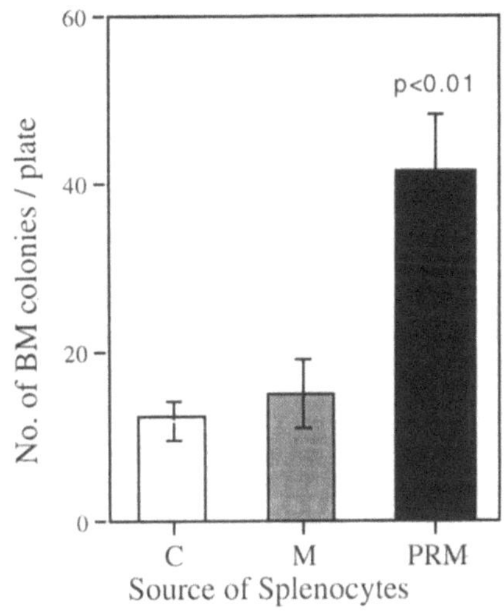

Fig. 1: Secretion of Factors from PRM and Control Splenocytes Stimulating CFU-GM Formation by Normal Bone-Marrow
10^6 splenocytes/ml from PRM (■); M controls (▒) or from C controls (□) in 0.3% agar were placed as a lower layer in culture dishes and overlayered by 10^5 normal bone marrow (BM) cells also in 0.3% agar. The values represent an average of 4 experiments ± S.D. The differences between BM colonies formed in the presence of PRM splenocytes and each of the control splenocytes was significant (P<0.01).

Next we determined the ability of PRM splenocytes to respond, by colony formation in soft agar, to cytokines present in WEH1 conditioned medium [mostly IL-3 and GM-CSF (17)] and to recombinant IL-3 and GM-CSF. Spleen cells in 0.3% agar were incubated with or without WEH1-conditioned medium, rIL-3 or rGM-CSF at 37°C for 7 days. Colonies (>20 cells) were then scored. Figure 2 shows that splenocytes from PRM had a significantly higher ability to respond to these cytokines than splenocytes from the 2 control groups.

Put together these data show that the production of and response to myeloid growth factors is significantly enhanced in PRM splenocytes. This situation could lead to an enhanced proliferation of myeloid cells transformed by a carcinogenic drug such as melphalan.

Fig. 2: Response (CFU-C Formation in Soft Agar) of PRM and Control Splenocytes to Myeloid Growth Factors
10^6 splenocytes/ml from PRM (■) from M controls (▒) or from C controls (□) were seeded in each plate in the presence of 10% conditioned medium of WEHI cells of rIL-3 (50U/ml) or of rGM-CSF (50U/ml). The differences between the number of colonies produced by PRM splenocytes and control splenocytes in the presence of these factors was significant (P<0.01). The results are of a representative experiment out of 4 performed.

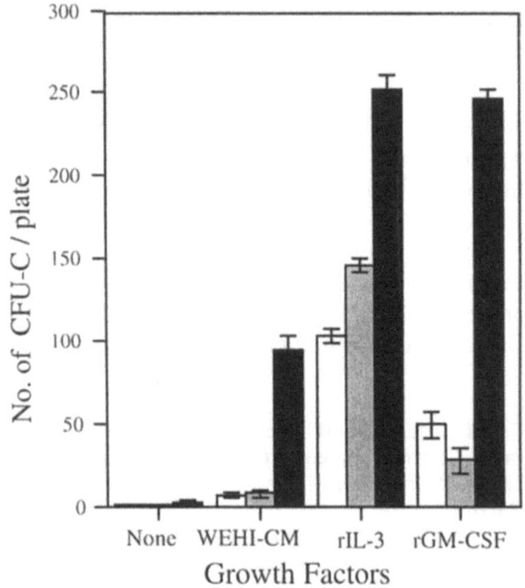

An Imbalanced TH1/TH2 Network in PRM

A common view prevailing among cancer researchers is that immune dysregulation may contribute to the progression of malignant diseases. One type of immune dysregulation associated with the progression of malignancy is an imbalance in the network of TH1 and TH2 type cytokines (18-20). In view of preliminary data showing that PRM splenocytes secreted less IL-2 than splenocytes from control mice (13) we set out to examine the TH1/TH2 network in PRM and in control mice.

Splenocytes from PRM or control spleens were stimulated by Con A. The cytokines secreted from these cells were measured by ELISA kits. T lymphocytes of PRM were found to be severely deficient in TH1 cytokine production. These splenocytes produced only 10-20% of the levels of IFNγ produced by control splenocytes. Another TH1 cytokine IL-2 was also decreased (about 2-3 fold). On the other hand PRM splenocytes showed a significant increase in the secretion of TH2-type cytokines. The amounts of IL-4 produced by T cells from PRM is 5-10 fold higher than that produced by controls and IL-10, another TH2 cytokine, was increased 2-3 fold. These results clearly show that plasmacytoma-regressors suffer from a TH1/TH2 imbalance manifested by a decreased synthesis of TH1 cytokines and an increased production of TH2 cytokines.

Concluding Remarks

It is widely accepted that therapy-induced genetic alterations are causally involved in the emergence of secondary neoplasms (3,5-9). We propose that above and beyond these genetic alterations which are necessary but insufficient for the induction of secondary preleukemia in plasmacytoma-regressor mice, a cytokine network imbalance plays a significant role in facilitating its development. We suggest that this hypothesis may be generalized to include secondary malignancies in humans.

The assumption that a cytokine imbalance is a necessary contributor for the generation of secondary preleukemia in PRM is supported by information published previously and by that provided in this study. Briefly, this information demonstrated that: **(a)** The proinflammatory cytokines IL-1α, IL-6 and TNFα are elevated in multiple myeloma patients and in plasmacytoma bearing mice (21-26). **(b)** Each of these cytokines is capable of regulating or modulating the expression of other cytokines or of their receptors (21-22,27-29). **(c)** PRM express higher levels of circulating TNFα than control mice (13). **(d)** PRM splenocytes secrete factors capable of stimulating the formation of GM colonies from normal bone marrow progenitors whereas control splenocytes do not. **(e)** PRM splenocytes respond to rIL-3 and rGM-CSF in GM colony formation, while control splenocytes do not. This finding coupled to the previous one may represent an autocrine loop facilitating myeloproliferation. **(f)** The secretion of TH1 and TH2-type cytokines from PRM splenocytes is dysregulated. There is a significant decrease of TH1 cytokines and a significant increase in TH2 cytokines. No such imbalance was seen in control mice. **(g)** PRM, but not control mice (i.e. normal mice treated with melphalan), harbor preleukemic cells (15).

The hypothetical scenario for the multifactorial mechanism by which the imbalanced cytokine network described above contributes to the development of secondary preleukemia is composed of 3 elements: **(1)** High levels of myeloid growth factors such as IL-3 and/or GM-CSF push myeloid progenitors into the cell cycle thus creating myeloproliferation. Proliferating myeloid cells would be more prone than resting cells to transformation by the mutagenic and carcinogenic alkylating agent melphalan used as an anti plasmacytoma chemotherapeutical agent. This could lead to the generation of premalignant myeloid clones. **(2)** A dysregulation in TH1 and TH2 subsets of $CD4^+$ T cells has been reported to occur in various types of cancer in animals and humans. The general finding was that a TH1 deficiency or malfunction and an expansion or a hyperfunction of the TH2 compartment occurs in cancer patients or tumor-bearing animals (18-20). Since TH1 cells are involved in cellular immune reactivities a downregulated function of such cells may account for deficient anti-tumor cellular activities (19). Similar circumstances may occur in PRM. A downregulated TH1 response may contribute to a deficient cellular anti leukemia immunity thus allowing for the proliferation and progression of the premalignant clones transformed by melphalan. An upregulated TH2 response may contribute to pro-tumor activities (30). **(3)** The proinflammatory cytokines IL-1α, IL-6 and TNFα having pleiotropic regulatory effects on many cells and on the expression and synthesis of their cellular products such as cytokines (21-22,27-29) may set the stage and put the above described aberrant cytokine cascade in motion.

Acknowledgements

This research has been supported by: The Rich Foundation, Lucerne, Switzerland; The Fainbarg Family Fund, Orange County, CA, USA; The Pikovsky Fund, Jerusalem, Israel; The James J. Leibman and Rita S. Leibman Endowment Fund for Cancer Research, New York, N.Y., USA; and by The Ela Kodesz Institute for Research on Cancer Development and Prevention, Tel Aviv University. I.P. Witz is the incumbent of the David Furman Chair in Immunobiology of Cancer, Tel Aviv University.

References

1. Bergsagel DE (1982) Plasma cell neoplasma and acute leukemia. Clin Haematol 11, 221-227
2. Levine EG and Bloomfield CD (1992) Leukemias and myelodysplastic syndromes secondary to drug, radiation and environmental exposure. Sem Oncol 19(1), 47-84
3. Ratain MJ and Rowley JD (1992) Therapy-related myeloid leukemia secondary to inhibitors of topoisomerase II: from the bedside to the target genes. Ann Oncol 3(2), 107-111
4. Travis LB, Curtis RE, Boice JD Jr, Platz CE, Hankey BF and Fraumeni JF Jr (1996) Second malignant neoplasms among long-term survivors of ovarian cancer. Cancer Res 56, 1564-1570
5. Mamuris Z, Prieur M, Dutrillaux B and Aurias, A (1989) The chemotherapeutic drug melphalan induces breakage of chromosomes regions rearranged in secondary leukemia. Cancer Genet Cytogenet 37, 65-77
6. Schneider NR, Bowman WP and Frenkel EP (1991) Translocation (3;21) (q26;q22) in secondary leukemia. Report of two cases and literature review. Ann Genet 34, 256-263
7. Tanaka K, Arif M, Eguchi M, Kyo T, Dohy H and Kamada N (1997) Frequent jumping translocations of chromosomal segments involving the ABL oncogene alone or in combination with CD3-MLL genes in secondary leukemias. Blood 89, 596-600
8. Felix CA, Hosler MR, Winick NJ, Masterson M, Wilson AE and Lange BJ (1995) AML-1 gene rearrangements in DNA topoisomerase II inhibitor-related leukemia in children. Blood 85, 3250-3256
9. Aplan PD, Chervinsky DS, Stanulla M and Burhans WC (1996) Site-specific DNA cleavage within the MLL breakpoint cluster region induced by topoisomerase II inhibitors. Blood 87, 2649-2658
10. Pedersen-Biergaar J, Larsen SO, Struck J, Hansen HM, Specht L, Ersboll J, Hansen MM and Nissen NI (1987) Risk of therapy-related leukemia and preleukemia after Hodgkin's disease. Lancet II, 83-86
11. Kaldor JM, Day NE, Clarke EA, Van Leeuwen FE, Henry-Amar, M and Fiorentino FE (1990) Leukemia following Hodgkin's disease. New Engl J Med 322, 7-14
12. Tura S, Fiacchini M, Zinzani PL, Brusamolino E and Gobbi PG (1993) Splenectomy and the increasing risk of secondary acute leukemia in Hodgkin's disease. J Clin Oncol 11, 925-930
13. Sagi O, Witz IP, Ramot B, Sahar E and Douer D (1988) Late immune and hematopoietic functions in plasmacytoma-bearing mice cured by melphalan. Br J Cancer 57, 271-276
14. Resnitzky P, Estrov Z and Haran-Ghera N (1985) High incidence of acute myeloid leukemia in SJL/J mice after X irradiation and corticosteroids. Leuk Res 9, 1519-1528
15. Sagi-Assif O, Trakhtenbrot L, Douer D and Witz IP (1998) Preleukemia in long-term plasmacytoma-regressor mice. Int J Cancer 76, 689-693
16. Sagi-Assif O, Douer D, Shaked N, Russell SW and Witz IP (1994) Myeloproliferation in long-term plasmacytoma regressor mice. Int J Cancer 56, 208-213
17. Nicola N (1989) Hematopoietic cell growth factors and their receptors. Ann Rev Biochem, 58, 45-77
18. Pellegrini P, Berghella AM, Del Beato T, Cicia S, Adorno D and Casciani CU (1996) Disregulation in TH1 and TH2 subsets of CD4+ T cells in peripheral blood of colorectal cancer patients and involvement in cancer establishment and progression. Cancer Immunol Immunother 42, 1-8

19. Lucey DR, Clerici M and Shearer GM (1996) Type 1 and type 2 cytokine dysregulation in human infectious, neoplastic, and inflammatory diseases. Clin Microbiol Rev 9, 532-562
20. Sredni B, Tichler T, Shani A, Catane R, Kaufman B, Strassman G, Albeck M and Kalechman Y (1996) Predominance of TH1 response in tumor-bearing mice and cancer patients treated with AS101. J Natl Cancer Inst 88, 1276-1284
21. Klein B (1995) Cytokine, cytokine receptors, transduction signals, and oncogenes in human multiple myeloma. Semin Hematol 32, 4-19
22. Dinarello CA (1996) Biologic basis for Interleukin-1 in disease. Blood 87, 2095-2147
23. Klein B and Bataille R (1992) Cytokine network in human multiple myeloma. Hematol Oncol Clin North Am 6, 273-284
24. Merico F, Bergui L, Gregoretti MG, Ghia P, Aimo G, Lindley IJ and Caligaris-Cappio F (1993) Cytokines involved in the progression of multiple myeloma. Clin Exp Immunol 92, 27-31
25. Hilbert DM, Kopf M, Mock BA, Kohler G and Rudikoff S (1995) Interleukin 6 is essential for in vivo development of B lineage neoplasms. J Exp Med 182, 243-248
26. Filella X, Blade J, Guillermo AL, Molina R, Rozman C and Ballesta AM (1996) Cytokines (IL-6, TNF-alpha, IL-1 alpha) and soluble interleukin-2 receptor as serum tumor markers in multiple myeloma. Cancer Detect Prev 20, 52-56
27. Neta R, Sayers TJ and Oppenheim JJ (1992) Relationship of TNF to interleukins. Immunol Ser 56, 499-566
28. Tracey KJ and Cerami A (1994) Tumor necrosis factor: a pleiotropic cytokine and therapeutic target. Annu RevMed 45, 491-503
29. Dinarello CA (1994) The biological properties of interleukin-1. Eur cytokine Netw 5, 517-531
30. Ghosh P, Komschlies KL, Cippitelli M, Longo DL, Subleski J, Ye J, Sica A, Young HA, Wiltrout RH and Ochoa AC (1995) Gradual loss of T helper 1 populations in spleen of mice during progressive tumor growth. J Natl Cancer Inst 87, 1478-1483

Discussion

Riccardo Dalla-Favera: What type of leukemia developed in the irradiated recipients of the regressor splenocytes?

Isaac Witz: This is now under investigation. It seems to be a very early progenitor cell. It shows, however, a mixed phenotype, such as T cell as well as myeloid cell markers, but the analysis is not finished yet.

Riccardo Dalla-Favera: I guess the alternative explanation is that you eradicated the plasmacytoma but you left a clonally related immature precursor that comes back with a different phenotype?

Isaac Witz: This may be possible but there is no evidence for that. For instance, in these cells we have not seen the typical immunoglobulin rearrangement that we saw in the plasmacytoma.

Heinz Jacobs: I disagree. The tissue damage in melphalan treated tumor mice is much higher than in melphalan-treated normal mice. Consequently, due to an inflammatory response, you have many more activated lymphocytes and that is why the tumor incidence in the melphalan tumor mice is higher; that is what one would expect because melphalan has a chance to introduce mutation into the genome of lymphocytes, whereas in the resting lymphocytes of normal mice it doesn't get a chance, and that is why you do not see any tumors. I do not think that one can say this has nothing to do with melphalan. The control should be that you also have to co-inject an antigen to activate the lymphocytes in the tumor-free control mice.

Isaac Witz: In fact, in the scheme I showed a very specific role for melphalan so I am saying exactly what you are saying. The first tumor creates the right milieu, for instance activated T and B cells, as well as inflammatory cells, and then the melphalan has a chance to work. In view of the involvement of such host factors I don't agree to call these types of tumors drug-induced. I think that I pointed out very clearly the contribution of host factors to the formation of secondary pre-leukemia. I think therefore that we are in total agreement.

The Role of Human Herpesvirus-8, (HHV-8), in Multiple Myeloma Pathogenesis

R.A. Vescio, MD and J.R. Berenson, MD
Veterans Affairs West Los Angeles Medical Center and Jonsson Comprehensive Cancer Center and Division of Hematology and Oncology, University of California School of Medicine, Los Angeles, California USA

The fate of any malignant cell is determined not only by its inherent genetic abnormalities but also by the environmental conditions in which the cell resides. Multiple myeloma is characterized by the accumulation of terminally differentiated plasma cells within the bone marrow. Even though malignant cells are readily detectable within the peripheral blood of these patients, the bulk of disease typically remains within the marrow cavity until the terminal stages of a patient's disease. Clearly, the microenvironment within the bone marrow is important for the growth of the myeloma cell. Within that bone marrow microenvironment is a complex network of cells which produce cytokines capable of supporting both malignant and normal hematopoietic cell growth. These supporting cells, primarily comprised of macrophages and fibroblasts, are collectively termed bone marrow stromal cells.

Bone Marrow Stromal Cells

Bone marrow stromal cells are often required to culture myeloma cells *ex vivo*. Only in rare cases, when the malignant cells are obtained from patients with plasma cell leukemia or from malignant effusions, will these malignant cells grow without stromal cell support. Investigators have found that even in these latter cases, the addition of interleukin-6 is often necessary for initial myeloma cell line growth [1]. Interleukin 6 (IL-6) is one of the primary cytokines produced by the bone marrow stromal cells. In addition, the production of IL-6 is enhanced by the adherence of malignant plasma cells, thus creating a symbiotic relationship between the bone marrow stromal cells and tumor cells in the myeloma patient [2]. While the stromal cells derived from normal patients can also sustain myeloma cells growth, many years ago Hamburger and Salmon suggested that a specific factor, present in bone marrow macrophages from myeloma patients, may be required to support the malignant clone [3].

Discovery of Human Herpesvirus 8

The existence of an infectious agent responsible for the development of Kaposi's sarcoma (KS) had been suspected for many years due to tumor epidemiology. Since KS was found more frequently in homosexual patients infected with HIV, compared to similarly infected hemophiliac patients, the causative agent was presumably sexually transmittable. In 1994, Chang and

Moore, applied a new technique, termed representational difference analysis (RDA), to search for DNA unique to the malignant cells of KS tissue [4]. Unique DNA sequences were isolated that when characterized were most homologous to genes known to be present within other members of the herpesvirus family. Further analysis revealed the existence of a new member of the gamma herpesvirus family coined Kaposi's sarcoma associated herpesvirus (KSHV). This new virus, now more commonly labeled Human herpesvirus-8 (HHV-8), has subsequently been sequenced and found to contain numerous homologues to human genes which could up-regulate cell growth and potentially lead to tumor development.

Following the initial discovery, other tumor types were assessed for viral infection. Interestingly, viral presence was found in just two relatively rare B-cell disorders, primary effusion lymphoma (PEL) and multicentric Castleman's disease [5,6]. Patients with multicentric Castleman's disease develop bulky adenopathy due to the accumulation of polyclonal B-cells and can respond to antibodies blocking the growth factor deemed responsible for tumor cell growth, IL-6. Interestingly, the virus itself contains an IL-6 homologue [7] and all three of these diseases share IL-6 as a major growth factor. Although the virus has been localized to the malignant cells in these three diseases, recently, HHV-8 has been found within circulating macrophages [8] and B-cells [9] of patients with KS.

HHV-8 Identification in Multiple Myeloma Bone Marrow Stroma

The malignant plasma cells derived from myeloma patients were also examined for HHV-8 presence since IL-6 is also the primary growth factor of this disease. Using the primers and conditions described in the original Science paper to amplify a portion of a viral minor capsid gene ($KS330_{233}$) [4], HHV-8 was not found by our group in the myeloma bone marrow aspirate material. Other groups, including another one based at UCLA, had similar negative results. We subsequently examined the long term marrow cultures established from the adherent cells of patients with myeloma. Using both the PCR assay with the viral specific primers derived from the $KS330_{233}$ fragment of ORF26, and in situ hybridization (ISH) with an HHV-8 specific probe, we demonstrated HHV-8 in all patients with myeloma except for one recently evaluated patient with early stage (Durie Salmon Stage IA) disease [10]. In addition, HHV-8 has been identified in a subset of patients with monoclonal gammopathy of undetermined significance (MGUS). By contrast, normal subjects and patients with other hematological malignancies did not contain HHV-8 in their identically cultured cells.

Although we had assumed that these adherent stromal cells were fibroblasts, immunohistochemistry was performed to characterize the HHV-8 infected cells. Surprisingly, the infected cells showed expression of CD68, CD83, and fascin all typically expressed by dendritic cells. CD1a, CD31 and CD34 were not expressed. Thus, these results are consistent with a dendritic cell phenotype without characteristics of a Langerhans cell [11] which is similar to the cell type found infected in cultures from the peripheral blood of Kaposi's sarcoma patients in one study [12]. Recently, the human cytomegalovirus has been shown to be similarly derived from long-term cultures of PBMCs bearing macrophage and dendritic cell markers [13]. Thus, dendritic cells may serve as a reservoir for a wide variety of different viruses.

HHV-8 in Fresh Bone Marrow and Blood Specimens

The original study demonstrated HHV-8 in stromal cells derived after long-term culture. To be certain these results were not due to an artifact of the culturing technique, fresh tissue was studied. Fresh bone marrow core biopsies were sectioned and stained for HHV-8 using ISH. Of 21 MM bone marrow core biopsies, 18 stained with a $KS233_{330}$ probe [14]. Viral presence was also identified in one of six core biopsies obtained from patients with MGUS yet in none of the specimens derived from normal subjects or patients with other hematological malignancies. The infected cells had a dendritic cell phenotype upon microscopic analysis and these cells comprised about 2% of the nucleated cells within the bone marrow. The long foot processes possessed by these cells may explain why the virus was not readily detectable in the bone marrow aspirates. We have subsequently performed PCR on these specimens and have identified HHV-8 in the DNA extracted from 12 of 17 bone marrow core biopsies derived from MM patients.

Using the $KS233_{330}$ primers, peripheral blood mononuclear cells only rarely contained detectable HHV-8. To increase the assay sensitivity, the PBMCs were enriched for cells expressing CD68 and CD83 using Dynal immunomagnetic beads. To date, HHV-8 has been detected within the circulating PBMCs of 51 of 74 MM patients. Only rarely (1 of 19) has the virus been detectable in patients with non-B cell malignancies or in normal subjects [15], Table 1. Interestingly, in these studies, most myeloma patients lacking the presence of virus in blood and/or bone marrow were in remission following high dose or conventional chemotherapy or were at an early clinical stage.

Table 1. HHV-8 in Peripheral Blood Mononuclear Cells Enriched for CD68 & CD83 expression*

Normal	Other Cancers	MGUS	MM
1/13	0/6	5/19	51/74

*using PCR with primers specific for the $KS330_{233}$ gene fragment

HHV-8 gene expression in multiple myeloma

In order to better understand how viral infection could perturb cellular growth, RT-PCR was performed to identify the genes expressed within the infected stromal cells. Expression was identified for most of the viral genes including vIL-6, vIL8-R, and vIRF [16]. The latter two genes have recently been identified as having oncogenic potential by their individual ability to cause NIH3T3 cell transformation [17,18]. To more directly compare gene expression in the HHV-8 infected cells, RDA was performed. Stromal cells cultured from a MM patient was used as the "tester" material while stroma cells derived from a normal patient served as the "driver" material. Two sets of experiments were performed using patient vs. control stromal cell RNA. After three rounds of amplification/selection, only one predominant cDNA product was detectable in one RDA set. This product was sequenced and matched the vIRF gene within the HHV-8 genome. The second RDA set yielded seven discrete cDNA products after three rounds of amplification. Each of these products were sequenced and five bands matched known germline genes such as HLA and elongation factor. Of the two remaining PCR products, one, again, matched HHV-8 vIRF while the second shared no known homology with any genes in GenBank. This final gene shared greatest homology with members of the melanoma associated tumor antigen gene (MAGE) family. This new gene, coined MAGE-D1, has subsequently been sequenced and encodes for a 574 amino acid protein. In contrast to other MAGE genes, this new gene is expressed in a wide range of normal tissues [19]. Current studies are underway to determine MAGE-D1 function and determine whether the gene is frequently overexpressed in multiple myeloma stroma.

Unique mutations of HHV-8 found in multiple myeloma specimens

Many groups have been unable to detect HHV-8 in MM patients [20,21,22], although supporting evidence also exists [23,24]. In particular, the majority of the serologically based studies have failed to find an association between MM and an HHV-8 antibody response [25,26]. In addition, since Kaposi's sarcoma and myeloma have now both been linked to the same virus, it is puzzling that myeloma and Kaposi's sarcoma are not linked epidemiologically.

Recent analysis of HHV-8 sequences derived from KS and PEL tumor tissue have revealed at least three unique viral strain types [27]. These strains (A, B and C) differ by approximately 1.5% within the three gene fragments most heavily studied. Compared to the original $KS330_{233}$ sequence reported by Chang et al. [4], all of the $KS330_{233}$ gene products amplified from multiple myeloma tissue harbor numerous base pair substitutions. Four mutations were universally found within the myeloma specimens (C to A, C to T, G to T, and A to C at base pairs 47631, 47632, 47654 and 47738 respectively) and confirms that the virus found in MM patients most closely matches strain B. In addition, a single base pair substitution from A to G at position 47731 in most of these specimens, suggests that the virus is most homologous to that found within the BC-2 cell line (subtype B'). This latter base pair substitution was confirmed since only the viral DNA products derived from multiple myeloma specimens cut with XmaI, verifying the 47731 A to G substitution. Finally, there were additional inter-patient but only rare intra-patient mutations within the $KS330_{233}$ sequences obtained. Thus, our results are unlikely to have occurred because of laboratory contamination (Fig. 1).

Conclusions

These early studies suggest that HHV-8 infection frequently occurs within patients with multiple myeloma. Although these results do not prove that the virus participates in multiple myeloma pathogenesis, significant circumstantial evidence suggests that this may be the case. Since the viral strain identified in the myeloma patients is restricted to a particular strain type, it seems unlikely that our findings could be explained by reactivation of a latent virus due to the immunosuppressed state of these patients. Furthermore, the virus is found in patients with MGUS who do not appear to be at greater risk for infections. The fact that the virus contains numerous human homologues to genes known to support cellular growth and potentially stimulate myeloma cell proliferation directly makes a compelling story. Hopefully, with further study, the role of HHV-8 in multiple myeloma pathogenesis will become clear. If the virus is indeed an important participant in disease development, it would permit a new avenue to either prevent or slow malignant plasma cell development.

```
KSHV  TCCACCATTGTGCTCGAATCCAACGGATTTGACCCCGTGTTCCCCATGGTCGTGCCGCAGCAACTGG
514-B ................G................AT.....................T..........
514-A ................G................AT.....................T..........
514-L .................................AT.....................T..........
MM-1  .................................AT.....................T..........
MM-4  ..................-....G.........AT.....................T..........
MM-14 ..................-..............AT.....................T..........

KSHV  GGCACGCTATTCTGCAGCAGCT-GTTGGTGTACCACATCTACTCCAAAATATCGGCCGGGGCCCCGG
514-B ......................-............................................
514-A ......................-............................................
514-L ......................-............................................
MM-1  ......................-............................................
MM-4  ......................T................................T...........
MM-14 ......................-............................................

KSHV  ATGATGTAAATATGGCGGAACTTGATCTATATACCACCAATGTGTCATTTATGGGGCGCACATATCG
514-B G......C......................................................C....
514-A G......C......................................................C....
514-L G......C......................................................C....
MM-1  .......C............-..............................................
MM-4  G......C...........................................................
MM-14 G......C...........................................................
```

***Nine clones from patient 514 were sequenced, only 1 bp difference noted (shown as 514-L)**

Fig. 1. $KS330_{233}$ gene segment sequences derived from MM patient samples compared to the original sequence in KSHV. Sequences for MM patient 514 were derived from the blood before (B), and after (A) mobilization chemotherapy and in the leukapheresis sample (L). Homology is indicated by a ".", while a deletion is indicated by a "-".

References

1. Zhang XG, Bataille R, Jourdan M, et al: Granulocyte-macrophage colony-stimulating factor synergizes with interleukin-6 in supporting the proliferation of human myeloma cells. Blood 1990; 76:2599.
2 Uchiyama H, Barut BA, Mohrbacher AF et al: Adhesion of human myeloma-derived cell lines to bone marrow stromal cells stimulates interleukin-6 secretion. Blood 1993, 82:3712-3720.
3 Salmon SE and Hamburger AW: Immunoproliferation and cancer: a common macrophage-derived promoter substance. Lancet 1978; 8077:1289.
4 Chang Y, Cesarman E, Pessin M, et al: Identification of herpesvirus-like DNA sequences in AIDS-associated Kaposi's sarcoma. Science 1994; 266:1865.
5 Cesarman E, Chang Y, Moore PS, Said JW, Knowles DM: Kaposi's sarcoma-associated herpesvirus-like DNA sequences in AIDS-related body cavity-based lymphomas. N Eng J Med 1995; 332:1186.

6 Soulier J, Grollet L, Oksenhendler E et al: Kaposi's sarcoma-associated herpesviurs-like DNA sequences in multicentric Castleman's disease. Blood 1995; 86:1276.
7 Moore P, Boshoff C, Weiss R, Chang Y: Molecular mimicry of human cytokine and cytokine response pathway genes by KSHV. Science 1996; 274:1739.
8 Sirianni MC, Vincenzi L, Fiorelli V, et al: gamma-Interferon production in peripheral blood mononuclear cells and tumor infiltrating lymphocytes from Kaposi's sarcoma patients: correlation with the presence of human herpesvirus-8 in peripheral blood mononuclear cells and lesional macrophages. Blood 1998; 91:968.
9 Kliche S, Kremmer E, Hammerschmidt W, Koszinowski U, Haas J. Persistent infection of Epstein-Barr virus-positive B lymphocytes by human herpesvirus 8. J Virol 1998; 72:8143.
10 Rettig M, Ma H, Vescio R, et al: Kaposi's sarcoma-associated herpesvirus infection of bone marrow dendritic cells from myeloma patients. Science 1997; 276:1851.
11 Hart DNJ: Dendritic cells: unique leukocyte populations which control the primary immune response. Blood 1997; 90:3245.
12 Uccini S, Sirianni MC, Vincenzi L, et al: Kaposi's sarcoma cells express the macrophage-associated antigen mannose receptor and develop in peripheral blood cultures of Kaposi's sarcoma patients. Am J of Pathology 1997; 150:929.
13 Soderberg-Naucler C, Fish KN, Nelson JA: Reactivation of latent human cytomegalovirus by allogeneic stimulation of blood cells from healthy donors. Cell 1997; 91:119.
14 Said J, Rettig M, Heppner K, et al: Localization of Kaposi's sarcoma-associated herpesvirus in bone marrow biopsy samples from patients with multiple myeloma. Blood 1997; 90:4278.
15 Rettig M, Vescio R, Moss T, et al: Detection of Kaposi's sarcoma-associated herpesvirus in the peripheral blood of multiple myeloma patients. Blood 1997; 90 (Sup. 1):587a.
16 Ma H, Vescio R, Der Danielian M, Schiller G, Berenson J: The HHV-8 IL-8R homologue and interferon regulatory factor genes are frequently expressed in myeloma bone marrow biopsies whereas the vIL-6 is rarely found. Blood 1998; 92(Sup. 1):515a.
17 Flore O, Raffi S, Ely S, O'Leary JJ, Hyjek EM, Cesarman E. Transformation of primary human endothelial cells by Kaposi's sarcoma-associated herpesvirus. Nature 1998; 394:588.
18 Bais C, Santomasso B, Coso O, et al. G-protein-coupled receptor of Kaposi's sarcoma-associated herpesvirus is a viral oncogene and angiogenesis activator. Nature 1998; 392:210.
19 Pold M, Zhou J, Chen G, Vescio R, Berenson J: Identification of a novel member of the MAGE tumor antigen family. Blood 1998; 92(Sup. 1):432a.
20 Tarte K, Olsen S, Lu Z, et al: Clinical-grade dendritic cells from patients with multiple myeloma are not infected with Kaposi's sarcoma associated-herpesvirus. Blood 1998; 91:1852.
21 Yi Q, Ekman M, Anton D, et al: Blood dendritic cells from myeloma patients are not infected with Kaposi's sarcoma-associated herpesvirus (KSHV/HHV-8). Blood 1998; 92:402.
22 Masood R, Zheng T, Tulpule A, et al: Kaposi's sarcoma-associated herpesvirus infection in multiple myeloma. Science 1997; 278;1970.
23 Chauhan D, Barati A, Raje N, et al: Detection of human herpesvirus-8 (HHV-8) sequence in multiple myeloma (MM) bone marrow stromal cells (BMSCs). Blood 1998; 92(Sup. 1):514a.
24 Gao SJ, Alsina M, Deng JH, et al: Antibodies to Kaposi's sarcoma-associated herpesvirus (human herpesvirus 8) in patients with multiple myeloma. J Infect Dis 1998; 178:846.
25 MacKenzie J, Sheldon J, Morgan G, Cook G, Schultz TF, Jarrett RF: HHV-8 and multiple myeloma in the U.K. Lancet 1997; 350:1144.
26 Marcelin AG Dupin N, Bouscary D, et al: HHV-8 and multiple myeloma in France. Lancet 1997; 350:1144.
27 Zong JC, Metroka C, Reitz MS, Nicholas J, Hayward GS: Strain variability among Kaposi's Sarcoma-associated herpesvirus (Human herpesvirus 8) genomes: evidence that a large cohort of United States AIDS patients may have been infected by a single common isolate. J Virology 1997; 71:2505.

Discussion

Richard Scheuermann: As you cannot detect HHV-8 in primary biopsies from multiple myeloma patients, the number of cells that contain HHV-8 must be very small, so they cannot be driving the proliferation of the myeloma cells. Maybe what that implies is that if they are involved, they are involved in a very early step in transformation.

Robert Vescio: We actually can find it routinely in bone marrow core biopsy specimens but it is less frequently detectable in bone marrow aspirates. We are doing quantitative measurements of KSHV and it ranges from patient to patient. Multiple myeloma is, obviously, a multifocal disease, so viral burden may differ in different regions of the bone marrow. It is hard to say how many viral copies one needs to cause a problem. My personal theory is that if there is chronic stimulation for many years, like one sees with pristane (or other environmental factors), this can lead to B-cell dysregulation and eventually oncogenesis.

Gary Rathbun: Does KSHV persist through bone marrow transplantation and treatment? Have you been able to track the patients and look at the dendritic cell expression of this virus over time?

Robert Vescio: It is still preliminary. Many of the patients who appear to be doing extremely well in complete remission do not have detectable KSHV, at least to the level of our assay sensitivity.

Gary Rathbun: What about relapse?

Robert Vescio: Many of those patients do have detectable KSHV at that point, but these results are really preliminary. In order to answer whether disease status correlates with viral load, a set experiment is needed rather than just collecting specimens from patients ad hoc. We have samples from a transplant study where we followed 200 patients over the course of a few years, so looking at those samples might be informative.

Subject Index

Current Topics in Microbiology and Immunology

Volumes published since 1989 (and still available)

Vol. 202: **Oldstone, Michael B. A.; Vitković, Ljubiša (Eds.):** HIV and Dementia. 1995. 40 figs. XIII, 279 pp. ISBN 3-540-59117-6

Vol. 203: **Sarnow, Peter (Ed.):** Cap-Independent Translation. 1995. 31 figs. XI, 183 pp. ISBN 3-540-59121-4

Vol. 204: **Saedler, Heinz; Gierl, Alfons (Eds.):** Transposable Elements. 1995. 42 figs. IX, 234 pp. ISBN 3-540-59342-X

Vol. 205: **Littman, Dan R. (Ed.):** The CD4 Molecule. 1995. 29 figs. XIII, 182 pp. ISBN 3-540-59344-6

Vol. 206: **Chisari, Francis V.; Oldstone, Michael B. A. (Eds.):** Transgenic Models of Human Viral and Immunological Disease. 1995. 53 figs. XI, 345 pp. ISBN 3-540-59341-1

Vol. 207: **Prusiner, Stanley B. (Ed.):** Prions Prions Prions. 1995. 42 figs. VII, 163 pp. ISBN 3-540-59343-8

Vol. 208: **Farnham, Peggy J. (Ed.):** Transcriptional Control of Cell Growth. 1995. 17 figs. IX, 141 pp. ISBN 3-540-60113-9

Vol. 209: **Miller, Virginia L. (Ed.):** Bacterial Invasiveness. 1996. 16 figs. IX, 115 pp. ISBN 3-540-60065-5

Vol. 210: **Potter, Michael; Rose, Noel R. (Eds.):** Immunology of Silicones. 1996. 136 figs. XX, 430 pp. ISBN 3-540-60272-0

Vol. 211: **Wolff, Linda; Perkins, Archibald S. (Eds.):** Molecular Aspects of Myeloid Stem Cell Development. 1996. 98 figs. XIV, 298 pp. ISBN 3-540-60414-6

Vol. 212: **Vainio, Olli; Imhof, Beat A. (Eds.):** Immunology and Developmental Biology of the Chicken. 1996. 43 figs. IX, 281 pp. ISBN 3-540-60585-1

Vol. 213/I: **Günthert, Ursula; Birchmeier, Walter (Eds.):** Attempts to Understand Metastasis Formation I. 1996. 35 figs. XV, 293 pp. ISBN 3-540-60680-7

Vol. 213/II: **Günthert, Ursula; Birchmeier, Walter (Eds.):** Attempts to Understand Metastasis Formation II. 1996. 33 figs. XV, 288 pp. ISBN 3-540-60681-5

Vol. 213/III: **Günthert, Ursula; Schlag, Peter M.; Birchmeier, Walter (Eds.):** Attempts to Understand Metastasis Formation III. 1996. 14 figs. XV, 262 pp. ISBN 3-540-60682-3

Vol. 214: **Kräusslich, Hans-Georg (Ed.):** Morphogenesis and Maturation of Retroviruses. 1996. 34 figs. XI, 344 pp. ISBN 3-540-60928-8

Vol. 215: **Shinnick, Thomas M. (Ed.):** Tuberculosis. 1996. 46 figs. XI, 307 pp. ISBN 3-540-60985-7

Vol. 216: **Rietschel, Ernst Th.; Wagner, Hermann (Eds.):** Pathology of Septic Shock. 1996. 34 figs. X, 321 pp. ISBN 3-540-61026-X

Vol. 217: **Jessberger, Rolf; Lieber, Michael R. (Eds.):** Molecular Analysis of DNA Rearrangements in the Immune System. 1996. 43 figs. IX, 224 pp. ISBN 3-540-61037-5

Vol. 218: **Berns, Kenneth I.; Giraud, Catherine (Eds.):** Adeno-Associated Virus (AAV) Vectors in Gene Therapy. 1996. 38 figs. IX,173 pp. ISBN 3-540-61076-6

Vol. 219: **Gross, Uwe (Ed.):** Toxoplasma gondii. 1996. 31 figs. XI, 274 pp. ISBN 3-540-61300-5

Vol. 220: **Rauscher, Frank J. III; Vogt, Peter K. (Eds.):** Chromosomal Translocations and Oncogenic Transcription Factors. 1997. 28 figs. XI, 166 pp. ISBN 3-540-61402-8

Vol. 221: **Kastan, Michael B. (Ed.):** Genetic Instability and Tumorigenesis. 1997. 12 figs.VII, 180 pp. ISBN 3-540-61518-0

Vol. 222: **Olding, Lars B. (Ed.):** Reproductive Immunology. 1997. 17 figs. XII, 219 pp. ISBN 3-540-61888-0

Vol. 223: **Tracy, S.; Chapman, N. M.; Mahy, B. W. J. (Eds.):** The Coxsackie B Viruses. 1997. 37 figs. VIII, 336 pp. ISBN 3-540-62390-6

Vol. 224: **Potter, Michael; Melchers, Fritz (Eds.):** C-Myc in B-Cell Neoplasia. 1997. 94 figs. XII, 291 pp. ISBN 3-540-62892-4

Vol. 225: **Vogt, Peter K.; Mahan, Michael J. (Eds.):** Bacterial Infection: Close Encounters at the Host Pathogen Interface. 1998. 15 figs. IX, 169 pp. ISBN 3-540-63260-3

Vol. 226: **Koprowski, Hilary; Weiner, David B. (Eds.):** DNA Vaccination/Genetic Vaccination. 1998. 31 figs. XVIII, 198 pp. ISBN 3-540-63392-8

Vol. 227: **Vogt, Peter K.; Reed, Steven I. (Eds.):** Cyclin Dependent Kinase (CDK) Inhibitors. 1998. 15 figs. XII, 169 pp. ISBN 3-540-63429-0

Vol. 228: **Pawson, Anthony I. (Ed.):** Protein Modules in Signal Transduction. 1998. 42 figs. IX, 368 pp. ISBN 3-540-63396-0

Vol. 229: **Kelsoe, Garnett; Flajnik, Martin (Eds.):** Somatic Diversification of Immune Responses. 1998. 38 figs. IX, 221 pp. ISBN 3-540-63608-0

Vol. 230: **Kärre, Klas; Colonna, Marco (Eds.):** Specificity, Function, and Development of NK Cells. 1998. 22 figs. IX, 248 pp. ISBN 3-540-63941-1

Vol. 231: **Holzmann, Bernhard; Wagner, Hermann (Eds.):** Leukocyte Integrins in the Immune System and Malignant Disease. 1998. 40 figs. XIII, 189 pp. ISBN 3-540-63609-9

Vol. 232: **Whitton, J. Lindsay (Ed.):** Antigen Presentation. 1998. 11 figs. IX, 244 pp. ISBN 3-540-63813-X

Vol. 233/I: **Tyler, Kenneth L.; Oldstone, Michael B. A. (Eds.):** Reoviruses I. 1998. 29 figs. XVIII, 223 pp. ISBN 3-540-63946-2

Vol. 233/II: **Tyler, Kenneth L.; Oldstone, Michael B. A. (Eds.):** Reoviruses II. 1998. 45 figs. XVI, 187 pp. ISBN 3-540-63947-0

Vol. 234: **Frankel, Arthur E. (Ed.):** Clinical Applications of Immunotoxins. 1999. 16 figs. IX, 122 pp. ISBN 3-540-64097-5

Vol. 235: **Klenk, Hans-Dieter (Ed.):** Marburg and Ebola Viruses. 1999. 34 figs. XI, 225 pp. ISBN 3-540-64729-5

Vol. 236: **Kraehenbuhl, Jean-Pierre; Neutra, Marian R. (Eds.):** Defense of Mucosal Surfaces: Pathogenesis, Immunity and Vaccines. 1999. 30 figs. IX, 296 pp. ISBN 3-540-64730-9

Vol. 237: **Claesson-Welsh, Lena (Ed.):** Vascular Growth Factors and Angiogenesis. 1999. 36 figs. X, 189 pp. ISBN 3-540-64731-7

Vol. 238: **Coffman, Robert L.; Romagnani, Sergio (Eds.):** Redirection of Th1 and Th2 Responses. 1999. 6 figs. IX, 148 pp. ISBN 3-540-65048-2

Vol. 239: **Vogt, Peter K.; Jackson, Andrew O. (Eds.):** Satellites and Defective Viral RNAs. 1999. 39 figs. XVI, 179 pp. ISBN 3-540-65049-0

Vol. 240: **Hammond, John; McGarrey, Peter; Yusibov, Vidadi (Eds.):** Plant Biotechnology. 1999. 12 figs. XII, 196 pp. ISBN 3-540-65104-7

Vol. 241: **Westblom, Tore U.; Czinn, Steven J.; Nedrud, John G. (Eds.):** Gastroduodenal Disease and Helicobacter pylori. 1999. 35 figs. XI, 313 pp. ISBN 3-540-65084-9

Vol. 243: **Famulok, Michael; Winnacker, Ernst-L.; Wong, Chi-Huey (Eds.):** Combinatorial Chemistry in Biology. 1999. 48 figs. VIII, 396 pp. ISBN 3-540-65704-5

Vol. 244: **Daeron, Marc; Vivier, Eric (Eds.):** Immunoreceptor Tyrosine-Based Inhibition Motifs. 1999. 19 figs. VIII, approx. 278 pp. ISBN 3-540-65789-4

MIX
Papier aus verantwortungsvollen Quellen
Paper from responsible sources
FSC® C105338

If you have any concerns about our products,
you can contact us on
ProductSafety@springernature.com

In case Publisher is established outside the EU,
the EU authorized representative is:
Springer Nature Customer Service Center GmbH
Europaplatz 3, 69115 Heidelberg, Germany

Printed by Libri Plureos GmbH
in Hamburg, Germany